Clinical Trials Dictionary

Terminology
and
Usage Recommendations

Curtis L. Meinert

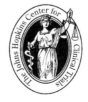

Clinical Trials Dictionary

Terminology
and
Usage Recommendations

Curtis L. Meinert

Baltimore, Maryland
The Johns Hopkins University
School of Hygiene and Public Health
Center for Clinical Trials

Edition 1.0

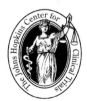

Copyright © 1996 by Curtis L. Meinert
All rights reserved

This document is protected under copyright laws and trade agreements. No part of it may be reproduced, stored in a retrieval system, or transmitted in any form or by any means electronic, mechanical, photocopying, recording, or otherwise without the express prior approval of the copyright owner.

Library of Congress Catalog Card Number
95-94294

ISBN 0-9646424-0-9

Ordering information
Copies of this document may be purchased through The Johns Hopkins Center for Clinical Trials, 615 North Wolfe Street, Baltimore, Maryland 21205 (phone 410/955-8198; fax 410/955-0932; E-mail cctmail@phnet.sph.jhu.edu)

Edition 1.0, 1st printing

Printed in the United States on acid free paper
by Harbor Duvall Graphics
Baltimore Maryland

C⚕D

Author

Curtis L. Meinert
Professor of Epidemiology and Biostatistics
The Johns Hopkins University
School of Hygiene and Public Health
615 North Wolfe Street
Baltimore, Maryland 21205

PhD, Biostatistics, 1964, University of Minnesota
Founding editor of *Controlled Clinical Trials*
Founding member, Society for Clinical Trials

Features

480 pages, hard back, cloth cover
4,300+ terms and 6,400+ definitions
Synonyms, antonyms, and related terms
500+ usage notes
Usage recommendations
Discourse on usage practices
Author and subject index

Orders

The Johns Hopkins Center for Clinical Trials
615 North Wolfe Street
Baltimore, Maryland 21205
Telephone: 410/955-8198 (voice); 410/955-0932 (fax)
E-mail: cctmail@phnet.sph.jhu.edu

Sample entries

collaborative *adj* - Characterization applied to work performed in concert with others, especially in relation to work requiring intellectual input. syn: **cooperative** rt: **multidisciplinary, multicenter** *Usage note*: Not recommended as a synonym for **multicenter** for reasons indicated in usage notes for **collaborative study** and **collaborative trial**.

collaborative trial *n* - 1. A **trial** involving two or more **clinics**; **multicenter trial** (preferred term). 2. A trial involving two or more **centers**; multicenter trial (preferred term). 3. A trial involving two or more **investigators**. See *trial* for list. syn: **cooperative trial** rt: **multicenter trial** *Usage note*: Avoid because of ambiguous uninformative nature. Most trials, even small ones carried out in a single center, require collaboration of various forms and types. Use other more informative adjectives to characterize nature or form of collaboration, such as **multidisciplinary** or **multicenter**.

database *n* - 1. A collection of related **data** or related **data files**, organized for ease and efficiency of use, especially in relation to activities such as those involving retrieving or updating specific files or **data fields**. 2. **analysis database** 3. **electronic database** rt: **centralized database, distributed database**

placebo *n* - [ME, fr L, I shall please, fr *placēre* to please; the first word of the first antiphon of the service for the dead, I shall please the Lord in the land of the living, fr Roman Catholic vespers] 1. A pharmacologically **inactive substance** given as a substitute for an **active substance**, especially when the person taking or receiving it is not informed whether it is an **active** or **inactive substance**. 2. **placebo treatment** (defn 1) 3. A sugar-coated pill made of lactose or some other pharmacologically inert substance. 4. Any medication considered to be useless, especially one administered in pill form. 5. **nil treatment** 6. An ineffective treatment. rt: **double placebo, homeopathic dose, multiple placebo, placebo treatment, sham, sham procedure** *Usage note*: Subject to varying use. Avoid in the sense of defns 4, 5, and 6. Not to be confused with **sham**; see note for that entry. The use of a placebo should not be construed to imply the absence of treatment, as in designs involving **null treatment**. Virtually all trials involve some care requirements. Investigators conducting them are obligated to meet care requirements, regardless of treatment assignment and whether masked or not. For example, that requirement in the case of the University Group Diabetes Program[156] obligated investigators to do their best in maintaining all patients enrolled on standard antidiabetic diets in addition to their assigned treatments. As a result, **control treatments** involving use of placebos are best thought of as **regimens** with placebos substituting for elements of the regimens. Labels, such as **placebo patient** or **placebo group**, obscure the true nature of the treatment process and create the erroneous impression that patients assigned to receive a placebo are left untreated when that is true of only one element of the regimen. Generic labels of this sort are wrong in the literal sense of usage (there is no such being as a placebo patient except, perhaps, for one coated with lactose) and have the potential for misleading when an assignment involving administration of a placebo also involves administration of other treatments (as in a **vaccine trial** where all infants enrolled receive vaccines for diphtheria and tetanus in addition to a pertussis vaccine or matching placebo).

Contents

Equations and functions

Graphic illustrations

Foreword

In writing an essay that celebrates the skills of the great German composer Johannes Brahms, Arnold Schönberg coined a pithy phrase of advice intended for other composers but relevant as well to writers: Say what you have to say with "precision and brevity". For authors reporting clinical trials, taking this advice could make the difference in getting your report published or not. If you take it, you are more likely to convince a journal's editor that your trial merits attention. If you ignore it, you run the risk of conveying an impression that you don't know the science of designing and running a first-rate trial. "Precision" lies in using terms that convey to others reading a trial report exactly how the trial was designed and exactly how it was carried out. "Brevity" lies in using terms and phrases that are succinct and effectively replacing wordy descriptions.

Giving writers, and their readers, precise terms with clear definitions is a main goal of compilers of dictionaries. An effective dictionary establishes an ample vocabulary of words and phrases that will leave no question as to what they stand for. Dr. Meinert has produced in this dictionary a treasure for those of you who aim to write about clinical trials with precision and brevity. It goes well beyond the general dictionaries of medicine in representing in detail and great accuracy the large and complex vocabulary needed to describe clearly the methods and results of clinical trials. It also provides a thorough index to the entries of its main section that facilitates the findings of terms associated with particular concepts and practical steps in trials. But perhaps its most extraordinary and admirable section is that on usage. Here Dr. Meinert gives us a deeply perceptive and strongly illuminating discourse on nuances in the rhetoric of scientific speech and writing as seen by him through his long and fruitful engagement with designing, running, reporting, and interpreting clinical trials.

For these reasons this new dictionary is going to be a classic at birth. It merits an audience far wider than just authors reporting clinical trials. That audience should include authors' editors, journal editors and their manuscript editors, indexers of clinical-trials papers, meta-analysts, teachers of clinical epidemiology, and anyone else who reads reports of trials and assesses their scientific strength and clinical value. I believe it will get that wide audience.

Edward J. Huth
Editor Emeritus, *Annals of Internal Medicine*

Preface

It is the fate of those who toil at the lower employments of life, to be rather driven by the fear of evil, than attracted by the prospect of good; to be exposed to censure, without hope of praise; to be disgraced by miscarriage, or punished for neglect, where success would have been without applause, and diligence without reward.

Among these unhappy mortals is the writer of dictionaries; whom mankind have considered, not as the pupil, but the slave of science, the pioneer of literature, doomed only to remove rubbish and clear obstructions from the paths of Learning and Genius, who press forward to conquest and glory, without bestowing a smile on the humble drudge that facilitates their progress. Every other author may aspire to praise; the lexicographer can only hope to escape reproach, and even this negative recompense has been yet granted to very few.

Preface to *A Dictionary of the English Language*
Samuel Johnson [1755][71]

One does not awake one morning and start writing a dictionary. The notion emerges out of the primordial ooze of musings while one is engaged in other pursuits, and has properties akin to a virus. For susceptibles, it is capable of producing a chronic condition without a known cure and with an unpredictable course. The condition can be in remission, some of them so long as to cause one to believe he is "cured", only to suffer a new bout more serious and prolonged than any in the past. Living with the virus is like having a camel in one's tent with the manners of a bull moose and the personality of an uninvited pushy relative who comes to stay.

From the outset, I have been plagued by a nefarious gremlin. I have learned to coexist with it but I have to confess to flashes of irritation and frustration even as recently as a few weeks ago after still another visit. I have to confess as well to the utterance of an expletive or two following its visits, especially after those resulting in trashed files. My wife has had her vocabulary enriched as a result of its visits. Perhaps, one day, she will write a dictionary of another sort as a result of this enriching experience.

The skeptics out there will doubt my evidence for existence of my gremlin because it is circumstantial. But how else do I account for the appearance of words, where they do not belong or for their absence where they once were? How else can I account for backup files of 0 bytes when days of work are at stake? What other explanation could there be for programs that suddenly malfunction after months of flawless operation? To be sure, I have done my best to undo what the gremlin has done, but given its devious nature the chance remains that it will be at work even as the presses roll.

The nearer one comes to the point of no return, the greater my hope, as with Johnson's, years before me, for the mere escape from recompense. But if Johnson failed in his hope, I am resigned to my fate. Hence, I expect to hear from readers about mistakes, things missing, and about definitions wrong, too broad, or too narrow. Who knows, having been born with some genetic abnormality, I might well be foolish enough to do this again. The feedback will be helpful. Old fashioned letter or high tech Fax or E-mail will do. My postal address, Fax number, and E-mail address are given elsewhere in this document (page iii).

This dictionary, in its various incarnations, has logged enough air miles to qualify for membership in the 100,000 mile club and has been a constant "companion" on summer vacations to the backcountry of upstate New York nigh onto a decade now. It has been rain soaked and charred at the campsite, "lost" in Denver, left on the subway in Atlanta, and "abandoned" at a rest stop on I 81.

It has been a source of frustration (especially when generating and printing — activities invented by the devil), but it has also served as the word equivalent of needlepoint and as a source of "entertainment" at meetings where discrete "doodling" is acceptable and as a safe and effective sedative on long flights and evenings in my easy chair.

Who knows? Maybe I was born with a fascination with words or the technical. Or maybe this work is simply the product of a literalist who, even at a young age, was content to resort to technicalities in "winning" arguments, when higher forms of victories were denied me.

Recognition of the need for language conventions emerged with the Coordinating Center Models Project, a study started in 1976 that involved the comparison of different trials with regard to design and operating features.[26] The establishment of the journal *Controlled Clinical Trials* and assumption of editorial responsibilities for it, reinforced that recognition [Meinert, 1980].[101] The creation of a dictionary began with a glossary developed for that project.[27] That glossary was refined and expanded for inclusion as an appendix in a book on clinical trials [Meinert and Tonascia, 1986].[102] Ultimately, it served as a starting point of sorts for this work.

I have had for a long time, an urge to produce a series of handbooks for trialists. I turned to that task after finishing the book on clinical trials in 1986, but kept hitting roadblocks because of an inadequate vocabulary to describe the features of trials. For a while, I was content to simply "add" to that glossary. Slowly, it grew into something resembling a dictionary, and gradually the amount of time devoted to it increased and the amount devoted to the handbook decreased until I was trapped, in a way like Murray, years ago, in his herculean effort to produce the first edition of the *Oxford English Dictionary*.

The language of clinical trials is the product of a living, dynamic process. It was evolving on board the Salisbury at sea in 1747 when Lind[91] did his experiment aimed at finding a treatment for scurvy and continues today. It is a mixture of the languages of medicine, biostatistics, epidemiology, computer science, and bioethics.

The entries contained in this Dictionary are the product of three related aims:

1. To produce a document having sufficient generality and coverage to satisfy the requirements of users from the various disciplines concerned with the design, conduct, and analysis of trials and with the utilization of results from them;

2. To introduce a vocabulary for the characterization and description of features and activities associated with trials;

3. To provide a document reflective of current usage practices and conventions in the field.

Achieving the first aim required the compilation of a dictionary overlapping the domains of medicine, statistics, epidemiology, computer science, and bioethics. Achieving the second aim required the development of nomenclature for features, elements, and activities of trials not described by existing vocabulary. Achieving the third aim required a review of books and journals to identify terms for inclusion and to note different uses of similar terms. Journals screened included the *British Medical Journal, Journal of the American Medical Association, Lancet, New England Journal of Medicine, Biometrics, Journal of the American Statistical Association*, and *Controlled Clinical Trials*. The screening process was akin to that used by Murray[110] in producing the *Oxford English Dictionary*.[109]

Inclusion and coverage principles are discussed elsewhere (*Explanatory notes*, page xix). One of the inclusion principles having pluses and minuses was one requiring inclusion of ordinary terms, such as **randomized**, **controlled**, **clinical**, and **trial** for the entry **randomized controlled clinical trial**. An obvious minus is the number of ordinary entries generated by the principle (about a third of the total). The pluses had to do with the nature of the document desired. The goal was to produce a dictionary that is self-contained and internally consistent.

A work of this kind is never finished. It continues to grow with limits nowhere in sight. I have learned, as Murray before me, that there is no escape from the web of words. Therefore, my only recourse is to declare it done and move onto the work that drove me to this folly in the first place. I hereby so declare (for now)!

16 October 1995

Curtis L. Meinert
Baltimore

In memory of Chris Klimt, the man who started me on the trail of trials and Helga Klimt — a wonderfully kind and gentle woman.

For one word a man is often set down as wise, and for one word he is often set down as a fool
Confucius: *Analects*, XIX, circa 500 BC

Contributors

Editors

Susan Tonascia	The Johns Hopkins University, Baltimore
Katheleen Bates	The Johns Hopkins University, Baltimore
Sandra Bryant	American Journal of Epidemiology, Baltimore
Christopher Dawson	The Johns Hopkins University, Baltimore
Jill Meinert	The Johns Hopkins University, Baltimore
Susan Meinert	Towson, Maryland
Susan Murray	American Journal of Epidemiology, Baltimore
Susan Vaupel	American Journal of Epidemiology, Baltimore

Graphics

Michele Donithan	The Johns Hopkins University, Baltimore
Jill Meinert	The Johns Hopkins University, Baltimore
Mark Van Natta	The Johns Hopkins University, Baltimore

Definitions

Patricia Belt	The Johns Hopkins University, Baltimore
Ronald Brookmeyer	The Johns Hopkins University, Baltimore
Joseph Canner	Blantyre, Malawi (International Eye Foundation)
Iain Chalmers	United Kingdom Cochrane Centre, Oxford
Betty Collison	The Johns Hopkins University, Baltimore
Kay Dickersin	University of Maryland, Baltimore
Adele Gilpin	The Johns Hopkins University, Baltimore
Steven Goodman	The Johns Hopkins University, Baltimore
Barbara S Hawkins	The Johns Hopkins University, Baltimore
Janet Holbrook	The Johns Hopkins University, Baltimore
Milana Isaacson	The Johns Hopkins University, Baltimore
Lisa Jacobson	The Johns Hopkins University, Baltimore
Helena Kraemer	Stanford University, Stanford, California
Harry Marks	The Johns Hopkins University, Baltimore
Elinor Miller	Memorial Sloan-Kettering Cancer Center, New York
Claudia Moy	The Johns Hopkins University, Baltimore
Steven Piantadosi	The Johns Hopkins University, Baltimore
Suresh C Rastogi	Food and Drug Administration, Rockville, Maryland
Evan B Siegel	Astra Pharmaceutical Products, Inc, Westborough, Massachusetts
Stephen Singer	Dedicated Response, Baltimore
James Tonascia	The Johns Hopkins University, Baltimore
Susan Tonascia	The Johns Hopkins University, Baltimore
Mark Van Natta	The Johns Hopkins University, Baltimore
Ina Wallace	University of North Carolina, Chapel Hill, North Carolina
O Dale Williams	University of Alabama, Birmingham
Marcelle Winget	The Johns Hopkins University, Baltimore
Scott Zeger	The Johns Hopkins University, Baltimore

Acknowledgments

I begin with a hearty Thank You! to all those persons listed on the preceding page for their contributions to this effort. They have come in the form of terms or definitions proposed for inclusion in the Dictionary and by way of critical comments regarding definitions.

Thanks are due to Iain Chalmers, O Dale Williams, and Barbara Hawkins who were kind enough and energetic enough to have read early versions of this work from cover to cover and to have provided detailed comments. Thanks are due as well to Claudia Moy for her efforts in combing the literature of clinical trials for candidate terms.

Thanks to Jim Tonascia for his active encouragement and help throughout this effort and for his critical comments and help on a fair number of definitions contained herein. Thanks as well to Mark Van Natta and Adele Gilpin for their help.

Special thanks are due to Susan Tonascia, an untiring collaborator throughout this project. It was she to whom I invariably turned for help in "researching" a term or in checking the accuracy of a definition. I have benefited from her advice and gentle, unrelenting, editing.

Thank you Susie (my wife) for your help as a "lay" reviewer and proofreader and for your forbearance in suffering the chronic paper clutter in and around my desk at home. Thanks Julie, Nancy, and Jill (our daughters) for the various tasks you performed over the years of this activity. And thanks to all four of you for your understanding and tolerance of the countless hours devoted to the Dictionary, many of them in the early morning before the house awakened, and for accepting the Dictionary as a traveling and camping partner!

Explanatory notes

Construction principles

This dictionary is similar to ordinary desk dictionaries to the extent to which it contains entries found in such dictionaries. The overlap arises from a construction principle requiring entries for the individual terms and phrases comprising compound terms. For example, the entry **randomized controlled clinical trial** leads to entries for **randomized**, **controlled**, **clinical**, and **trial** and for the phrase **controlled clinical trial**. While adherence to the principle has increased the number of entries, it is useful in constructing and deconstructing definitions for compound terms.

Definitions for elemental terms may be less or more extensive than those found in ordinary dictionaries, depending on need. For example, the definition for **down** *adj* in *Webster's Ninth New Collegiate Dictionary*[159] has four definitions compared to one herein. **Baseline** *n* has four definitions in Webster and six herein. Similarly, the definition for **random** *adj* is more detailed herein than in Webster.

A similar approach has been followed for modifiers, prefixes, and function words appearing in entries.

Order and place of entries

Entries are arranged alphabetically. Hence, terms such as **publication bias** and **selection bias**, having **bias** as a base are found in different letter sections of the Dictionary. The index contains lists of entries containing key base terms such as **bias, treatment,** and **trial**.

Defined and blind entries

Boldface print denotes defined entries. Generally, only the first use of such terms is bolded in the body of a definition. Terms in regular-face print in the listing of entries (pages li through xcv) correspond to blind entries. Blind entries in the dictionary are used to indicate locations of definitions and preferred terms.

Antonyms, synonyms, and related terms

A term is listed as an antonym (ant) if it is complementary, in some sense, to the entry. A term is listed as a synonym (syn) if it is considered to have uses identical or nearly identical to the entry. Other terms related to an entry, eg, **pseudorandom** and **quasirandom** for the entry **random** *adj, scientific*, are designated as related terms (denoted rt).

Spellings and hyphenation

Spelling and hyphenation conventions are, in large measure, similar to those in *Webster's Ninth New Collegiate Dictionary*.[159] Notable exceptions are **close-out** *n*, **database** *n*, and **followup** *n* (closeout, data base, and follow-up in *Webster's Ninth New Collegiate Dictionary*). Most prefixes such as **pre-**, **non-**, and **un-**, as in Webster, are affixed to the words they modify without hyphens.

Parts of speech and homographs

The part of speech represented by an entry is denoted in italic following the entry. The designation *v* denotes verb regardless of form. Homographs — terms with the same spelling and pronunciation but different meanings (eg, **study** *n* and **study** *v*) — are defined to the extent necessary.

Language and usage conventions

The default language of the Dictionary is that of **clinical trials**. Hence, the designation for a person enrolled into a trial is **patient**, except in references to trials involving healthy people or a mix of sick and healthy people. Medically neutral terms such as person, human being, or individual are used when the connotation of illness is inappropriate. Designations such as **enrollee**, **participant**, or **subject**, while devoid of connotations of illness, have been avoided. The term **enrollee** is bland and nondescript. The term **participant** has the potential of being confused with the one who is performing the trial. The most commonly used generic term in experimental settings is **subject**. Indeed, it is less bland than **enrollee** and avoids the confusion associated with **participant**. However, its use in the setting of trials carries connotations of subjection that are at odds with the notions of informed and voluntary consent and partnership, as discussed in a usage note for that entry (see page 263).

The term **treatment** *n* has been used throughout to refer to the experimental variable in a trial. This usage is consistent with the language of experimental design and with the definition of treatment in *Webster's Ninth New Collegiate Dictionary*, namely *the act or manner or an instance of treating someone or something: handling, usage; the techniques or actions customarily applied in a specified situation*. The term does, to be sure, carry medical implications when used in clinical settings in relation to patients.

The possibility of using another term such as **intervention** to designate the experimental variable in trials involving well people was considered but rejected because of the cumbersome nature of such terms, including **intervention**. While that term is largely devoid of the clinical connotation of treatment, it has connotations at odds with trials. None of the definitions of the root term **intervene** *v* in *Webster's Ninth New Collegiate Dictionary* are consistent with that usage, strictly speaking. The term, as defined therein, means *to occur, fall, or come between points of time or events; to enter or appear as an irrelevant or extraneous feature or circumstance*. The implication of irrelevance or of being extraneous is hardly a connotation to be conveyed when referring to the most important variable of a trial.

The modifier **clinical** is routinely dropped, except in usages in which there is a need or desire to emphasize the clinical or medical nature of a trial or class of trials (see definition for **clinical trial** for additional comments). Modifiers such as **data** in **data analysis** and **study** in **study patient** are dropped for most uses as well, except when they are considered necessary for clarity.

The general applicability of a term beyond the field of trials is conveyed by language in the definition. For example, an activity or procedure that relates to a class of designs larger than represented by trials is defined with that generality in mind by reference to the larger class of designs or by use of the term **study**, instead of a design-specific term such as **trial**.

Sources and references

Webster's Ninth New Collegiate Dictionary[159] served as the base dictionary for this work. In addition, many of the definitions for base or modifier terms are adapted or taken verbatim from Webster. Other desk dictionaries used include those represented by citations 2, 10, 108, 109, 147, as found on pages 303 through 313. Medical dictionaries used include those represented by citations 38, 148, and 153. Specialty and discipline-specific dictionaries and glossaries in the areas of mathematics and statistics, epidemiology, and computer science include those represented by citations 24, 54, 69, 76, 80, 84, 85, 99, 100, 143, 149, and 162. The dictionaries by James and James in mathematics, Freund and Williams in statistics, and Last in epidemiology were invaluable as reference sources and as guides for domains of coverage (citations 69, 54, and 84, respectively).

Texts used in statistics, epidemiology, and related fields include those denoted by citations 4, 14, 25, 43, 46, 56, 58, 67, 74, 79, 86, 88, 90, 106, and 138. Texts in clinical trials include those by Buyse, Staquet, and Sylvester,[18] Friedman, Furberg, and DeMets,[56] Leventhal and Wittes,[87] Meinert and Tonascia,[102] and Pocock.[126] The *Encyclopedia of Statistical Sciences*[82] and the *International Encyclopedia of Statistics*[83] were also used.

Adages

Adages appearing on the lead page of the various letter sections of the dictionary are admixtures of "everyday" utterances of farmer friends and neighbors back there in Sleepy Eye and of fellow trialists, colleagues, and acquaintances from various fields and disciplines. A few have elements traceable to *Muench's Postulates, Laws, and Corollaries* (JE Bearman, RB Loewenson, and W Gullen, Biometrics Note, No 4, April 1974; Office of Biometry and Epidemiology, National Eye Institute, Bethesda Md). Laws ascribed to Muench (Hugo, 1894 - 1972; professor of Biostatistics, Harvard University) are:

No full-scale study confirms the lead provide by a pilot study

Results can always be improved by omitting controls

In order to be realistic, the number of cases promised in any clinical study must be divided by a factor of at least ten

Referencing format and style

References are numbered and listed on pages 303 through 313 and are arranged in alphabetical order by author and in ascending order by year of publication by author. Citations are by number or by author and year of publication.

Biographical sketches

The Dictionary includes biographical sketches for deceased persons noted for their contributions to the field of clinical trials. It also contains sketches for a few other persons to the extent to which their names appear in defined entries. See the index entry, *biographical sketch*, for listing.

Usage notes

Confusing or troublesome terms are followed by notes indicating the nature of the confusion or trouble. Recommended usages and practices are also indicated via notes. See the index heading, *usage note*, for a listing of terms having such notes.

Etymologies

Etymologies for base and modifier terms are, for the most part, taken verbatim from *Webster's New Ninth Collegiate Dictionary*.[159] See pages xlvii through l for abbreviations used.

Abbreviations and designations

Pages xlvii through l provide a list of abbreviations and designations used in the body of this work. The listing includes shorthand designations used to denote organizational and operating units of trials, as well as designations used by various governmental agencies for designation.

Entry listing

Entries represented in the Dictionary are listed on pages li through xcv. See page xix, **Defined and blind entries**, for print conventions.

Indexes

The Dictionary contains a combined subject and author index. Terms or phrases in italic in a definition or related usage note refer to index headings, as in, See *bias* for list, in the entry for **bias**.

Entries dealing with or related to a particular topic or subject are indexed to that topic or subject. Some of the index headings serve the dual purpose of being both concatenation and subject headings. Hence, the contents of headings such as *bias* are composites of entries having the index term as a base and of terms related to that heading as a subject, eg, **Hawthorne effect** or **Heisenberg effect** in relation to the heading *bias*.

All authors listed in references appearing on pages 303 through 313 are indexed. Only the specific authors listed in text citations are indexed. For example, only Jones is indexed in a text citation of the form [Jones et al, 1990].

Studies cited are indexed under the heading *study index*. Page numbers cited correspond to mentions of those names or shortened forms of those names in a reference citation or in the text of a definition or usage note.

Entries defining an agency, institution, or place, such as the **American National Standards Institute** or the **Food and Drug Administration**, are indexed to the heading *agency and place index*.

Entries with usage notes are indexed to *usage note*.

Biographical sketches included in the Dictionary are listed under the index heading *biographical sketch*.

Headings without content, which simply refer users to the appropriate headings — blind entries, eg, *blind, see mask* and *endpoint, see outcome* — are interspersed throughout the index. Terms not recommended for usage or not preferred appear as blind entries. Headings with content related to others, eg, the headings *treatment assignment* and *randomization*, are interconnected by inclusion of "see also" instructions in each such heading.

The page numbers following entries in the reference list (pages 303 through 313) correspond to citations of those entries in the body of the Dictionary.

Usage practices, cautions, and recommendations

We use different words to mean the same thing. We vary our verbiage to reduce monotony and add zest and color to what we say or write. We expect variation and are taught to deal with it. A child learns that 10:45, quarter to eleven, 15 minutes to eleven, 15 minutes till eleven, and forty-five minutes after ten are the same. As adults, we understand when a radio announcer tells us that the *Yankees trounced the Red Sox, the Athletics pummelled the Angels, the Indians squeaked by the Tigers, and the Orioles were triumphant over the Twins,* though we would have learned as much if the announcer had used *beat* in place of *trounced, pummeled, squeaked by,* and *were triumphant over.*

We not only tolerate the variation but in some measure are enriched by it. Imagine Mark Twain or Robert Frost with the staid writing style of a scientist.

As in ordinary discourse, we accept minor variations in the discourse of a researcher without difficulty. We accept that an author is using the same basic trick as the sports announcer when discussing the work of others by referring to *Smith's findings and the work of Harrison and coworkers,* or by indicating that *Jones found, Franklin indicates,* and *Green et al concluded.*

However, our tolerance for variation diminishes as we move up the scale of required precision. Lawyers, responsible for drafting wills or contracts, are more interested in producing documents that will stand up to court challenges than in interesting reading. Variation of language in the discourse of research, even if not "fatal" in the same sense as for legal documents, is, nonetheless, undesirable to the extent that it confuses or obscures. For example, a reader is more likely to be confused than entertained by reference in one place to **baseline examinations**, in another to **screening examinations**, and in still another to **eligibility examinations**, when the three terms all refer to the same examinations. The emphasis should be on uniformity and precision, even if to the disadvantage of style and prose.

No self-respecting researcher sets about producing documents that are vague or confusing, although much of what we write is vague and confusing. Why? In part, because of haste and failure to refine, reiterate, and edit, ad nauseam, and in part because the language for a single project, even if carried out over a relatively short period of time, evolves — changes that may go unnoticed in the same way that most other gradual changes escape our notice. Most of the research efforts involving trials, even if followup is of short duration, measured in days or weeks, will extend over a period of months, if not years. Hence, thought must be given at the outset to terminology. Conventions should be established and maintained over the life of the project. The careful worker will establish a glossary of accepted terms and their definitions, including lists of accepted synonyms when applicable, and maintain and update it over the course of the activity.

Recommended and preferred usages

Terms in the table below are classified as follows:

R   Recommended
NR Not recommended
P   Preferred
NP Not preferred
A   Avoid
CC Caution, may be confusing or contradictory in some settings
CR Caution, may be redundant or unnecessary
CP Caution, presumptive
CW Caution, weasel term

Preferred is a weaker categorization than *Recommended* and is used when there are reasons for the preference but when they are not convincing enough to warrant a *Recommended* categorization. Most of the categorizations are supported in usage notes for listed terms or their complements (see index heading *usage note* for list). The categorization *Avoid* is used for terms with contradictory definitions or having high potential for confusion in other regards. Terms in the category *Caution, redundant* are likely to be redundant or unnecessary in most usages. The categorization *Caution, presumptive* is used for terms usually implying underlying facts, conditions, or assumptions. Those facts, conditions, or assumptions should be made explicit if terms in this class are used. The category *Caution, weasel* is used for terms used primarily for qualification or **weaseling** (see **weasel term**, page 297, for note).

Word or term	Category	Comment
allocation (defn 2)	NP	Use **assignment**, see **assignment** for usage note (pg 13)
allocation ratio	NP	Use **assignment ratio**
analysis by intention to treat	NP	Use **analysis by treatment assignment**
assignment	R	
arm (defn 2)	NP	Use **group**
average	NP	Use **mean**
baseline	CC	
bi- (meaning twice)	A	Use twice or **semi-**
biannual	A	Dual meaning; twice a year or once every other year
bias	CP	
bimonthly	A	Dual meaning; twice monthly or once every other month
biweekly	A	Dual meaning; twice weekly or once every other week
blind, blinded	NP	Use **mask** or **masked**
careful	CR	See **careful** for usage note (pg 33)

Word or term	Category	Comment
case-comparison study	NP	Use **case-control study**
case-compeer study	NP	Use **case-control study**
case-history study	A	Contradictory meanings
case-referent study	NP	Use **case-control study**
co- (prefix)	CC	co-principal investigator; contradictory meanings in certain usages; see **co-** for usage note
co-principal	CC	See usage note for **co-** and **co-principal**
co-principal investigator	A	Dual meaning; see usage note for **co-** and **co-principal**
collaborative	CR	collaborative trial; not a suitable synonym for multicenter
compeer	NR	case-compeer study; use **case-control study**
confounded	CP	See usage note for **confounded** (pg 52)
cooperative	CR	Not a suitable synonym for multicenter
double-blind, double-blinded	NP	Use **double-mask** or **double-masked**
double-mask, double-masked	P	
drop-in	A	Subject to confusion
early stopping	CP	See usage note for **early** *adj*
endpoint	NR; CC	See usage note for **endpoint**
experimental trial	CR	See usage note **experimental trial** (pg 93)
fraud	CP	See usage note (pg 104)
gold standard	CP	See usage note (pg 108)
informed consent	CP	Use **consent**; see usage note for **informed consent** (pg 127)
intention to treat	CP	Use more informative terminology such as analysis by original treatment assignment; see usage note (pg 129)
intervention	NP	Use treatment; see pg xx
mask, masked	P	
meta-analysis	R	
monthly	CC	See usage note for **month** (pg 161) and **time measure** (pg 274)
multicenter	R	See usage note for **multicenter** (pg 162)
open	CW	Not informative when used as an adjective in relation to trial (eg, open trial) or treatment administration (eg, open label); see usage note for **open** (pg 179)
open label	A	Uninformative and subject to confusion with **open trial**; use **unmasked**
open label trial	NR	Use **unmasked trial**
open trial	A	Subject to confusion; avoid; see usage note for **open trial** (pg 180)
oral consent	R	Use in conjunction with consents obtained without benefit of a written statement; not a synonym for **verbal consent**
outcome	P	See usage note for **endpoint** *n* (pg 86)
overmatch	CW; CP	See usage note for **overmatch** (pg 182)
overrepresent	CP	See usage note for **underrepresent** (pg 288)
overstudy	CP	See usage note for **understudy** (pg 288)
overview analysis	A	Synonym for **meta-analysis**; avoid, use **meta-analysis**
pre- (prefix)	CC	Use sparingly and with caution; see usage note for **pre-** (pg 203)

Word or term	Category	Comment
preclinical	CC	Meaning dependent on context; use with caution; see usage note (pg 203)
principal investigator	NP	Often not a useful designation, especially in multicenter settings; see usage note for **principal investigator** (pg 207); use only as an administrative label
randomness	CP	See usage note (pg 222)
run-in	NP	Use **lead-in**
semi- (prefix)	P	semiannual, semimonthly, semiweekly; preferred to **bi-**; see usage notes for **semi-** (pg 245) and **bi-** (pg 24)
side effect	CP	See usage notes for **side effect** (pg 248) and **drug reaction** (pg 79)
single-blind, single-blinded	NP	See usage note for **mask, masked** *adj* (pg 152)
single-mask, single-masked	P	See **mask, masked**
subject	NP	See usage note for **subject** (pg 263) for reasons to avoid or limit use
toxic drug reaction	CP	See usage note for **drug reaction** (pg 79)
toxic side effect	CP	See usage notes for **side effect** (pg 248) and **drug reaction** (pg 79)
treatment	P	Preferred label for the experimental variable in a trial; see usage notes for **treatment** (pg 276) and for **intervention** (pg 132)
treatment arm	NP	Use treatment group or regimen; see usage note for **treatment arm** (pg 277)
treatment failure	CP	See usage note for **treatment failure** (pg 280)
triple-blind, triple-blinded	NP	See defn for **blind** and usage note for **mask, masked** *adj* (pg 152)
triple-mask, triple-masked	P	See usage note for **mask, masked** *adj* (pg 152)
trohoc study	NR	Jocular; avoid
undermatch	CW; CP	See usage note for **overmatch** (pg 182)
underrepresent	CP	See usage note for **underrepresent** (pg 288)
understudy	CP	See usage note for **understudy** (pg 288)
verbal consent	NP	Use **oral consent** or **written consent**
withdrawal	CP	See usage note for **withdrawal** (pg 298)

Comparative and relative terms

Clinical trials, by definition, are comparative and concerned with ascertaining relative truth. As a consequence, the language of trials is laden with the language of relativity and comparison.

Comparative terms such as *large*, *early*, or *long* have meaning only in relation to explicitly defined or implied standards. The tendencies in everyday discourse to use such terms as if they have intrinsic meanings of their own is not acceptable in discourse when those terms are used or intended to have an explicit meaning. The careful user in such settings will take care to be explicit as to the meaning of comparative terms used in relation to some method, process, or result in which meanings are important.

Words such as *more* or *less* are in and of themselves comparative terms. They should not be used in relation to states or conditions not amenable to such quantification. For example, one is either

Comparative and relative terms   Comparative and relative terms

pregnant or not pregnant there are no other states. Similarly, it is pointless to think of or characterize one position or stand as *more* ethical than another. If one is ethical, there is no way to be *more* ethical.

For the most part, the language of comparison is symmetrical and should be thought of and used in that way. Hence, one should not use *early*, as in *early stopping*, unless there is a notion of what it means to stop on time or to be *late* in stopping. Similarly, the notion of *big* or *bigger* should have counterparts related to *small* or *smaller*, and the notion of *easy* has meaning only in contrast with *difficult* or *hard*.

Our everyday usage abounds in the use of relative terms as absolutes. To be convinced one need only count the number of times one is expected to make a decision or choice without the information needed for doing so. For example, at the fast food lunch counter, one is expected to answer the question: *Small, medium, or large?* without any idea of the sizes involved. Merchants are adept at wooing us into their stores by notice of *sale* or *discount* or by announcing *Everything 30% off*. We rush to spend to "save".

Often the norm or standard for comparison is implicit, as in *tall* or *short*, *fat* or *thin*, and *early* or *late*. We usually know what is meant when somebody tells us that *Johnny is tall, Darlene is fat*, or *Henry is late*. The standard implied for Johnny is the average height of other boys about the same age and general heritage as Johnny.

Our everyday language is laced with terms indicative of change, such as *more* or *less*, *up* or *down*, *high* or *low*, and *better* or *worse*. To make an assessment of change, one has to have observations of the condition or variable of interest at two or more points in time. Ordinarily, one is careful to indicate the point of comparison, eg, *We are better off financially now than we were a year ago*. Exceptions arise when the previous time point is implied, eg, *the patient is worse today*, or where there is a desire or value to being vague as to the actual point of comparison, eg, advertising claims such as *better than ever, new and improved, save more than ever*, or *Now, more than ever* (NBC television voiceover boast following their evening news show).

Change measures are the result of differencing operations and, hence, are signed. The direction of the comparison must be made explicit for proper interpretation of the measure. Typically, changes are measured relative to baseline or relative to a specified study treatment (usually a control treatment) in the case of trials. Changes relative to baseline are presented as a signed difference (eg, *the mean weight loss after 6 months of treatment was + 8.9 lbs*) or with sufficient information to allow the reader to do the differencing (eg, *the mean body weight was 156.5 lbs at baseline and 147.6 lbs after 6 months of treatment*). Changes relative to a specified treatment are presented in similar fashion (eg, *the 6 month mortality rates were 17.6% and 22.8%, for the test and control treatment groups, respectively*, or *the test-control difference in mortality was - 5.2%*).

Some changes will involve changes of changes (eg, *laser treatment produced a net intraocular pressure (IOP) drop of 3.1 mmHg relative to baseline and the control treatment as measured at the 6-month followup visit*). Net changes (defn 2) are differences of differences. The value, in the example, 3.1 mmHg, is in fact the result of two different differencing operations. The first one involves deriving the net IOP change for the two treatment groups being compared, done by subtracting the 6-month value for a patient from the patient's baseline value and deriving the mean of those differences for the eyes represented in the two treatment groups. The value for the laser-treated eyes is then subtracted from the corresponding value for control-treated eyes to yield the net laser treatment effect, $(16.5 - 22.1) - (19.4 - 21.9) = - 5.6 - (- 2.5) = - 3.1$.

Comparative and relative terms   **Comparative and relative terms**

The potential for confusion is great in all differencing operations. Confusion as to the way in which the differences were obtained, when they are large, has the potential of causing readers to indicate the wrong treatment. Hence, signed differences, such as the + 8.9 or - 3.1 in the paragraphs above should be accompanied by sufficient detail (via example or definitional verbiage) to minimize the chance of readers being confused about meaning of the sign in relation to the treatment favored or disfavored.

Redundancies, repetitions, and unnecessary words

The habit of repeating what we say for emphasis or "clarity" carries into what we write. In case of doubt, delete every other sentence in a prized draft. Most of the message survives with half the words. Early drafts of most things are long and wordy because of repetition and poor organization. The amount of redundant and repetitious material provided may go unnoticed until one is faced with the need to shorten or edit by edict of editors. It is sobering, at such times, to note the number of awkward or wordy parses or sentences that can be "fixed" simply by deleting them. Usually the editor's requirement to cut the length, sometimes by as much as 50%, though painful, results in a better, more informative paper.

Our spoken language, by the same token, is wordy, repetitious, and redundant. We repeat because we seemingly abhor silence and because we want to make certain we are "getting through". We use throwaway declaratives such as, *you know* in place of pauses, and we ask for reassurance in the form of questions such as *OK?* or *Understand?* — questions we ask repeatedly and usually without even pausing for an answer. Though our written word is devoid of such annoying fillers, it is certainly not free of redundancies and needless repetition.

The emphasis in scientific writing should be on conciseness and on word economy. Saying the same thing with different words in different places in the manuscript can cause a careful reader to assume that difference in language is purposeful and intended to convey difference. Consider the following sentences, intended by the writer to be equivalent: *Baseline information was collected at baseline visits* and *Entry data were collected during screening examinations.* The only way they will be recognized as being equivalent is if the reader is clever enough to equate *baseline information* and *entry data* and *baseline visits* and *screening examinations.*

Ralph Waldo Emerson reminds us that *A foolish consistency is the hobgoblin of little minds*, and indeed it may be so. However, the consistency of nomenclature and terminology within a manuscript and across related manuscripts is neither foolish nor is it likely to be the product of small minds.

Redundant words or phases should be avoided, if for no other reason than for word economy. Some words are unnecessary simply because they are obvious or implied in the context of usage, eg, *human* in *human subject, prospective* in *prospective followup*, and often *clinical* in *clinical trial.* Other examples are *primary* in *primary purpose* and *overall* in *overall aim.*

Other words, though technically unnecessary, are nonetheless required, for example, *female* in *pregnant female.*

Most adverbs (*ly* words) are unnecessary. Many can be deleted simply because they are implied in the context of usage, for example, *carefully* in *carefully measure.* One assumes care on the part of the researcher hence, there is nothing to be gained by its use in this context. If the writer believes it is important for the reader to know how something was done then details should be provided and the writer should leave the characterization to the reader. Other examples include *extremely* as in *extremely high* (use *high*), *highly* as in *highly important* (use *important*) or as in *highly significant* (use *significant* and state the p-value), *really* as in *really low* (use *low*), or *actually* as in *actually determined* (use *determined*).

Words expressing desire, such as *want* or *like*, are also unnecessary. For example, rather than writing *we want to point out* write *we point out*. Similarly, rather than writing *we would like to thank*, write *we thank*. As a reader one is more interested in what authors do than in what they would like to or want to do.

Many of the words or phrases of transition, deduction, conclusion, or exception, such as *however*, *generally*, *moreover*, *therefore*, *in general*, *in summary*, or *nonetheless*, can be eliminated from the finished written product. Use should be limited to places where they are needed to warn of breaks in flow, of exceptions to what is being said, or of a conclusion or deduction. Avoid redundant usage, as in *therefore, we conclude ...* (use *therefore* or *conclude*) or as in *In general, usually ...* (*usually* serves the same function as *in general*; use *usually* — one word and fewer letters than for *in general*).

Various other excesses are:
> *actively reinforce* (use *reinforce*)
> *careful monitoring* (use *monitoring*)
> *careful review* (use *review*, one assumes all reviews are carefully done)
> *comprehensive system* (use *system*; let the reader judge as to comprehensiveness)
> *effective solution* (use *solution*, all solutions are effective in the literal sense of that term)
> *formal system* (use *system*, one assumes a system has structure and hence is formal in that sense)
> *further clarification* (use *clarification*, let the reader decide if it is "further")
> *overcomplier* (jargon; avoid; it is not possible to "*overcomply*")
> *planned schedule* (use *schedule*, the term implies *planned*)
> *quite good* (jargon; avoid; describe and let the reader judge as to "goodness")
> *regularly review* (use *review* and indicate the schedule of review)
> *strict method* (use *method* and let the reader decide if it is "strict")

Not saying what we mean

Often we do not mean what we say or ask. The practice arises from our desire not to offend and from carelessness in the way we talk and write. Often the questions we are asked are not to be interpreted as questions at all, such as the *May I help you?* question of a building sentry (usually better interpreted as *Halt, who goes there?* or *What do you want?*). The proper answer to *May I bother you for the time?* is *yes* (assuming one is willing to be bothered) or *no*.

As a literalist, I find that there is a certain mischievous satisfaction in answering the question asked rather than the one intended. My usual answer to sentries at my institution is *Yes* to *Do you have an ID?* Depending on the sentry, I am from two to a half dozen strides beyond the sentry post before I am actually asked to produce my ID. On the phone, the proper response to *May I ask who is calling?* is *yes* (or *no*) and wait in silence for the proper question such as *Who may I say is calling?*, a less polite *Who is calling?*, or a curt *Who is this?*

One need merely read such childhood favorites as *Amelia Bedelia* to appreciate that what we say is not what we mean, especially when it comes to instruction. The adage *when everything else fails read the instructions* is as much a reflection of the usefulness of most instructions as of our own impatience in dealing with them. Surely any parent who has had to assemble a child's toy can attest to the "usefulness" of written instruction. Often, it is after one has managed to assemble the toy, largely by trial and error, that one manages to understand the instructions — an understanding most assuredly not enhanced by the desire of manufacturers to make one set of instructions work for 17

Not saying what we mean

versions of the toy and by the fact that your version is "new and improved" and is not mentioned in the instructions.

Amelia Bedelia's only "failing" was that she followed Mrs. Rogers' instructions to a T. So when she was told to dust the furniture she did — with powder — and when she was told to change the towels in the bathroom she did — by cutting them in half. The problem was in the instruction not with Amelia. Nevertheless, it was Amelia who suffered the embarrassment of "her" mistakes, not Mrs. Rogers for hers.

One need merely read the instructions in the manuals we write to discover that we are not necessarily any better at instructing than Mrs. Rogers. Similarly, we have the same potential as the sentry or the person on the other end of the phone for asking the wrong question when it comes to designing our data collection forms. It is certain that our instructions and data forms will be vague, confusing, and even misleading unless they are written and rewritten and tested and retested before being put to use.

Humanizing the inanimate

We learn as children to attribute human qualities to inanimate objects. Children's stories such as the *Little Engine That Could*, and TV shows such as *Sesame Street* are filled with objects that have human qualities. As children we are thrilled by fantasies of dancing sugarplums, steam engines with personalities, and scarecrows that come alive. As adults we come to realize that there are no talking scarecrows or engines that can, while at the same time offering encouragement to Betsy, the family car, as she struggles up a hill or cursing our computer for being so obstinate. We speak of Mother Nature, Father Time, Old Man River, winds that are calm or restless, stock markets that react, and economies that recover.

Some of the attributions are useful. It is more efficient (and colorful) to say that the *wind is calm* than to say that the *wind velocity is 0* or that the *computer tells us* instead of *our analysis indicates*.

We are likely to write that *the trial found, the study concluded*, and *the results tell us*. It is people who find, conclude, and tell us, not trials, studies, and results. Those processes are distinctly human and should not be attributed to the object of interest in what we write.

Pre- and post- words

The prefixes *pre-* and *post-* are used as modifiers to denote order or sequence in relation to some event or action, eg, pre- or post-war. Of the two, *pre-* is the more common and more objectionable. There is no doubt that if the Big Dictionary Writer in the Sky suddenly banned all *pre-* words a few would be missed, such as *preview* and *preamble*, but overall there would be more celebrations than wakes. Would anyone miss those vacuous congratulatory salutations of letters from credit card companies notifying us that our applications — applications never made or desired — have been *pre-approved*? Would anyone be upset if the airlines simply offered early boarding instead of the opportunity to *preboard*? Would we care if cooks suddenly stopped *pre-heating* their ovens and were content to simply heat them?

The creation of a *pre-* or *post-* word by affixing the prefix to a verb creates some of the most objectionable uses, for example, *preboarding* a plane or a *prerecorded* show. How is it possible? What is the state of being *preboarded*? Does it involve being beamed aboard in the "Star Trek" sense? Or does it involve boarding the plane on the tarmac before it has arrived at the gate? Similarly, what are we to make of the claim *prerecorded before a live audience*? How does a TV network manage to do that? Does it mean they recorded the show before the audience arrived? Does it mean that they did the recording before the audience died?

Pre- and post- words   **Pre- and post- words**

The best practice is to avoid all *pre-* and *post-* words, except those found in ordinary desk dictionaries. Use beyond the ordinary should be limited to instances in which such terms are used as forms of shorthand expressions for more complicated phrases, if at all. The finished written product should be scanned for jargonistic usages, undefined uses, and usages in which the terms can be avoided by use of other words or modifying phrases. In fact, most uses can be avoided with *before* or *after* as in *before randomization, after randomization, before screening, after screening* (instead of *pre-randomization, post-randomization, pre-screening,* and *post-screening*).

Small troublesome words

Prepositions such as *by, for, from, on, to,* and *through* are often used in relation to measurements or time designations. Hence, we may read that all patients were seen **by** *the middle of the year, measurements cover a range of values **from** 42 **to** 89, all patients are to be seen **on** the 1st of the month, the last interval includes values **through** 423,* or *patients were instructed to take their medication* **for** *a period of 10 days.* All of the words have varied usages, as is readily seen by the number of definitions and the length of the entries for those terms in any standard desk dictionary.

By in relation to time means up to, up to and beyond, close to, past, in the period of, not later than. *On* in the same context means occurrence at a given time or at an exact moment in time. Hence, the two words have different connotations and are not interchangeable, though they are often used as if they are. Perhaps the best example of such presumed interchangeability is in the 1990 National Census. Instructions on the outside of the packet mailed to every household in the United States prior to April 1, 1990 were to *complete your form and return it by April 1, 1990*; but the first item on the form asked the recipient to *list on the numbered lines below the names of each person living here on Sunday, April 1.* Clearly, no one at the Census Bureau had any concern regarding the logical inconsistency involved in expecting recipients to complete and return the form *by* April 1 while at the same time asking them to report the number of people living in the household *on* April 1. Clearly, as a literalist, I had to either guess as to my whereabouts on April 1 and comply with the instruction on the outside of the packet or ignore the instruction and wait until or after April 1 to fill out the form. For all we know, some of the undercounting was due to literalists being driven to inaction by contradictory instruction.

On in relation to time should refer to a point in time and *for* to an interval of time. *On* is sometimes confused with *for* and used instead of *for.* For example, baseball announcers, for reasons that remain a mystery to me, invariably speak of batting average *on* the year, eg, *Cal Ripkin is batting 287 on the year.* Why not *for the year?*

To means reaching or extending as far as, reaching or extending to some point or limit. *Through* means from the beginning to the end, in or during an entire period or interval, to and including. *For* is a function word for indicating amount, extent, or duration. *To,* in relation to a time point or continuous measure, may include the point indicated or may be inclusive of all points or measures up to but not including that point. Hence, its use leaves room for confusion. For example, does the statement *applications accepted up to January 15* mean the 14th is the last day they will be taken or will they be accepted through the 15th? The situation is not helped much by using *by* in place of *to.* A reasonable operational rule is to assume, unless one is told or otherwise indicated, that the use of *to* excludes the point of reference, and, hence, in the example above, plan on being done with the application by the 14th. The IRS avoids use of *by* or *on* with an instruction telling us that our tax returns must be filed *not later than April 15.* Does it mean we must file before April 15 or do we have until the midnight separating April 15th and 16th? Even a casual observer of activities on April 15 learns the answer. We should avoid such confusions by being explicit about whether the designated time point is included or excluded from permissible time points, eg, by indicating that *applications will be accepted through January 15th* or that *applications will be accepted up to and including January 15th* and that we have *through April 15* to file our tax return.

From is used as a function word to indicate a starting point, eg, ***from** this day forward* or ***from** January 16th on*. The term is subject to ambiguities when used as a reference point, eg, *people having weights from 150 lbs and greater*. The reader is in doubt about whether the statement is intended to include or exclude the value of 150. The problem is avoided by writing *people with a weight of 150 or greater*.

The language of praise, implied value judgment, and presumption

We have a variety of words and terms for expressing or intimating praise or value judgment. They are useful in everyday discourse but have a limited role in the discourse of science, where emphasis is on fact rather than on praise or value. The responsibility of the writer is to convey the necessary information to enable readers to reach their own conclusions. It is pointless, if not bad form, to coach readers as to the values they should adopt, except on editorial pages of journals or perhaps on the discussion pages of a manuscript.

A dispassionate writer avoids use of qualitative labels or characterizations such as *good, careful, accurate,* or *precise* in relation to his or her methods or procedures. They are what they are and laudatory characterizations do not make them better.

The use of self-laudatory language in relation to one's own work is foolhardy. It is presumptuous, pompous, and short-sighted to label one's own work original, unique, or innovative; likewise, it is a sign of consummate naivete to characterize work still in planning or execution as *definitive*, eg, *we are carrying out a trial to provide a definitive answer to the question*. Typically, *definitive* is a characterization applied in retrospect by others, years hence. By the same token, one should avoid characterizations such as *modern*, as in *we used modern methods to determine concentrations of the compound*. Modern is in the eye of the beholder, and the mere application of a label does not serve to make a method modern nor does absence of the term imply antiquation. Ditto for *easy* or *simple*.

Implied praise by use of laudatory language in relation to the work of others should be genuine. Avoid it as fluff or as a prelude to a wilting attack or criticism.

The clinical trialist should take pains to avoid implied conclusions or presumptions in the nomenclature used for key measures, variables, or phenomena. One reason for doing so has to do with the need to avoid confusion when doing the trial, for example, as discussed in a usage note for *endpoint* (page 86) as a synonym for *outcome*. Reaching an *endpoint* implies cessation or completion. Its use as a synonym for *outcome* may be justified when the event being referenced is death or some other event that, when it occurs, means the end of treatment or followup, but not in other uses.

Another reason has to do with the need for avoiding implied conclusions, for example, in most usages of *treatment failure* when applied to individual patients, eg, *the patient was considered to be a treatment failure because of the side effects associated with the treatment* or *patients having an MI were considered to be treatment failures* (see usage note for the term, page 280). Both uses imply cause and effect relationships. For the first use to be justified, one should be convinced that the side effects being referenced are unique to the indicated treatment. Even placebos have side effects. The second use implies that the treatment is known to prevent MI — an implication, which in all probability, presupposes more knowledge of the drug and its mode of action than actually exists.

Language of presumption

Language of presumption

Most uses of *treatment failure* are as implied indictments of a treatment arising because of the "failure" of the treatment to have prevented or delayed some adverse health event or outcome. Study personnel should be taught to use operationally neutral language (eg, event or outcome) in place of the characterization. In addition, they should be taught to avoid use as a collective label for an aggregate of events or outcomes having various explanations (as in a table entitled *Treatment failures by treatment group* with counts of a heterogeneous collection of events or outcomes observed in the different treatment groups). The term is meaningless in settings where used without regard to treatment assignment.

It is meaningless as well in settings where one of the study treatments is a placebo or null treatment. Use in such settings is indicative of a certain sloppiness of language and will likely cause discerning readers mild befuddlement as to ways in which placebo or null treatments could "fail".

The term *drug reaction* carries a cause and effect connotation as well. Similarly, many uses of *side effect* in relation to drugs imply such a relationship. Both terms should be avoided when the relationship is in question, or when they are used in settings where only some of the uses are justified (eg, a placebo-controlled trial where some of the "drug reactions" are due to placebo or in which some of the "reactions" occur in the absence of any drug).

Qualitative labels such as *mild*, *moderate*, or *severe* carry implied judgments that should be made explicit. Except when obvious, the implied rationale behind the labeling should be explained (eg, by indicating the sense in which something is considered to be *mild*, *moderate*, or *severe*).

For the most part, a label such as *toxic drug reaction*, should be avoided because of what it implies. For the use to be justified, one should be convinced that the reaction is in fact due to the drug and that the reaction is serious and life-threatening. Whenever possible the label should be replaced by neutral, more descriptive, and less presumptive language.

Many of the everyday examples of presumptive uses arise from erroneous assumptions (as in assuming that a woman answering the phone at a place of work is a secretary, that the captain of a plane is a man, and that a nurse is a woman). Uses based on presumption should be avoided.

Euphemisms

Our everyday language is filled with euphemisms that shield us from the harsh reality of life. Hence, a person "passes away" rather than dies. A veterinarian "puts a dog to sleep" instead of killing the animal, and the laboratory scientist "sacrifices" his rabbits. We know what these terms mean, so to that extent they are acceptable. Such expressions are troublesome only when used to purposefully obscure, eg, when telling a child that her "mommy has gone away" rather than that she has died.

The medical profession has its own form of euphemism to the extent that some of the most obnoxious procedures or treatments can have innocent sounding names or labels. Hence, as a patient I may not realize what is being proposed when I am told that they want to give me a retro-vulvar injection or that they want to enucleate my eye. The technical jargon of the medical profession has its place in classrooms, textbooks, and manuscripts but not in dialogues with patients and most assuredly not in dialogues carried out as part of a consent process. Investigators have a responsibility to ensure that the consents they obtain are ***informed***. They are not, by definition, if the person being asked to consent does not understand what is being proposed.

Trialists have their own euphemisms to obscure and confuse. As a group, they are more likely to label trials in which the physician or patient chooses the treatment to be administered as **open trials** (defn 1) than as **nonrandomized trials** and to speak of **open label trials** instead of **unmasked trials** when the study treatments are administered in unmasked fashion. The careful writer avoids euphemisms in favor of more informative terminology. Failing that, uses should be in conjunction with sufficient supporting detail to make their meanings clear.

Currency words

A currency word or phrase is one that implies use of an underlying process or procedure, eg, *validation was carried out by monitors, the study involved **documented** data collection procedures, patients gave their **informed** consent*. Words, such as *documented, validated*, or *informed* should not be used without supporting detail to indicate sense of use. Words such as *demonstrate, shown*, or *proven* become currency words when used in declarative statements, eg, *the results demonstrate the cost efficiency of the approach*. The writer should indicate the basis for the conclusion, or delete the claim from the finished manuscript.

Randomize, as in *patients were randomized*, is a currency word and should not be used in simple declarative statements without supporting detail about the process or procedure used to randomize. Failure to provide such supporting details has the potential of leaving readers uncertain about whether the use is in the formal or the lay sense of that term (see usage note for **random**, page 219).

Informed, as in **informed** *consent*, is an important currency word in trials. Use of the modifier *informed*, in relation to *consent* as in *patients gave their informed consent to be randomized*, should be limited to cases involving explicit steps or procedures to ensure that the consents were truly informed or where data are presented to indicate the degree to which consents were informed. Without such detail or supporting data, the writer should use *consent* without the modifier (see usage note for **informed consent**, page 127).

The careful writer will avoid unsupported use of currency words. Manuscripts should be read prior to submission to identify them. Those that are not supported by accompanying detail or data should be deleted.

The language of criticism

The language of criticism is negative by definition and for that reason it is usually flavored with suitable praise and accolade. Critics who are sensitive to the feelings of those being criticized will try to deliver their message as gently as possible and with as little personal harm as possible. Hence, we come to be apprehensive of meetings with our bosses that start with perfunctory praise for fear of what is to follow.

We follow the same practice when writing a critique. We start with the positive and proceed to the negative. Hence, we might start with laudatory preambles followed by wilting critiques.

Trials producing "bad news" are more likely to be viewed with suspicion and doubt than those producing "good news". The "bad news" may be in the form of results challenging an accepted treatment or in the form of results running counter to prevailing beliefs. When the medical community at large is presented with such challenges, there is a tendency for its members to question the results and integrity or competence of investigators rather than their treatments or prevailing beliefs.

There is a tendency to regard any study failing to produce the "right" result as being *flawed*. Hence, we have grown accustomed to critics, especially when in front of audiences or on camera, who characterize a controversial result as being the product of a *flawed study*. Such claims, unless supported by detail that justifies use of the characterization, are vacuous and should be viewed as forms of empty rhetoric. A responsible critic does not use the claim without supporting facts and ignores flaws having little or no bearing on the issue at hand.

In our everyday life, we are exposed to a bewildering array of half truths and lies and to an unending chain of denials and claims of innocence or ignorance. Hardly a day passes without hearing or seeing such words or phrases as *categorically deny*, *absolutely innocent*, or *no knowledge of* in relation to some event or activity. We become increasingly skeptical of all such claims as we age and may eventually, with sufficient age, quietly translate the categorical denial of a politician into tacit admission of guilt.

It is no wonder, therefore, that claims of researchers are greeted with skepticism, not so much because we expect them to have lied, but because we are uncertain of their motivation and their competence. Hence, we may be inclined to accept a criticism of a trial as valid without much thought if it jibes with our biases, and reject it as irrelevant or invalid if it does not.

The form and language of criticism depend on the underlying motivation of the critic. All criticism is in some sense constructive, even if devastating and "destructive". Hence, an archenemy can provide constructive criticism even if the intent was to discredit or destroy. Similarly, a review undertaken by a person to better understand the limitations of a study and its finding may end up destroying the study by highlighting weaknesses.

We are familiar with language aimed at discrediting and increasing doubt for the purpose of blunting the effect of a result. One need merely watch a few interviews with opponents of a finding to learn the language of this form of criticism. One can anticipate what critics employed by tobacco companies will say of the next study on passive smoking if the results are suggestive of harm. The study design and method of conduct will be characterized as *flawed* and the results will be labeled as *equivocal*, *inconclusive*, or *not definitive*.

Every study is imperfect and, hence, *flawed*. The issue therefore is not whether the study is flawed, but rather whether the flaws detected are so serious as to warrant rejection of the results.

Results are usually *equivocal*, *inconclusive*, or *not definitive* in that they leave room for doubt. Hence, the label can be applied to findings of any study, including those considered to have produced convincing results. These terms should be used sparingly and more as conclusions than as labels. Use should be supported by a detailed recitation of the facts and features of the study leading to the characterization.

The clever critic has a collection of universal criticisms that apply to all settings. One of those, in the case of trials, has to do with the fact that only persons consenting to enrollment can be studied. All randomized trials involve populations that are, by definition, select and not necessarily representative of the general population of interest. Hence, the statement that *the trial involved a highly select study population* is more a statement of fact than a criticism, though it is often used to leave the impression that the selectivity is the result of a bad study design or of improper study practices. It is used to suggest that the results are useless because they cannot be applied to the general population of interest. The critic is either unaware of the difference between **generalizability** and **validity** or is content to confuse the two issues (see pages 107 and 294).

A characteristic shared by both types of critics is in regard to the nature of their conclusion. Both are likely to underscore the need for more research on the issue at hand though their motivations for the statement are different. The statement from the constructive critic arises from a genuine desire for more information on the question at issue, whereas the destructive critic uses it more as a ploy than as an expression of desire for more information. The call is used to suggest that the current results are *equivocal* or *inconclusive* and as a tactic to dissuade groups or bodies from taking action in relation to the results. Critics with a vested interest in maintaining the status quo can be expected to achieve that end by whatever means possible, including use of the clarion call for more research to provide a "*definitive* answer" to the question or to resolve the issue.

Serious critics avoid grandstanding. They forego the use of cute tricks and clever phrases aimed at creating impressions without supporting substance. They stick to the facts and avoid use of generic claims as if they were unique to the study at hand. They concentrate on the issues that matter and ignore inconsequential "flaws". They avoid the use of value-laden words in favor of describing the features considered to be sources of concern.

The language of exception

Words such as *only*, *unless*, and *otherwise* are difficult to understand when they are used to indicate exception, as in the following from the Code of Federal Regulation for IRBs:

> *Unless otherwise required by Department or Agency heads, research activities in which the only involvement of human subjects will be in one or more of the following categories are exempt from this policy* (45 CFR 46, § 46.101; 18 June 1991 revision) (33 words)

Part of the problem is with the exception, *unless otherwise*. The statement is improved slightly by rewriting so the exception follows the rule:

> *Research activities in which the only involvement of human subjects will be in one or more of the following categories are exempt from this policy, unless otherwise required by Department or Agency heads* (33 words)

Only is a difficult word when used as an indicator of exception. One way to reduce use of the word is by elimination from constructions where it is unnecessary, as in *only once* or *only when*, and by deletion of only in the example above so as to read:

> *Research activities in which the involvement of human subjects will be in one or more of the following categories are exempt from this policy, unless otherwise required by Department or Agency heads* (32 words)

Only, when it precedes the main point, may be indicative of constructions that require more than the simple fix suggested above. For example, the better fix for the example above is to eliminate the clause *involvement of human subjects will be in one or more of the following categories* — a clause made necessary by use *only* in the example. Elimination of the clause would have allowed the drafters to have written:

> *The following categories of research are exempt from this policy, except where otherwise indicated by Department or Agency heads* (19 words)

The elimination would have reduced the word count from 33 to 19 and increased clarity of exposition.

The language of intimidation, implication, and position

We have various tricks to establish positions of superiority and for telegraphing our mental prowess. Hence, statisticians are likely to sprinkle their discourse with telltale signs of their skill or mental prowess by use of words such as *obviously*, *elementary*, *trivial*, *easily*, and *clearly* in relation to their mathematics and proofs. They are used as if the characterizations are useful to the receiver when, more often than not, they serve only to remind receivers of their own limitations, especially when confronted with things labeled as *trivial* or *easily shown* that are obscure and imponderable. Nor is it useful for the sender to "explain" by simply repeating that already stated or written, except to underscore one's own state of dementation.

Some of the signaling of standing and position occurs naturally and is useful in its proper context. For example, it may be appropriate and even useful for the statistician to describe something as *easily shown* when speaking to other statisticians, but not when speaking to members of another profession.

The setting of clinical trials involves people from different disciplines, each with their own peculiar language conventions and terminology. Much of the language of medicine will be foreign to others from different disciplines. The same is true for the language of the statistician as heard by others in the group.

People coming to this setting must be sensitive to the general state of knowledge of others in the group. They must be willing to adapt their language and methods of communication to the setting and must be willing to explain and educate as needed over the course of the trial. The vernacular of "household" terms within a discipline will be confusing and uninformative to others in the group not of that discipline. Members of the majority discipline need to recognize that use of esoteric lingo and jargon has the potential of being perceived by members of minority disciplines in the group as subtle forms of intimidation. The risk of intimidation exists whenever something complicated or esoteric is passed off as elementary or obvious.

Most forms of posturing, positioning, or intimidation via language are subtle and often the product of unconscious behavior. It arises as a natural consequence of the use of discipline-specific language in multidisciplinary settings such as those represented in clinical trials. The physicians, in a collaborating group, may use language and terminology foreign to other collaborators simply as a means of excluding them from the discussion or as a subtle reminder to keep their mouths shut. The statisticians may appear to speak in tongues and may converse without explanation as to how what they are saying relates to issues at hand.

Those in the majority in any setting have special needs to guard against the tyranny of numbers and assumption that it is they who represent the core of the activity. In the setting of trials, the majority of those involved in a multicenter trial will be MDs. Researchers from other specialties, including biostatisticians, will be in a distinct minority.

The language of division

We have various ways of communicating division or separation. When they are personal, we speak of we and they. When they are dispassionate, we have other means.

Taxonomies are based on divisions defined by mutually exclusive classes. Hence, the trialist may speak of randomized and nonrandomized trials and be content that the two classes cover the waterfront and that they are mutually exclusive.

Binary classification involving a seemingly well-defined characteristic, eg, in regard to one's gender, is straightforward. Problems arise when the line of demarcation is ill-defined, eg, with the characterization black or white as a surrogate for "race".

Problems also arise when a division is created with overlapping boundaries. For example, an epidemiologist may find it useful to classify studies as *observational* or *experimental*. The problem with the division is twofold. One has to do with the fact that the complement of *observational* is *nonobservational* and it is difficult to envision studies not involving observation of some sort. A second problem has to do with the fact that all members of the class *experimental study* are also members of the other class, *observational study*, to the extent that the class involves observation.

Problems are compounded when the applied labels also carry implied value judgments. A case in point is in the use of *basic* and *applied* in relation to the categorization of research. *Basic*, as an adjective and as defined in *Webster's Ninth New Collegiate Dictionary,*[159] means *of, relating to, or forming the basis or essence; fundamental; constituting or serving as the basis or starting point.* *Applied* as an adjective and as defined therein means to *put to practical use; especially applying general principles to solve definite problems.* The two terms are not complementary, and it is a mistake to use them as if they are.

That said, the fact is that many of the uses are as if the two terms are complementary. Such uses are unfortunate because, whether so intended or not, they have the potential for being divisive, if for no reason other than that they have the possibility of being viewed by those not in the valued class as degrading or as forms of "putdowns".

In the broad definitional sense, trials are as "basic" to medicine as bench research is to the laboratory sciences. Yet it is invariably those sciences that are designated or regarded as "basic" and those related to clinical medicine as "applied" and thereby labeled as being something less.

The trouble with the categorization is with the notion of basic. The complement of basic, if meant to mean *essential* or *important*, is *nonessential, unnecessary,* or *irrelevant.* Hence, the term has unfortunate connotations, especially in settings where it is used to set the work of one profession apart from that of another profession. Use in this way can be demeaning to the work of the profession not qualifying for the label. The characterization may have the effect of suggesting that its work is of less import than that of the profession characterized as basic.

Usurpative language

Societies have a propensity for usurpative usage. For example, *African-American* in the United States has come to be used in place of negro or black in reference to the cultural or racial heritage of peoples with negro ancestry, even though not all peoples of Africa are black. On a broader scale, we use *American* to mean peoples of the United States to the exclusion of all others living in the Americas. From the perspective of geography, a Canadian is as American as "Americans", but neither we nor they (in large measure) refer to peoples of Canada as Americans. They prefer, instead, to be called Canadians and thereby tacitly surrendering the term to us. Colin L. Powell (Chairman of the US Joint Chiefs of Staff in the Bush Administration), in remarks on 19 September 1994 following his return from Haiti, observed that we had only narrowly averted the prospect of *American youngsters killing Haitian youngsters and Haitian youngsters killing American youngsters.* He could just as well have spoken of Americans killing Americans, since Haiti is part of the Americas.

The language of usurpation arises from the use of a general term or label in a specialized circumstance that has the effect of usurping all other interpretations or implying that there are no other interpretations, for example, use of the labels *pro-life* and *pro-choice* as used in the abortion rights struggle. The alternative to *pro-life* is *anti-life* and *anti-choice* for *pro-choice.* The terms are used to paint people into corners by suggesting that a person labeled as *pro-choice* favors abortion on demand and that a person in the other corner opposes all abortions when, in fact, most people are likely to be both pro-life and pro-choice in the broad sense of those terms.

Most everyday forms of usurpation arise from failures to adopt usage patterns learned in one setting to a new and unfamiliar setting. The biggest "culprit" in the setting of clinical trials is likely to be the MD investigators: because they are at the top of the "pecking" order in the medical setting and because of their number. As a rule, the majority of people represented in any trial are MDs.

Clinical trials involve forms of clinical research, and most such research is, by definition, performed by MDs. Hence, the clinical investigator is prone to assuming that all investigators engaged in such activities are members of the medical profession and that the label *doctor* is synonymous with MD. Other members of the group with doctorates in other fields may feel slighted by uses implying that the only people in the setting with such a degree are MDs, eg, *the doctors doing the study recruited and enrolled a total of 400 patients.*

There is also need for care in the use of the label *investigator.* Often in the case of clinical trials, the label is used to imply that investigatorship status is limited to those in the group with an MD degree, eg, *investigators doing the trial saw patients every 3 weeks over the duration of the trial.* Other members of the group, as key to the investigation as those treating patients, may be peeved by the slight.

The designation *principal investigator* has varying interpretations, as discussed in a usage note for that term (page 207). Usages of this term in the multicenter trial are especially troublesome where there are, in effect, multiple principal investigators. The best advice is to avoid the use of the term in that setting. If it is used at all, it should be used to apply to all persons of equal standing in the group, regardless of degree or area of activity. For example, if it is used to denote heads of centers, then it should apply to all heads of centers and not simply to heads of clinics. The more common practice is to reserve the term for heads of clinics in that setting, eg, *we need to poll the PIs* (meaning clinic directors) *as to their preference regarding the proposed treatment modification.* Those usages imply that other people who play equally important roles (eg, the head of the coordinating center is not *principal*), have lesser standing in the group.

A form of usurpation arises in the multicenter trial when *center* is used as a synonym for clinic (see usage note for **center**, page 36), eg, *the 11 centers in the trial recruited a total of 842 patients.* People at other centers in the trial not responsible for recruiting patients may resent being written out of the study.

The language of implied subjugation, as in the use of *subject* (see usage note, page 263), though technically not usurpative, also should be avoided. That language is inconsistent with the notion of partnership as required for success in trials. The language of ownership is to be avoided for the same reason, as in *my statistician* or *my programmer.* The statistician or programmer is not likely to be warmed by usages that suggest that he or she is the property of a person or group. The same is true for persons enrolled in trials being referred to as *subjects.*

The language of positivity and negativity

Much of what we say or write is intended to express acceptance or rejection, generality or exception, inclusion or exclusion, presence or absence, permission or prohibition, approval or disapproval, or affirmation or rejection. Terms such as *yes* or *no, present* or *absent, certain* or *uncertain,* or *known* or *unknown* are used for characterizing or stating binary choices or states. The language of exception is expressed with qualifiers such as *only, few,* or *many.* Terms such as *not* or *no* are used for negation or for expressing some negative condition or state.

Binary states or conditions such as those covered with use of terms such as *all* or *none, yes* or *no,* or *present* or *absent* can be thought of as positive or negative and to that extent can be viewed as having arithmetic signs. Similarly, one can think of terms of exception or exclusion such as *only* or *closed* as negative, and terms of acceptance or inclusion such as *most* or *open* as positive.

The notion of signing in the mathematical sense is useful when analyzing or interpreting sentences containing several signed terms, and especially when the sentences involve terms of opposite sign or when they involve two or more negative terms. The rules of sign management for arithmetic operations apply to signed language. Crossing a positive with a positive produces a positive product. Crossing a negative with a positive produces a negative product, and crossing a negative with a negative produces a positive by negation of the negatives.

We are inclined to accentuate the positive and for that reason tend to use positive words in tandem, eg, *most certainly, absolutely sure*, or *Yes, we are open*. We have no trouble understanding the message conveyed, but it would have been conveyed as well (and with fewer words) by *certainly, sure*, or *open*.

Some double positives are crude and grammatically incorrect. For example, we know what is meant when someone tells us that *A is more better than B*, though it would have been less jarring to the ear had we simply been told that *A is better than B*.

Some uses of double positives are downright confusing. For example, what does it mean when Tariq Aziz, Deputy Prime Minister of Iraq, tells the world (Baghdad, Saturday 16 January 1993; prepared statement) that Iraq has complied with *"more than most"* of the UN stipulations? The statement is vacuous in the absence of definitions for *most* and *more*.

Most positive x positive crossings are unnecessary and, hence, are to be avoided. If a state or condition is positive, adding a positive descriptor does not make it "more" positive.

The two other kinds of crossings are more problematic. Of the two, positive x negative (or negative x positive) crossings are less objectionable than negative x negative crossings.

Many of our road signs involve the graphic equivalent of positive x negative crossings. Examples involve the use of recognized positive indicators, eg, P for parking or a right or left turn arrow to indicate that such turns are allowed, and a negator graphic, usually a diagonal line overlying the positive sign for the opposite message. Typically, it takes the brain a millisecond or two longer to inform the driver that such signs are proscribing the indicated activity as opposed to allowing it.

The arithmetical equivalent of this kind of crossing occurs with signed differences where a negative difference corresponds to something beneficial and a positive value corresponds to something bad, eg, a graphic display where values to the left of the y-axis denote improvement and values to the right of the y-axis denote worsening.

Our written language abounds in examples. Brewster Higley's familiar refrain *where seldom is heard a discouraging word and the skies are not cloudy all day* (Home on the Range, 1904) involves crossing a positive with a negative. The line is confusing because of the use of *not* and *all*. As a result, we remain uncertain as to whether he was telling us that the skies are clear all day or just part of the day. Higley could have avoided the confusion with the refrain *where words are usually encouraging and the skies are clear all day* (assuming that is what is meant by the line). Fortunately for us, Higley's concern was more with the sound and rhythm of words than with precision or efficiency of language.

As in Higley's line, most positive x negative crossings are subject to conflicting interpretations, for example, *No smoking is permitted* (announcements on commercial flights prior to takeoff). Does it mean no smoking or does it mean it is all right not to smoke? (The instruction *Please observe the no smoking sign when illuminated*, is no less obtuse. In a strict literary sense, a puffer could be in compliance with the instruction by fixating on the sign while puffing away.)

Positives and negatives

The announcement on Metroliners entering Union Station in Washington DC that *All doors will not open* has the same defect. Does it mean that only some of the doors on the right or left will open or that none will open? Imagine the panic of foreigners, unfamiliar with such constructions, if their conclusion is that none will open. Strictly speaking, the announcement applies to all stops, since egress is always from the right or left, depending on the location of the platform.

Other crossings of this form include expressions such as *busy doing nothing, driver carries no cash, no data were collected,* and *found no difference.* The problem in all these cases arises from crossing an active positive verb with a negator. The crossings lead to logical inconsistencies. How is it possible to be *busy* doing nothing? How does one *carry* nothing? How does one *collect* nothing? And how does one *find* nothing? Many of these apparent inconsistencies can be avoided, or at least made less jarring, by different constructions. For example, instead of *no data were collected,* write *data were not collected,* and instead of *driver carries no cash,* write *driver has no cash.*

Variations on the same theme have to do with the crossing of value terms, eg, *higher weight loss, lower weight gain, higher rate of loss, lower rate of gain,* or *survival as an endpoint.* A careful writer works to avoid such usages by various tricks. An obvious one involves a change in the base of comparison to enable the writer to express the difference in positive terms. For example, instead of *patients assigned to test treatment had a higher rate of weight loss than patients assigned to control treatment,* write *patients assigned to control treatment had a higher rate of weight gain than patients assigned to test treatment.* As noted previously, changes stated in positive terms are easier to understand than are negative changes.

Superfluous crossings can be avoided by expeditious editing. For example, use *none* instead of *none at all* (*none* is sufficient, *at all* is clutter). Similarly, use *not* or *no* instead of *absolutely not* or *positively no* (*not* or *no* is sufficient; *absolutely* and *positively* are unnecessary, except when used, for example, in a parent to child interaction, to distinguish this usage from others where something other than *not* or *no* is implied). Use of positive augmentations of negative terms is bad form in scientific writing in that they are unnecessary and tend to have the same effect on readers as on children when used by a parent — ie, it causes them to wonder whether unaugmented uses mean something less categorical than implied by the augmented terms.

The potential for confusion is greatest with negative x negative crossings. Some of these crossings can be avoided simply by deleting one of the negatives. For example, consider *Nobody can see the Great Oz, not nobody, not no how.* The guard making the pronouncement to Dorothy and her three companions at the entry to the Wizard's castle in the film version of the Wizard of Oz could just as well have proclaimed that *Nobody can see the Great Oz, nobody, no how* or simply *Nobody can see the Great Oz.*

The pronouncement of the guard, even if wordy, is clear. However, that is not usually the case with most double-negatives. For example, does the statement *Nobody doesn't like Sara Lee* mean that everyone likes Sara Lee or that no one likes Sara Lee? We know what the advertiser wants us to believe so why not claim *Everybody likes Sara Lee*? A good point, except that the latter statement is not as catchy as the former and, hence, not as revenue enriching — so much for literary accuracy.

We have been taught from grade school onward to avoid constructions involving double-negatives. Our parents and teachers corrected us when we said, *I don't want no food* or *I don't have no money.* With that kind of training and conditioning, one would expect our writing to be free of such constructions. They are, to be sure, free of vulgar constructions such as the two listed, but not of more subtle and sophisticated versions of the same thing. Many of the double-negatives in the discourse of trials arise from the practice of stating things in the negative as a means of indicating a measure of uncertainty. Hence, we speak of a patient as *not worse* because we are uncertain about whether the patient is better.

Other forms of the construction arise as a result of a desire to emphasis an unexpected result. Hence, the trialist describing results of a trial involving the use of a chemoprophylactic agent expected to cause weight loss, when presented with data showing no weight change, is more likely to write, *patients did not lose weight* than *patients did not experience a weight change*.

Another reason for such constructions has to do with our innate desire as researchers to maintain a measure of caution and conservatism in the interpretation given to results. Hence, we are usually more comfortable understating than overstating.

One has to be on constant guard for double-negatives with an eye toward elimination whenever possible. One means of elimination is by using complementary language (eg, by speaking of gain rather than loss). Others can be eliminated simply by using a different tack in the way results are presented or discussed. Those that remain should be analyzed to make certain that they are supported by sufficient discussion or detail to make their meaning clear. One way to do so in relation to a statement such as *patients assigned to the test treatment had lower weight losses than patients assigned to the control treatment* is by referring readers to the table or tables providing the basis for the statement or by following the statement with one containing results, eg, *Patients assigned to the test treatment had a mean weight loss of 3.4 pounds compared with a 5.3 pound weight loss for patients assigned to the control treatment.*

Pronouns

The practice in scientific writing is to avoid using the personal pronoun *I* in favor of the collective *we* or using impersonal references to the collective whole, such as *research team*, *research group*, or *investigators*. The practice is reasonable to the extent that most products are the result of collective efforts. However, there are instances where *I* is indicated, eg, in cases where a personal opinion is being expressed or stated. *We* should not be used as a synonym for *I*.

Persons enrolled into trials are broadly referred to as *subjects* or as *research subjects*. That characterization, as indicated in a usage note for the term (see page 263), is not well suited to treatment trials or other trials where enrolled persons stand to benefit from the participation. *Patient* is the preferred term for such trials and for most secondary prevention trials. Some other term such as *participant*, which is free of the connotations of patient, is preferred for primary prevention trials and for other types of trials involving healthy people.

The language of equivocation and weaseling

Every profession has language for equivocation and for weaseling (see weasel term for derivation note, page 297). Some of the language of equivocation is intentionally disguised. Hence, when the geneticist speaks of incomplete penetrance we are likely to believe the term is intended to describe a basic biological process. We are not likely to recognize it as a fudge factor for forcing data to fit an assumed mode of inheritance. Similarly, as patients we will not appreciate the nuances of what we are being told when we are told we have had a silent MI, or understand when the epidemiologist explains findings from a case-control study (or failure to find the obvious) as a result of "overmatching".

Some of the language of equivocation and weaseling is more universal. Virtually every discussion will contain words such as *perhaps*, *maybe*, *possibly*, *likely*, and *potentially*. Our conclusions are likely to be tentative and punctuated with caveats and reminders about the limits of the study and to end with the universal *more research on the subject is needed.*

Equivocation is equivocation, and once a clause is equivocated, adding other words of equivocation does not add to the degree of equivocation. Hence, it is sufficient to write *perhaps the results are due to* instead of *perhaps there is a possibility that the results are due to*. *Perhaps* and *possibly* mean the same thing.

Vacuous language and claims

A vacuous term (page 293) is one devoid of meaning in the context of usage. Everyday examples include the following:

> country (as in *country ham*)
> fresh (as in *fresh eggs*)
> home (as in *home cooking*)
> light or lite (as in *light butter, lite beer*)
> live (as in *live from New York*)
> natural (as in *all natural* or *natural food*)
> open (as in *Yes, we are open*; sign on door of gas station with pumps entombed by tumbleweeds)

Examples more germane to research include the following:

> careful (as in *careful observation*)
> comprehensive (as in *comprehensive system*)
> modern (as in *modern technique*)
> user friendly (as in *user friendly computer*)

A term or phrase is vacuous if it can be deleted without affecting the thought or notion being expressed. Manuscripts should be scoured for excess baggage of this sort. If a sentence works just as well without a word or phrase, the word or phrase should be deleted.

Jargon

Jargon in the 2nd edition of the American Heritage Dictionary[2] is defined as:

> *nonsensical, incoherent, or meaningless talk; a hybrid language or dialect; pidgin; the specialized or technical language of a trade, profession, or similar group*

Our everyday vocabulary is littered with jargon. We speak freely of *prioritizing, conceptualizing, defunding,* and *policy relevance*. Publications from governments and administrations are filled with it, and much of it is unintelligible.

All specialized activities involve the use of language having the characteristic features of jargon. The pages of protocols, manuals, and handbooks of trials are filled with jargon understandable to those doing the trial but not to others. A writer has an obligation to avoid the specialized jargon of the trial in manuscripts submitted for publication. That obligation should be met by repeated readings and editing for jargon prior to submission.

The detection of our own jargon is not so easy. The repeated use of jargonistic expressions over the course of the trial causes those expressions to become part of everyday speech. That familiarity increases the likelihood of use without notice in manuscripts produced from the trial. Therefore, repeated readings by authors for detecting jargon may not be sufficient. Readings by others outside the trial may be needed to aid in the identification of the strange and esoteric.

A good writer will define terms with specialized meanings key to understanding the manuscript. The definitions will be in the body of the manuscript or in a glossary appended to the manuscript. Terms needing definition include those basic to the trial such as *baseline, followup, loss to followup,* and *dropout.* The same is true for shorthand labels or abbreviations and for letter designations for terms or phrases.

Some expressions, when taken literally, are amusing. A case in point, relevant to trials, has to do with references to *placebo patients,* as in *placebo patients were seen on the same schedule as all other patients in the trial.* There is no such patient (except for one coated with sugar) nor is there a *placebo group.* The proper designation for a patient assigned to the placebo treatment is to refer to the assignment in relation to the patient or group, as in *placebo-assigned patient* or *placebo-assigned group.*

Truth by declaration and repetition

Much of what we do proceeds on the basis of trust. As a rule, we do not demand proof for the claims or statements made by a colleague. Generally, the closer the relationship the greater the trust. At the same time, however, we also recognize that the mere repetition of a claim, no matter how often or loudly proclaimed, does not constitute substantiation of the claim. Nor do protestations against a claim, no matter how vehement, render the claim false or vacuous. If so, we would not have overcrowded prisons and politicians being forced from office because of wrongdoing. Conversely, one cannot establish a truth by mere repetition of a claim. If so, we would still believe the earth to be flat and to be the center of the universe.

Data are needed to establish a claim as fact. Beliefs and perceptions, no matter how convincing or logically plausible, are different from data. For example, there are many who believe that women have been systematically excluded from trials. The perception is widely held and has helped to propel the US Congress to write legislation regarding how trials are designed, carried out, and analyzed.[154] The fact that the perception is widely held and perceived to be "plausible" because it jibes with our beliefs does not elevate the perception to fact. The perception cannot be established or dispelled by claim or counterclaim.

The researcher is trained to avoid jumping to conclusions and to respect data. Hence, one should expect that what they write is devoid of unsubstantiated claims, statements, or conclusions. However, the reality is that the researcher has the same difficulties as the politician in differentiating between what is believed to be true and what is known to be true. Hence, researchers are capable of proceeding on the basis of an unsubstantiated claim simply because it is plausible. Their prior beliefs and opinions will color the way they view a new set of results. They are more likely to embrace claims of others, even if not substantiated, if those claims support their own views or beliefs.

The amount of critical analysis we do before accepting or rejecting the work of others will depend, in part, on the way those results fit with our views or positions. We are more likely to accept a negative criticism of someone else's work if the results run counter to our view than when they support our view.

We form opinions about the work of others by criticisms read or heard without ever bothering to check original sources to determine whether the claims or conclusions of critics are justified. Hence, it is enough to read a critical review of a trial offered by someone else for us to form our opinion about that trial without ever reading the original article. Worse yet, we may do so without even realizing that the information being supplied is from sources with interests in promoting a particular point of view.

Though trained as researchers, as people we want to believe the things that fit our views and beliefs and reject, or at least question, those things that run counter to our views or beliefs. As a rule, we demand less evidence to support a belief than to change a belief. Further, though so trained, we are capable of trying to maintain an attitude of objectivity while espousing a particular point of view or promoting a cause we believe in by trying to justify the behavior on scientific grounds. Often we are not capable of recognizing the obvious dangers in mixing advocacy with research. The two notions are in large measure incompatible. Hence, as a rule, one must choose between being an advocate for some cause or approach and researching the merits of that cause or approach. Trying to do both at the same time will lead to "schizophrenia" and confusion.

Similarly, we must recognize the difference between the need for social reform and research that may lead to social reform. Social reform is social reform, and research is research. Research may lead to social reform, but it should not be undertaken as an instrument of social reform. Hence, the clinical researcher has to differentiate between that known to be true from research and that believed to be true from a social perspective.

In research, data speak. A scientific paper should be short on claims and long on data and facts.

Glossary of abbreviations and designations

A

abbr	abbreviation
ACTUP	AIDS Coalition to Unleash Power
AD	anno Domini
adj	adjective
adv	adverb
AF	Anglo-French
Afrik	Afrikaans
AIDS	acquired immune deficiency syndrome
Alb	Albanian
alter	alteration
ANDA	Abbreviated New Drug Application
AnoCo, AoC	analysis of covariance
ANOCO, AOC	analysis of covariance
AnoVa, AoV	analysis of variance
ANOVA, AOV	analysis of variance
ANSI	American National Standards Institute
ant	antonym
Ar	Arabic
Arab	Arabian
ARC	advisory-review committee
ARTEMC	advisory-review and treatment effects monitoring committee
ASCII	American Standard Code for Information Interchange
attrib	attributed, attributive

B

b	bit
B	byte
BC	before Christ
Brit	British

C

CATLINE	Catalog Online
CASS	Coronary Artery Surgery Study
CAST	Cardiac Arrhythmia Suppression Trial
CBER	Center for Biologics Evaluation and Research
CDER	Center for Drug Evaluation and Research
CDRH	Center for Devices and Radiological Health

CFSAN	Center for Food Safety and Applied Nutrition
CC	coordinating center
CDC	Centers for Disease Control and Prevention
CDP	Coronary Drug Project
CFR	code of federal regulations
CL	central laboratory
CO	chair's office
constr	construction
CPU	central processing unit
CRADA	Cooperative Research and Development Agreement
CRO	contract research organization
CRT	cathode ray tube
CV	curriculum vitae
CVM	Center for Veterinary Medicine

D

dat	dative
DCC	data coordinating center
defn	definition
defns	definitions
deriv	derivative
DCRT	Division of Computer Research Technology
DES	Drug Efficacy Study
DESI	Drug Efficacy Study Implementation
df	degrees of freedom
DHEW	Department of Health, Education, and Welfare
DHHS	Department of Health and Human Services
dial	dialect
DMC	data monitoring committee
DRG	Division of Research Grants
DRS	Diabetic Retinopathy Study
DSMC	data and safety monitoring committee

E

E	expected
EC	executive committee
ECG	electrocardiogram
ELA	Establishment License Application

F

F	French
FDA	Food and Drug Administration
fem	feminine
fr	from
freq	frequentative
FY	fiscal year

G

gB, GB	gigabyte
Ger	German
Gk	Greek
GLT	Glaucoma Laser Trial
gm	gram
Gmc	Germanic
Goth	Gothic
Gr Brit	Great Britain
GRASE	generally recognized as safe and effective

H

Heb	Hebrew
HEX	human experimentation, as in HEX committee

I

ID, Id	identification
ID	infectious dose
IDE	Investigational Device Exemption
IDEA	Investigational Device Exemption Application
IG	investigative group
IND	Investigational New Drug
INDA	Investigational New Drug Application
IRB	institutional review board
irreg	irregular
ISAM	indexed sequential access method
ISV	International Scientific Vocabulary
It, Ital	Italian

K

k, K	thousand
kB, KB	kilobyte

L

L	Latin
LAN	local area network
LGk	Late Greek
LD	lethal dose
lit	literally, literary
Lith	Lithuanian
LL	Late Latin

M

masc	masculine
mB, MB	megabyte
ME	Middle English
MEDLARS	Medical Literature Analysis Retrieval System
MEDLINE	MEDLARS Online
MF	Middle French
MGk	Middle Greek
MHG	Middle High German
MIr	Middle Irish
ML	Middle Latin
MLE	maximum likelihood estimate
MoP, MOP	manual of operations
MPS	Macular Photocoagulation Studies
MTD	maximum tolerable dose

N

n	noun
NCHGR	National Center for Human Genome Research
NCHS	National Center for Health Statistics
NCI	National Cancer Institute
NCRR	National Center of Research Resources
NCTR	National Center for Toxicological Research
NDA	New Drug Application
NDI	National Death Index
NEI	National Eye Institute
NHLBI	National Heart, Lung, and Blood Institute
NHANES	National Health and Nutrition Examination Survey
NHIS	National Health Interview Survey
NIA	National Institute on Aging
NIAAA	National Institute on Alcohol Abuse and Alcoholism

NIAID	National Institute of Allergy and Infectious Diseases
NIAMS	National Institute of Arthritis and Musculoskeletal and Skin Disorders
NICHD	National Institute of Child Health and Human Development
NIDA	National Institute on Drug Abuse
NIDCD	National Institute on Deafness and Other Communication Disorders
NIDDK	National Institute of Diabetes and Digestive and Kidney Diseases
NIDR	National Institute of Dental Research
NIEHS	National Institute of Environmental Health Sciences
NIGMS	National Institute of General Medical Sciences
NIH	National Institutes of Health
NIMH	National Institute of Mental Health
NINDS	National Institute of Neurological Disorders and Stroke
NINR	National Institutes of Nursing Research
NL	New Latin
NLM	National Library of Medicine
NTIS	National Technical Information Service

O

O	observed
obs	obsolete
OE	Old English
OF	Old French
OHG	Old High German
OIt	Old Italian
OL	Old Latin
OMB	Office of Management and Budget
OProv	Old Provencal
OPRR	Office for Protection from Research Risks
ORI	Office of Research Integrity
ORWH	Office of Research on Women's Health

OSlav	Old Church

P

PC	personal computer
pdf	probability distribution function
PDQ	Physician Data Query
PHS	Public Health Service; also USPHS
PHS	Physicians' Health Study
PI	principal investigator
pl	plural
PLA	Product License Application
PMA	Pre-Market Approval Application
PMR	proportionate mortality rate; proportionate mortality ratio
PO	project office, project officer
POSCH	Program on the Surgical Control of the Hyperlipidemias
pp	past participle
prep	preposition
prob	probably
Prov	Provencal
prp	present participle

R

RAM	random access memory
RC	reading center
RCT	randomized clinical trial; randomized control trial; randomized controlled trial
RFA	request for application
RFP	request for proposal
ROC	receiver operating characteristic
rt	related term

S

SC	steering committee
Scand	Scandinavian
SD, sd	standard deviation
SE, se	standard error
Sem	Seminary, Semitic
sing	singular
SHEP	Systolic Hypertension in the Elderly Program
Skt	Sanskrit
SMR	standardized mortality ratio
SoP, SOP	standard operating procedure
superl	superlative

syn	synonym

T

TEMC	treatment effects monitoring committee
TOXLINE	Toxicology Information Online
TOXNET	Toxicology Data Network
trt	treatment

U

USPHS	United States Public Health Service; also PHS
UGDP	University Group Diabetes Program

V

v	verb
VA	Veterans Administration
VACSP	Veterans Administration Cooperative Studies Program
VDT	video display terminal
vi	verb intransitive
VL	Vulgar Latin
vt	verb transitive

W

WHO	World Health Organization
WYSIWYG	what you see is what you get

X, Y, and Z

A flaw in a piece of white jade may be ground away, but a word spoken amiss may not be called back

Confucius: *The Book of Poetry*, circa 500 B.C.

Clinical Trials Dictionary

**Terminology
and
Usage Recommendations**

To make dictionaries is dull work
Samuel Johnson [1755][71]
Preface to *A Dictionary of the English Language*

A

a-, an- *prefix* - Without, not, as in asexual.

a posteriori *adj* - [L, lit, fr the latter] Related to or derived by reasoning based on **observed** facts or **data**; inductive, empirical. rt: **a priori**

a posteriori odds *n* - **posterior odds**

a posteriori probability *n* - **posterior probability**

a priori *adj* - [L, lit, fr the former] Relating to or derived by reasoning from presumptions or self-evident propositions; deductive. rt: **a posteriori**

a priori probability *n* - 1. A **probability** deduced or **estimated** from theory or belief. 2. A probability deduced or derived **prior** to the start of a **study**, ie, prior to the observation of **data**; **prior probability**.

abbreviate, abbreviated, abbreviating, abbreviates *v* - [ME *abbreviaten*, fr LL *abbreviatus*, pp of *abbreviare*] To shorten or reduce in length or size.

Abbreviated New Drug Application (ANDA) *n* - An **application** submitted to the **Food and Drug Administration** by the manufacturer or marketing **agent** of a proposed **generic drug** for permission to market that drug for the indication specified in the application; application must be approved by the FDA for marketing to proceed; application is similar in purpose to a **New Drug Application** but requires less supporting **data** than its namesake. Data required are those needed to demonstrate **bioequivalence** of the proposed generic drug to an **approved drug**, especially an approved **proprietary drug**. rt: **new drug, Investigational New Drug Application, Pre-Market Approval Application**

abscissa *n* - [NL, fr L, fem of *abscissus*, pp of *abscindere* to cut off, fr *ab-* + *scindere* to cut] 1. **x-coordinate** 2. **x-axis** rt: **ordinate**

abscissa axis *n* - **x-axis**

absolute *adj* - [ME *absolut*, fr L *absolutus*, fr pp of *absolvere*, to set free, absolve] 1. Pure, not mixed. 2. Having no qualifications, restrictions, or exceptions.

absolute deviation from mean *n* - **mean absolute deviation**

absolute value *n* - Numerical value ignoring sign (eg, the absolute value of +2 or -2 is 2); denoted by a vertical line or bar preceding and following the number or symbol, eg, |a|.

acceptance region *n* - The set of values for a **test statistic** which, when **observed** for a given set of **data**, leads to acceptance of the **null hypothesis**; regions defined by a single **critical value** for **one-tailed tests** and by an upper and lower critical value for **two-tailed tests**. The critical value(s) is (are) picked such that the region corresponds, in a **probability** sense, to 1 minus the specified **type I error** level for the test statistic. ant: **rejection region**

access *n* - [ME, MF & L; MF *acces* arrival, fr L *accessus* approach, fr *accessus*, pp of *accedere* to approach] Permission, liberty, or ability to enter, approach, communicate with, or pass to and from; a way or means of access.

access, accessed, accessing, accesses *v* - To get at; to gain entry.

accident *n* - [ME, fr MF, fr L *accident-*, *accidens* nonessential quality, chance, fr prp of *accidere* to happen, fr *ad-* + *cadere* to fall] 1. An unforeseen or unanticipated **event** or circumstance; **chance** occurrence. 2. An unfortunate or bad effect resulting from carelessness or ignorance. 3. A nonessential quality, quantity, or circumstance.

accidental *adj* - 1. Arising from extrinsic causes; incidental, nonessential. 2. Occurring unexpectedly as if by **chance**. 3. Happening without intent. 4. Happening through carelessness, especially such a happening with unfortunate result or consequence.

accidental bias *n* - **Bias** introduced due to **chance** into an **estimator** in an **experiment**, eg, bias in the estimated **treatment effect** of a **clinical trial** due to **imbalance** in the **distribution** of a **baseline covariate** among the **study groups** [Efron, 1971].[42]

accrual *n* - The action or process of **accruing**; something that is or has accrued; **patient accrual**.

accrue, accrued, accruing, accrues *v* - [ME *acreuen*, prob fr MF *acreue* increase, fr *acreistre* to increase, fr L *accrescere*, fr *ad-* + *crescere* to grow] To come about or to grow or increase as a direct result of some action, process, or procedure.

accuracy *n* - 1. Free of **error** or mistake; correctness. 2. Conformity to a truth, **standard**, or **model**; exactness. 3. The tendency of an **estimator** to be close to the true underlying value. rt: **veracity, precision**

accurate *adj* - [L *accuratus*, fr pp of *accurare*, to take care of, fr *ad-* + *cura* care] 1. Free from **error**; errorless. 2. Conforming exactly to a truth or **standard**; deviating only slightly or within acceptable limits from a specified standard.

achieve, achieved, achieving, achieves *v* - [ME *acheven*, fr MF *achever* to finish, fr *a-* (fr L *ad-*) + *chief* end, head] To carry out successfully, to accomplish; to get or attain as the result of effort; reach; to attain a desired end or aim.

achieved sample size *n* - **observed sample size**

acknowledge, acknowledged, acknowledging, acknowledges *v* - To express gratitude or obligation for; to take notice of; to make known the receipt of.

acknowledgment *n* - 1. An expression of appreciation or thanks for something done or contributed or for a kindness given. 2. A written expression of such appreciation or thanks, eg, as appearing in a **published manuscript**. rt: **credit**

acquire, acquired, acquiring, acquires *v* - [ME *aqueren*, fr MF *aquerre*, fr L *acquirere*, fr *ad-* + *quaerere* to seek, obtain] To obtain; to come into possession or **control** of; to come to have, eg, acquired immune deficiency.

acquisition *n* - [ME *acquisicioun*, fr MF or L; MF *acquisition*, fr L *acquisistion-*, *acquisitio*, fr *acquisitus*, pp of *acquirere*] The act of **acquiring**; something gained or **acquired**.

acronym *n* - [*arc-* + *-onym* (as in *homonym*)] A pronounceable word formed from the initial letter or letters of successive words or major parts of a compound term or phrase, eg, GRASE (**generally recognized as safe and effective**), radar (radio detecting and ranging), snafu (situation normal, all fucked up; of GI World War II origin). *Usage note*: Not to be confused with mere letter designations for places, agencies, units, or activities, eg, as is the case for most of the letter designations for commercial airports, and as is the case with most of the letter designations listed in the Glossary (page xlvii).

acrostic *n* - [MF & Gk; MF *acrostiche*, fr Gk *akrostichis*, fr *akr-* arc- + *sitchos* line; akin to steichein to go] Letters taken in some sequence from an ordinary sentence or verse that form a word, phrase, motto, or message; **acronym**.

active *adj* - [ME, fr MF or L; MF *actif*, fr L *activus*, fr *actus*, pp of *agere* to drive, do] Capable of acting or reacting; capable of producing some **effect**. ant: **inactive**

active agent *n* - **agent**; **active substance**

active control *adj* - [trials] Of or relating to a **control** that is or is intended to be **active**. ant: **inactive control** rt: **negative control, positive control**

active control treatment *n* - [trials] A **negative** or **positive control treatment** that is capable of producing a **treatment effect** in excess of that produced with an **inactive control treatment**. ant: **inactive control treatment** rt: **negative control treatment, positive control treatment**

active dose *n* - **active treatment dose**

active substance *n* - 1. A **substance** (such as a **drug**) that has biological activity. 2. In **trials**, a substance producing a **treatment effect** in excess of a **placebo treatment effect**. ant: **inactive substance**

active treatment *n* - A **treatment** that is capable of producing, a **positive** or **negative treatment effect** that is in excess of a **placebo treatment effect**; includes **standard care** when that care involves an active treatment process. ant: **inactive treatment**

active treatment dose *n* - 1. A **treatment dose** that is capable of producing a **positive** or **negative treatment effect** that is in excess of a **placebo treatment effect**. 2. A **dose** of a **test treatment**. ant: **inactive treatment dose** rt: **treatment dose**

acute *adj* - [L *acutus*, pp of *acuere* to sharpen, fr *acus*, needle; akin to L *acer* sharp] 1. Having a sudden onset or rapid change. 2. Lasting a short time. ant: **chronic**

acute disease *n* - 1. A **disease** characterized by sudden onset. 2. A disease having a short duration; not **chronic**. ant: **chronic disease**

acute study *n* - 1. A **study** involving the **collection**, **analysis**, or interpretation of rapidly changing **data**. 2. A **study** involving **short-term treatment** and **followup**. 3. A study involving **short-term followup**. syn: **short-term study** ant: **chronic study, long-term study**

ad- *prefix* - [ME, fr MF, OF & L; MF, fr OF, fr L, fr *ad*] Near; adjacent to.

ad hoc *adj* - Concerned with a specific end or purpose; formed, or used for a specific purpose.

ad hoc *adv* - [L, for this] For the particular end, case, or situation at hand without consideration of wider applications or implications.

ad hoc meta-analysis *n* - A **meta-analysis** based on two or more studies done in the past and without any plan for use in a meta-analysis when designed. ant: **designed meta-analysis**

ad hoc review group *n* - [research] A **group** created for the sole purpose of reviewing a designated set of **research proposals** for scientific merit and for advising the **sponsor** regarding funding of the proposals; also **ad hoc study section**, especially if the proposals are for support from the NIH. rt: **ad hoc study section**

ad hoc study section *n* - [research] A **study section** (especially one appointed by the **NIH**) created for the sole purpose of reviewing a designated proposal or set of **research proposals** for scientific merit and for advising the **sponsor** regarding funding. rt: **ad hoc review group**

adapt, adapted, adapting, adapts *v* - [F or L; F *adapter*, fr L *adaptare*, fr *ad-* + *aptare* to fit, fr *aptus* apt, fit] To make fit by modification or **change**.

adaptation *n* - The act or process of **adapting**; the state of being adapted.

adaptive *adj* - Serving to **adapt**; showing **adaptation**.

adaptive random treatment assignment *n* - **Adaptive treatment assignment** involving an element of **chance**, as introduced by **randomization**.

adaptive randomization *n* - **Adaptive treatment assignment** involving **randomization**. syn: dynamic randomization

adaptive treatment assignment *n* - Any method of **treatment assignment** in which the **treatment assignment ratio** changes as a function of previous assignments, **baseline data**, or observed **outcomes** [Simon, 1977].[142] Types include:

baseline adaptive treatment assignment, biased coin treatment assignment, minimization, minimum likelihood treatment assignment, number adaptive treatment assignment, play-the-winner treatment assignment, outcome adaptive treatment assignment, and **urn model treatment assignment**. syn: dynamic treatment assignment ant: **fixed treatment assignment**

adaptive treatment assignment design *n* - A **treatment assignment design** in which the **treatment assignment ratio** is allowed to change over the course of **patient enrollment**. See **adaptive treatment assignment** for types. ant: **fixed treatment assignment design**

adaptive treatment assignment schedule *n* - A **treatment assignment schedule** in which **treatment assignment probabilities** change (ie, are not fixed) over the course of **enrollment** as a result of some adaptive process. ant: **fixed treatment assignment schedule**

add, added, adding, adds *v* - [ME *adden*, fr L *addere*, fr *ad-* + *dere* to put] 1. To join or unite so as to bring about an increase or improvement. 2. To combine **numbers** into an equivalent simple quantity or number. 3. To perform **addition**; to come together or unite by addition. ant: **subtract**

addition *n* - [ME, fr MF, fr L *addition-*, *additio*, fr *additus*, pp of *addere*] 1. The result of **adding**. 2. The act or process of combining **numbers** into an equivalent simple quantity or number. ant: **subtraction**

adequate *adj* - [L *adaequatus*, pp of *adaequare* to make equal, fr *ad-* + *aequare* to equal] Sufficient for a specific purpose or function; sometimes with the connotation of being just barely sufficient or satisfactory.

adequate and well-controlled *adj* - Vernacular of the **Food and Drug Administration** used to characterize **trials** or **studies** considered suitable for or required in relation to approval of a **New Drug Application**. The expectation is that the evaluation is to be based on a **concurrent control group**, though there may be circumstances in which **historical controls** will suffice. Types of **control treatments** mentioned in FDA documents include **active treatment**, eg, an already approved treatment, **inactive treatment**, eg, **placebo treatment** when **masking** is possible, or **nontreatment**. rt: **adequate and well-**

controlled trial

adequate and well-controlled trial *n* - A **trial** characterized as or considered to have been **adequate and well-controlled** in relation to some stated purpose or end, such as in relation to a **new drug application.**

adhere, adhered, adhering, adheres *v* - [MF or L; MF *adhèrer*, fr L *adhaerēre*, fr *ad-* + *haerēre*, to stick] To commit to observance; to follow or **observe.**

adherence *n* - The act or quality of **adhering** to some system, procedure, or **protocol.** syn: **compliance** rt: **protocol adherence, treatment adherence**

adjust, adjusted, adjusting, adjusts *v* - [ME *ajusten*, fr MF *ajuster* to gauge, adjust, fr *a-* (fr L *ad-*) + *juste* right, exact] To **change** or modify so as to fit, **match,** or make correspond.

adjusted *adj* - Modified or accommodated to a set of conditions or specifications; of or relating to **adjustment.** ant: **raw, unadjusted**

adjustment *n* - 1. The act or process of **adjusting;** the state of being **adjusted.** 2. The **control** of extraneous **sources of variation** during **data analysis** that affect, or are believed to affect, some **comparison** by use of an **adjustment procedure.** Those procedures for **trials** traditionally involve the use of **baseline variables,** especially those considered to have **distributions** that differ by **treatment group** and that influence, or are suspected of influencing, **treatment** or **outcome.**

adjustment procedure *n* - Any of a variety of procedures performed during **data analysis** intended to remove the effect of one or more extraneous **sources of variation** that could affect, or are believed to affect, a particular **result.** Procedures include **direct** and **indirect rate adjustment, subgroup analysis, analysis of covariance,** and **linear** and **nonlinear regression analysis.** rt: **standardization, stratification**

adjustment variable *n* - A **variable,** such as age or gender, used for **adjustment** via some **analysis procedure;** in **trials,** usually a **baseline variable** or a demographic characteristic such as sex, race, or age on entry.

adjuvant *adj* - [F or L; F, fr L *adjuvant-, adjuvans,* prp of *adjuvare* to aid] Serving to aid or contribute, as in an **adjuvant treatment.**

adjuvant *n* - [**medicine**] Something that enhances the effectiveness of a **medical treatment.**

adjuvant treatment *n* - A **treatment** given in conjunction with another and that is administered with the knowledge or expectation that the **benefits** accruing to the **patient** will be greater than those expected with the use of either treatment alone, eg, immunotherapy as an adjuvant to chemotherapy for the treatment of a cancer.

administer, administered, administering, administers *v* - [ME *administren,* fr MF *administrer,* fr L *administratre,* fr *ad-* + *ministrate* to serve, fr *minister,* servant] 1. To manage or supervise execution, use, or conduct of. 2. To dispense or to give, as with a **treatment.**

administered treatment *n* - The **treatment** or **sequence** of **treatments** actually **administered** to a **treatment unit** in a **trial,** regardless of **treatment assignment.** syn: treatment administered rt: **assigned treatment**

administration *n* - 1. The act or process of **administering;** the act or process of performing specified functions or procedures. 2. Performance of executive duties or functions; management. 3. A governmental agency or board.

administrative *adj* - Of or relating to **administration** or an administration.

administrative review *n* - [**trials**] 1. An **ad hoc interim review** of **performance** of some activity to determine whether it is practical to continue a trial unaltered; especially a review considering costs. 2. **performance review** (defn 1) 3. **performance monitoring** *Usage note*: Note that defn 1 has a different operational meaning than defn 3; defn 1 refers to an **ad hoc** evaluation, whereas defn 3 refers to an ongoing process; not to be used interchangeably (see note for **performance monitoring** *n*). Not to be confused with reviews involving evaluations of **treatment results** as in **safety review, efficacy review,** or in **treatment effects monitoring.** Do not use in contexts where the review includes a review of **treatment results.** Use is ordinarily limited to review of performance where there is a desire or need to distinguish such a review from one involving an **interim look,** as in relation to **treatment effects monitoring, efficacy monitoring,** or **safety monitoring.** See also notes for **performance monitoring, efficacy monitoring, safety monitoring,** and **treatment effects monitoring.**

administrator *n* - One who administers, as in a government office, school, or business.

adolescent *n* - [F, fr L *adolescent-, adolescens,* prp of *adolescere* to grow up] 1. One who is in the **period** of pubescence and who has not yet reached the **age of majority**. 2. One who is immature or not yet mature, but is no longer considered a **child**.

adult *adj* - [L *adultus,* pp of *adolescere* to grow up, fr *ad-* + *olescere* (fr *alescere* to grow)] Fully developed and mature; grown up. rt: **mature**

adult *n* - 1. One who is fully developed or mature. 2. One who has reached a specified age and is no longer regarded as a **child** or **minor**, eg, one who has reached the **age of majority**.

adverse *adj* - [ME, fr MF *advers,* fr L *adversus,* pp of *adverstere*] Acting against or in a contrary direction.

adverse drug experience *n* - As defined in the Code of Federal Regulations for the **Food and Drug Administration**: *Any adverse event associated with the use of a drug in humans, whether or not considered drug related, including the following: An adverse event occurring in the course of the use of a drug product in professional practice; an adverse event occurring from drug overdose, whether accidental or intentional; an adverse event occurring from drug abuse; an adverse event occurring from drug withdrawal; and any significant failure of expected pharmacological action.* (page 22)[48] rt: **safety report, serious adverse drug experience, unexpected adverse drug experience**

adverse drug reaction *n* - A **drug reaction** that results in hospitalization, a prolongation of hospitalization, or that otherwise has **negative** health implications for the **patient** having such a reaction. rt: **toxic drug reaction, serious adverse drug experience** *Usage note*: See **drug reaction**.

adverse side effect *n* - A **side effect** that has adverse health implications for the **patient** having such a side effect. rt: **toxic side effect** *Usage note*: See **side effect**.

adverse treatment effect *n* - A **treatment effect** that has **negative** health implications; a **treatment effect** contrary to the one intended or desired. ant: **beneficial treatment effect**

advise, advised, advising, advises *v* - [ME *advisen,* fr MF *aviser,* fr *avis*] To give counsel or advice.

advisory *adj* - Having or exercising power to **advise**.

advisory board *n* - **advisory-review committee**

advisory committee *n* - **advisory-review committee**

advisory-review and treatment effects monitoring committee (ARTEMC) *n* - A **committee** that performs the functions of both the **advisory-review committee** and **treatment effects monitoring committee**. A **key committee** in the organizational structure of **multicenter treatment trials**. See *committee* for list.

advisory-review committee (ARC) *n* - A **committee** in the organizational structure of a **trial** that is responsible for reviewing the design and operations of the trial for the purpose of advising the **steering committee** and **sponsor** on matters related to the trial; voting members usually not involved in the execution of the trial or associated with any of the participating **centers** or **sponsor** of the trial. Selected **investigators** from the trial may serve as nonvoting members. A **key committee** in the organizational structure of some **multicenter treatment trials** with method of appointment and route of reporting similar to that described for **treatment effects monitoring committee**. syn: advisory board, advisory committee, policy-advisory board, policy-advisory committee, policy board, policy committee See *committee* for list.

advocate *n* - [ME *advocat,* fr MF, fr L *advocatus,* fr pp of *advocare* to summon, fr *ad-* + *vocare* to call] One who pleads the cause of another, especially before some body or tribunal. rt: **patient advocate**

affiliate *n* - An **affiliated** person, **organization**, or **institution**. rt: **associate**

affiliate, affiliated, affiliating, affiliates *v* - [ML *affiliatus,* pp of *affiliare* to adopt as a son, fr L *ad-* + *filius,* son] To bring into close connection, as a member or a branch; to associate.

affiliate center *n* - A **center**, established or adopted by a **parent center**, that is responsible for performing specified functions in affiliation with or as an **agent** of the **parent**; may or may not receive financial support from parent. See *center* for list. rt: **associate center, daughter center,**

satellite center, sibling center, sister center

affiliate clinic *n* - A **clinic**, established or adopted by a **parent clinic**, that is responsible for performing specified functions in relation to **patient enrollment**, **treatment**, or **followup** in affiliation with or as an **agent** of the parent clinic; may or may not receive financial support from parent. See *center* for list. rt: **associate clinic, daughter clinic, satellite clinic, sibling clinic, sister clinic**

after *adj* - Later in time. ant: **before**

age *n* - [ME, fr OF *aage*, fr (assumed) VL *aetaticum*, fr L *aetat-, aetas*, fr *aevum* lifetime] A **measure** of **time** marked from the occurrence of some event, such as birth, to the present or some event or date in the past. When reported, recorded, or treated as **years of age**, a count of the number of **birthday anniversaries** observed since birth; eg, 25 for a person born over 25 years ago but less than 26 years ago. rt: **birthdate, date of birth, years of age**

age of assent *n* - In **research**, the **age** at which **assent** is required before proceeding with any of the procedures, tests, or treatments involved in the research; usually at or around the age 5. See **assent** for added detail. rt: **age of consent**

age of consent *n* - In **research**, the **age** at which **consent** is required before proceeding with any of the procedures, tests, or treatments involved in the research; usually the **age of majority** or less, eg 16 in some cases or less for **emancipated minors**. See **assent** and **consent** for added detail. rt: **age of assent, age of majority**

age of majority *n* - The **age** at which full civil rights are accorded to a person; age 18 in the United States.

agency *n* - An administrative **unit** through which power or influence is exerted to achieve some stated end or to perform some specified function. See *agency and place index* for listing.

agent *n* - [ME, fr ML *agent-, agens*, fr L, prp of *agere* to drive, lead, act, do; akin to ON *aka* to travel in a vehicle, Gk, *agein* to drive, lead] 1. Something that produces or is capable of producing an **effect**; a chemically, physically, or biologically **active** component. 2. One who acts for or in place of another by granted authority; one that acts or executes power.

aggregate *adj* - [ME *aggregat*, fr L *aggregatus*, pp of *aggregare* to add to, fr *ad-* + *greg-, grex* flock] Formed by or characterized by the **collec-**tion or assemblage of **units** or entities into a body, mass, amount, or whole; existing as a combined entity or totality. rt: **group**

aggregate *n* - 1. The **total** amount or **sum**. 2. A collective mass or body of **units** or parts loosely associated with one another.

aggregate data *n* - **Data** characterizing a **group** in the absence of **data** for individual units or elements comprising the group, such as that used in **ecological studies** for measuring **exposure** to some known or presumed **risk factor**; **group data**. *Usage note*: Not to be confused with **grouped data**.

agree, agreed, agreeing, agrees *v* - [ME *agreen*, fr MF *agreer*, fr *a-* (fr L *ad-*) + *gre* will, pleasure, fr L *gratum*, neut of *gratus* pleasing, agreeable] 1. To be similar, to correspond, to be in accord. 2. To come to terms, to accept. ant: **disagree**

agreement *n* - 1. The act or fact of **agreeing**; similarity of action, course, or character. 2. An arrangement or compact as to course of action. ant: **disagreement**

aim *n* - [ME *aimen*, fr MF *aesmer* & *esmer*; MF *aesmer*, fr OF, fr *a-* (fr L *ad-*) + *esmer* to estimate, fr L *aestimare*] A stated intent or **purpose**; the directing of effort toward a goal. rt: **specific aim, objective, purpose**

alert *adj* - [It *all' erta*, lit, on the ascent] Watchful and prompt to respond to danger.

alert *n* - 1. The state of readiness of those warned by an **alert**. 2. An alarm or other signal of danger or of concern, as in a **clinical alert**. 3. The period during which an alert is in effect.

alert limit *n* - 1. A **limit** specified for a **treatment difference** that, when exceeded, serves to alert investigators to the possibility of stopping the **trial** or a **treatment** in it. 2. A limit specified for a laboratory test, that, when exceeded, causes it to be called to the attention of medical personnel or causes it to be repeated, or to have other tests or procedures performed to determine the medical importance of the **result** observed. rt: **normal limit, monitoring limit**

algorithm *n* - [alter of ME *algorisme*, fr OF & ML; OF, fr ML *algorismus* fr Ar *al-khuwārizmi*, fr *al-Khuwārizmi*, Arab mathematician, circa 825 AD] 1. A procedure for solving a mathematical problem in a step-by-step sequence. 2. Any step-by-step procedure for solving a problem or accomplishing some end.

alias *n* - [L, otherwise, fr *alius* other; an assumed or additional name] In **experimental design**, a **contrast** that has the same form as another and, hence, indistinguishable from the other form. rt: **confounded effect**

aliquot *adj* - [ML *aliquotus*, fr L *aliquot* some, several, fr *alius* other + *quot* how many] Contained an exact **number** of times in something else; fractional.

aliquot *n* - A portion or fraction of a substance, such as serum or blood.

allocate, allocated, allocating, allocates *v* - [ML *allocatus*, pp of *allocare*, fr L *ad-* + *locare* to place, fr *locus* place] To apportion or distribute among persons or things, or for a specific purpose.

allocation *n* - 1. A designated or specified apportionment or **distribution**. 2. **treatment assignment** *Usage note*: Not recommended in the sense of defn 2; use **treatment assignment** instead for reasons indicated in usage note for **assignment**.

allocation ratio *n* - **treatment assignment ratio**

allusion *n* - [LL *allusion-*, *allusio*, fr L *allusus*, pp of *alludere*] 1. The act of alluding or hinting at. 2. An implied or indirect reference.

alpha *n* - [ME, fr L, fr Gk, of Sem origin, akin to Heb *āleph* aleph] 1. The 1st letter of the **Greek alphabet**, uppercase A, lowercase α. 2. **type I error**

alpha error *n* - **type I error**, **significance level**

alphabet *n* - [ME *alphabete*, fr LL *alphabetum*, fr Gk *alphabētos*, fr *alpha* + *bēta* beta] 1. A set of letters or other characters that form the basis for a written language. 2. A system of **signs** or signals that serve as equivalents for letters or **characters** of an alphabet.

alternate *adj* - [L *alternatus*, pp of *alternare*, fr *alternus* alternate, fr *alter*] Occurring or succeeding in turn; every other.

alternate *n* - One or something that **alternates** or substitutes for another or something else.

alternate, alternated, alternating, alternates *v* - To perform or succeed by turns; to cause to alternate.

alternation *n* - The act or process of **alternating** or causing to **alternate**, eg, a **treatment assign-**ment scheme in which every other person **enrolled** is **assigned** to the **test treatment**.

alternation treatment assignment *n* - Any **systematic nonrandom** method of **treatment assignment** in which assignments **alternate**, eg, a scheme in which every other person **enrolled** in a **trial** is assigned to the **test treatment**; see also **odd-even method of treatment assignment**.

alternative *adj* - Of or relating to an **alternative**

alternative *n* - Choice, option, or proposition offered or proposed in opposition to some other choice, option, or proposition.

alternative hypothesis *n* - 1. A **hypothesis** stated as an **alternative** to the **null hypothesis** in which the **parameters**, functions, traits, **characteristics**, or effects of interest are assigned values that differ from those assigned for the null hypothesis. 2. The hypothesis that is accepted when the null hypothesis is rejected in a **test of hypothesis**. 3. **Alternative treatment hypothesis**. syn: **research hypothesis**, working hypothesis ant: **null hypothesis** rt: **one-tailed alternative hypothesis, two-tailed alternative hypothesis**

alternative treatment hypothesis *n* - A **hypothesis** that states that the true underlying effect of the **test treatment**, as expressed in terms of a specified **outcome measure**, is different from that associated with the **control treatment** or **comparison treatment**. ant: **null treatment hypothesis** rt: **one-tailed alternative hypothesis, two-tailed alternative hypothesis**

American National Standards Institute (ANSI) *n* - An **organization** responsible for promoting, establishing, and promulgating **standards** in various areas; standards established by the organization are referred to as **ANSI** standards. Activities include establishing and promulgating standards for **computer hardware** and **software**.

American Standard Code for Information Interchange (ASCII) *n* - (pronounced *askee*) A **standard** set of **codes**, consisting of 8 **bits** (7 information bits and one parity bit or 8 information bits), allowing for 128 (7 information bits) or 256 (8 information bits) code combinations. The different combinations are used to represent or transmit information denoting **characters**, such as upper and lower case letters, numeric characters, and punctuation marks, as well as nonprintable machine commands, in **computers**

and related **software** packages. For the 128-code set (7 information bits), the first 32 codes are used to represent uppercase letters and a few punctuation marks; the next set of 32 codes are used to denote numbers, spacing, and additional punctuation, the third set is used to denote lower case letters and rarely used punctuation, and the last set of 32 is used to denote nonprintable machine commands, such as line feed and carriage return.

analog *adj* - Being or related to a mechanism in which **data** are expressed or represented by a **continuous** physical **variable**, function, or process, such as the movements of the hands of a clock to represent the progression of time; **analogue**. ant: **digital**

analog computer *n* - 1. A **computer** that performs its operation by use of **analogs** in the operations, such as voltages to represent digital **data**. 2. Any **device** that is used to perform mathematical operations through the use of physical **variables** or **measures**, eg, a slide rule. ant: **digital computer**

analogue *adj* - [F *analogue*, fr *analogue* analogous, fr Gk *analogos*] Something that is similar to or bears a **relationship** to something else; **analog**.

analysis *n* - [NL, fr Gk, fr *analyein*, to break up, a releasing, fr *ana-* + *lyein* to loosen] 1. An examination of a whole, its parts, and interrelationships; a **statement** of such an analysis. 2. **data analysis**

analysis by administered treatment *n* - **Data analysis** in which **tabulations** and summaries are by the **administered treatment** (as opposed to the **assigned treatment**), eg, done by grouping **results** for **patients** who were assigned to the **test treatment** but refused the treatment with those for patients assigned to and receiving the **control treatment** in the case of a **placebo-controlled trial**. Not recommended as the primary method of analysis (see **analysis by assigned treatment**). ant: **analysis by assigned treatment** rt: **analysis by level of treatment adherence**

analysis by assigned treatment *n* - **Data analysis** in which **tabulations** and summaries are by **assigned treatment** regardless of **administered treatment**. Recommended primary method of analysis. syn: **analysis by intention to treat** ant: **analysis by administered treatment**

analysis by intention to treat *n* - **analysis by assigned treatment** *Usage note*: Not preferred usage; use **analysis by assigned treatment** instead to draw attention to defined operational aspects of the **assignment** process, rather than to what is or was intended in the treatment process.

analysis by level of treatment adherence *n* - **Data analysis** in which **tabulations** and summaries are by level of **treatment adherence**; typically done by performing **treatment comparisons** within defined **subgroups** of **patients** created using **measures** of observed **treatment adherence** or via **regression models** using measures of adherence for deriving adjusted treatment comparisons. Not recommended as a primary method of analysis (see **analysis by assigned treatment**). rt: **analysis by administered treatment**

analysis center *n* - 1. **data center** 2. **data coordinating center** 3. **coordinating center** See *center* for list.

analysis committee *n* - 1. A **committee** having responsibility for **analysis** of **data**, eg, a committee concerned with use of data from a **trial** to describe the **natural history** of the **disease** process being treated in the trial or one charged with performing analyses aimed at assessing the quality of the data collected. 2. A committee within the organizational structure of a multidisciplinary collaborating **group** charged with or having responsibility for analysis of one or more aspects of the data generated by the group. rt: **committee, performance monitoring committee, treatment effects monitoring committee, writing committee**

analysis database *n* - The subset of **data** contained in the **study database** that is available for **data analysis**. Generally limited to data that have been **coded, keyed, edited**, and stored electronically for retrieval and manipulation.

analysis of covariance (AnoCo, ANOCO, AoC, AOC) *n* - An **adjustment procedure** involving **regression procedures** to remove the effect of a **variable** (eg, age in a **trial** not involving age **stratification**) not **controlled** for in the **design** that may be related to the **classifications, factors**, or **variables** of interest in an **analysis of variance**. rt: **multiple regression analysis, analysis of variance**

analysis of principal components *n* - **principal component analysis**

analysis of variance (AnoVa, ANOVA, AoV, AOV) *n* - A method of **data analysis** for determining the contribution of **classifications** or **factors** (eg, **treatment** in a **clinical trial**) by partitioning the observed **variance** (**sum of squares**) into component parts related to those **classifications** or **factors**. rt: **analysis of covariance**

analysis principle *n* - [**trials**] A **principle** or **guideline** for **data analysis**. Those principles for **trials**, as discussed by Meinert and Tonascia [1986],[102] include: 1) The **primary analysis** should be by original **treatment assignment** (regardless of course of treatment); 2) The analyses should account for all **patients** (**observation units**) **enrolled**; 3) All **outcomes** or **events** occurring after **enrollment** should be counted regardless of when they occur relative to the start of **treatment**; 4) **Comparison** of higher order outcomes or events (eg, death) should be performed before performing comparisons for lower order outcomes or events (eg, cause-specific mortality or fatal or nonfatal MI); 5) The component parts (eg, death and nonfatal MI) of a **composite outcome** or **event** should be analyzed separately; a composite outcome or event should not serve as the basis for a primary analysis if the analysis of the component parts yield conflicting or offsetting differences (eg, a difference favoring one treatment group for death and a difference favoring the other treatment group for nonfatal MI). rt: **counting rule**

analyst *n* - One who analyzes or who is skilled in **analysis**.

analyst mask *n* - **data analyst mask**

ancillary *adj* - Subordinate, subsidiary, auxiliary, supplementary, subpart of.

ancillary publication *n* - [**research**] 1. A **publication** containing original **ancillary results**. 2. A publication bearing on an ancillary **aim** or **objective** of a specific **research project**; in the case of **trials**, usually publications devoted exclusively to results form **ancillary studies**. rt: **primary publication, secondary publication**

ancillary result *n* - [**research**] A **result** obtained from an **ancillary study**. rt: **primary result, secondary result**

ancillary study *n* - 1. A **study** that is subsidiary to, but not a required part of, the **parent study** and that is carried out using or relying on resources of the parent study. 2. A study arising from the parent study and done by personnel associated with the parent study. 3. **daughter study** rt: **sister study**

ANDA *n* - **Abbreviated New Drug Application**

anniversary *n* - [ME *aniversarie*, fr ML *anniversarium*, fr L neut of *anniversarium* returning annually, fr *annus* year + *versus*, pp of *vertere* to turn] 1. The **annual** recurrence of a date marking a notable **event**. 2. The celebration of an **anniversary**.

anniversary close-out *n* - **common followup period patient close-out**

annual *adj* - [ME, fr MF & LL; MF *annuel*, fr LL *annualis*, blend of L *annuus* yearly (fr *annus* year) and L *annalis* yearly (fr *annus* year); akin to Goth *athnam* (dat pl) years, Skt *atati* he walks, goes] Covering the **period** of a **year**; occurring or happening every year or once a year. rt: **biannual, semiannual, anniversary**

AnoCo, ANOCO *n* - **analysis of covariance**

AnoVa, ANOVA *n* - **analysis of variance**

ANSI *n* - **American National Standards Institute**

antagonist *n* - A **substance**, such as a **drug** or food type, that opposes the action of another substance (eg, milk opposing the action of tetracycline) ant: **synergist**

antagonistic treatment effect *n* - A **treatment effect** produced by the simultaneous use of two or more **substances** (eg, two different **drugs** or a drug and a food type) that is less than the **sum** of the effects of those substances acting alone. ant: **synergistic treatment effect**

antecedent *adj* - **prior**, before

antecedent *n* - [ME, fr ML & L; ML *antecedent-, antecedens*, fr L, logical antecedent, lit, one that goes before, fr neut of *antecedent-, antecedens*, prp of *antecedere*, fr *ante- + cedere* to go] A preceding **event**, condition, or cause; one's preceding significant life events, conditions, and traits.

anti-, ant-, anth- *prefix* - [anti- fr ME, fr MF & L; MF, fr L against, fr Gk, fr *anti*; ant- fr ME, fr L, against, fr Gk fr *anti*; anth- fr L against, fr Gk, fr *anti*] 1. Of the same kind, but having the opposite effect or meaning, eg, **antilogarithm**. 2. Opposing in practice, view, or opinion; opposing in effect or activity. 3. Serving to **prevent**, alleviate, or cure, as in antihypertension treatment; combating or defending against.

antilog *n* - **inverse logarithm, antilogarithm**

antilogarithm *n* - **inverse logarithm, antilog**

AoC, AOC *n* - **analysis of covariance**

AoV, AOV *n* - **analysis of variance**

applicant *n* - 1. One who applies; a person who prepares and submits a **funding proposal** for a **research project**. 2. A **group** of persons, **agency**, or **institution** that prepares and submits a **funding proposal** for a **research project**. syn: **offerer, proposer**

application *n* - [ME *applicacioun*, fr L *application-, applicatio* inclination, fr *applicatus*, pp of *applicare*] 1. A request or petition. 2. The form used in making such a request or petition. 3. **funding application** rt: contract application, **grant application**

approval *n* - An act or instance of **approving**.

approve, approved, approving, approves *v* - [ME *approven*, fr MF *approver*, fr L *approbare*, fr *ad-* + *probare* to prove] To accept as satisfactory; to give formal acceptance; to ratify.

approved drug *n* - 1. A **drug** and use proposed in a **New Drug Application approved** by the **Food and Drug Administration**. 2. A drug approved via other mechanisms in place at the **Food and Drug Administration**, eg, via the **Drug Efficacy Study Implementation** (DESI).[48] 3. Drugs listed in the *Physicians' Desk Reference*. 4. A drug listed in a recognized pharmacopeia or formulary and available for use. 5. **licensed drug**

approximate *adj* - [LL *approximatus*, pp of *approximare* to come near, fr L *ad-* + *proximare* to come near] 1. Nearly correct or **accurate**. 2. Located close together.

approximate, approximating, approximated, approximates *v* - 1. To bring near or close together. 2. To come near or to be close in **position**, value, **characteristic**, or trait.

approximation *n* - 1. The act or process of drawing together. 2. The quality of being close or near the true **position** or **standard**. 3. A mathematical quantity or expression, eg, an **estimator**, that is near, but not exactly equal to, the true underlying value or **standard**.

ARC *n* - **advisory-review committee**

arc- *adj* - **inverse**

archive *n* - [F &L; F, fr L *archivum*, fr Gk *archeion* government house, fr *archē* rule, government] A place where **documents** are stored for future access and use; **repository**. rt: **bank, repository** *Usage note*: See **repository**.

archive, archived, archiving, archives *v* - To **file** or collect **documents, records, data**, etc, into an **archive**.

arcsine, arc sine *n* - **inverse sine**

arcsine transformation *n* - **inverse sine transformation**

area *n* - [L, piece of level ground, threshing floor, fr *arēre* to be dry; akin to L *ardor*] The scope of a concept, operation, or activity.

arithmetic *n* - [ME *arsmetrik*, fr OF *arismetique*, fr L *arithmetica*, fr Gk *arithmētikē*, fr fem of *arithmētikos* arithmetical, fr *arithmein* to count, fr *arithmos* number; akin to OE *rim* number, Gk *arariskein* to fit] A branch of mathematics dealing with real **numbers** and the application of **addition, subtraction, multiplication**, or **division** to them.

arithmetic mean *n* - The **sum** of a set of numeric values divided by the number of values in the set; usually denoted by $\bar{x}$ or $\bar{y}$ for **sample means** and by μ for **population means**. syn: **average** See *mean* for list.

arm *n* - [ME, fr OE *earm*, akin to L *armus* shoulder, Gk *harmos* joint, L *arma* weapons, *ars* skill, Gk *arariskein* to fit] 1. A subpart or division of a **group**, structure, or activity. 2. **treatment arm**

ARTEMC *n* - **advisory-review and treatment effects monitoring committee**

ASCII *n* - **American Standard Code for Information Interchange**

assay *n* - [ME, fr OF *essai, assai* test, effort] Any procedure that is used to determine the presence or absence of a substance, eg, a **drug** or an enzyme in blood or urine, or to **estimate** the amount present. rt: **bioassay**

assay, assayed, assaying, assays *v* - To perform an **assay**.

assent *n* - 1. The act of **assenting**; a permission granted. 2. An expression of acquiesce in relation to something proposed after explanation of that proposed and its consequences. rt: **consent, assent form, assent statement, oral assent, signed assent, preassignment consent, post-assignment consent, signed consent, oral consent** *Usage note*: Generally in **research** settings, **assent** in addition to **consent** is required whenever consent is given by someone else on behalf of the person to be enrolled in a research undertaking, and where the person to be so **enrolled** has sufficient mental capacity to understand the nature and extent of what is being proposed. The starting age at which assent is required may vary, but is usually 5, or thereabouts, for most **institutional review boards**. For persons unable to read, the assent may be given orally after the person has been presented with a simple **oral** explanation of what is involved. For persons able to read (eg, children aged 7 or 8 to the **age of majority**), the process may require the use of a written **assent form** and a **signed assent** before proceeding. The process, while used primarily in relation to children, extends as well to **adults** with limited but sufficient mental capacities to allow them to assent.

assent, assented, assenting, assents *v* - [ME *assenten*, fr OF *assenter*, fr L *assentari*, fr *assentire*, fr *ad-* + *sentire* to feel] To express willingness to accept in relation to some proposal or plan, especially such expression after discussion and thoughtful consideration; permission granted. rt: **age of assent, assent form, consent** *Usage note*: Not to be confused with **consent** as used in research settings. One requires the assent of a **child** and the **consent** of the child's parent or guardian to enroll the child into a **study**. The *American Heritage Dictionary*[2] lists agree, accede, acquiesce, accept, consent, concur, and subscribe as synonyms and indicates: *These verbs mean to go along with another's views, proposals, or actions. Assent implies saying "yes" in a formal, somewhat impersonal manner. Agree and accede are loosely related in the sense of assenting after discussion or persuasion. But agree suggests mutual accommodation in a meeting of minds, whereas accede implies yielding on the part of one person or group. Acquiesce suggests agreeing, despite reservations, because of unwillingness to oppose. Accept may indicate agreement with some reluctance. Consent indicates complete and voluntary personal commitment to a proposal or desire. Concur refers to agreement with another's position, and may suggest that one has reached the same conclusion independently. Subscribe indicates hearty consent or approval.* See **assent** *n* for additional comments.

assent form *n* - A written **document** presented to a **child** above the **age of assent** or to an **adult** with diminished mental capacity who is asked to **enroll** into a **research project** and having the intended function of providing a written description (in language consistent with the age of the child or mental capacity of the adult) of the proposed **research**, of the nature of the commitment required, of the procedures to be performed and of the reasons for them, of the purpose of the research and why the person is being approached for enrollment, of the potential **risks** and **benefits** associated with participation, and of the right of the person to refuse to enroll and of the right to **withdraw** at anytime after **enrollment** without prejudice in regard to the nature or amount of care or treatment available to the person at the research site.

assent statement *n* - 1. **Assent form**, especially one that bears the signature of the assenting individual indicating a willingness on the part of that individual to **enroll** into a **research project**, or to submit to some **test** or procedure. 2. **signed assent** 3. A signed **document**, devoid of details regarding the nature and extent of the undertaking, indicating **assent** and that information regarding the undertaking was imparted orally. rt: **assent form, consent statement**

assess, assessed, assessing, assesses *v* - [ME *assessen*, prob fr ML *assessus*, pp of *assidēre*, fr L, to sit beside, assist in the office of a judge] To determine the value, size, or importance of.

assessment *n* - 1. The act or an instance of **assessing**. 2. The amount assessed.

assign, assigned, assigning, assigns *v* - [ME *assignen*, fr OF *assigner*, fr L *assignare*, fr *ad-* + *signare* to mark, fr *signum* mark, sign] To fix or specify in correspondence or **relationship**.

assigned to treatment *n* - The state of having been **assigned** to a **treatment** in a **trial**.

assigned treatment *n* - The **treatment**(s) assigned to a **treatment unit** in a **trial**. syn: **treatment assignment** rt: **administered treatment**

assignment *n* - 1. Something assigned or designated, as a duty, task, or **regimen**. 2. The act of **assigning**. 3. **treatment assignment** *Usage note*: Preferred to **allocation**, though not strongly, in references to treatment assignment. Allocation in that setting has a slightly more passive tone than assignment and, hence, assignment more accurately characterizes the process implied than does allocation.

assignment examination *n* - **treatment assignment examination**

assignment probabilities *n* - **treatment assignment probabilities**

assignment ratio *n* - **treatment assignment ratio**

assignment strata *n* - **treatment assignment strata**

assignment unit *n* - **treatment assignment unit**

assignment visit *n* - **treatment assignment visit**

assist, assisted, assisting, assists *v* - [MF or L; MF *assister* to help, stand by, fr L *assistere*, fr *ad-* + *sistere* to cause to stand; akin to L *stare* to stand] To give supplementary support or aid to.

associate *adj* - Closely related or connected, as in function, with another; having a secondary or subordinate status to another.

associate, associated, associating, associates *v* - [ME *associat* associated, fr L *associatus*, pp of *associare* to unite, fr *ad-* + *sociare* to join, fr *socius* companion] To join as partners; to combine or join. rt: **relate**

associate center *n* - A **center**, established or adopted by a **parent center**, that is responsible for performing specified functions in association with or as an **agent** of the **parent**; may or may not receive financial support from the parent. rt: **affiliate center, daughter center, satellite center, sibling center, sister center** See *center* for list.

associate clinic *n* - A **clinic**, established or adopted by a **parent clinic**, that is responsible for performing specified functions, such as **patient enrollment, treatment,** or **followup**, in association with or as an **agent** of the parent clinic; may or may not receive financial support from the parent. See *center* for list. rt: **affiliate clinic, daughter clinic, satellite clinic, sibling clinic, sister clinic**

association *n* - 1. [general] The state of being **associated**. The act of associating. 2. [general] An **organization** of persons having a common interest; **society**. 3. [**statistics**] An **observed** or postulated pattern of change of one **variable** (**event, factor**) to another, typically identified through **exploratory data analysis**, and noted or assessed using statistical methods; **dependence**. An association is considered to be present if the **probability** of occurrence of an **event, trait,** or **characteristic** depends on the occurrence of one or more other events, the presence of one or more characteristics, or on the value of one or more other variables. The **relationship** of two variables is characterized as **positive** if the change of one variable is associated with a change in the same direction for the other variable, and **negative** if the change of one variable is associated with a change in the opposite direction of the other variable. rt: **independence, relationship, correlation, dependent, statistical association** *Usage note*: Often used interchangeably with **relationship** without loss of meaning, especially in uses in the sense of defn 3. See also notes for **correlation** and **cause and effect**.

assume, assumed, assuming, assumes *v* - [ME *assumen*, fr L *assumere*, fr *ad-* + *sumere* to take] 1. To take as granted or **true**. 2. To suppose; to pretend to have or be. 3. To take up or in.

assumption *n* - [ME, fr LL *assumption-*, *assumptio* taking up, fr L *assumptus*, pp of *assumere*] A supposition that something is **true**; a fact or **statement** (proposition, **axiom, hypothesis,** or notion) taken for granted or as given.

attack *n* - An occurrence of illness or **disease**, especially, an active episode of a **chronic** or recurrent disease.

attack, attacked, attacking, attacks *v* - [MF *attaquer*, fr (assumed) OIt *estaccare* to attach, fr *stacca* stake, of Gmc origin; akin to OE *staca*] 1. To set upon forcefully. 2. To set to work on.

attack rate *n* - The **number** of new **cases** of an illness, **disease,** or condition observed over a defined **time period**, divided by the number at **risk** of developing that illness, disease, or condition during that time period.

attribute, attributed, attributing, attributes *v* - To **assign** to a particular cause or source; ascribe.

attribution *n* - 1. The act of **attributing**. 2. The ascribing of a particular work to an **author** or artist.

attribution of authorship *n* - **authorship attribution**

attrition *n* - [L *attrition-*, *attritio*, fr *attritus*, pp of *atterere* to rub against, fr *ad-* + *terere* to rub] Reduction in **number** or amount, as in the number of people lost from a **study** as a result of dropping out.

audit *n* - [ME fr L *auditus* act of hearing, fr *auditus*, pp] 1. A systematic **examination** or review of an **organization**, activity, or procedure. 2. A careful step by step review of some method or process. 3. **record audit** rt: **desk audit**, **off-site audit**, **on-site audit**, **record audit** *Usage note*: Subject to varying usage; accompany with sufficient detail to make sense of usage clear. Take care to distinguish usages having legal implications from those devoid of such meanings, such as audits done primarily as a part of **quality assurance** processes. See also **record audit**.

audit, **audited**, **auditing**, **audits** *v* - To examine, verify, or correct. *Usage note*: Not to be used interchangeably with **monitor** *v*. As a rule, **audit** *v*, implies a more detached and passive process than is the case with **monitor** *v*; see note for that entry. See also notes for **record audit** and **record monitor**.

audit trail *n* - The sequence of transactions linking two **events** or actions. In **data processing**, the sequence of transactions linking **data** in a finished **dataset** to those recorded in **source documents**, such as **data collection forms** or **medical records**.

auditor *n* - 1. One authorized to examine and verify **records** or accounts. 2. One who **audits**. 3. **record auditor** rt: **monitor** *Usage note*: See notes for **audit** *v*, **record auditor**, and **record monitor**.

aut- auto- *prefix* - [Gk, fr *autos* same, *-self*, self] 1. Self, same, one. 2. Automatic; self acting; self regulating.

author *n* - [ME *auctour*, fr ONF, fr L *auctor* promoter, originator, author, fr *auctus*, pp of *augēre* to increase] 1. The writer or one of the writers of a **document**, such as a **manuscript**. 2. The source or originator of a notion or concept.

author, **authored**, **authoring**, **authors** *v* - To write or originate.

author citation *n* - 1. The listing of authors in the **masthead** or title page of some **document**, **manuscript**, or work; **conventional author citation**, **corporate author citation**. 2. The citing of authors in relation to a document, manuscript, or work of the authors, eg, in a **reference citation**.

authorship *n* - 1. The source of a work, such as a **manuscript**. 2. The state or act of creating or writing, especially in relation to something written.

authorship attribution *n* - The persons, **group**, or **agency** to which a work is **attributed**. See **conventional authorship** and **corporate authorship**.

autocorrelation *n* - 1. The internal **relationship** or **correlation** of **repeated measures** ordered over time in a parent **population**. 2. **serial correlation**

availability *n* - The state or quality of being **available**.

available *adj* - Present or ready for use.

average *adj* - 1. Of, pertaining to, or equaling a mathematical **average**. 2. Common, ordinary.

average *n* - [modification of MF *avarie* damage to ship or cargo, fr OLt *avaria*, fr Ar *'awāriyah* damaged merchandise] 1. **arithmetic mean** 2. An **estimation** of or approximation to the arithmetic mean, such as provided by the **median** or **mode** or some other **central tendency measure**. 3. A typical or usual level, degree, or kind. rt: **median**, **mode** *Usage note*: Avoid in scientific writing, especially when referring to results based on a known measure of central tendency; use the proper, more precise, term.

average, **averaged**, **averaging**, **averages** *v* - 1. To bring to or arrive at an **average**. 2. To find or calculate the **mean**. 3. To proportionately divide or apportion.

average deviation *n* - **mean deviation**

award *n* - 1. Something that is conferred or bestowed, especially on the basis of need or merit. 2. **funding award**

axis *n* - [L, *axis* axle; akin to OE *eax* axis, axle, Gk *axōn*, L *axila* armpit, *agere* to drive] A reference **line** in a coordinate system, eg, the **x-** or **y-axis** in a plane **Cartesian coordinate system**.

B

back *adj* - 1. Not current. 2. To or toward a former state. 3. Being in or at the rear; in or into the past. 4. Moving or operating **backward**.

backup *n* - Any person, thing, or **procedure** that is or can be used to maintain an operation or activity in the event of a failure, malfunction, or absence of the primary person, thing, or procedure.

backward *adj* - Done or arranged in **reverse** order. ant: **forward**

backward stepwise regression *n* - **Stepwise regression**, that is typically performed by proceeding from the entire set of **regressors** to a smaller subset, by selectively removing regressors from the set in some ordered process with the ultimate goal of finding an appropriately restricted set. As distinct from **simultaneous regression**. See **stepwise regression** for more details. See **forward stepwise regression** for alternative approach.

balance *n* - [ME, fr OF, fr VL (assumed) *bilancia*, fr LL, *bilanc-*, *bilanx*, having two scale pans] 1. A property of **counts** or **totals** such that they are **equal** to or proportionate to one another. 2. A property of counts or totals such that they are approximately equal to or proportionate to one another; a property were the departures from equality or proportionality are not large. 3. A property of counts or totals such that the departures from balance are small enough so as to be consistent with having arisen from an underlying **distribution** having balance. *Usage note*: See **balanced**.

balance, balanced, balancing, balances *v* - To arrange, **adjust**, or proportion parts symmetrically or according to some preordained **ratio**; to bring to or hold in equilibrium. Used in **trials** to characterize **treatment assignment designs** that are intended to provide, or that have provided, assignments satisfying a specified **treatment assignment ratio**; treatment assignment designs calling for or providing equal numbers of assignments to the various **study treatments** or a specified proportionate mix. *Usage note*: See **balanced**.

balanced *adj* - Relating to or having a quality of symmetry, equality, or proportionality; not being **unbalanced**. In **trials** usually that quality in regard to **distributions** of counts across **treatment groups** for **baseline variables**. ant: **unbalanced** *Usage note*: The quality of balance is elusive in regard to the **baseline composition** of **treatment groups**. Variation in the numbers represented in the different treatment groups is to be expected, except for those variables **controlled** in the **assignment process**. Hence, most uses in this context are of a qualitative rather than quantitative nature. Use with caution in relation to a claim or assertion in regard to the distribution of baseline variables across treatment groups. See **unbalanced** for additional comments.

balanced block *n* - 1. A **block** in which a given **treatment** (or level of a **factor** or **variable**) is or is to be represented the same number of times relative to another treatment (or level of a factor or variable). 2. A block in which a given treatment (or level of a factor or variable) is or is to be represented in some specified **proportion** to another treatment (or level of a factor or variable) (eg, a block in which treatment A is represented twice as often as B for a **treatment design** with an assignment ratio of 2:1). ant: **unbalanced block** rt: **partially balanced block**

balanced block design *n* - A **design** (eg, as pertaining to the arrangement of **treatments** in a **trial**) involving **balanced blocks**. ant: **unbalanced block design** rt: **balanced incomplete block design**

balanced complete block *n* - **complete block**

balanced complete block design *n* - **complete block design**

balanced complete treatment assignment block *n* - **complete treatment assignment block** (defn 1)

balanced complete treatment assignment block design *n* - **complete treatment assignment block design**

balanced design *n* - 1. **balanced treatment design** 2. **balanced block design**

balanced incomplete block *n* - A **block** that is **incomplete** but **balanced** with regard to the **treatments** or levels of a **factor** or **variable** represented.

balanced incomplete block design *n* - An **experimental design** involving **balanced** but **incomplete blocks**. rt: **complete block design**

balanced incomplete treatment assignment block design *n* - A **treatment assignment design** involving **incomplete** but **balanced blocks**, eg, a **trial** involving three **treatments**, A,B, and C, 6 **blocks**, and two treatments per block arranged: Blk 1: A,B; Blk 2: B,A; Blk 3: B,C; Blk 4: C,B; Blk 5: A,C; Blk 6: C,A — incomplete because only two of the three treatments are represented per block and balanced because each treatment is represented the same number of times relative to any of the other treatments across the 6 blocks. syn: **balanced incomplete block design** rt: **complete treatment assignment block design**, **incomplete treatment assignment block design**

balanced randomization *n* - **Randomization** in which the **number** of **treatment assignments** made or to be made is **balanced**.

balanced randomization list *n* - 1. A **randomization list** that is constructed to provide **balance** in the number of **treatment assignments** made to the various **treatment groups**. 2. A randomization list that has provided such balance, regardless of method of construction.

balanced treatment assignment block *n* - A **treatment assignment block** that is **balanced**. syn: **balanced block** ant: **unbalanced block**, **unbalanced treatment assignment block**

balanced treatment assignment block design *n* - A **treatment design** involving **treatment assignment blocks** that are **balanced**. syn: **balanced block design** ant: **unbalanced block design**, **unbalanced treatment assignment block design**

balanced treatment assignment design *n* - A **treatment assignment design** that provides **balance** in the number of **treatment assignments** made to the various **treatment groups**. syn: **balanced treatment design** rt: **balanced treatment assignment block design**

balanced treatment design *n* - A **treatment design** that provides for or that has provided **balance** in the **treatment assignments**, especially as produced via designs involving **complete blocks**. syn: **balanced treatment assignment**

design ant: **unbalanced treatment design**

balanced trial *n* - 1. A **trial** employing a **balanced treatment assignment design**. 2. A trial in which the **treatment assignments** are **balanced**.

balancing interval *n* - **block size**

bandit *adj* - [**statistics**] Of, relating to, or concerned with a **stochastic process**.[82]

bandit *n* - [It *bandito*, fr pp of *bandire* to banish, of Gmc origin; akin to OHG *bannan* to command] [general] One or something that takes unfairly or robs. [**statistics**] Something that has or is based on an underlying **stochastic process**. rt: **one-armed bandit**, **two-armed bandit**

bank *n* - [ME, fr MF or OIt; MF *bangue*, fr OIt *banca*, lit, bench, of Gmc origin; akin to OE *benc*] 1. A facility that serves as a **site** for the collection and storage of biological specimens. 2. **data bank** syn: **repository** rt: **archive** *Usage note*: Generally usage should be reserved for settings in which the facility is established for ongoing deposits and withdrawals, as in blood or organ banks. If the primary function of the facility is to store specimens, such as blood or serum, for possible future **analyses** in relation to heretofore unspecified **hypotheses**, use **repository**.

bar *n* - [ME *barre*, fr MF] A vertical or horizontal rectangle or **line** whose height or length denotes a **measure** such as a **count**, **relative frequency**, or some other measure.

bar chart *n* - **bar diagram**

bar diagram *n* - A **method** of **display** for **discrete** or **categorical data** that involves a series of noncontiguous **bars** (one for each data **class**) arrayed on a common horizontal or vertical **axis** in which height or length denotes **count**, **frequency**, **proportion**, or some other **measure**. See *graphic display* for list.

base *adj* - Constituting or serving as a **base**.

base *n* - [ME, fr MF, fr L *basis*, fr Gk, step, base, fr *bainein* to go] 1. The fundamental part of something. 2. Foundation; a supporting part or layer. 3. The starting point of something. 4. A number (x in the expression $x^{2.65}$) that is raised to a **power**; especially such a number (eg, 10 in the base 10 number system) that when raised to a power equal to the **logarithm** of some number (eg, 100) produces that number ($10^2 = 100$). 5. The number that is raised to successive powers

Bar diagram

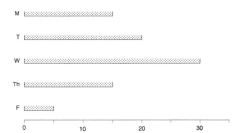

to generate the principal counting units of a number system, eg, the number 287 in the base 10 system is represented as $2(10^2) + 8(10^1) + 7(10^0)$.

baseline *adj* - 1. Of, relating to, or concerned with that which has occurred or is to occur just prior to or in conjunction with some act or **event**. 2. Of, relating to, or concerned with that which has occurred or is to occur in close proximity prior to or following some act or event. *Usage note*: Unqualified use should be limited to the sense of defn 1. Strictly speaking, uses in the sense of defn 2 represent mild debasements of the term to the extent that the references are to occurrences following the triggering act or event. Such uses are not consistent with the strict interpretation of **baseline** in that the term implies something timed in conjunction with or prior to the act or event of interest. See also notes for **baseline** *n* and **baseline period**.

baseline *n* - [general] 1. A **time point** or **period** (as in **baseline period**) from which subsequent **measurements** or activities are timed. 2. A **point** or **measure** for assessing subsequent **change**. 3. An observation or series of observations made on an **observation** or **treatment unit** at a designated point in **time** or within a designated **time interval** that serves as a basis for gauging change from that point forward in time for that unit. [trials] 4. **baseline period** 5. An observation or set of observations made or recorded on an observation or treatment unit just prior to or in conjunction with **treatment assignment** or initiation of treatment that serves as a basis for gauging change for that unit over the course of the trial. 6. An observation or set of observations made or recorded on an observation or treatment unit at a time point after the close

of the baseline period that serves as a basis for gauging change for that unit from that time point forward over the course of the trial (eg, an eye trial involving the use of photocoagulation for treatment of microhemorrhages by use of readings from a set of fundus photographs taken on a **patient** just having received an additional course of treatment for such a condition to provide a new baseline for assessing future changes in the eye). *Usage note*: Subject to varying uses in the context of trials, especially in relation to uses in the sense of defns 5 and 6. Most uses are in the sense of defn 5 but may, on occasion, be in the sense of defn 6. Typically, in the context of trials, unless otherwise indicated, the term should be reserved for characterizations that are appropriately thought of as being at baseline in the sense of defn 5 (see note for **baseline** *adj*) or in the sense of defn 1 for **baseline period**. However, even if the user is careful to limit usage to observations made prior to treatment assignment or initiation, ambiguities can still arise when the term is used as if always applying to a single time point (eg, as implied by the phrase *at baseline*) when that is not the case. Baseline observations in most trials arise from a series of **baseline examinations**, separated in time by days, weeks, or, in some cases, months (see **baseline period**). Hence, the time of observation for one baseline variable, relative to another, may be different (eg, as would be the case with baseline blood pressure measured at the **randomization visit** and baseline body weight measured one week prior to that visit at a prior baseline examination). The user is responsible for making the time differences among the variables represented in the baseline **dataset** known when describing the trial and its results. A certain amount of variability in the timing of one baseline observation or measurement relative to another and in the amount of time preceding the point of treatment assignment or initiation is unavoidable (except in cases where all required observations can be made at the same **clinic visit** and where that visit also serves as the **treatment assignment visit**). Unacceptably large variation is typically avoided by use of **time windows** specifying permissible **time intervals** within which the different observations are to be made one to another and the maximum permissible separation allowed for any single observation relative to the point of treatment assignment or initiation. The size of permissible separations will be a function of the importance of proximal linkages of one observation to another and of the individual observations to the point of treatment assignment or initiation. Observations considered to be highly correlated and where the **correlations** are important for establishing **valid** baselines will be required to be more closely linked in time than where such correlations are modest or unimportant. Similarly, observations subject to wide variation from one time to another for the same person may be observed several times at different time points in the **baseline period** and averaged, or may be required to have been made in a narrow time window with its upper limit affixed to the act of treatment assignment or initiation.

baseline adaptive randomization *n* - **Baseline adaptive treatment assignment** that involves **randomization**.

baseline adaptive treatment assignment *n* - A method of **treatment assignment** in which **treatment assignment probabilities** change over the course of the **trial** as a function of observed differences among the **treatment groups** for a designated **baseline variable** (or **variables**) so as to achieve comparable **treatment groups** with regard to the distribution of that variable or variables. rt: **adaptive treatment assignment**

baseline characteristic *n* - 1. A distinguishing property, feature, **attribute**, trait, or quality **measured** or **observed** or to be **measured** or **observed** at **baseline**. 2. Any such characteristic except one that is time-independent (eg, place of birth, ethic origin, gender). 3. **baseline variable** rt: **baseline data, baseline observation** *Usage note*: See **baseline** *adj* and **baseline** *n*.

baseline comparability *n* - [**trials**] 1. The absence of a notable **baseline difference** for a designated **variable** or set of such variables. 2. Similarity at **baseline**. 3. The extent to which **groups**, eg, **treatment groups** in a **trial**, are **comparable** with regard to a designated baseline variable or set of such variables. rt: **baseline composition, baseline difference**

baseline composition *n* - [**trials**] 1. The **composition** of a **treatment group** as assessed using **baseline data**. 2. The composition of the different treatment groups in a trial as assessed using baseline data, especially composition as indicated by **frequency distributions** for selected **baseline**

variables. rt: **baseline comparability, baseline difference**

baseline data *n* - **Data** collected or to be collected at **baseline**; in **trials**, usually the set of **data** collected or to be collected on a **study patient** or set of such patients during the **baseline period**. *Usage note*: The term is subject to ambiguities in settings where baseline data are collected over a period of time. **Precision** of communication in such settings requires specification of the amount of time separating the **observations** and the act or event defining the end of the baseline period, usually **treatment assignment** or **treatment initiation** in the case of trials. See **baseline** for additional comments.

baseline difference *n* - [**trials**] A **difference** in the **baseline composition** of the **treatment groups** with regard to a **baseline variable** or set of such variables; especially a difference considered **statistically significant** or a difference considered large enough to explain a portion of the **treatment effect** observed. rt: **baseline comparability, baseline composition**

baseline examination *n* - 1. A **patient examination**, carried out or to be carried out during the **baseline period**, that provides or is to provide **baseline data**. 2. Such an examination that is used as well to assess a patient's eligibility for **enrollment** into a **trial** or **followup study**. See **baseline** *adj* and **baseline** *n* for usage notes.

baseline observation *n* - An **observation** or recording of a **baseline variable** made on an **observation unit** or **treatment unit**; usually a **patient** in **trials**. See **baseline** *adj* and **baseline** *n* for usage notes.

baseline observation period *n* - 1. **baseline period** 2. **lead-in period, run-in period** See **baseline** *adj* and **baseline** *n* for usage notes.

baseline period *n* - [general] A **period** of **time** that is used or is to be used to perform procedures needed to assess the suitability and eligibility of a **study candidate** for **enrollment** into a **study** and, when applicable, to collect required **baseline data** and carry out the **consent process**. [**trials**] 1. A period defined by the start of the first **data collection visit** and ending with **assignment** to **treatment** or with the start of treatment. 2. A period defined by the start of the first data collection visit and ending with a **visit** or time point occurring shortly after **enrollment** or soon after initiation of treatment. 3. A period defined by some event or condition during the course of a trial. 4. **enrollment period** rt: **baseline observation period, lead-in period, run-in period** *Usage note*: Avoid in the sense of defn 2 without qualification (see note for **baseline** *adj*) and in the sense of defn 4. Provide accompanying detail for uses in the sense of defn 3 to avoid confusion with uses in the sense of defns 1 or 2. Traditionally, the point defining the end of the **baseline period** is marked either by the act of **treatment assignment** or initiation of **treatment**. Technically, the term should not be used to characterize observations made after that point without qualification. Confusion arises where the user mixes observations made at or before that time point of interest with those made after that time point. The practice arises from a desire, on the part of the user, to reduce the amount of missing **baseline data** by extending the period within which such observations can be made or within which observations made can be used for establishing baselines (as in the practice of considering any observations made within four weeks of **randomization** as constituting a **baseline observation**, even if the observation is after the initiation of treatment). Clearly, the utility of an observation serving as a baseline in the strict sense of that term is diminished if there is any possibility of the observation being influenced by treatment. Hence, the practice is not recommended, even if the permissible time interval following treatment assignment or initiation is small and if the likelihood of treatment having had an effect on the **variable** being observed is small. See also notes for **baseline** *adj* and for **baseline** *n*.

baseline study *n* - 1. A **study**, characterized by designated **observations** and **measurements**, designed to provide **baseline data**, usually as a prelude to administration of some experimental procedure or **treatment**. 2. **baseline examination** *Usage note*: See **baseline** *adj* and **baseline** *n* for usage notes.

baseline variable *n* - A **variable** to be measured, observed, or assessed at **baseline**. *Usage note*: See **baseline** *adj* and **baseline** *n* for usage notes.

baseline visit *n* - 1. A **visit** that is scheduled to take place or that has taken place during the **baseline period**. 2. A visit at which **baseline data** are collected. [**trials**] 3. Any of the baseline visits up to the one at which treatment is assigned; any such visits through the one in

which **treatment assignment** is issued. 4. Any of the baseline visits that take place up to the one at which treatment is initiated; any such visits through the one at which treatment is initiated. See assignment visit, **preassignment visit, pretreatment visit, treatment assignment visit, treatment initiation visit**. *Usage note*: See **baseline** *adj* and **baseline** *n* for usage notes.

baud *n* - A **measure** of speed for the electronic **transmission** of **data** equal to one pulse or code per second; usually one **bit**; **baud rate**. Named after JME Baudot, French inventor, 1845 - 1903.

baud rate *n* - The **rate** of electronic **data** transmission, as measured in the number of signals or **codes** transmitted per second. rt: **baud**

Bayes, Thomas - (1702 - 1761) English clergyman and mathematician; work included *An Essay Solving a Problem in the Doctrine of Chances* (published 1763)[6] containing the basis for what has come to be known as **Bayes' theorem**.

Bayes' theorem *n* - A **probability** theorem, developed by **Thomas Bayes**,[6] of the form:

$$P(E|C) = \frac{P(C|E) \times P(E)}{P(C|E) \times P(E) + P(C|\overline{E}) \times P(\overline{E})}$$

where P(E|C) is the **posterior probability** of the **event** E, given condition C, and is expressed as the product of the **prior probability** for the event, P(E), and the posterior probability of the condition given the event, P(C|E), divided by the sum of that product and the one for the prior probability when the event is absent, P($\overline{E}$), and the posterior probabilities for the condition when the event is absent, P(C|$\overline{E}$).

Bayesian *adj* - 1. Being or relating to a school of thought in which a **prior probability** distribution is assigned to **parameters** (**hypotheses**) fashioned from **observed data** by application of **Bayes theorem**. The resulting **posterior probabilities** can be viewed as measures of existing evidence and prior opinion, a result of logical reasoning, or subjective degree of belief. 2. One who performs a **Bayesian analysis**.

Bayesian analysis *n* - Any **method** of or approach to **data analysis** in which **prior** information or belief concerning some condition (expressed in the form of a **prior probability distribution**) is used in conjunction with **data** obtained from a **study** or **experiment** (expressed in the form of a **likelihood function**) to draw **inferences** concerning that condition [Cornfield, 1969;[28] 1966[29]]. See **frequentist analysis** for alternative approach. rt: **Bayesian, Bayes' theorem**

Bayesian estimate *n* - An **estimate** derived from a **posterior probability distribution** of a **parameter** and based on a **prior probability distribution** of the parameter and **likelihood function** of the **observed data**.

Bayesian inference *n* - A form of **inference** in which a **parameter** is considered a **random variable** having a **distribution** of values and involving both a **prior** and **posterior probability distribution** of the parameter.

Bayesian statistics *n* - 1. A branch of **statistics** incorporating **prior** objective or subjective collateral information concerning a **parameter** into the **estimation** process for that parameter. 2. Broadly, any statistical method using prior information or **probabilities** in the estimation process employed.

before *adj* - [ME, adv & prep, fr OE *beforan*, fr *be-* + *foran* before, fr *fore*] At an earlier time; previously. ant: **after**

before and after observation *n* - A comparative **observation** based on conditions existing before and after a certain change, planned or unplanned.

before and after study *n* - A type of **observational study** in which **observations** are made **after** a change and **compared** with those made or available before the change for the purpose of assessing the impact of the change on some process, procedure, or **outcome**, eg, a study involving a **comparison** of lengths of hospitalizations before and after implementation of a change in a care or treatment procedure. The study may rely on existing **data** for the comparison or may require collection of data. *Usage note*: Generally, the term is reserved for studies involving an active process of observation or assessment done in relation to the change. Use other terms, such as **fortuitous experiment** or **natural experiment**, when that process is passive.

behavior *n* - [alter of ME *behavour*, fr *behaven*] The manner of conducting oneself.

behavioral science *n* - A multidisciplinary **science**, involving psychology, sociology, and anthropology, that focuses on identifying etiologies and determinants of human behavior and on the utilization of such information in developing

and testing methods to be used in modifying **behavior**.

bell *n* - [ME *belle*, fr OE; akin to OE *bellan* to roar] A smooth, metal, cylindrically shaped, object, having a flared open bottom and rounded closed top that vibrates and gives forth a ringing sound when struck.

bell-shaped *adj* - Something having the shape or profile of a **bell**.

bell-shaped curve *n* - 1. A **curve** having the profile of a **bell**. 2. **normal curve**

Bell-shaped curve

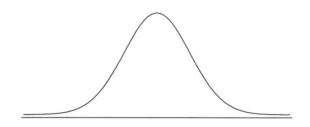

bell-shaped distribution *n* - 1. A **distribution** having the profile of a **bell**. 2. **normal distribution**

beneficence *n* - [L *beneficentia*, fr *beneficus*] 1. The quality or state of being **beneficent**, as evidenced by acts of kindness or by doing or producing good. 2. **beneficence, principle of**

beneficence, principle of *n* - A **principle** in **medical ethics** that asserts that the options available in treating or caring for one's fellow human beings is limited to that set which is justifiable on the basis of **beneficence**. Translated to research settings involving human beings, the principle means that only those acts, procedures, and **treatments** that meet this test are justifiable [Levine, 1986].[88] See also **medical ethics, principles of**.

beneficent *adj* - Doing or producing good; performing acts of kindness.

beneficial *adj* - [L *beneficium* favor, benefit] Conferring benefit; conducive to personal or social well-being; receiving or entitling one to receive advantage.

beneficial effect *n* - An **effect** that is, or is considered to be, of **benefit** to its recipient. In relation to a **patient**, an effect produced by a **treatment** or care procedure that has, or is considered to have, **positive** implications for the health or well-being of that **patient**.

beneficial treatment effect *n* - A **treatment effect** that has **positive** health implications. ant: **adverse treatment effect**

benefit *n* - [ME, fr AF *benfet*, fr L *bene factum*, fr neut of *bene bactus*] Something that promotes well-being or that provides an advantage.

benefit factor *n* - A **factor** or level of a factor considered or known to confer **benefit**; especially such a factor or level of a factor in the complementary sense of defn 2 for **risk factor**. ant: **risk factor** *Usage note*: See note for **risk factor**.

Berkson, Joseph - (1899 - 1982) Statistician-epidemiologist known for his challenges to established views and theories in **statistics** and **epidemiology** (USA; MD 1927, ScD 1928, Johns Hopkins; Head of the Division of Medical Statistics, Mayo Clinic, 1934 - 1964).

Berksonian bias *n* - 1. A type of **selection bias**, characterized by **Berkson** [1946][8] in the context of hospital-based **case-control studies**, in which the measurement of **association** between two **binary variables** (eg, presence or absence of two **diseases**, such as cholecystitis and diabetes) is biased due to differential rates of selection or entry for people having the conditions represented by the variables. 2. Broadly, any instance in which the **probabilities** of selection or entry of **observation units** into a study differ for the groups being compared.

Bernoulli, Jakob (Jacques) I - (1654 - 1705) Swiss mathematician and probabilist; the first of a line of famous mathematicians spanning several generations and all descendants of Niklaus Bernoulli (prominent merchant of Basel).

Bernoulli random variable *n* - A **random variable** that is capable of assuming just one of two values (eg, 0 or 1) with fixed probabilities, P and 1 - P, respectively [Feller, 1968;[46] Bernoulli, 1713[9]]. See also **binary variable**.

Bernoulli trial *n* - A single **replication** of an experimental procedure that has only one of two possible **outcomes**, as characterized by a **Bernoulli random variable** [Bernoulli, 1713].[9]

best *adj* - [ME, fr OE *betst*; akin to OE *bōt* remedy] 1. Most favorable in relation to a stated **hypothesis** or position. 2. Excelling all others. 3. Most productive of good or of advantage, utility, or satisfaction. ant: **worst**

best case *n* - The **case** (defn 1) that is **best** in some sense or aspect. ant: **worst case**

best case analysis *n* - An **analysis** based on a **best case assumption**, eg, an analysis of mortality from a **followup study** in which one **assumes** that all persons not known to be alive at the time of the analysis were in fact alive; an analysis of a **drug effect** in which one assumes that none of the observed or reported **events** are due to the drug when in doubt as to etiology. ant: **worst case analysis**

best case assumption *n* - **Assumption** of the **best** in regard to some event, condition, or **dataset** having varying interpretations or meanings, eg, assumption that **events** observed during the course of **treatment** with an **experimental drug** are not due to the **drug**. ant: **worst case assumption** rt: **best case analysis**

best medical judgment *n* - [**trials**] 1. A **medical judgment** regarding course of **treatment** that is at odds with the **treatment protocol**. 2. A medical judgment as to the appropriate course of treatment after the **sequence** of treatment steps or procedures specified in the treatment protocol have been followed and failed to produce the desired result or state. rt: **medical judgment**

best-worst case analysis *n* - Separate **analyses** involving a **best case assumption** and **worst case assumption**, especially those performed as a means of assessing the **robustness** of a finding or **conclusion** under different **assumptions**, eg, an analysis of **data** from a **followup study** of mortality assuming all persons whose **vital status** is unknown to be alive at the end of followup, and another in which they are assumed to be dead to determine whether the two analyses lead to different conclusions. rt: **best case analysis**, **worst case analysis**

bet *n* - Something that is laid, pledged, or wagered between two parties concerning the occurrence of some **event** or **outcome**.

beta *n* - [Gk *bēta* of Sem origin; akin to Heb, *bēth*, beth] 1. The 2nd letter in the **Greek alphabet**, uppercase B, lowercase β. 2. **type II error**

beta error *n* - **type II error**

betting odds *n* - 1. **odds** (defn 2) 2. **relative betting odds**

between *prep* - [ME *betwene*, prep & adv, fr OE *betwēonum*, fr *be-* + *twēonum* (akin to Goth *tweihnai* two each); akin to OE *twā*, two] In intermediate relation to; from one to the other of; serving to connect or unite in a relationship (as in regard to **difference**, likeness, or **proportion**).

between-patient *adj* - **between-person**

between-person *adj* - Relating to that done or **observed** between or across persons; of or relating to **designs** and **analyses** involving a **person** as the **experimental** or **observational unit**. ant: **within-person**

between-person study *n* - 1. A **study** with **persons** as the **experimental unit**; a study with persons as the **observational unit**. 2. A **study** in which the **comparisons** made or to be made are based on **results** from different **persons** or groups of persons. ant: **within-person study**

between-person trial *n* - A **trial** with a **parallel treatment design**. syn: **parallel group trial** ant: **within-person trial**

bi- *prefix* - [ME, fr L] Prefix, meaning two, as in **binary**, or twice, as in **biannual**. rt: **semi-** *Usage note*: Avoid in time designations, such as **biweekly**, **bimonthly**, or **biannually**, because of potential for confusion as to whether the prefix denotes count within the designated time interval, meaning twice (as in twice weekly), or frequency across the designated time interval, meaning once every other (as in once every other week). See also usage note for **semi-**.

biannual *adj* - 1. Occurring twice a year. 2. Occurring once every other year. rt: **bimonthly**, **biweekly**, **semiannual** *Usage note*: Avoid because of uncertainty as to whether defn 1 or defn 2 applies. See usage notes for **bi-** and **semi-**. Use **semiannual** for usages in the sense of defn 1, or state frequency, as in *twice a year* or as in *once every other year*. See usage note also for **semiannual**.

bias *n* - [fr OF *bias*, oblique, fr OProv, perhaps from Gk, *epikarsios*, oblique] 1. An inclination of temperament, state of mind, or action based on perception, opinion, or impression as opposed to fact, that serves to reduce rational thought or action, or the making of impartial judgments; a specified instance of such an inclination. 2. A tendency toward certain **measurements** or

outcomes over others as a result of a conscious or subconscious mind set, temperament, or the like; a specific expression of such a tendency. 3. **Deviation** of the **expected value** of an **estimate** of a **statistic** from its true value. See *bias* for list. *Usage note*: Distinguish between uses in which **bias** (defn 1 or 2) is being proposed in a speculative sense as opposed to an actual instance of bias. Usages in the latter sense should be supported with evidence or arguments to substantiate the claim. Usages in the former sense should be preceded or followed by appropriate modifiers, explanatory clauses, or statements to make it clear that the user is speculating rather than stating a fact. Similarly, since most undifferentiated uses (in the sense of defns 1 or 2) are in the speculative rather than fact sense, prudent readers will treat all uses of the term as being in the sense of speculation, except where accompanied by data, evidence, or arguments to establish bias as a fact.

bias control *v* - The exercise of restraint to reduce or eliminate the influence of **bias** on some process or procedure; such restraint as arising from **masking**, **standardizing**, **training**, and **certifying**. rt: **variance control**

bias free treatment assignment *n* - 1. **Treatment assignment** arising from any **scheme** having procedures designed to ensure that the decision as to whether or not a person should be **enrolled** for treatment assignment is **independent** of the assignment to be made. 2. **masked treatment assignment**

bias potential *n* - A **potential** for **bias** that may arise or be seen in the future, as in relation to a **conflict of interest**.

biased *adj* - 1. Exhibiting or characterized by **bias**. 2. Tending to yield one **outcome** more frequently than others. 3. Having an **expected value** not equalling the quantity or value of the **parameter** in question. ant: **unbiased**

biased coin randomization *n* - **Biased coin treatment assignment** involving **randomization**.

biased coin treatment assignment *n* - An **adaptive** method of **treatment assignment** for **trials** having **parallel treatment designs** in which **treatment assignment probabilities** are modified as a function of the observed difference in the **number** of **patients** already assigned to the various **study treatment groups** represented.

biased estimator *n* - An **estimator** having an **expected value** not equalling the **parameter** or quantity it is intended to **estimate**. ant: **unbiased estimator**

bibliographic citation *n* - **reference citation**

bibliography *n* - [prob fr NL *bibliographia*, fr Gk, the copying of books, fr *biblio-* + *-graphia* -graphy] The list of **references** cited in a scholarly work.

big *adj* - [ME, prob of Scand origin; akin to Norw dial *bugge* important man; akin to OE *byl* boil, Skt *bhūri* abundant] Large in dimension, bulk, extent, or number. *Usage note*: Use with caution; avoid as a generic label; when so used, as in **big trial**, provide accompanying detail to indicate sense of usage. ant: **small** rt: **large**

big and simple trial *n* - 1. A **data simple trial** that is also **big** in an absolute or relative sense in regard to **sample size**, eg, the Physicians' Health Study.[66] 2. A trial that is in some sense both **big** and **simple**. syn: large and simple trial rt: **big trial**, **data simple trial**, **simple trial** *Usage note*: Avoid as a generic label without accompanying detail to indicate sense of usage for both **big** and **simple**. Note that use in the sense of defn 1 does not necessarily imply ease of execution. Avoid such connotation when not appropriate, especially in trials involving major costs and efforts concentrated in the **coordinating center** or other core facilities having responsibilities for organizing and executing the trial. Many trials carrying the label of **simple** are merely **data simple**. See **simple trial** for added comments.

big trial *n* - 1. A **trial** having a **sample size** of 1,000 or more per **treatment group**; a trial having a per treatment sample size severalfold larger than that of similar trials heretofore done or reported. 2. A trial having a large **number** of **centers**, a large number of investigators, or involving a large outlay of money compared with other related trials. syn: large trial rt: **big and simple trial** *Usage note*: Avoid as a generic label without accompanying detail to indicate sense of usage. Often that which is **big** or **large** from one perspective is ordinary from another perspective; hence, the term is not informative by itself without explanation. Note as well that defn 2 has a different connotation than defn 1. Defn 1 relates to sample size, whereas defn 2 relates to other dimensions of the trial and may be used even if the sample size is not big in the

sense of defn 1. See **big and simple trial** for additional comments.

bimodal *adj* - Having two **modes**. rt: **multimodal**

bimodal distribution *n* - A **distribution** with two **modes**. rt: **multimodal distribution**

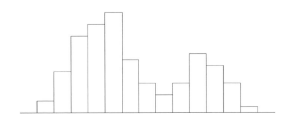

Bimodal distribution

bimonthly *adj* - 1. Occurring twice a month. 2. Occurring once every other month. rt: **biannual**, **biweekly**, **semimonthly** *Usage note*: Avoid because of ambiguity of meaning. See usage notes for **bi-** and **semi-**. Use **semimonthly** for usages in the sense of defn 1, or state frequency, as in *twice a month* or as in *once every other month*. See also usage note for **semimonthly**.

binary *adj* - [LL *binarius*, fr L *bini*] 1. Relating to or belonging to a system of **numbers** having 2 as its **base**. 2. Having one of two states (on, off; yes, no); involving a choice or **outcome** having one of two complementary states.

binary digit *n* - 1. **binary number** 2. **bit**

binary number *n* - A 0 or 1; represented by the absence or presence of an electrical signal or pulse in electronic circuits, such as in **computers**, for processing and storing **data**. rt: **binary digit**

binary number system *n* - A **number system** involving the **base** 2 in which any **number** can be represented by a particular arrangement of 0's and 1's (eg, 01000111, as the 8 **digit binary** representation of 71) and are viewed as corresponding to a sum of products of terms consisting of the binary value (0 or 1) at a designated position in the sequence multiplied by 2 raised to the power corresponding to that position; position number determined by counting from left to right with the 1st position corresponding to position zero. For example, the sum $0 \cdot 2^7 + 1 \cdot 2^6 + 0 \cdot 2^5 + 0 \cdot 2^4 + 0 \cdot 2^3 + 1 \cdot 2^2 + 1 \cdot 2^1 + 1 \cdot 2^0 = 71$ corresponding to the binary number 01000111. rt: **binary digit**, **decimal number system**, **hexadecimal number system**

binary outcome *n* - [**followup studies**] 1. A **binary variable** with one of its values denoting the desired state and the other denoting the complementary state, with all persons or **observation units** having the desired state on **entry** or at the starting point of observation, and capable of a single unidirectional transition over the course of observation (eg, transition from life to death for **vital status** or from being disease-free to a state of disease). 2. A variable as characterized in defn 1, but for each of a series of contiguous **time intervals**. 3. A binary variable capable of assuming either value upon entry or at the start of observation and capable of a single bi-directional transition (as in the transition from negative to positive or from positive to negative). 4. A variable as characterized in defn 3, but for each of a series of contiguous time intervals. 5. **binary variable**

binary outcome measure *n* - An **outcome measure** that assumes only one of two values or states (eg, present or absent; alive or dead; yes or no) over a defined course of **observation**.

binary variable *n* - A **variable** that is capable of assuming only one of two possible values (eg, 0 or 1, or more generally, E_1 or E_2) over a defined period of **observation**; equivalent to a **Bernoulli random variable** if the **probabilities** of E_1 and E_2 are fixed.

binomial *n* - [NL *binomium*, fr ML neut of *binomius*, having two names, alter of L binominus, fr *bi-* + *nomin-*, *nomen* name] A **polynomial** consisting of two terms, eg, x + y.

binomial coefficient *n* - The **coefficient** (numeric multiplier) preceding a specified term in the expansion of $(x + y)^n$, eg, 2 for the 2nd term and 1 for the 1st and 3rd (last) terms in the expansion for n = 2.

binomial distribution *n* - A **probability distribution** of the form:

$$f(k) = \binom{n}{k} p^k (1-p)^{n-k} \text{ for } k = 0, 1, 2, \cdots, n$$

that gives the **probability** of n **independent Bernoulli trials** resulting in k successes and n-k failures, where **success** or **failure** is defined by presence or absence of some condition or **event** (eg, drawing or failing to draw a red ball from an **urn** containing red and blue balls) and where the probability is p for success and 1 - p for failure.

binomial theorem *n* - A **theorem** that specifies that the expansion of the **binomial**, $(x + y)^n$, yields n + 1 terms of the general form:

$$[n!/(k!(n-k)!] x^k y^{n-k}$$

bioassay *n* - A procedure for determining the relative strength of a substance, such as a **drug**, by comparing its effect, as **measured** or **observed** in some organism or substrate, with that of known amounts, as measured or observed in the same organism or substrate.

bioavailability *n* - The degree to which something ingested (**drug**, nutrient) is **available** at some physiological site of activity; the state of being **bioavailable**.

bioavailability study *n* - A **study** (typically involving administration of a substance, such as a **drug** or drugs, in different **dosages**, routes of administration, or formulations) done for the purpose of determining the **bioavailability** of a substance.

bioavailable *adj* - 1. The **rate** and extent to which an administered substance, such as a **drug**, enters the general circulation of the body. 2. A **characteristic** attributed to a substance, such as a drug, that, when ingested or administered in sufficient quantity, produces a measurable effect, as evidenced by some observation, measurement, laboratory test, **bioassay**, or the like.

bioequivalence *n* - The state or property of being **bioequivalent**. rt: **equivalence**

bioequivalent *adj* - **Equivalent** in amount or action as **measured** by or in some biological system or process; producing the same effect in a biological organism or system; **drugs** are said to bioequivalent in a defined biological setting if specified amounts of those drugs produce the same effect in that setting. rt: **equivalent**

biologic *n* - A **drug** derived from a biological source or product; **biological product**.

biological, biologic *adj* - Of, pertaining to, caused by, or affecting life or living organisms; of or relating to **biology** or to a living process.

biological marker *n* - A naturally occurring substance or entity in body parts, fluids, or tissues that is associated with some condition or **characteristic** and, as a result, is used to help identify individuals with that condition or characteristic. rt: **biological tracer substance**

biological product *n* - 1. Any product of a biological process used for the **prevention**, **treatment**, or cure of **disease** or injuries; includes **vaccine**, virus, therapeutic serum, toxin, antitoxin, hormone, antibiotic, or analogous products. 2. (As defined in section 351 (a) of the Public Health Service Act, 42 USC 262 (a), for the purpose of regulation of the use of biological products in human beings): Any virus, therapeutic serum, toxin, antitoxin, vaccine, blood and blood component or derivative, allergenic product, or analogous product applicable to the **prevention**, **treatment**, or cure of **diseases** or injuries of human beings. Hormones and antibodies are examples of "biologics" not identified in the Public Health Service Act, and, hence are not subject to the provisions of the Act. Biological products are also considered **drugs**, and therefore many of the provisions of the Food, Drug, and Cosmetic Act applying to **new drugs** apply to biological products as well. syn: **biologic**

biological tracer substance *n* - A substance (eg, a breakdown product of a **drug**) produced as a result of some biological process, that is used as a **tracer substance**. rt: **biological marker**

biology *n* - [Ger *biologie*, fr *bi-* + *-logie* -logy] 1. A branch of **science** concerned with understanding life processes of living organisms; including the study of structure, functioning, growth, origin, evolution, and **distribution**. 2. The life processes or **characteristic** phenomena of a **group** or **category** of living organisms.

biometrician *n* - One trained in **biometry** or who uses the **methods** and procedures of **biometry** for **collection** or **analysis** of **data** related to the biological sciences. syn: **biostatistician**

biometrics *n* - **biometry**

biometry *n* - A discipline of the biological sciences concerned with the application of mathematical-statistical theory, principles, and practices to the **observation**, **measurement**, and **analysis** of biological **data** and phenomena. syn: **biostatis-**tics

biostatistical *adj* - Of or relating to **biostatistics**.

biostatistical center *n* - 1. **data center** 2. **data coordinating center** 3. **coordinating center** syn: **statistical center**

biostatistician *n* - One who is trained in **biostatistics** or who uses the methods and procedures of biostatistics for the **collection** or **analysis** of **data** related to the biological sciences. syn: **biometrician**

biostatistics *n* - A discipline of the biological sciences concerned with the application of mathematical-statistical theory, principles, and practices to the **observation**, **measurement**, and **analysis** of biological phenomena. syn: **biometry**

birth *n* - [ME, fr ON *byrth*; akin to OE *beran*] The emergence of a new being from the body of its **parent**. The state of having newly emerged or come into being.

birth cohort *n* - A **group** of people born within the same **time period**, eg, those born in 1960. rt: **cohort, cohort effect, generation effect**

birthdate *n* - 1. The **date** a person is or was born. 2. The date something comes into being. 3. **birthday** rt: **date of birth** *Usage note*: Use only in the sense of defn 1 or 2 in formal scientific writings or presentations. Avoid as a synonym for **birthday anniversary**

birthday *n* - 1. **birthdate** (defns 1 or 2) 2. **birthday anniversary**

birthday anniversary *n* - The **anniversary** of one's **birthday**; **birthday** (defn 2)

bit (b) *n* - 1. **binary digit**; formed from the contraction of **b**inary and dig**it**; denoted by b in numerical or mathematical expressions, eg, 2^{20}b. 2. A unit of information in a **computer** expressed in binary form, typically expressed by presence or absence of some condition or state or by something indicative of an on or off condition. 3. A representation of a single binary digit, eg, by presence or absence of a pulse of current. 4. A unit of **storage** capacity capable of containing or representing a binary digit. rt: **byte**

bivariate *adj* - Of, relating to, or having two **variables**. rt: **multivariate**, **univariate**

bivariate analysis *n* - **Analysis** involving two **variables** aimed at assessing their interrelationship.

bivariate density function *n* - A **joint density function** involving two **random variables**.

bivariate distribution *n* - The **joint distribution** of two **random variables**. rt: **univariate distribution**

bivariate normal distribution *n* - The **joint distribution** of two **random variables**, x and y, for which the **marginal distribution** of y on x (and x on y) is **linear**, and the **conditional distribution** of y, given x (or of x, given y), is **normal** with **variance** independent of x (or y) and having the general form:

$$f(x,y) = \frac{1}{2\pi\sigma_x\sigma_y\sqrt{1-\rho^2}}\exp[-\frac{1}{2(1-\rho^2)}w]$$

where w is defined as follows:

$$w = \frac{(x-\mu_x)^2}{\sigma_x^2} - \frac{2\rho(x-\mu_x)(y-\mu_y)}{\sigma_x\sigma_y} + \frac{(y-\mu_y)^2}{\sigma_y^2}$$

and where the **parameter** ρ corresponds to the **correlation coefficient** for x and y and is a value of or bounded between 1 and - 1, σ_x and σ_y correspond to the **standard deviations** of the variables x and y, respectively, and μ_x and μ_y correspond to the **means** for the variables x and y, respectively.

biweekly *adj* - 1. Occurring twice a **week**. 2. Occurring once every other week. rt: **biannual**, **bimonthly**, **semiweekly** *Usage note*: Avoid because of uncertainty as to whether defn 1 or defn 2 applies. State **frequency** explicitly, eg, *twice a week* or *once every other week*. See usage note also for **semiweekly**.

blind, blinded *adj* - [ME, fr OE; akin to OHG *blint* blind, OE *blandan* to mix] 1. Being without sight; unable to see; having vision measuring less than an amount considered to constitute blindness. 2. Being unable or unwilling to discern. 3. Of or relating to something considered to be the product of stupidity or of ignorance, eg, *blind stupidity*. 4. Being unaware or uninformed of some fact or condition; not recommended usage, use **mask** or **masked**. rt: single-blind, double-blind, triple-blind *Usage note*: Not recommended for usage in sense of defn 4; see usage note for **mask** for reasons.

blind *n* - 1. Something to hinder sight or keep out light. 2. A place of concealment. 3. Something

put forward or done for the purpose of misleading or concealing. 4. **mask** *Usage note*: Not recommended as a synonym for **mask**; use **mask** rather than **blind** for reasons stated in usage note for **mask**.

blind, blinded, blinding, blinds *v* - 1. To hide or conceal. 2. To **mask** (make **blind**) by withholding, hiding, or concealing some fact. *Usage note*: Not recommended as a synonym for **mask**; use **mask** rather than **blind** for reasons stated in usage note for **mask**, **masked** *adj*.

blind experiment *n* - **masked experiment**

blind randomization *n* - **masked randomization**

blind treatment assignment *n* - **masked treatment assignment**

blind trial *n* - **masked trial**

block *n* - [ME *blok*, fr MF *bloc*, fr MD *blok*; akin to OHG *bloh* block, MIr *blog* fragment] 1. [general] A group, quantity, section, or segment that is considered as a **unit** for some specified purpose, procedure, process, or action; **stratum**. 2. [trials] A grouping of **treatments** or of **treatment assignments** administered or to be administered in the order listed; especially a grouping of assignments in a **parallel treatment design** that satisfy the **assignment ratio**. 3. The **experimental unit** or collection of units receiving the treatments represented in a block; a single unit in the case of **crossover designs** and as many units as there are treatment assignments represented in a block in **parallel treatment designs**. syn (trials): **treatment assignment block** rt: **blocked treatment assignment**, **blocked randomization** *Usage note*: Not to be confused with **stratum** (although often so confused, especially in lay usage, as suggested by defn 1); see note for **stratification**. The **block size** may be the same for all blocks, eg, as required for a **crossover treatment design** and as arising in **parallel treatment designs** involving blocks of the same size. The size will be equal to the number of **study treatments** in the case of **complete crossover designs**. The size for parallel treatment designs will be the sum of the numbers represented in the assignment ratio (eg, 2 for a design involving two study treatments and a **uniform treatment assignment ratio** and 15 for a design involving 6 study treatments and an assignment ratio of 1:1:1:1:1:2.5) or multiples thereof. The usual strategy in parallel treatment designs is to have a mix of blocks of different sizes, themselves randomly ordered, with all blocks being some multiple of the smallest possible block size. The purpose of blocking is to ensure **balance** in the mix of the **treatment groups** with regard to time of enrollment. The blocking helps to eliminate the risk of differential **secular trends** in the make-up of the treatment groups. Time-related shifts in the nature of persons **enrolled** over the course of a trial can be a **confounding variable** for **treatment comparisons**, in the absence of blocking, if the mix of persons represented changes over time and is different by treatment group.

block design *n* - An **experimental design** involving **blocks**.

block effect *n* - The amount of **variance** (as in an **analysis of variance**) that is accounted for by **blocks** in an **experimental design**. rt: **treatment assignment block effect**

block size *n* - 1. The number of **experimental units** comprising or to comprise a **block**. 2. **treatment assignment block size**

block treatment design *n* - A type of **fixed treatment assignment design** in which **treatments assignments** are arranged in **blocks** having a specified **treatment assignment ratio**. rt: **complete block treatment design, incomplete block treatment design**

blocked *adj* - Of, relating to, or being the result of **blocking**.

blocked, blocking, blocks *v* - The process of establishing defined **groups**, as in a **block treatment design**.

blocked randomization *n* - 1. **Blocked treatment assignments** in which the assignments are the result of some **randomization** process. 2. **Randomization** constrained by **blocking**. rt: **restricted treatment assignment**

blocked treatment assignment *n* - A **treatment assignment** that has been or is to be constrained in such a way so that when a **block** is filled (ie, when the number of assignments equals the number called for in a block) those assignments satisfy some specified condition (eg, the number of assignments for each treatment are **equal** or are in some specified **ratio** one to another). rt: **blocked randomization, restricted treatment assignment**

blocking interval *n* - **block size**

board *n* - [ME *bord* piece of sawed lumber, border, ship's side, fr OE; akin to OHG *bort* ship's side, Skt *bardhaka* carpenter] A **group** of persons having managerial, supervisory, investigatory, or advisory powers. syn: **committee** (in some contexts)

body *n* - [ME, fr OE *bodig*; akin to OHG *botah* body] A **group** of people organized for some purpose.

bogus *a* - [*bogus* (a machine for making counterfeit money)] Not genuine; counterfeit; fake; **sham**.

bogus data *n* - 1. **falsified data** 2. unreliable data rt: **scientific misconduct**

Bonferroni's inequality *n* - A **statement**, developed by Carlo E Bonferroni (Italian, 1892 - 1960), that expresses the upper bound **probability** of one or more of **k independent events**, each with probability **p**, occurring simultaneously, as the **product** of **k** and **p** [Feller, 1968, pages 110 and 111].[46] For example, suppose one wishes to perform 10 **independent** tests such that the **type I error** for any one of the tests does not exceed 0.05, then each test should be performed at a type I error level of 0.05/10 = 0.005.

book *n* - [ME, fr OE *bōc*; akin to OHG *buoh* book; perhaps akin to OE *bōc* beech, probably fr early Germanic practice of carving runic characters on beech wood tablets] A set of ordered bound pages containing written or **graphic** material.

booklet *n* - A pamphlet or small **book**.

bootstrap *adj* - Of or relating to something **robust** or rough and ready.

bootstrap estimate *n* - An **estimate** derived from a single **bootstrap sample** or from a series of such samples. rt: **bootstrap method, bootstrap sample, jackknife estimate**

bootstrap method *n* - A largely **nonparametric method** of assessing the **accuracy** of an **estimate** of a **statistic** (defn 1) by use of the **distribution** of the estimate as determined by repeated sampling from a **population** created using multiple copies of the **observed data**. Each sample (of the same size as the original) is used to produce an estimate of the statistic of interest. The distribution of estimates (as obtained from the different samples) is used to produce a measure of the accuracy of the estimate. The method derives it name from its rough and ready qualities as expressed by the notion of pulling oneself up by one's bootstraps. See Diaconis and Efron [1983][36] for review. rt: **bootstrap estimate, bootstrap sample**

bootstrap sample *n* - A **sample** drawn from a **population** of **observed data**, as created for sampling for use in a **bootstrap method**. rt: **bootstrap estimate, bootstrap method**

boundary *n* - Something that indicates or fixes a **limit**.

box *n* - [ME, fr OE, fr LL *buxis*, fr Gk *pyxis*, fr *pyxos* box tree] A closed rectangular space denoted by rules or borders used for displaying printed matter or other graphic information.

box plot *n* - A **plot** or **graphic display** of the **distribution** of a set of **observed data**; typically used for comparing several related sets of data, such as **patients** in a **trial** observed at various time points over the course of **treatment**. Each plot consists of a **box** having length or width determined by designated **percentile** points (typically, the 25th and 75th) and a line (**tail** or **whisker**) connecting the lower end or left side of the box to the smallest value observed (or such a value ignoring those considered to be **outliers**) and a corresponding line for the upper end or right side of the box for the largest value observed. The **midpoint** of the distribution (**median**) is typically denoted by positioning a mark or symbol within the box at the midpoint.

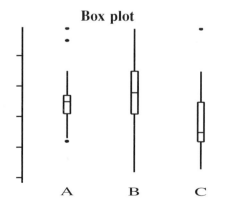

Box plot

break *n* - An interruption in continuity or sequence.

break, broke, broken, breaking, breaks *v* - [ME *breken*, fr OE *brecan*; akin to OHG *brehhan* to

break, L *frangere*, MIr *braigid* he breaks wind] To **stop**, **terminate**, or interrupt.

breakdown *n* - 1. The act or process of breaking down or failing to function; the condition resulting from such breakdown or failure. 2. Departure from an accepted **norm**, process, or procedure, as in **randomization breakdown**.

brochure *n* - [F, fr *brocher* to sew, fr MF, to prick, fr OF *brochier*, fr *broche*] Pamphlet or booklet, especially one containing descriptive or advertising material. rt: **investigator's brochure**, patient brochure, **patient information booklet**

budget *n* - [ME *bowgette*, fr MF *bougette*, dim of *bouge* leather bag, fr L *bulga*, of Gaulish origin; akin to MIr *bolg* bag; akin to OE *bœlg* bag] 1. A plan for the use of a fixed amount of money or of a specified resource. 2. A **statement** of the anticipated financial **position** of an administration or specified activity for a defined forthcoming **time period** based on **estimates** of income and expenditures. 3. The amount of money available for or assigned to a particular purpose.

bug *n* - 1. A hidden defect, fault, flaw, or imperfection in the **hardware** or **software** of a **computer** or associated system or **program** that causes or is capable of causing disruption, malfunction, or **error**. 2. A defect, fault, or flaw in some **design**, **plan**, process, or system. rt: **virus**

business *n* - 1. Commercial activity engaged in or pursued as a means of livelihood. 2. Commercial or industrial enterprise; trade.

business office *n* - 1. The place or **office** within an **institution** or **business** considered to be the seat or headquarters of the institution or business. 2. The place or office of an institution or business firm where financial records are processed and kept. 3. The office in an investigator's institution having legal responsibility for receipt of **research funds** from a **sponsor** and overseeing the expenditure of those funds under specified ground rules and direction of the **investigator**.

byte (B) *n* - A **group** of adjacent **bits** (eg, 8 and usually fewer than in a **word**) used in a **computer** to represent alphabetic, numeric, and other special characters, that are treated as a unit of information by a **computer**. Eight information bits are needed to represent the 256 ($=2^8$) characters in the **ASCII** extended character set.

C

calculate, calculated, calculating, calculates *v* - [L *calculatus*, pp of *calculare*, fr *calculus* pebble (used in reckoning), dim of *calc-*, *calx* stone used in gaming lime] To determine by a mathematical process, especially in relation to arithmetic operations involving numerical values.

calculated *adj* - 1. Determined by mathematical **calculation**. 2. likely

calculated sample size *n* - The **sample size** desired or required for a **study**, as derived from a **sample size calculation**.

calculation *n* - The process or act of **calculating**.

candidate *n* - [L *candidatus*, fr *candidatus* clothed in white, fr *candidus* white; fr the white toga worn by candidates for office in ancient Rome] One that aspires to or is under consideration for some office, post, membership, or **enrollment**; **study candidate**.

cardinal *adj* - Of basic or fundamental importance.

cardinal number *n* - An **integer** such as 7 or 1,589, that indicates **count** or number in some group or assemblage. rt: **ordinal number**

care *n* - [ME, fr OE *caru*; akin to OHG *kara* lament, L *garrire* to chatter] Painstaking or watchful attention or application.

careful *adj* - Exercising care; marked by wary caution or prudence. *Usage note*: usually unnecessary when describing one's own work or that of a group with which one is associated, especially when referring to some process or procedure performed, as in *data were carefully analyzed*, or as in *patients were carefully examined*. One assumes that the work was carefully done. In any case, the word carries little content, since judgment regarding the amount of care exercised in some procedure or activity derives from the quality of the methods and procedures used in performing the procedure or activity, not from declaration. Further, its use in relation to one activity and not in regard to other equally important activities may have the effect of causing readers to assume that those activities were done with less care or even carelessly.

Cartesian *adj* - [NL *cartesianus*, fr *Cartesius* Descartes] Of or relating to the René Descartes or his philosophy.

Cartesian coordinate *n* - 1. Either of two **coordinates** that locate a point on a plane and **measure** its distance from either of two intersecting straight-line axes along a line **parallel** to the other **axis**. 2. Any of three coordinates that locate a point in space and measure its distance from any of three intersecting coordinate planes measured parallel to that one of three straight-line axes that is the intersection of the other two planes.

case *n* - [ME *cas*, fr OF, fr L *casus* fall, chance, fr *casus*, pp of *cadere*, to fall] 1. A circumstance or set of conditions. 2. A person who has the **disease** or condition of interest; a person with the disease of interest in a **case-control study**. 3. **incident case** 4. A person requiring medical or surgical care because of some disease, medical condition, injury, or the like. 5. **patient** 6. A person presenting with **symptoms** or **observed** in a circumstance that draws attention to some **incident** or **event** suspected of being related to or causing the symptoms. 7. An incident or event that is the subject of an **investigation**, eg, a group luncheon in relation to an outbreak of sore throats.

case finding *v* - Detection, by means of tests or other procedures, of the presence of a **disease** or health condition in persons not heretofore known to have that disease; **screening**.

case history *n* - 1. A collection of facts and observations concerning past conditions and **diseases**, health states, and environmental exposures of a **patient**, as compiled and assembled by a physician, physician's assistant, or some other medically qualified person; usually compiled in conjunction with a **workup** for **diagnosis** or **treatment** of some health condition or disease, or as a prelude to implementation of **preventive** procedures for a person at risk of some disease or **adverse** health condition, or as part of the **data collection** activities for a **re-**

search **project**. 2. The **document** containing such facts and **observations**.

case record *n* - 1. The collection of **records** and **documents** related to a **case**. 2. **medical record** 3. **case report**

case report *n* - 1. A series of facts and narrative statements, generally presented in written form, that describes a **case** (defn 6) and circumstances related to it; **case record** (defn 1). 2. A report of circumstances surrounding a case (defn 7). 3. **case report form**

case report form *n* - The collection of individual **data forms** related to a **case enrolled** into a **study**, especially when arranged in order of use and completed in totality before submission to the **center** or **sponsor** responsible for receiving such forms. syn: **case report**

case study *n* - An evaluation of a **case** or series of cases for the purpose of drawing conclusions regarding the **natural history** or etiology of a condition. See *study* for list.

case-cohort study *n* - 1. A **study** involving a **case-cohort study design**; usually a subpart of a larger **followup study**. 2. The use of techniques similar to those used in a **case-control study** for analysis of **data** from a **follovup study**; eg, see Prentice [1986][127] and Mantel [1973].[96] See *study* for list. syn: **nested case-control study**, synthetic case-control study, synthetic retrospective study

case-cohort study design *n* - A type of **followup study design** in which the generation, collection, or **analysis** of **data**, especially data for **covariate analyses** is restricted to a subset of individuals experiencing the **event** or **outcome** of interest (eg, breast cancer) and to a selected (usually random) subset of individuals free of that event or outcome; employed to reduce the cost or complexity of data collection or analysis associated with a conventional followup study. rt: **case-cohort study**

case-comparison study *n* - **case-control study**

case-compeer study *n* - **case-control study**

case-control *adj* - Of or relating to **cases** and **controls**; of or relating to a **comparison** of cases and controls in a **case-control study**.

case-control study *n* - 1. A **study** that involves the identification of persons with the **disease** or condition of interest (**cases**) and a group of persons free of the disease or condition of interest (**controls**) and in which cases and controls are compared with respect to some attribute or **exposure** believed or suspected of being causally related to that disease or condition (eg, see Schlesselman, 1982). 2. An **analysis** of existing **data**, eg, as collected from a **cohort study**, of the form and nature of that performed in a case-control study. syn (not recommended): case-comparison study, case-compeer study, **case-history study**, case-referent study, **retrospective study**, trohoc study[44] *Usage note*: See **retrospective study**.

case-control study design *n* - A type of **study design** involving the identification and **comparison** of **cases** and **controls**, as in a **case-control study**.

case-history *adj* - Of, related to, or concerned with a **case history**.

case-history study *n* - 1. A **study** based on information obtained from **case histories**; often done as a prelude to a more extensive **epidemiological study**. 2. **case-control study** See *study* for list.

case-referent study *n* - **case-control study**

catch, caught, catching, catches *v* - [ME *cacchen*, fr ONF *cachier* to hunt, fr (assumed) VL *captiare*, alter of L *captare* to chase, fr *captus*, pp of *capere* to take] 1. To capture or seize. 2. To become affected by.

catchment *n* - The action of catching or of gathering.

catchment area *n* - The geographical **area** or **region** served by an **institution**; in regard to **studies** involving **recruitment** of **study subjects**, the area or region from which they come or are recruited.

categorical *adj* - [LL categoricus, fr Gk katēgorikos, fr katēgoria] 1. Of, relating to, or involving a **category**. 2. certain; **absolute** (defn 2); unqualified

categorical data *n* - **Nonmetric data**, such as gender, race, or marital status, that indicate **class** or **category** but are not amenable to ordinary arithmetic operations. rt: **discrete data** See *data* for list.

categorical variable *n* - A **variable** that is used to indicate or identify **category** or **classification**.

categorization *n* - The act or process of arranging (persons, objects, numbers) into **categories** or **classes**; **classification**. rt: **classification**

categorize, categorized, categorizing, categorizes *v* - To put into **categories**; **classify**.

category *n* - [LL *categoria*, fr Gk *kategoria* predication, category, fr *kategorein*, to accuse, affirm, predicate] A division or **class** within a system of **classification**. rt: **class**

category matching *v* - [**epidemiology**] To cause two or more groups of **observation units** to correspond within the **limits** or **range** of some **category** or **classification**, eg, all having the same occupational classification, all residing within the same geographical area, or all being within the same decade of life. rt: **frequency matching, group matching, individual matching, pair matching**

cathode *n* - [Gk *kathodos* way down, fr *kata-* + *hodos* way] The electron-emitting electrode of an electron tube.

cathode ray *n* - A stream of electrons emitted from the **cathode** of a vacuum tube when heated and propelled by a strong electric field.

cathode ray tube (CRT) *n* - A vacuum tube in which **cathode rays** are projected onto a fluorescent screen to form images (such as those displayed on the screen of a **computer terminal**). rt: **video display terminal**

causal *adj* - Expressing or indicating **cause**; of, relating to, or constituting a cause; involving causation; arising from a cause.

causal relationship *n* - A **relationship** in which there is a known **effect** for a given **cause**; **cause and effect**. rt: **Henle-Koch's postulates** *Usage note*: See **cause and effect**.

causality *n* - A **relationship** between **cause and effect**; a relationship between regularly occurring events; **causal relationship**; **cause and effect** rt: **Henle-Koch's postulates** *Usage note*: See **cause and effect**.

cause *n* - [ME, fr OF, fr L *causa*] Something that produces or brings about an **effect** or a **result**.

cause and effect *n* - A linkage between a **cause** and its **effect**, eg, tubercle bacillus as the cause of tuberculosis, or hypertension as a cause of stroke. rt: **Henle-Koch's postulates** *Usage note*: Avoid as a statement or claim, except where the linkage is recognized as established, or where the user provides supporting **data** for its existence. See Last [1988][84] and Rothman [1988][133] for a discussion of **necessary and sufficient conditions** for claims of **causality**.

Used with varying degrees of rigor, depending on setting and user. For example, a microbiologist may restrict use to instances where **Henle-Koch's postulates** apply, whereas a physician or epidemiologist may use the term as a probabilistic expression of relationship in which there is evidence that presence of a **factor** is associated with an increased **incidence** of **disease** and absence of the factor is associated with a reduced incidence of the disease.

CBER *n* - **Center for Biologics Evaluation and Research**

CC *n* - **coordinating center**

CDC *n* - **Centers for Disease Control and Prevention**

CDER *n* - **Center for Drug Evaluation and Research**

CDRH *n* - **Center for Devices and Radiological Health**

cease, ceased, ceasing, ceases *v* - [ME *cesen*, fr MF *cesser*, fr L *cessare* to delay, fr *cessus*, pp of *cedere*] To cause to come to an end; to bring an activity or action to an end.

censor, censored, censoring, censors *v* - To delete, suppress, or eliminate. rt: **mask**

censored data *n* - 1. **Data** that are the result of **censored observations** or that have been censored. 2. Data that are subject to **censorship**.

censored followup observation *n* - 1. A **followup observation** subject to **censorship**. 2. Absence of followup observation (defn 1 or 2) because of censorship. 3. Inability to continue followup because of censorship; usually because of the existence or occurrence of some **event** or condition, such as death, **loss to followup**, or **withdrawal** (defn 1) precluding observation. rt: **censored observation, left censored observation, right censored observation**

censored observation *n* - 1. Absence of **observation** (defn 1) because of censorship. 2. An observation subject to **censorship**. 3. Inability to observe because of censorship; usually because of the existence or occurrence of some **event** or condition, such as death, **loss to followup**, or **withdrawal** (defn 1) precluding observation. rt: **left censored observation, right censored observation**

censoring condition *n* - 1. A condition (eg, termination of **followup**) or **event** (eg, death in an eye **study** with change in visual acuity as the

primary outcome) that makes it impossible to continue observing an **observation unit** for the **outcome**(s) of interest. 2. **censoring variable**

censoring variable *n* - A **variable** that represents the presence or absence of a **censoring condition**. See *variable* for list.

censorship *n* - The act or process of **censoring**.

census *n* - [L, fr *censēre*] 1. A complete (without **sampling**) enumeration, or one that is designed to be complete, of a **population**; the enumeration and related **data collection** typically performed by query using face-to-face or telephone interview, or mailed questionnaire and **followup** mailings, with or without direct contact of **nonrespondents**. 2. **count**, tally rt: **survey**

center *n* - [ME *centre*, fr MF, fr L *centrum*, fr Gk *kentron* sharp point, center of a circle, fr *kentein*, to prick; akin to OHG *hantag* pointed] [general] 1. The middle **point** or part, as in a **distribution**. 2. A point or focus around which things are organized. 3. The focus of attention or interest. 4. core 5. The source or focus of an influence, action, or force. 6. **study center** (defn 4) 7. A place, such as a **study clinic**, where **study candidates** and study **enrollees** are seen for evaluation and **treatment** in a trial; **study center** (defn 1). syn: **site** *Usage note*: In **multicenter trials**, often used in the sense of defn 7 to the exclusion of associated **resource centers**, as in the statement *the trial has 8 centers*, when in fact it has 12 centers, 8 of which are clinics and the other 4 of which are **resource centers**. Avoid such usage because of lack of precision and insensitivities to those in the resource centers of such trials. See **study center**, **investigator**, and **principal investigator** for added comments. Avoid by reserving the term, **center**, for uses in the collective sense of that term; use **study clinic** or some other appropriate term, such as **field site** or **data collection site**, in references to the subset of centers responsible for **data collection**.

center director *n* - 1. One who heads a **center**. 2. **study center director**

Center for Biologics Evaluation and Research (CBER) *n* - See **Food and Drug Administration**.

Center for Devices and Radiological Health (CDRH) *n* - See **Food and Drug Administration**.

Center for Drug Evaluation and Research (CDER) *n* - See **Food and Drug Administration**.

Center for Food Safety and Applied Nutrition (CFSAN) *n* - See **Food and Drug Administration**.

Center for Veterinary Medicine (CVM) *n* - See **Food and Drug Administration**.

Centers for Disease Control and Prevention (CDC) *n* - Part of the **United States Public Health Service** (USPHS) and located in Atlanta, Georgia. Responsibilities include investigation of outbreaks of infectious **diseases** and establishment and maintenance of reporting and surveillance procedures for various diseases.

centile *n* - A contiguous **range** of values that accounts for one one-hundredth of the **total counts** represented in a **frequency distribution**. See *quantile* for list.

central *adj* - [L *centralis*, fr *centrum* center] 1. Containing or constituting a **center**. 2. Of major or primary importance. 3. Situated near the center. 4. Holding to the middle or center between two extremes. 5. Controlling, directing, or performing local or branch activities. rt: **local**

central laboratory (CL) *n* - 1. A **study center** in the structure of a **multicenter study**, such as a **multicenter trial**, responsible for performing specified **tests** (defn 2) on specimens collected by participating **field centers** or **clinical centers** from people enrolled or considered for **enrollment** into the **study**; as distinct from **local laboratory** (defn 1). 2. A facility within an **institution**, such as a hospital, responsible for performing a variety of tests or analyses, as ordered by and received from staff of the various departments or units of the institution having access to its services. rt: **local laboratory** See *center* for list.

central limit theorem *n* - A general **theorem** in **probability** and **statistics** having to do with the conditions under which the **distribution** of the sum of n **independent random variables** (as **observed** from repeated **samplings** of a specified **population**) is ever more closely approximated by a specified **normal distribution** as n increases. For example, the theorem is the basis for the fact that the **sampling distribution** of the **means** of n independent observations, drawn from a population with finite **variance**, approaches a normal distribution as n increases.

central limit theorem of the mean *n* - A specific expression of the **central limit theorem** for the (arithmetic) **mean** that states that the **distribution** of the **mean** of a **variable** observed in **random samples** derived from a specified **population** with finite **variance** is approximated by a **normal distribution** as **n** becomes large.

central processing unit (CPU) *n* - The part of a **computer** that contains the electronic circuitry controlling the interpretation and execution of program instructions and that performs arithmetic and logical operations.

central repository *n* - A **repository** that is centrally (as opposed to locally) located; a place that serves as a repository for some aspect of a collective activity or collaborating group. In **multicenter** structures, an operational or administrative **unit** that is a repository for **documents** or specimens that are generated by units in that structure, eg, the **coordinating center** as the repository for **study forms** generated at **data collection sites** or a **central laboratory** responsible for receiving and storing blood samples collected from **study subjects** seen at **study clinics**. See **bank** and **repository** for usage notes.

central tendency measure *n* - A **measure**, such as the **mean**, **median**, or **mode**, serving to **estimate** the central **point** of a **distribution**. syn: measure of central tendency

centralize, centralized, centralizing, centralizes *v* - 1. To bring under a common control or administration. 2. To bring together around a **center** or common point.

centralized data analysis *n* - An arrangement in **multicenter** settings where all **data analyses** are carried out at a single **site**, eg, the **data coordinating center** in a **multicenter trial**. ant: **distributed data analysis** rt: **centralized data entry**

centralized data entry *n* - A form of **data entry** in which **data**, generated and recorded at different **sites** are sent to a **central** facility for conversion to machine-readable form by **coding** and **keying** for **storage** in a **database**. ant: **distributed data entry** rt: **centralized data analysis**

centralized data system *n* - A **data system** that is established and maintained at a central site (eg, the **data coordinating center**) in a **multicenter** structure; **site** is responsible for performing defined tasks in relation to maintaining that system. ant: **distributed data system**

centralized database *n* - A **database** residing and maintained at a **central** facility, eg, at the **data coordinating center** in a **multicenter trial**. ant: **distributed database**

centralized funding *n* - A method of funding **centers** in a **multicenter** structure in which funds are awarded to a **center** for **distribution** to other centers in the structure. ant: **distributed funding** rt: **consortium funding agreement**, **consortium funding award**

certificate *n* - [ME *certificat*, fr MF, fr ML *certificatum*, fr LL, neut of *certificatus*, pp of *certficare* to certify] A **document** containing a specified statement or **certification**, especially one attesting to the truth or veracity of something.

Certificate of Confidentiality *n* - A **certificate**, issued by the Secretary of **Health and Human Services** (or designees of the Secretary) having the purpose of protecting **study records** and **forms** from subpoena in criminal, civil, administrative, or legislative hearings at the federal, state, or local level. The protection provided is void to the extent waived in writing by a study subject. The protection does not preclude access to study records by the **Food and Drug Administration** in relation to **audits** or reviews performed by that **agency**. The protection provided is not time limited. It remains up to and beyond the time of death of individual research subjects. Certificates are granted only on request and then only when the applicant makes a case as to need (usually stated in terms of the likely negative impact on the degree of cooperation likely absent the protection provided with a certificate). Typically, issue is limited to research involving the collection of **data** on persons which, if revealed, could be embarrassing or in some way injurious to such persons. Use generally limited to studies involving study of aberrant or illegal behaviors or involving the collection of intimate information having to do with highly personal and private life styles.

certification *n* - 1. The act or process of **certifying**, eg, through exposure to defined training and completion of defined tasks. 2. The state of being certified.

certify, certified, certifying, certifies *v* - [ME *certifien*, fr MF *certifier*, fr LL *certificare*, fr L *certus*, certain] To attest to or confirm, as in meeting a specified **standard** or **norm**.

cessation *n* - [ME *cessacioun*, fr MF *cessation*, fr L *cessation-*, *cessatio*, delay, idleness, fr *cessatus*, pp of *cessare* to delay, be idle] A temporary or final **ceasing**; stop.

CFSAN *n* - **Center for Food Safety and Applied Nutrition**

chair *n* - [ME *chaiere*, fr OF, fr L *cathedra*, fr Gk *kathedra*, fr *kata- cata-* + *hedra* seat] 1. The presiding **officer** of a **group** or **organization**. 2. The head position in an organizational structure. syn: **chairperson** rt: **chairman, chairwoman, vice-chair** *Usage note*: Note that defn 1 refers to the person holding the position and that defn 2 refers to the position itself. **Chair** preferred for both usages because of emphasis on the position and neutrality regarding gender. See also usage notes for **chairman, chairperson,** and **chairwoman.**

chair of study *n* - **study chair**

chair's office (CO) *n* - The **office** of the **study chair**.

chairman *n* - 1. A male **chair**. 2. A male or female chair. rt: **chairperson, chairwoman, vice-chairman** *Usage note*: Not recommended; use **chair** (see usage note for **chair** for reason), except in the sense of defn 1, and then only when the corresponding term, **chairwoman**, is used when indicated. See also usage notes for **chairperson** and **chairwoman.**

chairperson *n* - **chair** rt: **chairman, vice-chairperson** *Usage note*: Acceptable, but cumbersome, gender-neutral term for **chair**. Avoid unbalanced use in which **chairperson** is used to designate position held by a female and **chairman** is used as the opposing term for reference to a position held by a male. See also usage notes for **chair, chairman,** and **chairwoman.**

chairwoman *n* - Female **chair**. rt: **chairman, vice-chairwoman** *Usage note*: Not recommended; use **chair** (see usage note for **chair** for reasons), except in opposition to **chairman** (defn 1). See also usage notes for **chair, chairman,** and **chairperson.**

chance *adj* - Of or relating to **chance**.

chance *n* - [ME, fr OF, fr (assumed) VL *cadentia* fall; fr L *cadent-*, *cadens*, prp of *cadere* to fall akin to Skt *śad* to fall] 1. Something that happens or is presumed to have happened without any apparent predictability or order. 2. The **probability** or **likelihood** of a designated **event** or **outcome**. rt: **lottery, random**

chance, chanced, chancing, chances *v* - To cause to come about or to happen by **chance**. rt: **randomization**

chance variable *n* - **random variable**

chance variation *n* - **random variation**

change *n* - 1. The act, process, or result of **changing**. 2. The value of some **variable** or **function** at one **point** in **time** subtracted from that at another point in time; **difference** (defn 2). rt: **net change**

change, changed, changing, changes *v* - [ME *changen*, fr OF *changier*, fr L *cambiare* to exchange, of Celt origin; akin to OIr *camm* crooked; akin to Gk *skambos* crooked] To make or become **different**; to undergo **transformation**, substitution, or transition; exchange.

changeover *n* - A conversion or transition to a different purpose, system, or function.

changeover design *n* - **crossover treatment design**

character *n* - [ME *caracter*, fr MF *caractère*, fr L *character* mark, distinctive quality, fr Gk *charakēr*, fr *charassein* to scratch, engrave] 1. A property, feature, attribute, **trait**, or quality that distinguishes a person, place, or thing. 2. A **graphic** symbol, such as a letter of an alphabet, used in writing or printing; **ASCII** character.

characteristic *adj* - Revealing, distinguishing, or typical of the individual **character**.

characteristic *n* - A distinguishing property, feature, attribute, **trait**, or quality.

chart *n* - [MF *charte*, fr L *charta* piece of papyrus, document] 1. A **document**, **page**, or sheet displaying information in tabular form; **graph**; **diagram**. 2. **patient chart**; **patient record**

check *n* - [ME *chek*, fr MF *eschec*, fr Ar *shah*, fr Per, lit, king; akin to Gk *ktasthai* to acquire, Skt *ksatra* dominion] 1. The act of testing or verifying. 2. Inspection or **investigation**. 3. A standard for testing or evaluation; criterion. rt: **criterion**

check, checked, checking, checks *v* - 1. To compare with some **standard**, source, or authority for **verification**. 2. To inspect for **errors** or deficiencies. 3. To mark with a check to indicate some action or condition. 4. To restrict, restrain, or stop.

check digit *n* - A **digit** that is affixed to a numeric identifier, eg, an **identification number**, typically the last digit of the identifier, that is used to identify recording or keying **errors**; done by comparing the value of the check digit, as computed for the identifier as issued, with the one computed for the identifier as recorded or keyed [Anderson et al, 1974;[3] Fellegi and Sunter, 1969;[45] Smythe, 1968;[145] Selmer, 1967[140]]. syn: self-checking digit

chi *n* - [Gk *chei*, chi] The 22nd letter of the **Greek alphabet**, uppercase X, lowercase χ.

chi-square, chi-squared *n* - 1. The symbol, X^2. 2. **chi-square test statistic** *Usage note*: May be written chi-square or chi-squared; chi-square preferred.

chi-square distribution *n* - A type of **probability density function** with **mean** equal to **degrees of freedom** (df) and **variance** equal to two times the number of degrees of freedom. Typically tabled or computed for small df (eg, 1 through 120) and approximated by the **normal distribution** for large df; distribution used to gauge the statistical likelihood of an **observed value** of the **chi-square test statistic**.

Chi-square distribution

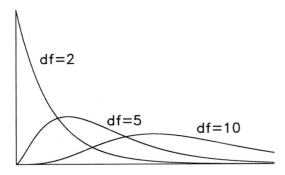

chi-square goodness-of-fit test *n* - A **goodness of fit test** based on the **chi-square distribution**. Due to **Karl Pearson** and used for assessing degree of discrepancy between **observed** and **expected counts** for a set of mutually exclusive **categories**; expected counts as derived or observed under a specified **hypothesis**.

chi-square test *n* - Any **statistical test** that produces a **test statistic** that is evaluated using a **chi-square distribution**.

chi-square test statistic *n* - A **test statistic**, consisting of the sum of two or more terms of the type, $(O - E)^2/E$, where E corresponds to an **expected** or hypothesized value and O to an observed value for a defined **class** or **category**. The statistic is used for comparing two or more **proportions** or for comparing an observed distribution to an expected or hypothesized one (**goodness of fit**). The value obtained is evaluated against a **chi-square distribution** with the specified **degrees of freedom** to provide an observed **p-value** for the test statistic.

child *n* - [ME, fr OE *cild*; akin to Goth *kilthei* womb, Skt *jathara* belly] 1. A person between infancy and adulthood. 2. A person between infancy and pubescence. 3. A person not yet at or beyond the **age of majority**.

chronic *adj* - [F *chronique*, fr Gk *chronikos* of time, fr *chronos*] Marked by long duration or repeated occurrences. ant: **acute**

chronic disease *n* - A **disease** that lasts a long time; incurable disease. ant: **acute disease**

chronic study *n* - 1. A **study** involving the **collection**, **analysis**, or interpretation of slowly changing **data**. 2. A **study** involving **long-term treatment** and **followup**. 3. A study involving **long-term followup**. syn: **long-term study** ant: **acute study**

circadian *adj* - [L *circa* about + *dies* day + E *-an*] Having the approximate property of occurring in a **daily** (24-hour) **period** or cycle. rt: **diurnal** *Usage note*: Limit usage to settings in which the period or cycle is or is presumed to be 24-hours.

circadian rhythm *n* - A **rhythm** or cycle that has a 24-hour period. *Usage note*: See **circadian**.

circadian variation *n* - **Variation** that is due to or associated with **time** of **day** (24-hours). rt: **diurnal variation** *Usage note*: See **circadian**.

circle *n* - [often attrib ME *cercle*, fr OF, fr L *circulus*, dim of *circus* circle, circus, fr or akin to Gk *krikos*, *kirkos* ring; akin to OE *hiring* ring] A closed plane **curve**, every point of which is equidistant from a fixed point within the curve; the plane surface bound by such a curve.

circle graph *n* - A method of **data** display in which portions of a **circle**, defined by radii, correspond to **frequencies**, **relative frequencies**, or **proportions** of the whole. See *graphic display* for list. syn: circular graph, pie chart

Circle graph

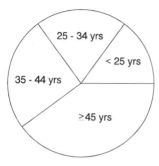

circuit *n* - [ME, fr MF *circuite*, fr L *circuitus*, fr pp of *circumire*, *circuire* to go around, fr *circum-* + *ire* to go] A route traveled or to be traveled, especially one encompassing a number of stops or stations.

circuit rider *n* - One who travels a **circuit**. In the setting of **multicenter trials**, typically a person from the **treatment coordinating center**, **data center**, **data coordinating center**, or **coordinating center** responsible for visiting participating **clinical centers** on a regular basis to **monitor**, **audit**, and trouble-shoot. rt: **study clinic monitor**, **clinical research associate**, **study clinic monitor**

circular *adj* - [ME *circuler*, fr MF, fr LL *circularis*, fr L *cirulus* circle] Having the form of a **circle**.

circular graph *n* - **circle graph**

citation *n* - 1. An act of quoting or referring to previous work, studies, or cases of one's own or of others. 2. **reference citation**

citation bias *n* - **reference bias**

cite, cited, citing, cites *v* - [MF *citer* to cite, summon, fr L *citare* to put in motion, rouse, summon, fr *citus*, pp of *ciēre*, to stir, move] 1. To quote by way of example, authority, or proof. 2. To refer to. 3. To bring forward or call to another's attention.

CL *n* - **central laboratory**

claim, claimed *n* - An assertion open to challenge; something asserted.

claim, claimed, claiming, claims *v* - [ME *claimen*, fr MF *clamer*, fr L *clamare* to cry out, shout; akin to L *calare* to call] To assert in the face of possible contradiction.

class *n* - [F *classe*, fr L *classis*, group called to arms, class of citizens; akin to L *calare* to call]

1. A **group** or set of persons or objects sharing a common **attribute** or **characteristic**. 2. The set of values represented in a **class interval**; the group represented in a class interval. syn: **category**

class frequency *n* - The **frequency** associated with a given **class**.

class interval *n* - The **interval** or **range** of values represented in a **class** of a **frequency distribution**; defined by the **difference** between the upper and lower values of the class.

classification *n* - 1. The act or process of arranging (persons, objects, numbers) into **classes** or **categories**; **categorization**. 2. A particular class or category. rt: **categorization**, **stratification**

classify, classifying, classified, classifies *v* - To arrange into or to assign (persons, objects, numbers) to **classes**.

clean *adj* - [ME *clene*, fr OE *clæne*; akin to OHG *kleini* delicate, dainty, Gk *glainoi* ornaments] **Free** or relatively free of imperfections or **errors**; not **dirty**. ant: **dirty**

clean data *n* - **Data** that have been subjected to **edit queries** and **editing** to reduce or resolve noted deficiencies due to missing information, **errors**, or inconsistencies. ant: **dirty data**

clearance *n* - [**medicine**] The process of eliminating a substance (eg, albumin, urea, or a **tracer substance**) from a biological organism or system, such as the human body; especially via excretory organs.

clearance rate *n* - [**medicine**] A **measure** of the speed at which an ingested or administered substance, such as a **drug**, is eliminated from a biological organism or system, such as the human body.

clearance study *n* - [**medicine**] A **study** designed to **estimate** the **rate** at which a substance is metabolized or excreted from some biological organism or system, such as the human body; characterized by the collection of **baseline data** for designated **measures** on the **observation units** followed by ingestion or administration of some substance, such as a **drug**, to those units and then a series of timed **observations** for those same measures to **estimate** rate of clearance. See *study* for list.

clinic *n* - [F *cliniquē*, fr Gk *klinike*, medical practice and pertaining to sick bed, fr fem of *klinikos* of a bed, fr *klinē* bed fr *klinein*] 1. A place where medical **care** is provided to ambulatory (nonresident) **patients**. 2. The instruction of medical students through **observation** of and participation in the **examination** and care of patients. 3. An assembly of students for such instruction. 4. A place of instruction for medical students. 5. **study clinic**

clinic coordinator *n* - 1. **study clinic coordinator** 2. **data coordinator** See *position* for list.

clinic director *n* - 1. The head of a **clinic**. 2. **study clinic director** See *position* for list.

clinic monitor *n* - **study clinic monitor**

clinic personnel *n* - 1. **Personnel** employed in a **clinic**. 2. **study clinic personnel**

clinic preference treatment design *n* - A **preference treatment design** in **multicenter trials** in which individual **clinics** are allowed to exercise a **preference** as to the **treatments** to be administered in the trial in that clinic, eg, one in which a clinic decides whether the **control treatment** to be used is **active** or **inactive**.

clinic visit *n* - 1. A **visit** that takes place at a **clinic**. 2. **study clinic visit** 3. **patient clinic visit**

clinical *adj* - 1. Relating to a **clinic** or sickbed. 2. Relating to care rendered at a clinic. 3. Relating to the **symptoms** or course of **disease**. 4. Relating to **observation**, impression, and opinion derived from experience; especially in relation to caring for **patients**. rt: **preclinical** *Usage note*: Often used simply to underscore or emphasize a setting or framework for an activity or observation. Frequently redundant or unnecessary, especially in contexts in which, without the modifier, it is clear that the reference is to a "clinical" setting. See also usage note for **clinical trial**.

clinical alert *n* - 1. An **alert** informing or forewarning of potential problems in relation to some **treatment** or procedure. 2. An alert based on **results** of a **study** or **trial** and mailed to pertinent members of the health care profession by a government agency, such as the **National Institutes of Health**.

clinical center *n* - 1. **clinic** 2. A **center** in the organizational structure of a **study**, such as a **multicenter clinical trial**, that is responsible for the **recruitment, enrollment, followup,** or **treatment** of **patients** and related **examinations** and **data collection** procedures as required in a

specified **study**; **study clinic**. See *center* for list.

clinical coordinating center *n* - 1. A **center** in a **multicenter clinical trial** that is responsible for addressing issues and questions relating to care of **patients** enrolled in a trial. Usually present only in **multicenter** trials involving seriously ill patients and complicated **treatment protocols**. 2. **treatment coordinating center** See also **coordinating center** and **data coordinating center**.

clinical disease *n* - **Disease** that is identifiable by characteristic **signs** and **symptoms**.

clinical epidemiologist *n* - 1. One trained in or engaged in the practice of **clinical epidemiology**. 2. A physician specializing in **clinical epidemiology**.

clinical epidemiology *n* - A subspecialty of **epidemiology** concerned primarily with **clinical disease**. rt: **descriptive epidemiology, experimental epidemiology**

clinical event *n* - An **event** (defn 1), in relation to one's state of health, that is considered to have **negative** or **adverse** implications (eg, diagnosis of cancer, hospitalization for a myocardial infarction, initiation of treatment for hypertension).

clinical investigation *n* - An **investigation** involving people having, or suspected of having, a **disease** (or related health condition) and in which physicians have a major role in diagnosing that disease (or related health condition) and for examining and treating those with the condition. rt: **clinical research**

clinical investigator *n* - One who carries out **investigations** on people in a **clinical** setting. *Usage note*: See **investigator**.

clinical monitor *n* - 1. One who **monitors patients** in a **clinical** setting. 2. **study clinic monitor**

clinical research *n* - 1. **Research** involving people having or suspected of having **clinical disease**. 2. **clinical investigation**

clinical research associate *n* - A person, usually in the employ of a **drug firm**, having responsibility for monitoring **data collection** in **trials**. syn: **study clinic monitor**, medical research associate rt: **circuit rider**

clinical significance *n* - A finding or **observation** considered to have relevance in determining the future course or prognosis of a specific **disease**

or related health condition; sometimes used in contradistinction to **statistical significance**.

clinical study *n* - 1. A **study** carried out in a **clinic** or hospital. 2. **clinical investigation** See *study* for list.

clinical trial *n* - 1. A **controlled experiment** (defn 1) having a **clinical event** as an **outcome measure** and done in a **clinic** or clinical setting and involving persons having a specific **disease** or health condition. 2. A controlled experiment involving the administration of different **study treatments** in a **parallel treatment design** to a defined set of **study subjects** having a given **disease** or related health condition and done to evaluate the **efficacy** and **safety** of a **test treatment** in ameliorating or curing that disease or related health condition; any such experiment, including those involving healthy people, undertaken to assess efficacy or safety of a treatment (eg, usefulness of **monitoring** fetal heart rate on pregnancy outcome; usefulness of different dietary schemes in the prevention of hypertension). 3. A controlled experiment involving human beings as **study subjects** (defn 1) and designed to have or having **clinical significance** or relevance. 4. An **uncontrolled trial** involving **treatment** and **followup** of people given a particular treatment. 5. (**MEDLINE** definition) preplanned, usually controlled, clinical study of the safety, efficacy, or optimum dosage schedule of one or more diagnostic, therapeutic, or prophylactic drugs, devices, or techniques in humans selected according to predetermined criteria of eligibility and observed for predefined evidence of favorable and unfavorable effects. 6. The first use(s) of a new treatment in human beings. rt: **crossover trial, natural experiment, n of 1 trial** *Usage note*: Subject to wide and varying usage; may refer to either a **controlled** or an **uncontrolled trial**. The term may be used for trials with either a **parallel** or **crossover treatment design**. Typically, however, the modifier, **crossover**, replaces the modifier, **clinical**, in uses related to **crossover trials**. Also, typically, the modifier, **clinical**, is reserved for experiments carried out in clinical settings involving clinical **disease** (see **clinic** for etymology). However, usage has been extended to include **prevention trials** and sometimes even **community trials** when they address health conditions or practices considered to have medical importance. The modifier, **clinical**, may be dropped in most

settings, except those in which there is a need to remind readers of the setting for the trial, or to avoid confusion with other types of trials (eg, court trials). Usage of the term, **clinical trial**, or more simply, **trial**, without other modifiers, should be limited to settings in which usage is consistent with the sense of defns 1, 2, or 3 and even then uses of modifiers, such as **randomized** or **controlled**, serving to make clear the conditions of usage, are advised for the first use of the term in a discourse. Most references herein are to **trials** as opposed to **clinical trials**. See page xx (*Language and usage conventions*) for additional comments. See *trial* for list.

clinically meaningful difference *n* - 1. An **observed difference** between two groups of **patients** considered to have medical importance. 2. An observed **treatment difference** considered to have medical importance. rt: **meaningful difference**

clinically significant *n* - A finding or **observation** that is considered to be important to the health of a person or group of persons.

close *adj* - [ME *clos*, fr MF, fr L *clausus*, pp of *claudere* to shut, close; akin to Gk *kleiein* to close, OHG *sliozan*, OE *hlot* lot] 1. Not **open**; closed. 2. ended 3. Having a limit or **boundary**, as in **closed sequential design**.

close, closed, closing, closes *v* - [ME *closen*, fr OF *clos-*, stem of *clore*, fr L *claudere*] 1. To cease or suspend operations. 2. To deny or limit access to; exclude. 3. To bring to an end; a coming or bringing to a conclusion or end.

close of trial *n* - 1. The point at which **treatment** (as dictated under the **treatment protocol**), **scheduled followup**, and **data collection** end — typically marked by completion of the **close-out stage** of the **trial**. 2. The **point** at which treatment is stopped or suspended in a trial (not recommended usage). 3. The point at which all activities related to the trial, including **data analysis**, end — typically marked by completion of the **termination stage** of the trial. 4. Termination of the **enrollment phase**. 5. Termination of funding for the trial. *Usage note*: Phrase subject to ambiguities, especially in settings in which **study treatments** are administered only once on **enrollment** or shortly thereafter and in which those so enrolled and treated are then simply followed for **outcomes** of interest. In one sense, in this setting, the trial is ended as soon as the last person enrolled has been treated, even though **followup** may continue for years thereafter. Usage should be restricted to settings in which all patient-related activities are terminated, including **scheduled followup visits** and related data collection. Avoid use in settings in which only specific activities or functions are terminated, such as enrollment but not followup; be specific in such settings about what has ended and what continues.

close out *v* - To cease or terminate some procedure or operation, such as **data collection** in relation to **patient close-out** in a **trial**

close-out *n* - 1. The process of ceasing operations or of terminating an activity or working relationship. 2. **patient close-out**

close-out examination *n* - An **examination** performed on separation of a person from a **study**; **patient close-out examination**

close-out followup visit *n* - A **followup visit** performed in relation to **close-out**; **patient close-out followup visit**. rt: **close-out examination**

close-out stage *n* - [trials] A **stage of trial** in which persons **enrolled** are separated from the trial in preparation for the **termination stage**; typically starts with the first such separation and ends with the last; **patient close-out stage of trial**.

closed class interval *n* - A **class interval** with both an upper and lower **end point**; not an **open class interval**.

closed randomization *n* - **masked randomization**

closed sequential design *n* - [trials] A **sequential design** with a **closed** (truncated) **region** defined by diverging boundary lines (upper and lower) positioned about the **x-axis** and extending to the right from the **y-axis** to points of intersection with lines extending from the x-axis; region defined by the y-axis and specified boundary lines referred to as region of indecision; considered closed because of boundary lines extending from x-axis; closed in order to impose an upper limit on the number of **observations** needed for a decision. An **observed treatment difference** that lies above the upper or below the lower boundary line favors an **alternative treatment hypothesis** in which the **test treatment** is considered to be superior or inferior (depending on the boundary crossed) to the **control treatment**. An observed difference lying to the right of boundary lines rising from the x-axis corre-

sponds to a result considered to favor the **null hypothesis**. Boundary lines extending from the x-axis do not exist for **open sequential designs**.

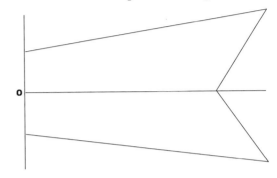

Closed sequential design

closed sequential trial *n* - A **trial** with a **closed sequential design**. See *trial* for list.

closed treatment assignment *n* - **masked treatment assignment**

cluster *n* - [ME, fr OE *clyster*; akin to OE *clott*, clot] 1. A **number** of similar things or persons collected, grouped, or found together. 2. An apparent concentration of people in a defined area or defined group of people having or having had a **disease** or an **adverse event** or **outcome** identified fortuitously or through systematic **analysis**. *Usage note*: Use with caution in the sense of defn 2 in a declarative fashion. When used in the sense of defn 2, provide comparative data from other areas involving similar **populations** and statistical arguments and **p-values** supporting the notion that the concentration is not a **chance event**. Keep in mind that conventional rules for interpretation of **tests of significance** and p-values do not apply, since the concentration was identified by fortuitous means or via **data dredging**. (Not to be confused with **subgroup**. Most usages of this term are in relation to a defined **denominator**.) As a rule, the actual denominator or **population base** for a cluster, as used in the sense of defn 1, is not explicitly defined or known. It is usually defined indirectly and only in rough terms, such as by the estimated population size of a defined geographical or political region or subdivision.

cluster randomization *n* - **group randomization**

cluster sample *n* - A **sample** in which the **sampling unit** is, or is to be, comprised of an aggregate of elements having a common characteristic (eg, all members of the same household, all people over age 18 residing in a defined region). rt: **cluster sampling**

cluster sampling *n* - A **method** of **sampling** in which the **sampling unit** is an aggregate (cluster) of elements defined by some common characteristic (eg, all members of the same household; all people over age 18 residing in a defined region). rt: **cluster sample**

cluster treatment assignment *n* - **group treatment assignment**

co- *prefix* - [ME, fr L, fr *com-*; akin to OE *ge-*, perfective and collective prefix, Gk *koinos* common] 1. In or of the same degree; with, together, **joint**, or jointly, as in **co-variance**. 2. One that is associated in action with another, **co-investigator**; one with such an **association** but having a lesser share of responsibility or authority such as a deputy or alternate. *Usage note*: Avoid when contradictory or incompatible with the term to which it is affixed, eg, **co-principal investigators** or co-primary investigators. Principal and primary connote being first; it is not possible for two persons or things to both be first.

CO *n* - **chair's office**

co-investigator *n* - Broadly, one who works with another in an **investigation**. In **research**, usually a **peer** but subordinate to the **principal investigator**.

co-principal *n* - 1. One who is second in line to the person designated as or considered to be principal, eg, a **co-principal investigator**. 2. One having the same importance or standing as another in relation to heading or directing some activity; eg, a **co-principal investigator**. *Usage note*: Avoid because of different meanings as represented by defns 1 and 2 and contradictory connotations as discussed in the usage note for **co-**.

co-principal investigator *n* - 1. One of two persons who share equally the duties and responsibilities of **principal investigator**. 2. One who is a **peer** of the principal investigator and who is designated to or who assumes the duties and responsibilities of the principal investigator in the absence or incapacitation of that person. 3. **co-investigator** *Usage note*: Avoid because of

contradictory connotations as discussed in the usage note for **co-**.

co-worker *n* - 1. One who works with another. 2. A member of the **investigative group** of a **study**.

code *n* - [ME, fr MF, fr L *caudex*, *codex*, trunk of a tree, tablet of wood covered with wax for writing on, book; akin to L *cudere* to beat] A signal or **symbol** used for communication or transmission of information.

code, coded, coding, codes *v* - To **transform** into **code** by use of a signal or **symbol**.

coefficient *n* - [NL *coefficient-*, *coefficiens*, fr L *co-* + *efficient-*, *efficiens* efficient] 1. Any of the numerical **constant** multipliers in an algebraic term or expression (eg, 2 in the term 2y or 0.4 and 1.2 in the expression $0.4x_1 + 1.2x_2$). 2. A number that serves as a **measure** of some property, **characteristic**, or **relationship**, as with a coefficient in a **regression model**.

coefficient of association *n* - A **measure** of **relationship** for **grouped data** arranged in a two-by-two **contingency table**; ranges from -1 for perfect **negative** relationship to +1 for perfect **positive** relationship.

coefficient of variation (CoV) *n* - The **ratio** of the **standard deviation** to the **mean** of a set of **data**, sometimes multiplied by 100 to express as a **percentage**.

cohort *n* - [MF and L; MF *cohorte*, fr L *cohort-*, *cohors*, enclosed yard, company of soldiers, multitude; one-tenth part of an ancient Roman legion] 1. A **group** of persons all having the same **factor**, **characteristic**, or trait (eg, the same age, **gender**, or **ethic origin**). 2. **followup cohort** rt: **birth cohort**, **subgroup** *Usage note*: Most usages in **trials** and **epidemiology** are in the sense of defn 2 in that the focus is on what happens or has happened to the cohort.

cohort analysis *n* - **Analysis** performed on a **cohort**; especially one performed as a means of **controlling** for some **variable** (eg, by restricting the analysis to the cohort of people enrolled before a **protocol** change in a **trial** to eliminate the change as a source of variation) or one to determine whether or not there is a **cohort effect**. *Usage note*: Note difference between this form of analysis and **cross-sectional analysis**, even in cases where results are presented over time, as in **followup studies**. For example, a plot of the **mean** of some **variable** (eg, fasting blood glucose, as reported by the University Group Diabetes Program Research Group [1970b][157]) over time in a trial for the two forms of analysis may look the same even though done differently and based on different datasets. For example, the cohort may be defined as those having had a specified number of years of followup and having been observed at each of the specified **data collection** time points over that **time period** (as done in the reference cited above). The plot for the cross-sectional analysis will be based on data available at each of the time points over the period of interest, regardless of representation at the other time points in the plot. In the former approach, the analysis is constrained to represent the same people at each of the time points. In the latter approach, even in instances where the **n** at designated time points is the same, the people represented may be different. Typically, the two types of analyses in trials yield similar results. Exceptions being instances (rare) in which there is a time related **cohort effect**.

cohort effect *n* - An **effect** due to, or attributed to, some **cohort** or cohort phenomenon, eg, a change in the **event rate** in a **trial** due to a change in the population enrolled over time. rt: **generation effect** *Usage note*: Use with caution, even in the speculative sense and especially in the declarative sense. If used in a declarative fashion, support with appropriate statistical arguments and temper with the conservatism needed for interpreting **p-values** arising from **tests of significance** suggested by **data dredging**; or identify the **trait**, **characteristic**, or constellation of traits and characteristics, that define the cohort. Note also that existence of a **cohort effect** in a trial is irrelevant in regard to **treatment comparisons** of interest, except where the effect is differential by **treatment group** (rare).

cohort study *n* - 1. A **followup study** of a defined **cohort**. 2. **followup study** See *study* for list. *Usage note*: All **trials**, by definition, involve a defined **cohort** and in this general sense are, therefore, members of this larger class of studies. However, the term is best reserved for the subset excluding trials to avoid confusing studies that are **observational** in nature with those that are **experimental**. See **followup study** for additional comment.

coin *n* - [ME, fr MF, wedge, coner, fr L *cuneus* wedge] A flat, thin, and usually round, metal object having opposing and differing faces (eg, a "Lincoln" penny with the face of Lincoln on one side and the Lincoln Memorial on the other side).

collaborate, collaborated, collaborating, collaborates *v* - [LL *collaboratus*, pp of *collaborare* to labor together, fr L *com-* + *laborare* to labor] To work jointly with others, especially in relation to intellectual endeavor.

collaborative *adj* - Characterization applied to work performed in concert with others, especially in relation to work requiring intellectual input. syn: **cooperative** rt: **multidisciplinary**, **multicenter** *Usage note*: Not recommended as a synonym for **multicenter** for reasons indicated in usage notes for **collaborative study** and **collaborative trial**.

collaborative group *n* - A **group** of people collaborating to achieve a common end, such as the design and conduct of a **study**.

collaborative study *n* - 1. A **study** involving two or more **data collection** sites; **multicenter study** (preferred term). 2. A study involving two or more **centers**; multicenter study (preferred term). 3. A study involving two or more **investigators**. See *study* for list. syn: **cooperative study** rt: **multicenter study** *Usage note*: Avoid because of ambiguous uninformative nature. Most studies involve collaboration of one form or another and, hence, the modifier, **collaborative**, is often unnecessary. Use other more informative modifiers, such as **multicenter** or **multidisciplinary**, depending on emphasis.

collaborative trial *n* - 1. A **trial** involving two or more **clinics**; **multicenter trial** (preferred term). 2. A trial involving two or more **centers**; multicenter trial (preferred term). 3. A trial involving two or more **investigators**. See *trial* for list. syn: **cooperative trial** rt: **multicenter trial** *Usage note*: Avoid because of ambiguous uninformative nature. Most trials, even small ones carried out in a single center, require collaboration of various forms and types. Use other more informative adjectives to characterize nature or form of collaboration, such as **multidisciplinary** or **multicenter**.

collect, collected, collecting, collects *v* - [L *collectus*, pp of *colligere* to collect, fr *com-* + *legere* to gather] To bring together into one place; to gather or exact from a number of persons or sources.

collection *n* - 1. The act or process of **collecting**. 2. Something collected, such as **data**, for **analysis** or **comparison**.

collection site *n* - 1. The **site** at which a **collection** is made, eg, blood for laboratory tests. 2. **data collection site**

collector *n* - One who **collects**.

column *n* - [ME *columne*, fr MF *colmne*, fr L *columna*, fr *columen* top; akin to L *collis* hill] 1. A vertical arrangement of items written printed on a page; such an arrangement as displayed electronically on a **video screen** of a **computer**. 2. One of two or more vertical sections of a printed page separated by a rule or blank space. rt: **row**

combination *n* - 1. A selection, **collection**, or arrangement of distinct entities without regard to order. 2. An ordered sequence or arrangement, eg, of letters or **numbers**. 3. The result or act of combining.

combine, combined, combining, combines *v* - [ME *combinen*, fr MF *combiner*, fr LL *combinare*, fr L com- + *bini* two by two] 1. To merge into one so as to lose or obscure individual **characteristics**; to unite into a single **number** or expression. 2. Intermix or blend.

combined modality *n* - [**medicine**] The combined use of different forms of **treatment** for a particular condition (eg, radiation therapy following surgery for breast cancer).

combined modality trial *n* - A **trial** involving use of two or more modes of **treatment** on the same person (eg, surgery and **drugs**). See *trial* for list.

committee *n* - A **group** of persons with responsibility for performing a designated function or set of functions on behalf of a larger body of people, group, or **agency**. See *committee* for list. syn: **board** (in some contexts)

common *adj* - [ME *commun*, fr OF, fr L *communis*] Same or similar to all.

common closing date *n* - [**trials**] 1. A **date** for the close of **followup** that is the same for all persons **enrolled**, as in a **common date patient close-out**. 2. A date common to all **sites** in a **multicenter trial** for ceasing or closing some function or activity, eg, the use of the same date

for **cessation** of **enrollment** regardless of when a clinic entered a trial.

common date patient close-out *n* - [**trials**] A method of **patient close-out** in which **patients** are separated from a trial on or about the same calendar date, regardless of when they were **enrolled**. Roughly equivalent to **common followup period patient close-out** when **enrollment** has occurred within a short period of time. rt: **common followup period patient close-out**

common followup period patient close-out *n* - [**trials**] A method of **patient close-out** in which **patients** are separated from a trial after a specified period of **followup** (eg, after two years). Roughly equivalent to **common date patient close-out** when **enrollment** has occurred within a short period of time. syn: anniversary close-out rt: **common date patient close-out**

community *n* - [ME *comunete*, fr MF *comunete'*, fr L *communitat-*, *communitas*, fr *communis*] 1. A **group** of people residing in a defined locale. 2. A group of people residing in a defined locale and served by a common government and having, in a broad sense, common heritage, interest, or culture. 3. The **area** in which such a group resides. 4. A social group sharing common **characteristics** or interest and perceived or perceiving itself as distinct in some respect from the larger society of which it is part.

community trial *n* - 1. An **experiment** involving two or more communities and having **community** (defns 1 or 2) as the **treatment unit**. 2. A **trial** carried out in a community (as opposed to a **clinic**) setting. 3. **field trial** rt: **demonstration trial** See *trial* for list. *Usage note*: Subject to varying usage. Avoid in the sense of defn 2; use **field trial**.

company *n* - [ME *companie*, fr OF *compagnie*, fr *compain* companion, fr LL *companio*] A **business** enterprise or firm; a business or firm engaged in trade or manufacture. rt: **drug company, industry**

comparability *n* - The state of being similar or **comparable**.

comparable *adj* - The state of being equal or similar or of being suitable for **comparison**.

comparative *adj* - Characterized by **comparison**.

comparative study *n* - Any of a class of **studies**, including **controlled trials**, involving two or more groups of people chosen or arranged so as to provide a basis for **comparison** of the **variable**(s) of interest. See *study* for list.

comparative trial *n* - 1. **controlled trial** 2. Any **trial** involving two or more **treatment groups**. See *trial* for list.

compare, compared, comparing, compares *v* - [ME *comparen*, fr MF *compares*, fr L *comparare*, to couple, compare, fr *compar*, like, fr *com-* + *par*, equal] 1. To **examine** or **analyze** to identify similarities and differences among different individuals, items, or objects. 2. To position two or more groups, items, or objects so as to be able to perform a **comparison** using some statistical procedure.

comparison *n* - [ME, fr MF *comparasion*, fr L *comparation-*, *comparatio*, fr *compartatus*, pp of *comparare*] 1. The act or process of **comparing**. 2. An **examination** or **analysis** of two or more individuals, items, or objects for the purpose of identifying similarities and differences. 3. An **observed difference** or **observed treatment difference**; **contrast**.

comparison group *n* - A **group** of **observational** or **experimental units**, designated in the **study design** or arbitrarily chosen, that was or is to be used as a basis for **comparisons** with other groups in the **study**; typically the **control-treated group** in a **controlled trial**. rt: **reference group**

comparison treatment *n* - The **treatment** against which others are evaluated or **measured**; typically the **control treatment** in **controlled trials**. rt: **standard treatment**

compassionate use *n* - Use of a **drug**, still controlled under **Investigational New Drug Applications** (INDs), on **patients** and under circumstances not provided for in the INDs. Permission for such use is granted by the FDA and is generally limited to cases of terminal illness, eg, patients in the terminal phase of acquired immune deficiency syndrome. rt: **emergency use, expanded availability**

compeer *n* - [modif of L *compar*, fr *compar*, adj like] 1. A person of equal **rank** or status; equal; **peer**. 2. A comrade, companion, or associate.

competence *n* - The quality or state of being **competent**.

competence, principle of *n* - A **principle** in **medical ethics** that asserts that the care and **treatment** performed or offered in a **research** setting involving human beings must be offered in a **competent** fashion, consistent with accepted standards of care [Levine, 1986].[88] See also **medical ethics, principles of**.

competent *adj* - [ME suitable, fr MF & L; MF, fr L *competent-*, *competens*, fr prp of *competere*] Having requisite and adequate abilities or qualities to perform within accepted **standards**.

competing risk *n* - A **risk** for an **outcome** that is not the focus of **study** that influences the risk of outcome of one that is the focus of study (eg, the risk of a person dying from cancer before the development of heart disease in a cardiovascular study).

complete *adj* - [ME *complet*, fr MF, fr L *completus*, fr pp of *complēre*] Having all the necessary parts or steps; full; finished. *Usage note*: Use with caution in scientific writing, especially in the absence of accompanying defining detail. Subject to ambiguities of meaning when the notion of completion or concept of completeness has different meanings or interpretation depending on perspective. See also notes for **complete** *v* and **completely**.

complete, completed, completing, completes *v* - 1. To bring to an end in a finished state. 2. To make whole or perfect. 3. To mark the end of. *Usage note*: Use with caution in scientific writing, especially in the absence of defining detail. May be subject to ambiguities of meaning when the notion of completion or completeness has different meanings, as in the *trial was completed*; complete in the sense of **enrollment**, in the sense of **treatment**, in the sense of **followup**, or in the sense of finished or done. See also notes for **complete** and **completely**

complete block *n* - 1. A **block** in which all **treatments** or levels of a **factor** or **variable** represented in an **experimental design** appear or are to appear the same **number** of times. 2. A block in which all treatments or levels of a factor or variable represented in the design appear or are to appear at least once and in the **proportion** or **ratio** to one another specified in the design. ant: **incomplete block**

complete block design *n* - An **experimental design** involving **complete blocks**.

complete block treatment design *n* - [trials] A **treatment design** involving use of **complete blocks** in the **treatment assignment design**. rt: **incomplete block treatment design**

complete crossover *n* - **complete treatment crossover**

complete crossover treatment design *n* - 1. A **crossover treatment design** that provides for **administration** of all of the **study treatments** to the **experimental units** (eg, **patients**) in the **trial**. 2. A crossover treatment design in which each of the individual **experimental units** receive all of the treatments represented in the design. rt: **incomplete crossover treatment design**

complete factorial *n* - 1. A **factorial design** or **factorial experiment** in which each **factor**, condition, or **treatment** appears or is administered in combination with every other factor, condition, or treatment represented in the design or experiment; eg, the combinations A$\bar{\text{B}}$, AB, $\bar{\text{A}}$B, and $\bar{\text{A}}\bar{\text{B}}$ in a **parallel trial** involving the **test treatments**, A and B, and **matching placebos**, $\bar{\text{A}}$ and $\bar{\text{B}}$. 2. A design or experiment in which a specified subset of the factors, conditions, or treatments represented appear or are administered in combination with every other factor, condition, or treatment within that subset; eg, the treatment combinations represented above as part of a larger set involving a third treatment, C, not used in combination with A or B or their matching placebos. syn: full factorial ant: **incomplete factorial** rt: **nonfactorial**

complete factorial treatment design *n* - A type of **parallel treatment design** in which each **study treatment** is represented in combination with every other study treatment, eg, a **double-masked placebo-controlled** design involving **drugs** A and B and four **treatment groups**: A$\bar{\text{B}}$, AB, B$\bar{\text{A}}$, and $\bar{\text{A}}\bar{\text{B}}$, where $\bar{\text{A}}$ and $\bar{\text{B}}$ correspond to **placebo treatments** matching drugs A and B, respectively. The treatments may involve different **drugs**, procedures, or levels of doses of the same treatment. syn: full factorial treatment design rt: **incomplete factorial treatment design**

complete mask *n* - [trials] 1. A **mask** in which all members of a designated **class** or **category** of people associated with a trial (eg, **patients**, **treaters**, **data collectors**, **readers**, or **monitors**) are **masked** to **treatment assignment** and **administration**. 2. A mask in relation to treatment assignment and administration imposed on patients and all study personnel having patient contact, as in a **double-mask trial**; such a mask

applying as well to all personnel responsible for **treatments effects monitoring**, as in a **triple-mask trial**. rt: **nonmask, partial mask, masking level** *Usage note*: Masking may be complete for one class of people and partial or none for another. For example, the masking would be complete for patients in a **single-mask trial** and none for **treaters**.

complete randomization *n* - **Randomization** not constrained by restrictions, such as those imposed by **blocking**. syn: simple randomization, unrestricted randomization

complete treatment assignment block *n* - 1. A **treatment assignment block** in which all **treatments** represented in the **design** appear or are to appear the same number of times; one in which all treatments represented in the design appear or are to appear at least once and in the **proportion** or **ratio** specified in the design. 2. A treatment assignment block that is filled. rt: **incomplete treatment assignment block**

complete treatment assignment block design *n* - A **parallel treatment design** involving **complete treatment assignment blocks** (eg, a design involving three **treatments**, A, B, and C, **assigned** in the **ratio** of 1:1:2 in **blocks** of size 4 or 8; sample block of size 4: A,C,B,C; sample block of size 8: C,A,C,B,C,C,A,B); so characterized even if **enrollment** is closed before a block is complete (as in the Coronary Drug Project [Coronary Drug Project Research Group, 1973][30] involving blocks of size 15, within each of two **strata** per **clinic**; generally the last block in each strata of most clinics was only partly filled when enrollment was completed). syn: **complete block design** ant: **incomplete treatment assignment block design**

complete treatment crossover *n* - 1. A treatment scheme in which a person receives or is to receive each of the **study treatments** in a designated order, as in a **treatment crossover trial**. 2. A treatment scheme in a treatment crossover design that is completed, ie, has the specified number of **treatment crossovers**. *Usage note*: Note that **complete** has different meanings in defns 1 and 2. The reference in defn 1 is to completeness whereas the reference in defn 2 is to completion. Hence, something can be complete in the sense of defn 2 but incomplete in the sense of defn 1, as in a completed sequence of treatment crossovers in a **incomplete crossover treatment design**.

complete treatment crossover design *n* - A **crossover treatment design** that provides for administration of all **study treatments** in some specified order to the **experimental units** (eg, **patients**) in a **trial**, examples include **Latin square** and **Greco-Latin square treatment designs**.

completely *adv* - In totality or a state of **completeness**. *Usage note*: Often best avoided; usually unnecessary or redundant, as in *completely obvious*, or subject to ambiguity, as in *completely randomized*. See also notes for **complete** *adj* and **complete** *v*.

completely confounded *n* - [**research**] A state in which there is a one-to-one relation between **variables** that can be used to explain an observed result. For example, the **treatment difference** observed in a **trial** involving two **clinics** is said to be completely confounded by **clinic** if there is a one-to-one correspondence between **clinic** and **treatment**, such that all **patients** receiving the **test treatment** are from one clinic and all those receiving the **control treatment** are from the other clinic. The difference observed can be explained either by treatment or clinic. See also **controlled variable**. rt: **confounded**, **partially confounded** *Usage note*: To be used as an explanation of an observed **result** there should be documented evidence of confounding, as demonstrated by the **joint distribution** of the variables considered to be confounded. Avoid as **weasel term**.

completely masked *adj* - [**trials**] 1. A condition in which all those to receive or receiving **treatment** in a trial, as well as all those involved in administering the **assigned treatments** and in **data collection** and **generation** are **masked** to **treatment assignment**; **double-masked**. 2. Such a condition but where those involved in **treatment effects monitoring** are also masked to treatment assignment; **triple-masked**. ant: **nonmasked** rt: **partially masked**

completely masked randomization *n* - Completely masked **treatment assignment** in which **assignments** are generated using **randomization** procedures. ant: open randomization, **unmasked randomization** rt: **partially masked randomization** *Usage note*: See note for **completely masked treatment assignment**.

completely masked treatment assignment *n* - 1. **Masked treatment assignment** (defn 1) in regard to **patients** and **clinic personnel**. 2. Masked treatment assignment (as above) including personnel issuing assignments. 3. Either of the schemes in defns 1 or 2 above, and in which treatment assignments remain masked to **study patients** and **clinic** personnel after issue, as in **double-masked** or **triple-masked trials**; **masked treatment assignment** (defn 2). ant: **open treatment assignment, unmasked treatment assignment** rt: **partially masked treatment assignment** *Usage note*: Subject to confusion; avoid by providing sufficient details to indicate sense of use. Masked treatment assignment, in the sense of defns 1 or 2, is an essential feature of any sound assignment scheme, regardless of whether or not the treatments also are to be administered in masked fashion, as in defn 3.

completely masked trial *n* - 1. A **trial** in which all of the **study treatments** are administered in a **single-** or **double-masked** fashion. 2. A trial in which all of the staff in a **clinic** are masked to **treatment assignment**. rt: **partially masked trial, unmasked trial**

completely randomized design *n* - Any type of **experimental design** in which the **treatments**, levels of a **factor**, or some other **experimental variable** are **assigned** to **experimental units** via **complete randomization**.

completely randomized treatment design *n* - A **treatment design** in which **treatments** are **assigned** to **experimental units** via **complete randomization**.

complex *adj* - [L *complexus*, pp of *complecti* to embrace, comprise (a multitude of objects), fr *com-* + *plectere* to braid] 1. Composed of two or more parts; **composite**. 2. Concerned with or being complex numbers. ant: **simple** (defn 1)

complex treatment *n* - A **treatment** having two or more **components**, eg, a treatment involving the use of two or more **drugs** in combination. ant: **simple treatment**

complex treatment design *n* - 1. A **treatment design** having **factorial structured treatments**. 2. A design in which the **treatment unit** receives a **complex treatment**. ant: **simple treatment design**

complex trial *n* - A trial having a **complex treatment design**. ant: **simple trial** *Usage note*: See note for **simple trial**.

compliance *n* - 1. The act or process of **complying** with a procedure or routine; conformity to rules or regulations. 2. **patient compliance** syn: **adherence** ant: **noncompliance**

compliant *adj* - **Complying** or a willingness to comply. ant: **noncompliant**

compliant person *n* - A person **complying** with a specified request, procedure, or routine; eg, in relation to accepting the **assigned treatment** regimen in a **trial**. ant: **noncompliant person**

comply, complied, complying, complies *v* - [It *complire*, fr Sp *cumplir* to complete, perform what is due, be courteous, fr L *complēre* to complete] To act in accordance with a set of **rules**, regulations, or procedures.

component *n* - [L *component-*, *componens*, prp of *componere* to put together] 1. A constituent part; ingredient. 2. Any one of the vector terms added to form a vector sum or resultant; a **coordinate** of a vector.

component analysis *n* - **principal component analysis**

components of variance model *n* - **random- effects model**

composite *adj* - [L *compositus*, pp of *componere*] Having multiple parts or **components**; **complex**.

composite event *n* - An **event** that is considered to have occurred if any one of several different events or **outcomes** are observed (eg, occurrence of an attack of angina pectoris, transient ischemic attack, or myocardial infarction). rt: **composite outcome**

composite hypothesis *n* - A **hypothesis** in which the **parameter** of interest assumes any one of an array of values. ant: **simple hypothesis**

composite outcome *n* - An **outcome** comprised of any of several different outcomes (eg, prolonged attack of angina pectoris, elevated bilirubin, or abnormal ECG tracing in a cardiovascular **trial**). rt: **composite event**

composition *n* - [ME *composicioun*, fr MF *composition*, fr L *compostion-*, *compositio*, fr *compositus*] 1. The general makeup or character of something. 2. The **product** or result of combining or mixing, as in **baseline composition**.

computer *n* - A programmable electronic **device** used to manipulate and store **data**. rt: **mainframe, minicomputer, microcomputer, supercomputer, superminicomputer** *Usage note*:

Subject to considerable misuse arising from failure to distinguish between operations performed on a computer, via a particular **program** or **software** package and the computer itself. Hence, *my computer isn't working*, more often than not, means that a piece of software malfunctioned, rather than the computer itself. Misuse also arises from the tendency to ascribe personal attributes or qualities to a computer, as in *the computer tells us*, or in affixing blame, as in *the computer managed to screw up my calculation*, when, more likely than not, it is something the user did (or failed to do) that caused the problem.

computer program *n* - A set of instructions or statements supplied to a **computer** for performing some defined task or function.

computer terminal *n* - Any device (**dumb** or **intelligent computer terminal**) that can be used for **input** or **output**; may be part of a network of terminals or may operate independently.

computer-assisted data collection *n* - Any system of **data collection** in which a **computer** is used either to facilitate data collection, eg, the use of computer-generated **video displays** to prompt and guide data collection, or as a substitutes for **paper forms**.

conclude, concluded, concluding, concludes *v* - [ME *concluden*, fr L *concludere* to shut up, end, infer, fr *com-* + *claudere* to shut] 1. To bring to an end, especially in a particular way or by a particular action. 2. To reach or come to a logical end or finish. 3. To finish or complete by reaching a reasoned decision or **inference**.

conclusion *n* - [ME, fr MF, fr L *conclusion-*, *conclusio*, fr *conclusus*, pp of *concludere*] 1. A reasoned judgment; **inference**; the necessary consequence of two or more propositions taken as premises. 2. The last part of something, such as a **result** or **outcome**.

concomitant *adj* - [L *concomitant-*, *concomitans*, prp of *concomitari* to accompany, fr *com-* + *comitari* to accompany, fr *comit-*, *comes* companion] Accompanying, especially in a subordinate or incidental way.

concurrent *adj* - [ME, fr MF & L; MF fr L *concurrent-*, *concurrens*, prp of *concurrere*] 1. Running **parallel**. 2. Occurring at the same time. ant: **nonconcurrent** *Usage note*: A comparative term that derives its meaning from the context of usage in relation to some implied

comparison. In the context of **followup studies**, the implied comparison relates to the different **study groups** represented in a study, as in *concurrent enrollment into the various treatment groups represented in a trial.*

concurrent cohort study *n* - 1. A **cohort study** in which the different cohorts represented are **enrolled** and **followed** over the same time period. 2. A cohort study in which all **data** are collected concurrently and prospectively in time; as opposed to **nonconcurrent cohort study**. See *study* for list. syn: **concurrent followup study**

concurrent control *n* - A **control** (defn 1) **concurrent** or **simultaneous** in time to that to which **compared**, eg, **control-assigned patients** in a **trial** involving a **parallel treatment design**. syn: **parallel control** ant: **nonconcurrent control, historical control**

concurrent control group *n* - A **control group** that was, is, or is to be observed over the same time period as the other **groups** in the **study**. ant: **historical control group**

concurrent enrollment *n* - Simultaneous **enrollment** of **observation units**, eg, typically **patients** in a **clinical trial**, into the various **study groups** represented in the **study design**. ant: **nonconcurrent enrollment**

concurrent followup *n* - [Studies with multiple study groups] **Followup** that takes place over the same time period for the different **study groups** represented in a **study design**; generally **prospective** and performed in real time.

concurrent followup study *n* - A **followup study** having two or more **study groups** and **concurrent followup** of those groups; generally assumed to be concurrent when the modifier **concurrent** is not used. See *study* for list. syn: **followup study, concurrent cohort study** (under some circumstances) ant: **nonconcurrent followup study**

concurrent prospective study *n* - **concurrent followup study**

condition *n* - [ME *condcion*, fr MF, fr L *condicion-, condicio*, terms of agreement, condition, fr *condicere*, to agree, fr *com-* + *dicere*, to say, determine] 1. Something essential to the appearance or occurrence of something else. 2. A state of being. 3. A restricting or modifying factor; qualification. 4. [**mathematics**] An assertion or assumption that must prevail for a statement to be correct. rt: **necessary condition, sufficient condition, necessary and sufficient condition**

conditional *adj* - Subject to; **dependent** upon. ant: **unconditional** rt: **restricted**

conditional distribution *n* - The **distribution** of a **variable**, given some **condition**, eg, the distribution of family size, given place of residence. ant: **unconditional distribution**

conditional life expectancy *n* - **Life expectancy** given some **condition** or combination of conditions, eg, survival to age 50 for conditional life expectancy at age 50. rt: **life expectancy, unconditional life expectancy, lifetable**

conditional power *n* - The **power** expected by the completion of a **study**, given the **results** up to some point in the course of a study. rt: **expected power, observed power, stochastic curtailment**

conditional probability *n* - The **probability** of an **event** or **outcome**, given some **condition**, eg, the probability of death in a specified **period** of **time**, given a prior myocardial infarction. ant: **unconditional probability**

conditional survival rate *n* - 1. The **number** of people entering a defined time **interval** alive at the end of the interval, divided by the number entering the interval. 2. The number of people entering a defined interval not having the condition of interest and free of that condition at the end of the interval, divided by the number entering the interval. rt: **cumulative survival rate, survival probability**

conditional type II error *n* - **Type II error** given **results** up to some point in an ongoing **study**, eg, as determined in **stochastic curtailment**. rt: **conditional power**

conditioning variable *n* - **moderator variable**

confidence *n* - 1. Belief or faith. 2. A relation of trust or intimacy. 3. The assurance that someone or some **agency** will keep designated information private.

confidence coefficient *n* - **confidence level**

confidence interval *n* - An **interval** of values, estimated from **observed data** presumed to include the **parameter** of interest (eg, the **population mean**) at a specified **confidence level**. For example, the 95% confidence interval for the **observed mean**, $\bar{x}$, of a **normally distributed variable**, estimated from a **sample** drawn from a larger underlying **population**, is centered at x̄ and has a lower **end point** of x̄ - 1.96·SE$_{(mean)}$ and an upper end point of x̄ + 1.96·SE$_{(mean)}$. Ninety-five percent of such intervals, constructed from **independent samples** from the larger underlying population, will contain the true population mean (**parameter**). However, there is no assurance that any given interval will do so. Typically the interval is defined by both a lower and upper end point, but it will have just one end point if the **type I error** represented in the confidence level is **one-tailed**.

confidence level *n* - One minus the specified **type I error** level for a **confidence interval**; often multiplied by 100 to express as a **percent**. rt: **p-value**

confidence limits *n* - The **end points** of a **confidence interval**.

confidential *adj* - 1. Being or relating to that which is private or secret; done or communicated in **confidence**. 2. Marked by intimacy or willingness to confide. 3. Entrusted with **confidence**. 4. Containing information which, if disclosed (except to designated persons or parties for specified uses), is or has the potential of being prejudicial, harmful, or embarrassing to the person or party to which the information pertains.

confidentiality *n* - 1. The state of being assured that that which is confided, obtained, or found in a specific setting will remain private and that it will not be revealed or disclosed to others, except as designated or implied, eg, the assurance given to a **study participant** on **entry** into a **study** that the information given by or obtained on the person will not be revealed to others outside the immediate confines of the study in ways in which it would be possible to identify the person. 2. The state of confiding.

confirmatory data analysis *n* - **Data analysis** aimed at verifying or confirming an **observation** or **conclusion** made or reached from prior data analyses.

conflate, conflated, conflating, conflates *v* - [L *conflatus*, pp of *conflare* to blow together, fuse, fr *com-* + *flare* to blow] 1. To bring together; fuse. 2. To confuse; mix up. 3. To combine into a **composite** whole.

conflation *n* - A blending or fusion of two or more things or effects, eg, a mixing of **effects** due to the **test** and **control treatment**.

conflict *n* - [ME, fr L *conflictus* act of striking together, fr *confictus* pp of *configere* to strike together fr *com-* + *figere* to strike] 1. Competitive or opposing actions. 2. Mental struggle resulting from incompatible or opposing needs or conditions.

conflict of interest *n* - Any **interest**, deriving from financial holdings, proprietorship in some **business** or in **relationship** to some product, a post or position held, or from a stand taken by a person, group, **agency**, **firm**, or **institution** that is acknowledged as constituting a **conflict** or that is perceived as having such a **potential** in relation to some activity performed, view espoused, judgment exercised, or action taken or performed by that person, group, agency, firm, or institution. See also **bias potential** and **potential bias**. *Usage note*: Most often used in relation to financial, business, or proprietary interests, but can be used in relation to one's post or employment, or more broadly in relation to a philosophical position or point of view that is considered to be in conflict with one's duty or to have influenced or to have the potential of influencing one's judgment or action in relation to some activity or function. Avoid as an implied charge or in speculative sense. Generally, unless supported with factual information detailing the nature of the interest considered to constitute a conflict, the term should not be used. Avoid, as well, suppositions as to effect. The direction or nature of the effect of a conflict of interest may be opposite to the one suggested by the conflict in cases in which the individual is aware of the conflict and overcompensates for it.

confound, confounded, confounding, confounds *v* - [ME confounden, fr ME *confondre*, fr L *confundere* to pour together, confuse, fr *com-* + *fundere* + to pour] To mix up or confuse.

confounded *n* - [**research**] A state in which the **effect** of one **variable** is confused, mixed up with, or obscured by the effect of another variable. See **completely confounded** and **partially confounded**. See also **controlled variable**. rt: **confounder, confounding variable, interaction** *Usage note*: To be used as an explanation of an observed **result**, there should be evidence of confounding, as demonstrated by differences in the **joint distribution** of the variables considered to be confounders in relation to the groups being compared. Confounding in trials occurs when the **distribution** of a **baseline variable** (or set of such variables) differs across the **treatment groups** being compared and when that (those) variable (variables) is (are) related to **outcome**. Technically, such a difference for a variable that is not related to outcome is not a **confounder**, although it is sometimes referred to as such (not recommended usage). Avoid using as a **weasel term**. Note also that confounding and **interaction** have different conceptual bases and implications and, hence, should not be confused. The variable in question must be related to outcome in both cases in trials. However, in the case of confounding, the variable must be differentially distributed by treatment group; in the case of interaction, the variable must influence the **treatment difference** observed. The existence of an interaction does not effect one's ability to compare among the treatment groups; the presence of a confounder does. Both types of conditions affect the way in which results are viewed and interpreted. Confounding influences one's certainty regarding the existence of a **treatment effect** since the difference can be explained either by the treatments applied or by the confounding variable. Interaction influences one's certainty as to the extent to which a result may be applied to a broader population, eg, does the treatment work in both males and females or only in males? See also usage notes for **confounding variable** and for **interacting variable**.

confounded effect *n* - An **effect** that is **confounded** with some other effect or **variable**. In the case of **trials**, the effect of one **treatment** in a **trial** is said to be confounded with the effect of another treatment if it is impossible to distinguish between the effects of the two treatments, eg, because both effects are estimated by the same **contrast**. A **treatment difference** is said to be confounded by a **baseline variable** if that variable has a different **distribution** in the treatment groups being compared and the variable also influences **outcome**. rt: **alias**

confounder *n* - 1. Something that **confounds**. 2. **confounding variable**

confounding *adj* - The state or process of being **confounded**.

confounding variable *n* - 1. [**epidemiology**] Broadly, a **variable**, causally related to some **event** or **outcome** (eg, development of a **disease**), that distorts an **association** between that outcome and some precursor **event** or **exposure**

by obscuring or falsely accentuating the **association**. Defined by Last[85] (1st edition) as *a factor that distorts the apparent magnitude of an effect of a study factor on risk. Such a factor is a determinant of the outcome of interest and is unequally distributed among the exposed and the unexposed.* 2. [**trials**] Any **variable**, especially one observed before or on **enrollment**, related to **treatment assignment** or that by **chance** turns out to be related to treatment assignment and that influences **outcome**, eg, a **baseline variable** that has a different distribution in the **treatment groups** being compared and that is related to outcome. See *variable* for list. rt: **interacting variable** *Usage note*: It is important, in the case of trials, to distinguish between variables observed before **treatment assignment** and those observed after assignment and initiation of treatment. Variables of the first kind are, by definition, **independent** of treatment assignment, whereas variables of the second kind may not be. The distinction is important in that variables of the first kind may help to explain the size, presence, or absence of a treatment difference, whereas variables of the second kind may themselves be confounded with treatment and, therefore, while perhaps useful in helping one to understand the nature of or extent of a **treatment effect**, cannot be used to explain a difference observed. For example, **compliance measures**, by definition observed after the initiation of treatment, may help explain how a treatment works but cannot be used to explain away an observed difference.

consent *n* - 1. Voluntary agreement or acquiescence by a person, or by that person's guardian or representative on their behalf, to undertake, submit to, or **comply** with an act or procedure that is to be done by another person, party, or **agency**. 2. **consent process** rt: **assent, deferred consent, consent statement, informed consent, preassignment consent, post-assignment consent, oral consent, signed consent** *Usage note*: Not to be confused with **assent** *n*.

consent, consented, consenting, consented *v* - [ME *consenten* fr L *consentire*, fr *com-* + *sentire* to feel] 1. To agree or to express a willingness to voluntarily proceed or comply to something planned or proposed, especially such agreement or expression of willingness after having been informed as to the nature and consequences of that planned or proposed. 2. The process of obtaining such agreement or expression of willingness. *Usage note*: Not to be confused with **assent** as used in research settings in relation to permissions. See note for **assent** *v* for differences. One requires the assent of a **child** and the **consent** of the child's parent or guardian to enroll the child into a **study**.

consent form *n* - 1. A **form** used for obtaining **consent**, especially one reviewed and approved by an **institutional review board** (or body with similar function), that has a place for the consenting person (or that person's parent or guardian) to sign to acknowledge consent; consists of a written statement read or presented to the person (or person's parent or guardian) asked to consent that indicates the reason for the request, the nature and extent of the commitment implied by consent, the methods and procedures to which the person will be exposed, and the likely **risks** and **benefits** accruing to the person by consenting. 2. **consent statement** syn: **disclosure form** (defn 2; not recommended), **disclosure and consent form** rt: **consent statement**, **consent process**, **disclosure statement**, **informed consent**, **preassignment consent**, **post-assignment consent**, **signed consent**, **oral consent**

consent process *n* - The methods and procedures used in obtaining **consent**, especially in relation to **enrollment** into a **study** or other forms of **research**; including description of the setting in which consent is requested, type of information to be presented prior to requesting consent, name of person or persons responsible for obtaining and documenting consent, and description of the nature and extent of opportunity offered for dialogue and query prior to requesting consent. In trials and other forms of research involving human beings, the process and related materials used for obtaining consent are to be reviewed and approved by the **institutional review board** (or similar board or committee) of record prior to use. The nature and complexity of the process proposed and related materials will depend on the type and setting of the research proposed. The process may be carried out in a single session (eg, in a simple, short-term, largely risk-free trial) or may extend over two or more sessions, conditions and circumstances permitting. Generally, all other things being equal, a process involving two or more sessions, separated in time by one day or more, is preferable to a single session, especially in trials where those

to be **enrolled** are expected to undergo complicated or risky procedures, are to be exposed to potentially risky treatments, or where **data collection** and followup are to continue over an extended period of time. rt: **consent, informed consent**

consent statement *n* - 1. A **consent form** with a signature block for the person **consenting**, typically placed at the end of the statement and used to **document** the fact of **consent** by the act of signing. 2. **signed consent** rt: **consent form**, **disclosure and consent form**, **consent process**, **disclosure statement**, **informed consent**, **preassignment consent**, **post-assignment consent**, **signed consent**, **oral consent**

consistency *n* - The property of a **consistent estimator**.

consistent *adj* - [L *consistent-, consistens*, prp of *consistere*] Marked by regularity of **performance**.

consistent estimator *n* - An **estimator** that has the property of yielding **estimates** that approach the true underlying value (**parameter**) as **sample size** increases.

consortium *n* - [L fellowship, fr *consort-, consors*] A structure, arrangement, or **group** formed to undertake some enterprise or activity that is beyond the capabilities or resources of the individual units or members.

consortium funding *n* - A type of **funding** in which monies received by a designated **center** are disbursed to other centers in a **multicenter study** according to terms set forth in a **consortium funding agreement** and involving **contracts** with (typically the case) or **grants** to those other centers. rt: **indirect distribution of funds**

consortium funding agreement *n* - A **funding agreement** between the **sponsor** and a **center** in a **multicenter study** in which funds are received by that center for disbursal to one or more other centers in the study, typically via contractual agreements.

consortium funding award *n* - 1. A **grant** or **contract** awarded to a **center** in a **multicenter study** that involves a **consortium funding agreement**. The center receiving the **award** assumes responsibility for **distribution** of **funds** to all other participating centers in the study. 2. Such an award except that it is for support of only certain centers in the study; remaining centers funded in other ways.

constant *adj* - [ME, fr MF, fr L *constant-*, *constans*, fr prp of *constare* to stand firm, be consistent, fr *com-* + *stare* to stand] Not **variable**, **uniform**; continually occurring or recurring.

constant *n* - 1. A **number** that has a fixed value; a number that is assumed not to change value in a given mathematical argument or discussion. 2. Something invariable or unchanging.

contact *n* - [F or L; F, fr L *contactus*, fr *contactus*, pp of *contingere* to have contact with] 1. The establishment or maintenance of communications with someone; **patient contact**. 2. A person exposed to an infectious agent by physical contact or proximate association with a person harboring the agent and considered capable of infecting others with it. rt: **direct contact**, **indirect contact**

contact, contacted, contacting, contacts *v* - 1. To touch or join. 2. To get in touch with for communication or interaction.

contaminant *n* - Something that **contaminates**.

contaminate, contaminated, contaminating, contaminates *v* - [L *contaminatus*, pp of *contaminare*; akin to L *contagio* contagion] To soil, stain, or corrupt; to make inferior by admixture.

contamination *n* - A process of being **contaminated**; the state of being contaminated. rt: **treatment cross-contamination**

contingency *n* - The quality of being **contingent**.

contingency table *n* - A **table** having two or more dimensions, each dimension corresponding to a **variable** having two or more mutually exclusive **discrete classes** or **categories**; the total **number** of cells in the table corresponds to the **product** of the numbers of classes or categories represented; each cell contains a **count** or **total** corresponding to the class or category represented for that cell; summing across the cells of a given variable provides the **marginal frequency distribution** for that variable. See **two-by-two table** for simplest case.

contingent *adj* - [ME, fr MF, fr L *contingent-*, *contingens*, prp of *contingere*, to have contact with, befall, fr *com-* + *tangere*, touch] Dependent upon or **conditioned** by something.

contingent variable *n* - **intermediate variable**

continual *adj* - [ME, fr MF, fr L *coninuus* continuous] Repeated regularly and often; not interrupted or broken in time or **sequence**.

continual assessment dosage design *n* - A **unit sequential Bayesian dosage design** involving aspects of the **up-down dosage design** but with the goal of exposing as many of the **observation** or **treatment units** to a **dosage** at or near the **maximum tolerable dose** (MTD) and in which the dosage used for the next unit to be exposed is based on an **estimate** of the MTD, as determined via a **Bayesian** method of **estimation** using **data** from all previously exposed units.[118] rt: **dosage design, traditional sequential dosage design, up-down sequential dosage design**

continual reassessment dosage design *n* - **continual assessment dosage design**

continue, continued, continuing, continues *v* - 1. To maintain without interruption in time, space, or sequence. 2. To remain in existence, place, or effect. 3. To resume an activity after an interruption or **suspension**.

continuity *adj* - Of, being, or having uninterrupted connection, succession, or union; of uninterrupted duration or continuation without major **change**.

continuity correction *n* - A **correction** applied when approximating the **distribution** of a **discrete variable** with a **continuous variable**, eg, **Yates' continuity correction**.

continuous *adj* - [L *continuus*, fr *continere*, to hold together] A property ascribed to a **function**, **variable**, or **measure** in which all values over a defined **range** are represented, ie, a property in which the **absolute difference** between two neighboring **points** can be made arbitrarily close to zero by ever increasing **precision** in the **measurement** process. ant: **discrete**

continuous data *n* - **Data** based on a **continuous variable**. See *data type* for list. ant: **discrete data**

continuous variable *n* - A **variable** that is capable of assuming any value over a specified **range**. See *variable* for list. ant: **discrete variable**

contract *n* - [ME, fr L *contractus*, fr *contractus*, pp of *contrahere* to draw together, make a contract, reduce in size, fr *com-* + *trahere* to draw] 1. [general] A binding **agreement** between two or more parties, especially one that is legally enforceable. 2. [**business**] A legally binding, usually written, agreement between one party desiring specified goods or services and another proposing to provide such goods or services; the contract specifies the nature of goods or services to be delivered, the schedule or duration of activities, and terms of payment for said goods or services, eg, an agreement between a **sponsor** and the **business office** of an **investigator's** place of employment in relation to performing a specified **research project**. rt: **grant, subcontract, cooperative agreement** *Usage note*: Both **grants** and **contracts** are used to fund **trials**, but the two mechanisms have different origins, administrative implications, and requirements, at least as applied by the **NIH** [Department of Health and Human Services, 1982;[34] Department of Health, Education, and Welfare, 1977[35]]. Hence, the term should not be used interchangeably or confused with grant. See notes for **grant** and **subcontract** for additional comments.

contract application *n* - **contract proposal**

contract office *n* - 1. The **office** in the **sponsoring agency** whose staff are responsible for negotiating, awarding, and funding **contracts**. 2. That office in a **lead center**, serving as a surrogate for the sponsoring agency, under the **consortium mode of funding** and involving use of contracts for dispersal of funds to the other centers. 3. **business office** (defn 3) *Usage note*: Care should be taken to distinguish between usage in the sense of defn 2 versus defn 1. Use in the sense of defn 3 not recommended in that those offices typically have responsibilities for **grants** as well as contracts. rt: **grants management office**

contract officer *n* - 1. The individual in the **sponsoring agency** who is responsible for negotiating, awarding, and funding **contracts** for specified projects. 2. Such a person in a **lead center** under the **consortium mode of funding** and involving the use of contracts for dispersal of funds to the other centers. rt: **grants management officer** *Usage note*: Care should be taken to distinguish between usage in the sense of defn 2 versus defn 1.

contract proposal *n* - A **funding proposal** that, if awarded, involves funding via a **contract**. rt: **grant proposal**

contract research organization (CRO) *n* - 1. A **research organization** funded in part or totality

via **contract**. 2. An **organization** in the **business** of contracting with **firms** developing **drugs**, **biologics**, or **devices** to perform **trials** on their behalf or to prepare materials (such as for an **NDA**) on their behalf for submission to the **FDA**.

contractor *n* - 1. One who **contracts** or is a party to a **contract**. 2. One who provides a service or a product in relation to a contract. 3. One who agrees to provide specified goods or services in return for specified payments or considerations from the payer. rt: **subcontractor, grantee** *Usage note*: See **contract** and **grant**.

contractsmanship *n* - The "art" or practice of applying for **contracts**, especially practices not directly related to the scope or nature of work proposed and that are considered by the **applicant** to increase the prospect of **funding**; generally having to do with the **organization** or **presentation** of material and **documentation** related to **budget** and **cost** projections; **grantsmanship** when applying for **grants**.

contrast *n* - 1. The **difference** or degree of difference between things having similar or comparable natures. 2. **Comparison** of similar things to set off differences. 3. The state of being **compared**. 4. The use of opposing elements to set off or to compare. 5. [**statistics**] A **linear combination** of **estimates** having known **constant coefficients** such that their **sum** is zero, eg, a **test-control treatment difference**.

contrast, contrasted, contrasting, contrasts *v* - [F *contraster*, fr MF, to oppose, resist] **Compare** or appraise in respect to **differences**; to set off in **contrast**.

control *adj* - Of or relating to a **control**. *Usage note*: See usage notes for **controlled** and for **randomized control trial**.

control *n* - 1. A **standard** of **comparison** for testing, verifying, or evaluating some **observation** or **result**. 2. Something that **controls** (defn 1 or 2). 3. A person or larger **observation unit** used for comparison, eg, a control in a **case-control study**; **control patient** 4. **control treatment**

control, controlled, controlling, controls *v* - [ME *controllen*, fr MF *contreroller*, fr *conterolle*, copy of an account, audit, fr ML *contrarotulus*, fr L *contra-* + *rotulus*, little wheel] 1. To exercise restraint or direction over. 2. To regulate or hold in check, as in the control of a process. 3.

To test, verify, or evaluate via **parallel** processes or via a standard of **comparison**.

control drug *n* - 1. The **drug** used as a **control treatment** in a **drug trial**. 2. A drug against which others are compared.

control experiment *n* - **controlled experiment**

control group *n* - 1. **comparison group** 2. **control-treated group**

control patient *n* - 1. A **patient** assigned to the **control treatment** in a **trial**. 2. A person in a **case-control study** free of the **disease** or health condition of interest but similar to cases in other regards and that, when taken together as a group (**control group**), form the basis for **comparisons** made in such a study.

control treatment *n* - A **treatment**, **active** or **inactive**, that serves as a basis for **comparison**, especially in a **clinical trial**. rt: **inactive control treatment, active control treatment, study treatment, test treatment** *Usage note*: Active treatments include **standard care** or use of a **study treatment** (defn 2) designed to produce a **positive** or **negative treatment effect**; inactive treatments include **placebo treatment, sham treatment, nontreatment**, and **null treatment**. See **study treatment** for additional comments.

control-assigned *adj* - [**trials**] Of, relating to, or being **assigned** to the **control treatment**. rt: **test-assigned, control-treated** *Usage note*: Used to characterize **assignment** to a control treatment, as in **control-assigned patient** or **control-assigned group**.

control-assigned group *n* - [**trials**] 1. The **group assigned** to the **control treatment**. 2. The group that received or is receiving a **control treatment**. rt: **test-assigned group, control-treated group, control-assigned patient** *Usage note*: Use in the sense of defn 2 not recommended because those receiving a control treatment may not have been **control-assigned**. See also note for **control-assigned**.

control-assigned patient *n* - [**trials**] 1. A **patient assigned** to the **control treatment**. 2. A patient who received or is receiving a **control treatment**. rt: **test-assigned patient, control-treated patient, control-assigned group** *Usage note*: Use in the sense of defn 2 not recommended. See notes for **control-assigned group** and **control-assigned**.

control-treated *adj* - [**trials**] Of, relating to, or being treated with a **control treatment**. rt: **test-treated, control-assigned** *Usage note*: Used to characterize a **patient** or group of patients, as in **control-treated patient** or **control-treated group**. Sometimes used as a synonym for **control-assigned**; not recommended because being so assigned is not equivalent to being control-treated. The reference is to **assignment** (without regard to **administered treatment**) in **control-assigned** and to administered treatment (without regard to assignment) in **control-treated**.

control-treated group *n* - 1. The group of **treatment units assigned** to receive a specific **control treatment**. 2. The group of treatment units that received or are receiving a specific control treatment, whether or not originally assigned to that treatment. syn: **control-assigned group** (in context of defn 1 for **control-treated group**) rt: **test-treated group, control-assigned group** *Usage note*: Not to be confused with **control-assigned group**. See usage note for **control-treated**. Use **control-assigned group** for uses in the sense of defn 1.

control-treated patient *n* - 1. A **patient assigned** to a **control treatment** in a **trial**. 2. A patient in a trial who is receiving or has received a specific control treatment, whether or not originally assigned to that treatment. syn: **control-assigned patient** (in context of defn 1 for **control-treated patient**) rt: **test-treated patient, control-assigned patient** *Usage note*: Not to be confused with **control-assigned patient**. See usage note for **control-treated**. Use **control-assigned patient** for uses in the sense of defn 1. Not recommended in the sense of defn 2 since that usage obscures the difference between an assigned and chosen or selected treatment; use other language to make the distinction clear.

controlled *adj* - 1. Constrained, monitored, or watched. 2. Any system of **observation** and **data collection** that is designed to provide a basis for **comparing** one group with another, such as provided in a **parallel treatment design** with **concurrent enrollment** to the different **study groups** represented in the design. ant: **uncontrolled** *Usage note*: Often unnecessary or redundant as a modifier, especially as a modifier of design terms that, in and of themselves, convey the notion of control, as in *randomized controlled trial*; the modifier **randomized** indicates the nature of the control implied and **controlled** adds nothing, except where to indicate other forms of control over and above those implied with **randomized**. Often redundant in the broader setting of trials as well, even if not randomized, since the notion of control is usually implicit in such usages, if not in the sense of defn 2 above, then certainly in the sense of defn 1. One can assume that the notion of **control**, as implied in defn 1, applies in all research settings involving experimentation. Hence, usage of the term should be limited to those in the sense of defn 2. However, it is conventional to use the term as a modifier of **trial**, especially if not preceded or followed by the modifier **randomized** (or some other design term implying control) simply to make clear that usage of **trial** is in the sense of defn 1. See also usage note for **randomized controlled trial**.

controlled clinical trial *n* - 1. A **controlled trial** involving **treatment** of a **clinical** condition. 2. **controlled trial** *Usage note*: See **clinical trial** and **controlled trial** for comments.

controlled experiment *n* - 1. An **experiment** involving two or more **study groups** and designed to provide a basis for **comparison** of those groups. 2. An **experiment** designed to **control** an **extraneous source of variation** to allow the experimenter to observe the effect of the **variable** of interest with more precision, eg, **treatment** in the case of a **trial**.

controlled randomization *n* - **Controlled treatment assignment** involving **randomization**. ant: **uncontrolled randomization** rt: **masked randomization**

controlled treatment assignment *n* - Any **assignment scheme** that includes safeguards designed to reduce the possibility of releasing **treatment assignments** before **treatment units** have been judged **eligible** for **enrollment** and ready for **treatment**. The safeguards may be maintained at a **clinic** or elsewhere (eg, at a **coordinating center**). They may consist of internally administered checks (eg, as performed by **clinic personnel** without any prompting or **monitoring** from outside the clinic in schemes involving a numbered file of sealed envelopes at the clinic) or of externally administered checks (eg, as administered from a coordinating center) before an assignment can be obtained or is released. ant: **uncontrolled treatment assignment** rt: **masked**

treatment assignment

controlled treatment assignment clinical trial *n* - A **clinical trial** involving **controlled treatment assignment**.

controlled trial *n* - 1. A **trial** involving one or more **test treatments**, at least one **control treatment**, and **concurrent patient enrollment**, **treatment**, and **followup**. 2. A trial involving two or more study treatments and concurrent patient enrollment, treatment, and followup. See *trial* for list. ant: **uncontrolled trial**

controlled variable *n* - 1. A **variable** that is constrained in some way. In **trials** usually a variable that is used for **stratification** during **treatment assignment** or for **adjustment** of the observed **treatment effect** during **data analysis**. 2. A variable that is **monitored** or watched during **data collection** (not recommended usage). See *variable* for list.

convention *n* - [ME, fr MF or L; MF, fr L *convention-*, *conventio*, fr *conventus*, pp] 1. agreement, compact 2. A general **agreement** about basic principles or procedures. 3. An established technique or practice; **rule**.

conventional *adj* - 1. Formed by **agreement** or compact. 2. ordinary, commonplace

conventional author *n* - A person responsible for writing some **document**, such as a **manuscript**, and who is identified as an **author** in the **masthead** or title of a work. ant: **corporate author**

conventional author citation *n* - 1. A form of **author citation** in which only individuals are named in the **masthead** or title of a work. 2. Such a citation in a **bibliography** or **reference list**. See *author/authorship* for list. ant: **corporate author citation** rt: **modified conventional author citation**

conventional authorship *n* - A form of **authorship** involving only individuals as named authors. ant: **corporate authorship** rt: **modified conventional authorship**

cooperative *adj* - 1. Marked by willingness and ability to work with others. 2. Of or relating to cooperation. 3. Relating to or comprising a structure of interrelated units dedicated to achieving a common end. syn: **collaborative** rt: **multidisciplinary**, **multicenter** *Usage note*: Not recommended as a modifier for study, as in **cooperative study** or **cooperative trial**, for reasons indicated in usage notes for those terms.

Also not a suitable synonym for **multicenter** as indicated in a usage note for that term.

cooperative agreement *n* - 1. An **agreement** between an institute of the **National Institutes of Health** and a set of **investigators** that provides a structure for sponsor-investigator cooperation in the **design** and execution of a research project that is funded by **grants** (as opposed to **contracts**). 2. Any written agreement between a **sponsor** and **investigator**(s) that provides a defined role for both parties in the design and conduct of a specified **research project**. 3. **Cooperative Research and Development Agreement**. rt: **contract, grant**

cooperative group *n* - **investigative group**

cooperative study *n* - 1. **multicenter study** 2. A **study** involving multiple **investigators**, whether in a **multicenter** setting or not. syn: **collaborative study** rt: **multicenter study** *Usage note*: Avoid because of ambiguous uninformative nature of the modifier **cooperative**. Most studies require cooperation and, hence, in this sense the term **cooperative** is unnecessary. Use other more informative adjectives, such as **multicenter** or **multidisciplinary**, depending on emphasis. See *study* for list.

cooperative trial *n* - 1. **multicenter trial** 2. A **trial** involving multiple **investigators**, whether **multicenter** or not. syn: **collaborative trial** rt: **multicenter trial** *Usage note*: Avoid because of ambiguous uninformative nature of the modifier **cooperative**. Most trials require cooperation and, hence, in this sense the term **cooperative** is unnecessary. Use other more informative adjectives, such as **multicenter** or **multidisciplinary**, depending on emphasis. See *trial* for list.

Cooperative Research and Development Agreement (CRADA) *n* - A **cooperative agreement** between an agency of the federal government and industry, a university, or foundation for development of a **product** or for bring a **proprietary product** to market. The agreements arise from the Federal Technology Transfer Act of 1986. The act was intended to facilitate interaction between government and the private sector of the economy for development and commercialization of products.

coordinate *n* - One of two or more **numbers** used to identify or locate a **point** on a **line**, surface, or in space, eg, the value x or y for the point (x, y) in a plane **Cartesian coordinate** system. rt:

x-coordinate, y-coordinate, xy-coordinate

coordinate, coordinated, coordinating, coordinates *v* - 1. To place in the same **order, class,** or **rank**. 2. To harmonize in a common action or effort.

coordinating center (CC) *n* - 1. A **center** in the structure of a **multicenter study** that is responsible for receiving, editing, processing, analyzing, and storing **study data** and for coordination of activities required for execution of the study. 2. A center having general responsibilities for coordination of activities required for execution of a study, without responsibilities for coordination of **data collection**. rt: **biostatistical center, data center, data coordinating center, statistical center, treatment coordinating center** See *center* for list.

coordinating center director *n* - **Director** of the **coordinating center**.

coordination *n* - [F or LL; F, fr LL *coodination-, coordinatio*, fr L *co-* + *ordination-, ordinatio* arrangement, fr *ordinatus*, pp of *ordinare* to arrange] 1. The act of **coordinating**. 2. The harmonious interaction and functioning of parts or units toward an effective end or result.

coordinator *n* - 1. The individual in the **data center, data coordinating center,** or **coordinating center** responsible for coordinating the receipt of **data** from **data collection** and **data generation sites** and for communicating with such sites regarding data flow; **study clinic coordinator** (defn 2), **data coordinator** (defn 1). 2. The **director** of the **data coordinating center** or **coordinating center**. 3. The director of the **study**.

Cornfield, Jerome - (1912 - 1979) US biostatistician/epidemiologist; made numerous contributions to methodology of **trials, case-control studies,** and **observational studies**. Contributions include introduction of **logistic regression** procedures in the **analysis** of **followup studies** and the estimation of **relative risks** and exposure-specific **rates** from case-control studies.

corporate *adj* - [L *corporatus*, pp of *corporate* to make into a body, fr *corpor-* corpus] Of or relating to a **group** of individuals formed into a united whole for some defined purpose.

corporate author *n* - A **corporate** entity, such as an **agency, institution,** or **collaborative group,** designated as **author** of some work; usually in the absence of named individual authors in the **masthead** of papers. See *author/authorship* for list. ant: **conventional author** rt: **corporate author citation**

corporate author citation *n* - 1. A form of **citation** in which only a **corporate** entity is named as **author** in the **masthead** or title of a work. 2. Such a citation in a **bibliography** or **reference list**. See *author/authorship* for list. ant: **conventional author citation** rt: **modified corporate author citation**

corporate authorship *n* - A form of attribution in which **authorship** is attributed to a **corporate** entity. ant: **conventional authorship** rt: **modified corporate authorship**

correct *adj* - [ME, corrected, fr L *corretus*, fr pp of *corrigere*] 1. Conforming to an approved **standard** or **convention**. 2. Conforming to or agreeing with logic or fact. 3. Conforming to a set amount or value.

correct, corrected, correcting, corrects *v* - [ME *correcten*, fr L *correctus*, pp of *corrigere*, fr *com-* + *regere* to lead straight] 1. To make or set right; to amend so as to set right. 2. To alter or **adjust**, especially so as to bring to some **standard** or required condition. 3. To point out for amendment or **correction**, as with an **error** or fault.

correction *n* - 1. The action or instance of **correcting**. 2. Amendment to bring into conformity with a **standard**. 3. Something substituted in place of that considered to be wrong or in question. 4. A quantity applied by way of correcting.

correlate, correlated, correlating, correlates *v* - To arrange or present so as to show **relationships**; to establish or demonstrate as having a **correlation**.

correlated *adj* - The state of being arrayed or presented so as to show a **relationship**. **Random variables** are said to be correlated if they are not **independent**.

correlated observations *n* - **Observations** or **measurements** that are **correlated**, eg, the height and age of children, one's body weight before and after a diet, the ages of husbands and wives. rt: **paired observations**

correlation *n* - [ML *correlation-, correlatio*, fr L *com-* + *relation-, relatio* relation] 1. A **relationship** known or presumed to be **causal** between

two things that is complementary, **parallel**, or **reciprocal**. 2. The act of **correlating**. 3. A **linear** interdependence between two **normally distributed variables** as expressed by a **correlation coefficient** or in some other mathematical sense. 4. Any of several different methods of correlation, such as **Kendall's tau**, **Pearson's product-moment correlation**, and **Spearman's rank correlation**. rt: **association, dependence, illusory correlation, relationship** *Usage note*: May be used in lay sense (defn 1), as in *there is a correlation between the state of the economy and rate of unemployment*; avoid lay usage by using **association** or **relationship** instead of correlation; limit use to sense conveyed in defns 3 and 4. The existence of a correlation between two **variables** does not imply the existence of a **cause and effect relationship**, nor does the absence of a correlation imply **independence** of the two variables (see note for **correlation coefficient**). Sometimes used interchangeably with **association** or **relationship**, as implied for uses in the sense of defn 1. See also notes for **association** and **cause and effect**.

correlation coefficient *n* - 1. A **function** or **number** that **measures** the **expected** or **observed relationship** existing between two **random variables**; equal to the **covariance** of the two variables divided by the **product** of their respective **standard deviations**. 2. Any of several different types of correlation coefficients, such as **Kendall's tau**, **Pearson's product-moment correlation coefficient**, and **Spearman's rank correlation** *Usage note*: A relationship involving two **variables** measured with a correlation coefficient is said to be **positive** if the value for the one variable or member of a pair of **observations** increases as the other increases, and is said to be **negative** if the value for the one variable or member of a pair of observations increases as the other decreases. The two variables or pairs of observations on those variables are said to have a perfect relationship (ie, a coefficient of -1 or +1) if the value for the one variable or member of a pair of observations can be **predicted** without **error** from the other. The variables are said to be uncorrelated if the value of the one variable or member of a pair of observations is of no value in predicting the other. A nonzero coefficient implies a **dependent** relationship between the variables, but a coefficient of zero does not imply independence, except where the variables have nonzero **variance** and are **normally distributed**.

correlation matrix *n* - A **matrix** corresponding to the **variables** in a **model** having **n** (≥ 2) **variables** in which the value for the element represented in the ith **row** and jth **column** corresponds to the **correlation** of the ith and jth variables. rt: **correlation matrix** rt: **variance-covariance matrix**

cost *n* - [ME *costen*, fr MF *coster*, fr (assumed) VL *costare*, fr L *constare* to stand firm, to cost] 1. The amount or equivalent paid or charged for something; price; the outlay of expenditure or effort made to achieve some end or object. 2. The loss or penalty, measured in monetary or other terms, incurred in gaining something.

cost, costing, costs *v* - [ME *costen*, fr MF *coster*, fr (assumed) VL *costare*, fr L *constare* to stand firm, to cost] 1. To cause someone or something to pay, suffer, or lose something. 2. To fix the **cost** of something.

cost-benefit *adj* - Cost versus **benefit**. rt: **cost-effective**

cost-benefit analysis *n* - [**medicine**] An assessment of the **costs** accruing to an individual exposed to some **treatment**, process, or procedure versus the **benefits** derived from undertaking or submitting to that treatment, process, or procedure. Cost may be measured in monetary terms or in broader terms; **risk-benefit analysis**. rt: **cost-effectiveness analysis, cost-utility analysis**

cost-effective *adj* - Economical in terms of benefits, especially tangible **benefits**, produced relative to monetary costs (or a broader measure of cost) incurred. rt: **cost-benefit**

cost-effectiveness analysis *n* - **Analysis** aimed at determining the **effectiveness** of different approaches or strategies for achieving a stated end or desired result (eg, reduction of blood pressure by a certain amount) relative to costs required to achieve that end or result; used to compare different strategies in terms of **benefit** per unit **cost** and used by planners or decision makers in setting priorities involving **allocation** of scarce **resources**. rt: **cost-benefit analysis, cost-utility analysis**

cost-reimbursement *adj* - Of or relating to **reimbursement** for monetary **costs** incurred in relation to some activity, duty, or responsibility; unlike **fixed-cost**.

cost-reimbursement contract *n* - A **contract** in which the amount of money paid is dictated by reasonable and allowable expenses for work performed; unlike **fixed-cost contract**. rt: **fee-for-service agreement**

cost-utility analysis *n* - An **analysis** of the **utility**, as measured against some **standard** or desired social value, of different approaches or strategies as a function of absolute or relative **cost**. rt: **cost-benefit analysis, cost-effectiveness analysis**

count *n* - [ME *countien*, fr MF *conter*, *compter*, fr L *computare* fr *com-* + *putare* to consider] A **total** obtained by counting or tallying; **frequency**.

counter *n* - [ME *countour*, fr MF *comptouer*, fr ML *computatorium* computing place, fr L *computatus*, pp of *computare*] 1. A **device** or instrument used in reckoning or recording **counts** of transactions or **events**. 2. A flat table-like surface over which business is transacted.

counting rule *n* - [**trials**] A **rule** related to the counting of persons (**observation units**) **enrolled** into a trial or **events** observed in relation to the **primary analysis**. The counting rules, discussed by Meinert and Tonascia [1986],[102] include: 1) All persons enrolled (**assigned** to **treatment**) should be counted in the **denominator** for the primary analysis. 2) All events should be counted regardless of when they occur after enrollment. 3) Events should be counted in the **treatment group** to which a person (observation unit) was assigned, regardless of degree of **compliance** to the assigned treatment. 4) Counts of subsets of events (eg, deaths due to cardiovascular causes) should not be used for analyses until counts and analyses of the higher order events (eg, deaths, regardless of cause) have been performed. rt: **analysis principle**

covariable *n* - A **variable** that is related to or varies with another variable. syn: **covariate**

covariance *n* - 1. The **expected value** of the **product** of **deviations** of two **random variables** from their respective **means**; 0 for **independent** variables. 2. The first **product-moment** about the **means** of two random variables, defined as the product of the expected **standard deviations** for the two variables multiplied by their expected **correlation coefficient**; estimated using observed standard deviations and correlation coefficients. rt: **variance**

covariant *adj* - Varying with something else so as to preserve a **relationship**.

covariate *n* - 1. **covariable** 2. The value assumed by a **covariable**.

Cox model *n* - **Cox proportional hazards regression model**

Cox proportional hazards regression model *n* - A **regression model** for **survival analysis** involving (possibly) **censored survival time** and for which one assumes proportional **hazard rates** across **baseline variables** and across time; due to DR Cox [1972];[31] used in trials to **adjust** observed **event rate ratios** of one **treatment group** to another for **baseline differences** among groups being compared in regard to important baseline variables believed to influence, or considered capable of influencing, the **distribution** of the time to the event of interest. Also referred to as **Cox's proportional hazards regression model**.

CPU *n* - **central processing unit**

CRADA *n* - **Cooperative Research and Development Agreement**

credit *n* - [MF, fr OIt *credito*, fr L *creditum* something entrusted to another, loan, fr neut of *creditus*; pp of *credere* to believe, entrust] 1. Recognition by name of some person, **group**, or **agency** for having performed specific functions or duties in relation to some activity, project, or production. 2. Such a recognition appearing in print in a published **manuscript** or at the start or end of a film. rt: **acknowledgment**

criterion (sing), **criteria** (pl) *n* - [Gk *kritērion*, fr *krinein* to judge, decide] 1. A characterizing condition, mark, or trait. 2. A **standard** on which a judgment or decision may be based.

critical *adj* - 1. Of, relating to, or being a turning point at an important juncture; crucial; decisive. 2. Relating to or being a state of importance, especially in relation to some decision or interpretation. rt: **critical region**

critical region *n* - The **rejection region** for a **test of significance** (corresponds in a **probability** sense to the **type I error** of the test); defined by a single **critical value** for **one-tailed alternative hypotheses** and an upper and lower critical value for **two-tailed alternative hypotheses**. syn: **rejection region** ant: **acceptance region**

critical value *n* - A value that represents the boundary between the **acceptance** and **rejection (critical) region** for a **test of significance**, eg, the value of 1.645 for a **one-tailed test of hypothesis** at the 0.05 **type error I** level for a **test statistic** having a **normal distribution**.

CRO *n* - **contract research organization**

cross *adj* - 1. Lying across from one another. 2. Mutually opposing or exclusive.

cross *adv* - Not **parallel**.

cross *n* - [ME, fr OE, fr ON or OIr; ON *kross*, fr (assumed) OIr *cross*, fr L *cruc-*, *crux*] A figure or mark formed by two intersecting **lines** crossing at or near their midpoints; the **symbols** X, x, or +; such a **symbol** when used to mark a **point** of interest or action.

cross, crossed, crossing, crosses *v* - 1. To lie or be situated across. 2. To go or pass from one side or condition to another.

cross, crossed *adj* - 1. Lying across or in opposition to. 2. Running counter to; opposite. 3. Involving mutual interchange; reciprocal. 4. joined ant: **uncrossed**

cross tabulation *n* - **cross-data tabulation**

cross-contamination *n* - **treatment cross-contamination**

cross-data classification *n* - **Classification** of **data** by two or more **variables**, as in a **contingency table**. syn: **cross-data tabulation**

cross-data stratification *n* - **cross-data classification**

cross-data tabulation *n* - A **tabulation** of **data** by two or more **variables**, as in tabulations for **contingency tables**. syn: **cross-data classification**

cross-reference *n* - A notation or **reference** at one place to pertinent information at another place.

cross-section *n* - 1. A cutting, slice, or piece of something taken from a whole. 2. A composite representation typifying the constituents or **relationships** of a whole.

cross-sectional analysis *n* - An **analysis** of time-related **data**, such as those in a **trial** arising from **observation** of people at designated time points over the course of **followup** by treating data at each time point as if they were **independent** of data at all other such time points. *Usage note*: Note the difference between this form of analysis and **cohort analysis**.

cross-sectional study *n* - 1. A **nonexperimental study** involving **observation** of a defined **population** at a single point in time or over a narrowly defined **time interval**. ant: **followup study** 2. **cross-sectional survey** 3. **cross-sectional analysis** (not a recommended synonym)

cross-sectional survey *n* - A **survey** involving **observations** made at a single time point or over a narrowly defined **time interval**. ant: **followup survey**

crossed treatment design *n* - 1. **crossover treatment design** 2. **factorial treatment design**

crossed treatments *n* - **Treatments** that are used in combination with one another, simultaneously or in sequence. rt: **crossover treatment design, factorial treatment design, treatment crossover**

crossover *n* - 1. An instance of crossing from one set or group to another. 2. **treatment crossover**

crossover design *n* - **crossover treatment design**

crossover study *n* - **crossover trial**

crossover treatment *n* - The **treatment** given after a **treatment switch** or **treatment crossover**.

crossover treatment design *n* - A **treatment design** that provides for the administration of two or more of the **study treatments**, one after another in a specified or **random** order, to **experimental units** in a **trial**; each administration may be followed by a **washout period**. ant: **noncrossover treatment design, parallel treatment design** rt: **multi-period crossover treatment design**

crossover trial *n* - A **trial** involving a **crossover treatment design**. See *trial* for list.

CRT *n* - **cathode ray tube**

crude *adj* - [ME, fr L *crudus* raw] 1. In an unrefined, natural state; **raw**. 2. Tabulated without being broken down into **classes**. 3. Not **adjusted**. ant: **adjusted** *Usage note*: Used primarily as a modifier to distinguish an **observed value**, such as a **rate**, from one that has been **adjusted**. While commonly used, the modifier has the disadvantage of connoting something that is rough, undesirable, or inaccurate, when in fact the term is used simply to label a value as an observed unadjusted value. Use **observed** or **unadjusted** to avoid the connotation.

crude rate *n* - **Rate** calculated or **estimated** from **observed data** prior to any **adjustment** or **standardization**. syn: **observed rate**

cumulative *adj* - To build or increase by the successive **addition** of individual items, parts, or **counts**.

cumulative frequency *n* - The **sum** of **frequencies** through a designated **point** for an ordered set of **class intervals**; the summation for "less than" cumulative frequencies are from lowest to highest class intervals and from highest to lowest class intervals for "greater than" cumulative frequencies; so named because frequencies have a value ≤ the upper value of the indicated class interval for summations from lowest to highest class interval and ≥ the lower value of the indicated class interval for summations from highest to lowest class interval, eg, for counts of people falling into age intervals 25 - 35, 35 - 45, and 45 - 55, if the observed frequencies are 7, 5, and 3, respectively, the corresponding "less than" cumulative frequencies are 7, 12, and 15 and 3, 8, and 15 for the "greater than" cumulative frequencies. rt: **cumulative frequency distribution**

cumulative frequency distribution *n* - A **frequency distribution** of **cumulative frequencies**; referred to as a "less than" cumulative frequency distribution (pictured below) when each successive frequency is the sum of frequencies for the class interval of interest and all others having lower values and to a "greater than" cumulative frequency distribution when each successive frequency is the sum of frequencies for the class interval of interest and all others having higher values. rt: **cumulative frequency**

Cumulative frequency distribution

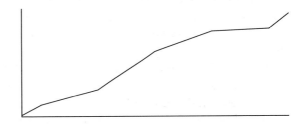

cumulative morbidity *n* - The total **number** of occurrences of an illness or **morbid** condition occurring over a designated **time** for a specified **followup cohort**.

cumulative morbidity curve *n* - A **morbidity curve** that displays the **cumulative** number of illnesses or **morbid events** (or **cumulative morbidity rate**) observed up to a designated **time** for a specified **followup cohort**. rt: **lifetable**

cumulative morbidity rate *n* - **Cumulative morbidity** expressed as a **rate**.

cumulative mortality *n* - The total **number** of deaths occurring over a designated **time** for a specified **followup cohort**.

cumulative mortality curve *n* - A **mortality curve** that displays the **cumulative** number of deaths (or **cumulative mortality rate**) observed up to a designated **time** for a specified **followup cohort**. rt: **lifetable**

cumulative mortality rate *n* - **Cumulative mortality** expressed as a **rate**.

cumulative percent *n* - **percentile**

cumulative survival rate *n* - **survival rate** (defn 1) rt: **conditional survival rate** *Usage note*: See **survival rate**.

currency *n* - 1. General use or acceptance. 2. A medium of **verbal** or intellectual expression.

currency term *n* - 1. A **term** having an underlying implied operational meaning or connotation (eg, terms such as **followup, mask,** or **randomize**). 2. A term having a precise meaning or definition (eg, **random** *adj, scientific,* **arithmetic mean,** and **variance**). 3. A term having an implied **scientific** or **research** value (eg, **case-control study, clinical trial,** or **experiment**). rt: **value laden term, vacuous term, weasel term** *Usage note*: The careful worker and writer takes pains to avoid debasement of currency terms. A common form of debasement arises from use of a currency term in a loose lay sense, such as in *we performed* **random** *blood sugar determinations* or *we selected patients at* **random** *when* **haphazard** is the more appropriate term. Debasement also occurs whenever the worker or writer intermingles lay and scientific usage of a term without distinction, as in *patients* **randomized** *to treatment had* **random** *blood sugars at each followup visit.* Such indiscriminate usage is, at best, likely to confuse readers, and worst yet, cause them to question the **accuracy** and

precision of that being reported. See also notes for **value laden term** and **vacuous term**.

curriculum vitae (CV) *n* - [L, course of (one's) life] A short, tabular-like listing; an account of an individual's life accomplishments, especially in relation to one's profession or work; typically contains selected demographic data, such as one's date of birth and place of birth, a summary of educational and training experiences, current and previous places of employment, honors and awards received, and a listing of pertinent **publications** and **presentations**. syn: vitae

curtail, curtailed, curtailing, curtails *v* - [by folk etymology; fr *curtal* to dock an animal's tail, fr *curtal, n*, docked-tailed animal, fr MF *courtault*] To make or cut short; to abbreviate.

curtailment *n* - The act of **curtailing**; the state of being curtailed.

curve *n* - 1. A **graphic display** consisting of a smooth continuous **line**, straight or curved, or a series of connected lines, that is the result of a plot or tracing arising from a mathematical equation or function, some process, such as **curve fitting**, or from simply joining the point in a plot by a series of straight lines. 2. A mathematical **relationship** that is capable of being displayed graphically, eg, **Gompertz's curve**. 3. A series of points not lying on a straight line; a smooth **continuous** curved line.

curve fit *n* - A **fit** of a straight **line** or smooth **curve** to a set of **data** points; the fit may be by eye, the method of **least squares**, or by some other method.

curve fitting *v* - The process of deriving a **curve** from **observed data** by an **empirical curve fit** or by use of some mathematical model or procedure, such as in a **least squares curve fit**.

cutpoint *n* - 1. The value (**point**) in an ordered **sequence** of **numbers** that is used to separate it into two subparts. 2. **subgrouping cutpoint**

CV *n* - **curriculum vitae**

CVM *n* - **Center for Veterinary Medicine**

Collect no more than 10 times the data needed to answer the question of interest

D

daily *adj* - 1. Occurring, made, or acted upon every **day**. 2. Occurring, made, or acted upon every **weekday**. rt: **day, weekly, monthly, yearly** *Usage note*: See **day** and also **time measure**.

data *n* - [L, pl of **datum**] Factual information, such as **measurements, observations,** or **statistics,** used as a basis for reasoning, discussion, or calculation. In **trials**, the term usually refers to information collected and recorded on **patients** considered for **enrollment** or actually enrolled. rt: **observed data, raw data** *Usage note*: Plural, but also singular, especially in reference to a set or mass of data, as in *data is collected at weekly intervals*. Though use in the singular form is increasingly common, such usage is not recommended.

data analysis *n* - The process of ordering, examining, synthesizing, and interpreting **data**, especially in relation to preparing a **report** or presentation. See *data analysis* for list.

data analysis mask *n* - A **mask** imposed on the process of **data analysis** as a means of keeping those who perform the analysis from knowing or learning of the values of some **variable**, data condition, or data state, to keep that information from influencing their actions or judgments in performing, presenting, or interpreting their analysis, eg, one imposed in the **data coordinating center** for a **clinical trial** in relation to **treatment assignment**. rt: **data analyst mask, data collection mask, reader mask, treatment mask**

data analyst *n* - One who analyzes **data**.

data analyst mask *n* - A **mask** imposed on **data analysis** by masking the **data analyst**. rt: **data analysis mask, data collector mask, reader mask, treater mask**

data and safety monitoring *v* - **Monitoring** of **performance** in relation to **data collection** and **quality** and for **treatment effects**. rt: **data monitoring, performance monitoring, safety monitoring, treatment effects monitoring**

data and safety monitoring committee (DSMC) *n* - 1. A **committee** that performs both **performance** and **treatment effects monitoring**. 2. **treatment effects monitoring committee** syn: **data monitoring committee**

data audit *n* - 1. The **comparison** of **data** in a **source document** with those in a **secondary document** as a means of checking for discrepancies. 2. A comparison of data in a **study form** with those recorded in a **medical chart** for discrepancies. 3. A comparison of specified **data elements** on an **original study form** with the corresponding elements in a **record** or **electronic file** produced from the original for discrepancies.

data bank *n* - 1. A collection of **computer** readable **databases** or **programs**. 2. A place for storing **data; archive; repository**.

data base *n* - **database**

data center *n* - 1. A **center** in a **study** structure that is responsible for receiving, **editing,** processing, **analyzing,** and storing **study data**, but that has few if any of the other responsibilities assumed by a **data coordinating center** or **coordinating center**. 2. **data coordinating center** rt: **biostatistical center, statistical center**

data classification *n* - The act or process of arranging **data** into **classes** or **categories**, eg, as needed for preparing a **frequency distribution**.

data coding *n* - A process involving the **assignment** and use of numeric and letter codes to denote **categories, classes,** or patterns of information represented on a **data form** or in a **record**, eg, the use of the letters M and F to denote the gender of a **study participant** or the assignment of number codes to the different wave forms on an electrocardiogram. rt: **data reduction, data transcription, data transformation**

data coding *v* - The act of transforming **data** into **codes**.

data collection *v* - 1. The act of observing, recording, or assembling **data** for some defined purpose, such as in a **research project**. 2. The act of observing and completing **data forms** on **observation units** of a **study**, as in relation to **patients** in a **trial** at a **clinic**; the act of mailing and receiving forms in the case of **surveys** or **followup** done by mail.

data collection form *n* - A **data form** used for **data collection**.

data collection instrument *n* - **data collection form**

data collection mask *n* - A **mask** imposed on a **data collection** process by masking the **data collector**. rt: **data analysis mask, data analyst mask, data collector mask, reader mask, treater mask, treatment mask**

data collection protocol *n* - 1. The **protocol** for **data collection**. 2. That portion of the **study protocol** concerned with data collection, especially that portion containing details of the **data collection schedule**, data collection procedures, and data to be collected. 3. The **data collection schedule** and associated **data collection forms**. rt: **study protocol, treatment protocol**

data collection schedule *n* - 1. The designated **time points** at which **data** will be collected in a **study**. The **schedule** may be specified by calendar time (as in a **trial** requiring **data collection** on all **study participants** every January and July) or relative to some starting point (as in a trial where data for each person are collected at **randomization** and at 7 and 14 days following randomization). 2. **data collection form** (not recommended usage)

data collection site *n* - 1. A **site** responsible for **data collection**, eg, a **clinic** in a **clinical trial** or a site that mails and receives forms in a **follow-up study** done by mail. 2. **data generation site** (defn 1) *Usage note*: Distinguish between data collection and data generation sites. A data collection site is, by definition, a data generation site, but a data generation site need not be a data collection site, eg, a **reading center** responsible for reading eye fundus photographs taken at a data collection site.

data collection visit *n* - 1. Any **visit** by a **study candidate** or **study participant** to a **study center** for **data collection**. 2. Any **visit** by study personnel to the home or place of residence of a **study candidate** or **study participant** for data collection.

data collector *n* - One who collects or assembles **data**.

data collector mask *n* - A **mask** imposed on **data collection** by masking the **data collector**. rt: **data analyst mask, data collection mask, reader mask, treater mask**

data coordinating center (DCC) *n* - 1. A **center** in a **multicenter study** structure that has the duties of a **data center** (defn 1), as well as duties for coordination of activities related to **data collection**. 2. **coordinating center** (defn 1) *Usage note*: The modifier, **data**, is used to emphasize the data functions of the center, especially in settings involving two or more centers with coordination responsibilities (as in a structure with a **data coordinating center** and **treatment coordinating center**).

data coordinator *n* - 1. An individual in the **data center, data coordinating center**, or **coordinating center** responsible for coordinating the receipt of data from **study centers** and for communicating with them regarding data flow. 2. **study clinic coordinator** (defn 1 or 2)

data dredging *v* - **Data analyses** done on an **ad hoc** basis, without benefit of prior stated **hypotheses**, especially those done with the aim or intent of trying to find noteworthy differences within or among different **subgroups**; **exploratory data analysis**; see **dredge**. *Usage note*: Often used in a pejorative sense, especially in reference to analyses in which it appears that only large differences are presented and where the number of **comparisons** made is not specified.

data editing *v* - 1. The process of reviewing **data** for the purpose of detecting deficiencies or **errors** in the way they are collected or recorded. 2. The actual process of detecting deficient or erroneous values on completed **data forms**. rt: **data query**

data element *n* - A unit of **data** recorded or to be recorded for a specific **data item** or **data field**; **datum**.

data entry *n* - 1. The process of entering **data**, **raw** or edited, into some **database** for storage and subsequent use; typically done by keying responses to queries appearing on a **computer terminal** or by transcribing information contained on a **data form** to produce a mechanically or electronically readable **database**; **data keying**. 2. The process of completing a **data form**. rt: **centralized data entry, distributed data entry, double data entry**

data field *n* - A space on a **data form** or in an **electronic record** designated to contain, or that actually contains, alphabetic and/or numeric characters of information recorded in response to a specific **data item** on the form.

data file *n* - A collection of **data records**, as contained on paper forms or in electronic **records**, arrayed or organized in some fashion.

data form *n* - 1. A collection of **data items** as contained on or in a **data record**. 2. A **form** containing **data**. 3. A form, **paper** or **electronic**, for **data collection**. rt: **case report form**

data freeze *n* - **Data** held in a fixed state, especially such a state imposed on an active **database** or **data file** in order to complete some task requiring a stable, nonchanging, database or data file (eg, as required for preparation of a **treatment effects monitoring report**). rt: **data snapshot**

data freeze *v* - The act or process of **freezing** an active **database** or **file** in order to hold in a fixed state, eg, as required for preparation of a **treatment effects monitoring report**.

data generation *n* - 1. **data collection** (defn 1) 2. The **generation** of **data** from specimens, documents, or materials collected by others, eg, data generated from blood samples received at a **laboratory** or from readings of fundus photographs made at a **reading center**.

data generation site *n* - 1. A **site** that generates **data** from existing **records**, eg, a **reading center**. 2. **data collection site** *Usage note*: See note for **data collection site**.

data item *n* - 1. A written **request**, usually in the form of an instruction, statement, or question, and associated **data field** for **response**, especially such a request and field as contained in a **data form**. 2. The response to such a request. 3. **data field**

data keying *n* - A process involving use of a keyboard and defined key strokes to represent observed **data**; **data entry**.

data management *n* - A constellation of activities, typically performed by a **data center**, **data coordinating center**, or **coordinating center**, related to receiving, editing, updating, storing, and retrieving **data** for some specified task or function.

data manager *n* - One who manages **data** or who is involved in **data management**.

data monitoring *v* - 1. **Monitoring** related to the process of **data collection**. 2. Monitoring related to the detection of problems in the execution of a **study** (**performance monitoring**) or for detecting **treatment effects** (**treatment monitoring**). rt: **data and safety monitoring, performance monitoring, safety monitoring, treatment effects monitoring**

data monitoring committee (DMC) *n* - A committee with defined responsibilities for **data monitoring**, eg, as required in **performance** or **treatment effects monitoring**. syn: **data and safety monitoring committee, performance monitoring committee, safety monitoring committee, treatment effects monitoring committee, treatment effects and performance monitoring committee, treatment effects monitoring and analysis committee** *Usage note*: Not recommended because of ambiguities regarding domain of responsibility. Use a more specific term denoting the area of responsibility of the committee, eg, **treatment effects monitoring committee** when the committee has responsibility for **treatment monitoring**.

data monitoring report *n* - 1. A **report** of some aspect of **data monitoring**. 2. A **report**, containing summary **tabulations** and **analyses**, prepared in relation to a data monitoring activity; such a report as seen by a **data monitoring committee**; **performance monitoring report**; **treatment effects monitoring committee**.

data processing *n* - 1. The constellation of activities related to **inventorying** and entering **data**. 2. Those activities performed subsequent to **data entry** in relation to **editing, updating**, and **analyzing**; especially activities performed in relation to the creation and maintenance of an **electronic database**.

data purge *n* - The removal of specified **data elements** from a **dataset** because of known or suspected deficiencies; eg, data known to have been or suspected of having been fabricated.

data query *n* - A **query** regarding a **data element** or **item**. rt: **data editing, edit query**

data record *n* - A collection of data **items**, as contained in a **paper** or **electronic form**, treated as a **unit** for some defined purpose or function.

data reduction *n* - The process of condensing **data**, by codification, grouping, summarization, and other means so as to make them more amenable to storage and processing.

data simple *adj* - Of, relating to, or characterized by **data collection** procedures and requirements that are **simple** (defn 2).

data simple trial *n* - A **trial** having a **parallel treatment design** and **simple** (defn 2) **data collection** procedures, especially one in which essential **baseline** and **followup data** are recorded on a few short, simple forms and having death or some other **clinical event** that can be reliably observed without use of elaborate diagnostic tests or procedures, as the **outcome** of sole or **primary** interest. rt: **big trial, simple trial, big and simple trial** *Usage note*: See **simple trial**.

data snapshot *n* - A **snapshot** of an active **database** or **file**; generally not preceded by any special effort to ensure **clean data**. rt: **data freeze**

data system *n* - A collection of interrelated procedures and routines (performed by hand or **computer**) that are used in the creation and maintenance of a **database** or some data-related function, such as **data analysis**. rt: **centralized data system, distributed data system**

data transcription *n* - 1. **Transcription** of **data** onto a **data collection form**. 2. Transcription of data already recorded on a data collection form to some other form, document, or list; not to be confused with **data coding** or **data editing**.

data transformation *n* - 1. A one-to-one mapping of **data** from one **measurement scale** to another; typically performed to simplify calculations for **data analysis** or to provide data having distributional or other properties better suited than the **original** to some form of display or statistical analysis. 2. Any form of **data reduction** or simplification, regardless of whether or not a one-to-one mapping, eg, the distillation of multiple **outcome measures** into a single **composite outcome**. 3. **data coding** rt: **inverse sine transformation, log transformation, square root transformation, standard score, T-score, Z-transformation, Z-score**

database *n* - 1. A collection of related **data** or related **data files**, organized for ease and efficiency of use, especially in relation to activities such as those involving retrieving or updating specific files or **data fields**. 2. **analysis database** 3. **electronic database** rt: **centralized database, distributed database**

database management system *n* - A collection of structured procedures and routines, usually involving **computers** and **programs**, used for entering, sorting, editing, storing, and retrieving **data**.

dataset *n* - 1. A collection of **information** organized and arrayed in some way for convenience of access and use. 2. **electronic dataset** *Usage note*: Subject to varying uses, often used in references to **electronic database** but may refer to collections of information not amenable to electronic processing or manipulation. In the setting of **trials**, often used in references to collections of **data** on defined **populations** observed at one or more **time points** over the course of **observation**, but may also refer to such collections for a single **variable**. rt: **database**

date *n* - [ME, fr ME, fr LL *data*, fr *data* (as in *data Romae* given in Rome), fem of L *datus*, pp of *dare* to give; akin to L *dos* gift, dowry Gk *didonai* to give] 1. The time at which an **event** occurred or occurs, eg, **date of birth**. 2. A statement of time of execution or completion, eg, the date a form is completed. 3. An appointment for a designated time, eg, as for a **clinic visit**.

date of birth *n* - 1. The **date** a person is or was born. 2. The date something comes into being. rt: **birthdate**

datum *n* - [L, fr neut, of *datus*] A single **data element**; singular of **data**. rt: **data** *Usage note*: Not in common usage. See note for **data**.

daughter *adj* - 1. Belonging to the first generation of offspring produced by reproduction, division, or replication. 2. A structure, unit, or organization created and nurtured by a **parent**.

daughter *n* - [ME *doughter*, fr OE *dohtor*; akin to OHG *tohter* daughter, Gk *thygater*] 1. Human female having the relation of a **child** to **parents**. 2. Something considered as a **daughter**.

daughter center *n* - A **center** that is established and nurtured by a **parent center**. rt: **affiliate center, associate center, satellite center, sister center**

daughter clinic *n* - A **clinic** that is established and nurtured by a **parent clinic**. rt: **affiliate clinic, associate clinic, satellite clinic, sister clinic**

daughter study *n* - A **study** that is established and nurtured by a **parent study**. rt: **ancillary study, sister study**

day *n* - [ME, fr OE *dæg*; akin to OHG *tag* day] 1. The time of light between one night and the next; that portion of a 24-hour period in which most work and business activities are performed, such as 9:00 AM to 5:00 PM. 2. The time required for the earth to make one revolution on its axis; a 24-hour period starting at midnight. 3. A specified day or **date**. rt: **daily, week, month, year** *Usage note*: Subject to confusion when used as a time measure in the sense of defns 1 or 2; avoid by being explicit as to nature of usage. Avoid use of the term **day** in the two senses without distinction. See also **time measure**.

DCC *n* - **data coordinating center**

death rate *n* - **mortality rate**

debug, debugged, debugging, debugs *v* - The process of locating and removing **errors** or malfunctioning parts or components, eg, in a **computer program**.

decile *n* - [L *decem* ten] A **range** (defn 2) that accounts for one-tenth of the total counts represented in a **frequency distribution**. See *quantile* for list.

decimal *adj* - [(assumed) NL *decimalis*, fr ML, of a tithe, fr L *decima* tithe] Numbered or proceeding by tens; based on the number 10, especially when expressed in or utilizing decimal notation as denoted by use of a **decimal point**. 2. Subdivided into 10th or 100th units.

decimal number system *n* - 1. A number system of base 10 in which **numbers** are represented by sums of terms corresponding to the digits in the number and where the term for a designated **digit** position (determined by counting from right to left starting with 0) of the number is the product of the digit occupying that position and of 10 raised to the power corresponding to its position, eg, 71 corresponds to $(7)(10^1)$ + $(1)(10^0)$. 2. Such a system in which numbers are expressed using decimal points to separate whole numbers from remaining decimal fractions. rt: **binary number system, hexadecimal number system**

decimal point *n* - A dot, similar in form and positioning on a line to a period, that separates a whole number from the remaining decimal fraction.

declaration *n* - The act of declaring; something declared; a document containing such a declaration.

Declaration of Helsinki *n* - **World Medical Association Declaration of Helsinki**

dedicate, dedicated *adj* - Given over to a particular purpose, function, or use.

dedicated computer *n* - A **computer** that is under the control of a single user (or a few users) and used for a specified **project**, function, or activity.

deduce, deduced, deducing, deduces *v* - [L *deducere*, lit, to lead away, fr *de-* + *ducere* to lead] 1. To determine by **deduction**; to **infer** from general **principles**. 2. To **trace** the course of.

deduct, deducted, deducting, deducts *v* - [L *deductus*, pp of *deducere*] 1. To take away from a **total**; **subtract** from. 2. To **deduce** or **infer**.

deduction *n* - 1. The derivation of a **conclusion** by reasoning; **inference** in which the conclusion about particulars follows necessarily from the general or universal. 2. Something **subtracted** or **deducted**. rt: **induction**

defer, deferred, deferring, defers *v* - [MF *deferren*, *differren*, fr MF *deferer*, *defferer*, fr LL *deferre*, fr L, to bring down, bring, fr *de-* + *ferre* to carry] 1. To delegate to another. 2. To postpone or put off to a future **time**.

deferred consent *n* - [trials] **Consent** delayed or postponed beyond the point of **treatment assignment** or start of **treatment** because of trauma causing unconsciousness or other conditions precluding consent before **enrollment** and treatment assignment; the actual **consent process** being deferred or delayed until the person (or that person's guardian) is in a position to give or withhold consent [eg, as reported by the Brain Resuscitation Clinical Trial II Study Group, 1991].[13] See Levine [1991][89] and Fost and Robertson [1980][53] for discussion of conditions of use. rt: **post-assignment consent**

definitive *adj* - [ME *diffinity*, fr MF *definitif*, fr L *definitivus*, fr *definitus*] Serving to provide a final solution or answer; authoritative and conclusive. *Usage note*: Best avoided, except in contradistinction to **preliminary**, or other modifiers suggesting something preliminary, such as **pilot** or **feasible**, or sometimes as a synonym for **full-scale**. Avoid as a characterization of one's own work; likely to be viewed as wishful thinking or arrogance. Even in settings where the term is justified, eg, usages in the sense of defn 1 for **definitive trial**, the term should be used with caution since the characterization is usually applied to things done in the past and considered to be important rather than as a promise of things to come. See **definitive trial** for additional comments.

definitive trial *n* - 1. A **trial** intended to answer an important question, especially one that is planned to have or one that has an adequate **sample size**, as measured by the **type I** and **type II error** protection provided. 2. **full-scale trial** (defn 1) 3. A **trial** done in the past, judged to have been **definitive** because of the results it produced or the impact it had or has on changing a practice or procedure. *Usage note*: Acceptable in the sense of defns 1 and 2, but best avoided even in these senses and replaced with some other more descriptive, less judgmental term such as **full-scale trial**. Usage is best reserved for characterizations of works by others done in the past and considered to have been of major importance.

degree *adj* - amount, extent

degree *n* - [ME, fr OF *degre*, fr (assumed) VL *degradus*, fr L *de-* + *gradus*] 1. A step or stage in a process, course, or order of **classification**. 2. A **measure** of damage to tissue caused by disease or injury. 3. The extent, measure, or scope of an action, condition, or relation. 4. One of the divisions or **intervals** marked on a **measurement scale** or on a measuring **device**. 5. Any of various **units** for measuring temperature. 6. A 360th part of the circumference of a circle. 7. The sum of the exponents of the **variables** in the term of highest degree in a polynomial, polynomial function, or polynomial equation.

degree of confidence *n* - **confidence level**

degrees of freedom (df) *n* - An integer number associated with a **statistic**, such as a **variance** or **test statistic**, corresponding to the number of **independent** and unrestricted values that are needed to determine its value.

Delaney Amendment *n* - [after chief sponsor, James J Delaney, Rep, D - NY; 1945 - 47; 1949 - 78] An amendment to the Food, Drug and Cosmetic Act requiring the **FDA** to prohibit the sale of any food additive shown to cause cancer in laboratory animals.

delta *n* - [ME *deltha*, fr Gk *delta*, of Sem origin; akin to Heb *dāleth* daleth] 1. The 4th letter of the **Greek alphabet**, uppercase Δ, lowercase δ.

2. **change** 3. A small increment in the value of a **variable**.

demographer *n* - One trained in **demography** or who uses the methods and procedures of **demography** for **collection** or **analysis** of **data** related to the study of human populations.

demographic *adj* - Of or relating to the nature, characteristics, and density of a **population**.

demographic data *n* - 1. Factual information on the size, density, distribution, and **vital statistics** of a human **population**. 2. Factual information such as age, gender, marital status, race, etc, collected or recorded for an individual or set of individuals.

demography *n* - [F *démographie*, fr Gk *dēmos* people + F *-graphie* -graphy] A **discipline** devoted to the study of human **populations** with respect to size, distribution, density, and **vital statistics**.

demonstrate, demonstrated, demonstrating, demonstrates *v* - [L *demonstratus*, pp of *demonstrare*, fr *de-* + *monstrare* to show] 1. To show clearly. 2. To **prove**. 3. To make clear by reasoning or evidence; to illustrate by example.

demonstration *n* - An act, process, or means of **demonstrating** by providing proof or derivation or by show of merit or function.

demonstration study *n* - 1. A **study** that is undertaken to **demonstrate** or establish the practicality or feasibility of some procedure or approach; sometimes also **pilot study** or **feasibility study**. 2. **demonstration trial**

demonstration trial *n* - 1. A **trial** that is undertaken to **demonstrate** the practicality or feasibility of administering some **treatment**; sometimes also **pilot trial** or **feasibility trial**. 2. A trial that is undertaken to establish or **prove** (defn 6) some treatment to be superior to another. rt: **community trial, effectiveness trial, field trial, management trial** *Usage note*: Best avoided in the sense of defn 1; use **feasibility trial** or **pilot trial** to avoid confusion with uses in the sense of defn 2. Generally, use in the sense of defn 2 is in regard to a trial of an **effective** treatment aimed **proving** its value so as to promote its use. **Demonstration** in the sense of defn 2 is likely to raise questions regarding the **ethics** underlying the trial to the extent that it is motivated by a desire to **prove** the value of a treatment in the absence of a legitimate state of **equipoise**.

denominator *n* - 1. The devisor of a fraction, eg, 7 in the fraction 5/7 (may also be written as 5 ÷ 7); the **number** by which the **numerator** of a fraction is divided. 2. The number of individual elements comprising a **total** or whole, such as the number of **patients** enrolled in a **trial**.

density *n* - 1. The quality or state of being dense. 2. The quantity per unit volume, unit length, or unit area, eg, the number of residents per square mile or number of dwellings per square mile.

density function *n* - **probability density function**

Department of Health and Human Services (DHHS) *n* - A **department** in the executive arm of the United States Government, responsible for agencies concerned with health and human services; includes the **United States Public Health Service** (USPHS) and the **National Institutes of Health** (NIH) as a part of the USPHS. Created in 1980 with the dissolution of the Department of Health, Education, and Welfare (DHEW).

Department of Health, Education, and Welfare (DHEW) *n* - See **Department of Health and Human Services**.

departure *n* - Divergence or **deviation** from a **standard**; the act or instance of departing.

dependence *n* - The state or quality of being influenced or determined by, or being subject to another. ant: **independence**

dependent *adj* - [ME *dependant*, fr MF, prp of *dependre*] 1. Something that is conditioned, determined, or fixed by another. 2. Not mathematically **independent**. ant: **independent**

dependent double data entry *n* - **Double data entry** with both entries performed by the same person at the same time. rt: **independent double data entry, quasi-independent double data entry**

dependent random variable *n* - A **random variable** subject to the influence of other variables in regard to the values it assumes; a variable that is not **independent**. ant: **independent random variable** rt: **dependent variable**

dependent variable *n* - A **variable** that is **dependent** on one or more other **variables**; typically the variable appearing to the left of the equal sign in an **equation**; often designated by **y** or **Y**, as in $y = a + bx + e$. ant: **independent variable** rt: **dependent random variable**

DES *n* - **Drug Efficacy Study**

describe, described, describing, describes *v* - [L *describere*, fr *de-* + *scribere* to write] 1. To represent or to give an account of in words, oral or written. 2. To represent or characterize by **data** or factual information. 3. To represent by a figure, **model**, or picture.

descriptive *adj* - 1. Serving to **describe**. 2. Referring to, constituting, or grounded in matters of **observation** or experience.

descriptive epidemiology *n* - 1. That subpart of **epidemiology** concerned primarily with the assembly of **data** for describing the occurrence of **disease** or other health conditions in human **populations** and the factors associated with those diseases or health conditions. 2. **epidemiological study** rt: **clinical epidemiology, experimental epidemiology**

descriptive statistic *n* - Any **statistic** that describes or that may be used to describe a **population**, process, or procedure, eg, **mean** and **variance** of a **dataset**.

descriptive study *n* - [epidemiology] A **study** undertaken primarily for the purpose of obtaining **data** intended to **describe** some **population** or aspect of a population. rt: **epidemiological study, observational study**

DESI *n* - **Drug Efficacy Study Implementation**

design *n* - 1. A plan or **protocol** for carrying out something, such as a **study** or an **experiment**. 2. **experimental design** 3. **treatment assignment design**

design, designed, designing, designs *v* - [MF *designer*, fr L *designare*, fr *de-* + *signare* to mark, mark out] To conceive, create, plan, or fashion, as in designing an **experiment**.

design unit *n* - [trials] 1. The **observation unit** used for **sample size calculations**, usually persons, but sometimes a smaller unit (eg, eyes) or larger unit (eg, members of a family). 2. **treatment unit**

design variable *n* - [trials] The **variable** used for **sample size calculations**. rt: **primary outcome variable**

designed meta-analysis *n* - A **meta-analysis** based on or to be based on **data** from two or more studies designed with the intent of pooling for meta-analysis; also **planned meta-analysis** (not recommended, see usage note for **planned meta-analysis**). ant: **ad hoc meta-analysis**

desk *n* - [ME *deske*, fr ML *desca*, modif of OIt *desco* table, fr L *discus* dish, disc] 1. A table, counter, stand, or booth at which one performs tasks involving reading and paper and pencil tasks. 2. A place of activity associated with a designated position or person.

desk audit *n* - 1. An **audit** performed at a desk of operation. 2. **off-site record audit**

destroy, destroyed, destroying, destroys *v* - [ME *destroyen*, fr OF *destruire*, fr (assumed) VL *destrugere*, alter of L *destruere*, fr *de-* + *struere* to build] To tear down or break up; demolish.

destructive *adj* - Designed or intended to disprove or discredit.

destructive data analysis *n* - **Analysis** aimed at challenging a finding or **conclusion**; done primarily as a means of assessing the **robustness** of a finding or conclusion prior to **presentation** or **publication** by use of an analysis approach or assumptions considered to be most likely to disprove or discredit the finding. rt: **worst case analysis, sensitivity analysis**

determinant *n* - 1. An element, condition, or **factor** that determines or causes the nature of something. 2. Something that fixes or conditions an **outcome**. 3. A square array of numbers, called the elements of the determinant, enclosed by brackets or by vertical straight lines, symbolizing the sum of certain products of those elements. The number of **rows** or **columns** in the array is called the order of the determinant. rt: **matrix**

develop, developed, developing, develops *v* - [F *développer*, fr MF *desveloper, desvoluper*, fr *des-* de- + *-veloper, -voluper* (as in MF *enveloper* to enclose)] 1. To realize the potential of. 2. To come to have gradually; to acquire. 3. To cause to unfold gradually. 4. To set forth or make clear by degree or detail. 5. To work out the possibilities of.

development *n* - 1. The act, process, or result of **developing**. 2. The state of being developed.

deviate *n* - The amount a **variable** differs from some standard point of location, usually the **mean**; often presented as a standardized value, eg, a **normal deviate**.

deviate, deviated, deviating, deviates *v* - [LL *deviatus*, pp of *deviare*, fr L *de-* + *via* way] 1. To stray or move away from. 2. To depart from a **plan, standard**, or **norm**.

deviation *n* - 1. An act or instance of deviating or departing from some value or **standard**. 2. The difference between a value of the **frequency distribution** and a fixed **number**, such as the **mean**. 3. **difference** (defn 1) 4. **protocol departure**

deviation from mean *n* - The **signed** amount a given value of a **variable** differs from the **mean** for that variable; derived by subtracting the value from the mean. rt: **absolute deviation from mean**

device *n* - [ME *devis, devise*, fr MF, division, intention, fr OF *deviser* to divide, regulate, tell] 1. Something devised or contrived, such as a plan, procedure, scheme, or strategy. 2. A piece of equipment or mechanism designed to serve a special purpose or perform a special function; **input/output device**. 3. **medical device**

df *n* - **degrees of freedom**

DHHS *n* - **Department of Health and Human Services**

diagnosis *n* - [NL, fr Gk *diagnōsis*, fr *diagignōskein* to distinguish, fr *dia-* + *gignōskein* to know] 1. The act or process of identifying a **disease** from **signs** and **symptoms**; the decision reached in such a process. 2. An **investigation** or **analysis** of the cause or nature of a condition, situation, or problem; the conclusion drawn from such an investigation or analysis.

diagnostic *adj* - Of or relating to **diagnosis**, especially of **disease**.

diagnostic trial *n* - A **trial** designed to evaluate the usefulness of some **diagnostic** procedure, tool, kit, or **device**.

diagram *n* - [Gk *diagramma*, fr *diagraphein* to mark out by lines, fr *dia-* + *graphein* to write] 1. A **graphic display** intended to explain rather than accurately represent, eg, a drawing showing arrangements and relations in a schematic fashion. 2. A line drawing displaying a mathematical relationship or made to display some process. rt: **figure, graph**

dial, dialed, dialing, dials *v* - To make a telephone call or connection.

dichotomous *adj* - [LL *dichotomos*, fr Gk, fr *dich-* + *temnein* to cut] 1. Dividing into two parts. 2. Relating to, involving, or proceeding from dichotomy.

dichotomous variable *n* - A **discrete variable** that may assume only one of two values. syn:

binary variable

differ, differed, differing, differs *v* - [ME *differen*, fr MF or L; MF *differer* to postpone, be different, fr L *differre*, fr *dis-* + *ferre* to carry] To be unlike or distinct in nature, form, or value.

difference *n* - 1. The amount by which a value departs or **differs** from another. 2. The amount by which a value or function differs from itself as measured at two distinct and different times points; **change** (defn 2). 3. An important or significant change, as in a **clinically meaningful difference**.

digit *n* - [ME, fr L *digtus* finger, toe] 1. One of the 10 Arabic numerals, 0 through 9. 2. Any numeral or character used in a number system, such as the **hexadecimal number system**, to form a **number**.

digit bias *n* - A **bias** associated with a **measurement** (such as that for blood pressure) that causes the **distribution** of the terminal **digit** of such **measurements** to depart from the one **expected**; typically the result of **digit preference** on the part of the person making or recording the measurement.

digit preference *n* - A tendency to favor some **digits** over others in a **measurement** or recording process, as in **digit bias**.

digital *adj* - [L *digitalis*] 1. Of or relating to the fingers or toes; done with a finger. 2. Of or relating to **calculation** by numerical methods or by discrete units. 3. Of or relating to **data** in the form of numerical digits. ant: **analog** 4. Providing a readout in numerical digits.

digital computer *n* - A **computer** in which information used in its operations is processed as if represented by **digits** of a **number system**, such as in the **binary number system**. ant: **analog computer**

digitize, digitizing, digitized, digitizes *v* - To convert **data** to **digital** form; the conversion of an **analog** tracing, eg, as represented on an oscilloscope or in a paper tracing made from the oscilloscope, to digital form.

direct *adj* - [ME, fr L *directus* straight] 1. Stemming or arising from a source without intervening conditions or constraints. 2. Proceeding from one point to another in time or space without deviation or interruption; proceeding by the shortest way. ant: **indirect**

direct contact *n* - 1. A **contact** of one person or party with another person or party directly, without the use or involvement of intermediary agents or parties, eg, **direct patient contact**. 2. **contact** (defn 2) ant: **indirect contact**

direct cost *n* - A **cost**, expressed in **relative** or **absolute** monetary terms, arising or incurred as a **direct** consequence of making a product or performing a service and exclusive of **indirect costs**; typically the costs of salaries and fringe benefits, machinery, supplies, and materials needed for making the product or performing the service. ant: **indirect cost** rt: **total cost**

direct data entry *n* - 1. **on-line data entry** 2. **Data entry** done from **paper forms** completed during the **data collection** process without any intermediate **coding** or **transcription**. 3. Data entry done at the **generation site**. ant: **indirect data entry**

direct distribution of funds *n* - **Distribution of funds** to **centers** in a **study** directly from the **sponsor** via **direct funding awards**. ant: **indirect distribution of funds**

direct funding award *n* - A **funding award** (**grant** or **contract**) received directly from the **sponsor**. ant: **indirect funding award**

direct patient contact *n* - [trials] The establishment of a **contact** between a **patient** and **study clinic**, usually arising as a result of an action by the clinic, eg, contacts that arise from a clinic reviewing its medical records to identify **candidates** for a trial, and then contacting those so identified without use of intermediaries or **surrogates**. ant: **indirect patient contact**

direct patient recruitment *n* - Any method of **patient recruitment** that involves **direct patient contact**. ant: **indirect patient recruitment**

direct rate adjustment *n* - A **method** of **adjustment** used for comparing **rates** observed in different **populations** having different **distributions** for a **variable** or combination of variables affecting, or presumed to affect, the rates, eg, such a method applied to **mortality rates** in populations having different age and gender distributions. The adjustment is done by specifying a **standard population** and calculating a **weighted mean** of the observed rates in each population for the distribution specified. The resulting rates are said to be adjusted for the variables represented in the standard population. See **indirect rate adjustment** for alternative method.[72] rt: **standardization, standardized rate**

direct research cost *n* - **Direct cost** expected or incurred in relation to a **research project** or activity. rt: **indirect research cost, total research cost**

direct standardization *n* - **direct rate adjustment**

director *n* - 1. The administrative or administrative and scientific head of an institution or organization, or of a **center**, department, or **group**. 2. **center director**

dirty *adj* - Contaminated; not clean or pure. ant: **clean**

dirty data *n* - 1. **Data** containing **errors** and deficiencies. 2. unedited data 3. Data with outstanding **edit queries** awaiting resolution. ant: **clean data**

disagree, disagreed, disagreeing, disagrees *v* - [ME *disagreen*, fr MF *desagreer*, fr *des-* + *agreer* to agree] 1. To be dissimilar or different. 2. To fail to **agree**. ant: **agree**

disagreement *n* - 1. The act or fact of **disagreeing**; dissimilarity of action, course, or character. 2. The state of being at **variance**; disparity. ant: **agreement**

disciplinary *adj* - Of or relating to a particular field of **study**.

discipline *n* - [ME, fr OF & L; OF, fr L *disciplina* teaching, learning, fr *discipulus* pupil] A field of **study**; a subject that is taught.

disclose, disclosed, disclosing, discloses *v* - [ME *disclosen*, fr MF *desclos-*, stem of *desclore* to disclose, fr ML *disclaudere* to open, fr L *dis-* + *claudere* to close] 1. To reveal; to make known or public. 2. To open for view.

disclosure *n* - 1. The act of revealing to or informing others of facts important or having the potential of being important in regard to some action planned or in regard to the meaning or interpretation to be given to presentations or representations of the person or party making the disclosure. 2. An act or instance of **disclosing**, revealing, or informing.

disclosure and consent form *n* - A **form** including narrative intended to **disclose** for the purpose of informing and for documenting the fact of **consent**. syn: **consent form** rt: **disclosure form**

disclosure form *n* - 1. A **form** used to solicit or record factual information regarding real or

potential **conflicts of interest**. 2. A **form** including narrative intended to **disclose** for the purpose of informing; **consent form** (not recommended usage)

disclosure statement *n* - 1. A **statement** presented to a person or party for the purpose of making known facts or information considered important for that person or party in making a decision or judgment in regard to some action planned or in the interpretation to be given to a representation or presentation by the person or party making the **disclosure**; especially such a statement, written or oral, presented as a prelude to an act, such as signing a legal document or enrolling in some activity. 2. A written signed statement disclosing facts and conditions (or absence thereof) considered to be of importance in understanding, interpreting, or using the document accompanying the statement or to which appended and that are not likely to be known or fully appreciated by intended recipients of the statement, eg, in the case of a **manuscript** from a **trial**, a statement affixed to or accompanying it disclosing the nature and extent of the proprietary or financial interests of its authors in the **treatment**(s) evaluated, or that attests to the absence of such interests. 3. **consent statement** (not recommended usage)

discrete *adj* - [ME, fr L *discretus*] Individually distinct, taking on or having a **finite** or countably **infinite** number of values; not mathematically **continuous**. ant: **continuous**

discrete data *n* - **Data** based on a **discrete variable**, such as **counts** of children in a family. See *data type* for list. ant: **continuous data**

discrete variable *n* - A **variable** that is capable of assuming only **discrete** values. ant: **continuous variable** rt: **dichotomous variable, polychotomous variable**

disease *n* - [ME *disese*, fr MF *desaise*, fr *des-* dis- + *aise* ease; literally, the opposite of ease] Broadly, an abnormal state or condition of an organism or of one of its parts or bodily systems that impairs normal function, especially a state or condition due to infection, weakness, or stress. In human beings, a **morbid** process, state, or condition having a characteristic presentation or course and distinguished from other forms of **morbidity** by a unique constellation of **signs** and **symptoms**.

disease natural history *n* - 1. The course of a **disease** left untreated. 2. The course of disease, treated or untreated. 3. The course of a disease treated with standard modes of therapy. syn: natural history of disease

disk *n* - [L *discus*] [**computer**] A circular rigid plate, coated with magnetic material and used for the electronic storage of **data**; done via an **input/output device** designed to read information from and write information to the disk when rotating at a specified speed.

diskette *n* - [**computer**] A round, thin, flat, flexible platter-like object, coated with magnetic material and used for electronic storage of **data**; done via an **input/output device** designed to read information from and write information to the diskette when rotating at a specified speed. Also floppy disk.

dispersion *n* - 1. The **scatter** of the values of a **frequency distribution** from its **average**. 2. The act or process of dispersing; the state of being dispersed.

distribute, distributed, distributing, distributes *v* - [ME *distributen*, fr L *distributus*, pp of *distribuere*, fr dis- + *tribuere* to allot] 1. To divide or apportion. 2. To spread out or **scatter**. 3. To give out or deliver.

distributed data analysis *n* - [**multicenter studies**] 1. An arrangement in which **investigators** at individual **data generation sites** have responsibilities for **analyses** of **data** generated at those sites; such a setting where investigators at each such site have the option of analyzing their own data if they so choose, eg, in an **unmasked multicenter trial** having a **coordinating center** responsible for analysis and having **distributed data entry** or a **distributed database**. 2. An arrangement in which investigators at the various **data generation sites** carry out or may carry out analyses of study data by having **direct** access, usually via some electronic linkage, to the **analysis database** of the **study**, or portions thereof; such an arrangement but where investigators at all centers, regardless of whether a data generation site, have such rights or responsibilities. ant: **centralized data analysis**

distributed data entry *n* - [**multicenter study**] A form of **data entry** in which **data** are keyed at the **collection** or **generation sites**. ant: **centralized data entry**

distributed data system *n* - A **data system** consisting of component parts that are established and maintained at individual **data collection** or **generation sites** in a **multicenter** structure and where those sites perform functions similar to those performed at the **data coordinating center** for creating and maintaining a **centralized data system**. ant: **centralized data entry**

distributed database *n* - A **database** assembled from component parts residing at different institutions or at different locations in the same institution, eg, a database comprised of **data** generated and keyed at the various **data generation sites** in a **multicenter study**. ant: **centralized database**

distributed funding *n* - A method of funding **centers** in **multicenter** structures in which funds are awarded to individual centers directly from the **funding agency**. ant: **centralized funding**

distribution *n* - 1. The act or process of distributing. 2. The position, arrangement, **dispersion**, or occurrence throughout space or over a defined space or time period. 3. **frequency distribution**

distribution center *n* - [**multicenter study**] 1. A **center** that is responsible for distributing funds, some product, or commodity to associated **centers**, especially one with that function as its primary or sole responsibility. 2. **procurement and distribution center**

distribution function *n* - 1. The count of elements in a **frequency distribution** for a **variable** at or below a specified value. 2. Such a function for unit total frequency; values correspond to **proportions** for $\leq$ x; **probability distribution function**.

distribution of funds *n* - The act or process of distributing **funds**, directly or indirectly, to the various **sites** within a structure for the purpose of performing some activity or function. rt: **direct distribution of funds, indirect distribution of funds**

distribution-free *adj* - [**statistics**] Of or relating to a **method** of **inference**, as in **hypothesis testing**, not **dependent** on the form, shape, or nature of the underlying **distribution** of the **variable** of interest; **nonparametric**.

distribution-free method *n* - [**statistics**] A method of **inference**, as in **hypothesis testing**, not **dependent** on the form, shape, or nature of the underlying **distribution** of the **variable** of interest; **nonparametric method**.

diurnal *adj* - [ME, fr L *diurnalis*] 1. Recurring every **day**; having a daily period or cycle. 2. Of, relating to, or occurring in the daytime. rt: **circadian** *Usage note*: Note that usages in the sense of defn 1 are subject to confusion in that the cycle or period could be one of 24 hours, or day (as opposed to night). Be explicit as to time reference; use circadian when the time reference is to a 24-hour period.

diurnal variation *n* - **Variation** that is due to or associated with **time** of **day**. rt: **circadian variation** *Usage note*: See **diurnal**.

divide, divided, dividing, divides *v* - [ME *dividen*, fr L *dividere*, fr *dis-* + *-videre* to separate] 1. To subject a number or quantity to the operation of finding how many times it contains another number or quantity; to perform mathematical division. 2. To separate into two or more parts, areas, or groups. ant: **multiply** rt: **subtract**

division *n* - [ME, fr MF, fr L *division-*, *divisio*, fr *divisus*, pp of *dividere* to divide] 1. One of the parts or groupings into which a whole is divided; **section**. 2. The act or process of **dividing**; the mathematical operation of dividing. ant: **multiplication** rt: **subtraction**

Division of Research Grants (DRG) *n* - A **division** within the **National Institutes of Health**; responsibilities include receipt of **research grant applications**, assignment to institutes of the NIH for **funding** (if ultimately approved for funding), assignment to **study sections** for review, and maintenance and direction of merit reviews as performed by study sections (standing or **ad hoc**).

DMC *n* - **data monitoring committee**

document *n* - [ME, fr MF, fr LL & L; LL *documentum* official paper, fr L *lesson*, proof, fr *docēre* to teach] 1. An **original** or official **record** offered or relied upon as a basis for an action, claim, or statement. 2. Any written work, such as a **manuscript** or **medical record**, that serves as a basis for an action, claim, or statement.

document, documented, documenting, documents *v* - 1. To provide documentary evidence. 2. To furnish with **documents**. 3. To provide with factual information such as exact references

or authoritative statements to substantiate a claim or statement.

documentation *n* - 1. The act or process of furnishing or authenticating with **documents**. 2. The use of **documents** in substantiating or authenticating a claim or statement. 3. The use of **reference citations** and notes to support statements or claims made in written works.

documented assent *n* - 1. Documented evidence of **assent** by the presence of a signed and dated **assent form** in the **file** of a **study subject**; **signed assent**. 2. **witnessed assent** (defn 1 or 2); as in the case of an **oral assent**, by presence of a **document** detailing the nature of the information imparted, the date assent was obtained, and bearing the signature of the person requesting assent and that of a witness. rt: **signed assent, witnessed assent**

documented consent *n* - 1. **Documented** evidence of **consent** by the presence of a signed and dated **consent form** in the **file** of a **study subject**; **signed consent**. 2. **witnessed consent** (defns 1 or 2); as in the case of an **oral consent**, by presence of a document detailing the nature of the information imparted, the date consent was obtained, and bearing the signature of the person requesting the consent and that of a witness. rt: **signed consent, witnessed consent**

dosage *n* - 1. The determination and regulation of **doses**. 2. The amount, **frequency**, and number of **doses** administered or to be administered to or taken by a **patient** over a specified **time period**. 3. The amount of something received. 4. **exposure** *Usage note*: Sometimes used as if synonymous with **dose**, as in the sense of defn 3 above and defn 2 for **dose**. However, the two terms have different primary meanings, as seen by comparison of their respective first definitions and, hence, should not be confused or interchanged when used together. For example, one prescribes a **dose** of 1.5 gms tid (three times a day), but the per day **dosage** is 4.5 gms.

dosage design *n* - [trials] 1. A **design** within the **study protocol** that specifies **dosage** for persons on **enrollment** and for changing or adjusting **dosage** after enrollment as dictated by observed **effect** or **outcome**. 2. A design in which two or more dosages of the same **drug** are tested in a trial. 3. The design or plan for choosing the dosages to be tested in **phase I/II drug trials** involving **parallel treatment designs**; **continual**

assessment dosage design, **traditional dosage design**, and **up-down dosage design**.

dose *n* - [F, fr LL *dosis*, fr Gk, lit, act of giving, fr *didonai* to give] 1. A **measured** quantity of a **drug**, substance, procedure, or routine **administered** or to be administered at one time; **treatment dose**. 2. The amount of something received, **exposure**. rt: **median dose** *Usage note*: Sometimes used as if synonymous with **dosage**, as in the sense of defn 2 above and defn 3 for **dosage**. However, the two terms have different primary meanings as seen by comparison of their respective first definitions and, hence, should not be confused or interchanged when used together. For example, one prescribes a **dosage** of 4.5 gms per day, to be taken in 1.5 gm **doses** tid (three times a day).

dose escalation *n* - The state or act of **escalating dose**, as in a **phase I dose ranging study** aimed at finding the highest dose that can be safely administered; **escalation** may be per **patient** (as in a cancer chemoprophylaxis setting with the aim of finding the **maximum tolerable dose** for a patient) or per group of patients (as in a **study** in which the first group of patients enrolled is exposed to dose D, the next group enrolled is exposed to dose 2D, etc, with each subsequent group being exposed to a higher dose up to some **maximum** or until some condition or **event** is observed in one or more members of a group). rt: **dose ranging study**, **maximum tolerable dose**

dose escalation design *n* - A **design** involving **dose escalation**. rt: **dose escalation**, **dose ranging study**

dose ranging study *n* - A **study** involving a series of different **dose** levels of a **treatment** (usually a **drug**) for the purpose of determining an appropriate dose for some use or purpose. rt: **dose escalation**, **maximum tolerable dose**

dose response *n* - An **association** in which change in **dose** is related to change in **response** or **outcome**.

double *adj* - [ME, fr OF, fr L *duplus* akin to Gk, *diploos*, fr *duo* two + *-plus* multiplied by; akin to OE *-feald* -fold] Having a twofold relation or character; dual; twice. rt: **single**, **triple**

double blind *n* - **double masked**

double data entry *n* - A method of **data entry** in which **data** are entered (keyed) twice by the same person (**dependent double data entry**) or

different persons (**independent double data entry**).

double dummy placebo *n* - **double placebo**

double entry *n* - Any method in which an item of information is recorded, entered, or keyed twice for the purpose of providing a basis for detecting or checking for **errors**, as in bookkeeping systems in which money transactions are accounted for on both the income and debit side of ledgers or in **double data entry**. rt: **independent double data entry**, **dependent double data entry**

double mask, **double masked** *n* - 1. An arrangement in which two different kinds of persons or groups of persons are or are to be **masked**. 2. A **mask** of **treatment assignment** imposed in a **trial** on persons receiving or to receive **treatment** and on those administering or who are to **administer** treatment. rt: **mask**, **single mask**, **triple mask**

double placebo *n* - A **placebo** having two different shapes or forms, eg, a tablet and a capsule, as needed in a **double placebo treatment design**; also double dummy placebo. rt: **single placebo**, **multiple placebo**

double placebo treatment design *n* - A **treatment design** that involves two **placebos**, eg, a **design** in which certain persons in a **trial** receive both placebos or one in which a person assigned to **control treatment** receives one or the other of the two placebos, but not both; also double dummy treatment design. The design arises in **single-** or **double-masked trials** that involve two (or more) **test treatments** that cannot be **masked** with a **single placebo** because of differences in the **treatment schedule**, in **dose** or **dosage**, or in route of administration, as in the University Group Diabetes Program.[157] rt: **multiple placebo treatment design**, **single placebo treatment design**

double-blind *adj* - **double-masked** See **blind** for usage note.

double-blind trial *n* - **double-masked trial**

double-mask, **double-masked** *adj* - [**experiments**] Of, relating to, or being a procedure in which neither the experimenters nor the people being experimented upon know the identity of the **treatments** being applied during the course of the experiment. syn: double-blind (not recommended; see **mask**, **masked** *adj* for reasons) rt: **single-mask**, **triple-mask**, **nonmask**

double-masked treatment *n* - [**trials**] A **treatment** that is or is to be administered such that neither the person receiving it nor the person(s) administering it is or is to be informed as to its identity. rt: **single-masked treatment**

double-masked treatment assignment *n* - [**trials**] A **treatment assignment** that is or is to be issued **double-masked**. rt: **single-masked treatment assignment**

double-masked trial *n* - A **trial** that has or is to have **double-mask treatments**. rt: **single-masked trial**, **triple-masked trial**

down *adj* - Directed or going from a higher to a lower position or from great to less. ant: **up**

down *adv* - [ME *doun*, fr OE *dūne*, short for *adūne*, of *dūne*, fr *a-* (fr *of*) *of* off, from + *dūne*, dat of *dūn* hill] To or toward a concentrated or effective state.

drawer *n* - A sliding box or receptacle for **storage**; opened by pulling and closed by pushing.

dredge, **dredged**, **dredging**, **dredges** *v* - [obs *dredge*, n, *sweetmeat*, fr ME *drage*, *drege*, fr MF *dragie*, modif of L *tragemata* sweetmeats, fr Gk *tragēmata*, pl of *tragēma* sweetmeat, fr *trōgein* to gnaw] To look or search, as in **data dredging**.

DRG *n* - **Division of Research Grants**

drop out *v* - To **withdraw** from participation or membership; to quit.

drop-in *n* - [**trial**] A person who has been **enrolled** in a trial and who receives a **study treatment** different from or in addition to the **assigned treatment**; especially when the **treatment** change occurs because of unanticipated problems with the assigned treatment or because of wishes or demands of the person. rt: **treatment crossover** *Usage note*: Avoid, except perhaps in settings where there is a desire or need to convey a certain looseness with regard to the administration of the **treatment protocol**. Do not use in relation to changes or switches that are part of the **treatment protocol**.

dropout *n* - 1. [**general**] One who terminates involvement in an activity by declaration or action or as deduced from an unbroken **sequence** of failed contacts or absences from scheduled activities; especially one who so terminates because of waning interest or for physical, practical, or philosophical reasons. 2. A person who **withdraws** (defn 2) from a **trial** or **followup study** by an announced unwillingness to continue to submit to the required procedures for **treatment**, evaluation, or **data collection** or as deduced in **retrospect** from an unbroken series of absences from scheduled contacts for such treatment, evaluation, or data collection. 3. A person who misses a **scheduled visit** or who is not contacted within the indicated **time window** for a scheduled contact. 4. [**trials**] One who refuses or stops taking the **assigned treatment**. 5. One who stops taking the assigned treatment and whose reason for doing so is judged not to be related to the assigned treatment. *Usage note*: Subject to varying usage. Use should be limited to that implied by defns 1 and 2. Most trials require continued **data collection** regardless of course of treatment. Hence, a "dropout" in the sense of defns 4 and 5 will continue to be an active participant in regard to scheduled data collection. Persons meeting the requirements of defns 4 or 5 are better characterized in relation to **treatment compliance**. Avoid uses in the sense of defn 5 because of difficulty in making reliable judgments regarding the reason a person stops taking the assigned treatment. The stated reason may not be the real reason and seemingly vague reasons, which on the surface do not appear to be related to treatment, may, in fact, be treatment related. Defn 2 includes those who actively refuse, those who passively refuse, as well as those who are simply unable to continue in a trial or followup study for physical or practical reasons, eg, because of having moved to a location where it is no longer possible or convenient to return for scheduled visits. Further, it allows for the possibility of a person being designated as a dropout as a result of failure, for whatever the reason, to return for scheduled contacts. Hence, one who misses a specified number of consecutive visits may be classified as a dropout. Similarly, the definition implies that the state is transitory. Most long-term trials will have provisions for reinstating persons classified as dropouts if and when they return to a **study clinic** for required data collection. Avoid in the sense of defn 3 in relation a single visit or contact in the absence of other reasons for regarding someone as a dropout. Use other language, such as **missed visit** or missed procedure, to avoid the connotation of dropout in the global sense of that term. The term should not be confused with **lost to followup**, **noncompliant**, **withdrawal**, or **endpoint**. A dropout (defn 2) need not be lost to **followup** if one can determine **outcome** without seeing or contacting the person (as in some forms of followup for survival) but will be if the outcome measure depends on data collected from **examinations** of the person. Similarly, the act of dropping out need not affect **treatment compliance** to the assigned treatment. A person will become noncompliant upon dropping out (or soon thereafter) in settings where dropping out results in discontinuation of an active treatment process (as in the case of a **drug trial** where patients are required to take a daily **dose** of a **drug** or matching **placebo** and where the process of supplying them with the assigned treatment depends on visits to the study clinic). However, there may be no effect on treatment compliance in settings where the assigned **test treatment** is administered only once on **enrollment** and where that treatment is not routinely available outside the trial, as in a surgery trial involving a special operation and where there is no established **standard treatment**, such as in the Program on the Surgical Control of the Hyperlipidemias [Buchwald et al, 1990].[17] Similarly, the term should not be confused with or used as a synonym for **withdrawal** (defn 2), since its meaning is different from that for dropout. See **withdrawal** and **endpoint** for additional comments.

drug *n* - [ME *drogge*, fr OF *drogue*, chemical material, possibly from MLG *droge*, dry goods] A chemical compound or noninfectious **biological** substance which is or may be administered to human beings or other animals as an aid in the **diagnosis**, **treatment**, or **prevention** of a **disease** or clinical condition for the relief of pain or suffering, or to control or modify a physiological or pathological condition. As stated in the Federal Food, Drug, and Cosmetic Act of 1938: *(1) articles recognized in the official United States Pharmacopœia, official Homœopathic Pharmacopœia of the United States, or official National Formulary, or any supplements to them; and (2) articles intended for use in the diagnosis, cure, mitigation, treatment, or prevention of disease in man or other animals; and (3) articles (other than food) intended to affect the structure or any function of the body of man or any other animals; and (4) articles intended for use as a component of any article specified in clause (1), (2), or (3); but does not include devices or their components, parts, or accesso-*

ries. *Usage note*: From the perspective of the FDA, the term is inclusive of **biological products** (including those used in-vitro for diagnostic purposes) and antibiotic and biological drugs.

drug company *n* - 1. A **company** involved in the development and marketing of **proprietary drugs**. 2. A company involved in the marketing of drugs. rt: **drug industry**

drug industry *n* - 1. A branch of manufacture and trade involving the development, testing, and marketing of **drugs**. 2. **drug company** rt: **industry**

drug interaction *n* - An **interaction** in which the effect of one **drug** is enhanced, diminished, or otherwise modified when used in conjunction with another drug. rt: **antagonistic treatment effect**, **synergistic treatment effect**, **treatment interaction**

drug lag *n* - 1. **Lag** between development of a **new drug** and **registration** (defn 4) [Kennedy, 1978].[77] 2. [**drug trial**] treatment lag *Usage note*: Avoid in the sense of defn 2; use **treatment lag** or some other appropriate term for use in the sense of defn 2.

drug reaction *n* - A **reaction** caused by a **drug**, especially one that is undesirable or annoying. rt: **toxic drug reaction**, **side effect** *Usage note*: Use with caution as a claim or assertion. The mere occurrence of some **event** or condition in a person taking a drug does not mean that it was the result of the drug. Accompany all uses implying drug-related cause with supporting evidence or argument as to the reasons for the presumption. Use cause-neutral language when in doubt as to cause. Avoid as a label for a collection of events or conditions having a variety of explanations and as a label spanning **treatment groups** receiving different drugs or treatments. Use of the term in relation to events or conditions observed in people not receiving a drug (except, perhaps, for a **matching placebo**) is misleading and invariably serves as an indicator of carelessness on the part of the user. It is illogical to view **control treatments** involving **nontreatment** or placebos as producers of "drug reactions" in the usual physiological sense of usage.

drug trial *n* - 1. A **trial** having a **drug** or combination of drugs as the **test treatment**; a trial having multiple test treatments, each of which involves use of a drug or combination of drugs.

2. **phase I**, **phase I/II**, **phase III**, or **phase IV** **drug trial**

Drug Efficacy Study (DES) *n* - A **study** of the **safety** and **efficacy** of **drugs**, authorized by the Commissioner of the **FDA** in response to the **Kefauver-Harris Act of 1962** and performed by the Division of Medical Sciences of the National Academy of Sciences-National Research Council; study involved assessing evidence of **safety** and **efficacy** of drugs introduced into the market from 1938 - 1962 as new drugs and classifying them as effective, effective with qualifications, probably effective, possibly effective, ineffective as a fixed combination, and ineffective; drugs considered to be unsafe or ineffective were subjected to actions by the FDA via the **Drug Efficacy Study Implementation**; study involved evaluation of 2,824 drug preparations (almost 4,000 drug formulations because many of the drugs were marketed in different doses and forms) from 237 different firms.[116] rt: **Drug Efficacy Study Implementation**

Drug Efficacy Study Implementation (DESI) *n* - **Implementation** of findings of the **Drug Efficacy Study** commencing with publication of Drug Efficacy Study Implementation Notices and Notices of Opportunity for Hearings;[52] **drugs**, via that study, judged lacking in evidence establishing **safety** and **efficacy** were subjected to additional review and requirements via the **Food and Drug Administration**, including the imposition of requirements for review as **new drugs** via submission of **New Drug Applications** and approval of same in order for said drug products to remain on the market; drugs judged to have adequate evidence for safety and efficacy were exempted from requirements of the new drug application process and regarded as approved.

dry *adj* - [ME, fr OE *drȳge*; akin to OHG *truckan* dry, OE *drēahnian* to drain] Not yielding what is expected or desired.

dry lab, **dry labbed**, **dry labbing** *v* - To make-up or create **data** with the intent of subterfuge or deception.

dry labbed data *n* - Made-up **data**; data **fabricated** from theory or based on expectation with the intent of subterfuge or deception, as in the case of a student dry labbing results of an experiment. syn: **fabricated data**, **falsified data**, **forged data** rt: **fudged data**, **scientific misconduct**

dry run *n* - A practice exercise; rehearsal; **trial** (defn 5). syn: **pilot test**, **pretest**, **test run** rt: **pilot study**

DSMC *n* - **data and safety monitoring committee**

dumb *adj* - [ME, fr OE; akin to OHG *tumb* mute, OE *dēaf* deaf] Not having any means of interacting; lacking in intelligence. ant: **smart**

dumb computer terminal *n* - A **terminal** that can serve as an **input/output device**, but that does not have **independent** processing capabilities. ant: **intelligent computer terminal**

dumb terminal *n* - **dumb computer terminal**

dummy *adj* - Having the appearance of being real.

dummy placebo *n* - **placebo**

dummy table *n* - A **table**, usually of two or more **dimensions**, displaying the format of data for analysis or presentation, especially such a table produced as a prelude to **data collection** or **analysis** and having empty cells or cells containing fictitious data. syn: **mock table**, **table shell** *Usage note*: Subject to mischievous use, eg, *dummy tables produced by dummies*; use **table shell** or **mock table** instead.

dummy variable *n* - A **binary variable** that is used to indicate the presence or absence of some condition or **factor**, usually in some **regression model**, but otherwise devoid of meaning.

duplicate *adj* - [ME, fr L *duplicatus*, pp of *duplicare* to double, fr *duplic-*, *duplex*] 1. To make **double** or twofold. 2. To make an exact copy of. 3. To produce something equal to.

duplicate *n* - Either of two things exactly alike; an identical copy.

duplicate, **duplicated**, **duplicating**, **duplicates** *v* - To make **double** or twofold; to reproduce; to repeat. rt: **repeat**, **replicate**

duplication *n* - The act or process of **duplicating**. rt: **repetition**, **replication** *Usage note*: Not to be confused with **replication**; see usage note for **replication**.

dynamic *adj* - [F *dynamique*, fr Gk *dynamikos* powerful, fr *dynamis* power, fr *dynasthai* to be able] Marked by continuing **change**.

dynamic randomization *n* - **adaptive randomization**

dynamic treatment assignment *n* - **adaptive treatment assignment**

dynamic treatment assignment schedule *n* - **adaptive treatment assignment schedule**

E

e *n* - [5th letter of the English alphabet] The **base** of the system of **natural logarithms** having a numeric value of 2.7182818284 ⋯. syn: **natural constant**

early *adj* - 1. Of or relating to occurrence before the usual **time**. 2. Of or relating to the beginning of a period of time, development, or series. *Usage note*: Not usually informative as a characterization unless accompanied by details indicating the sense of usage. Usages without qualification or added explanatory detail reflect judgments on the part of the user. For example, early morning may be 5:00 AM to one person and 9:00 AM to another, but 7:00 AM will be understood by both, whether viewed as early or late (see usage note for **early stopping** for additional comments).

early *adv* - [ME *erly*, fr OE *ǣrlice*, fr *ǣr* early, soon] 1. Before the usual **time**. 2. Near the beginning of a period of time, a development, or a **series**; near the beginning of a course, process, or series. *Usage note*: See **early** *adj*.

early stop *n* - [**trials**] An instance in which a trial is stopped prior to its scheduled end, especially because of accumulated **data** from within the trial suggesting **benefit** or harm associated with one of the **study treatments**. syn: **premature stop** *Usage note*: See comment for **early stopping** and **trial stop**.

early stopping *n* - [**trials**] 1. A condition or provision incorporated into the **design** of a **trial** for terminating **enrollment** and **treatment** (or simply treatment where enrollment is already completed) if accumulated **data** are considered to merit such an action; usually because of an **adverse** or **beneficial treatment effect**. 2. **early stop** rt: **stopping rule** *Usage note*: For reasons indicated in the usage note for **early** *adj*, accompany with sufficient detail to indicate sense of usage.

early stopping rule *n* - **stopping rule**

early termination of trial *n* - 1. **Trial termination** before achieving the desired or required **sample size**; especially a termination due to **data** indicating **benefit** or harm of a **study treatment**.

2. A termination that occurs prior to the scheduled end of the **trial**, although the desired or required sample size has been achieved; especially a termination due to **data** indicating benefit or harm of a **study treatment** (eg, terminations that occurred in the University Group Diabetes Program because of the possibility of harm [University Group Diabetes Program Research Group, 1975;[155] 1970b[157]] or in the Macular Photocoagulation Studies because of benefit [Macular Photocoagulation Study Group, 1983;[92] 1982[93]]). 3. Any **termination** of a **trial** that occurs before the time anticipated when planned, regardless of the reason, including reasons unrelated to **treatment results**, such as those having to do with funding or other practical considerations. *Usage note*: See **early stopping** for cautionary note.

EC *n* - **executive committee**

ecological *adj* - Of or relating to **ecology**.

ecological fallacy *n* - A **relationship** derived or observed using **aggregate data** assembled from various **populations** erroneously assumed to imply that the relationship holds at the elemental or individual level, eg, (ala Last[84]) assuming that a relationship between hardness of water and mortality due to heart disease across various population implies that the risk of death from heart disease is a function of hardness of water. Colorfully defined by Michael and coworkers[104] as *a foxy, two-faced beast who lurks in the darkened corners of large population studies and tricks unwary readers into accepting unwarranted conclusions. This fellow can often be found infesting so-called ecologic research, in which* **groups** *of people in selected geographic areas, census tracts, or other specified locations are the units of study. Crafty and shy, he presents conclusions that may be valid or may be false, depending on the mouth from which he chooses to speak. To abort his trickery, you must remember that studies of groups can lead to spurious conclusions when uncritically applied to individuals.*

ecological study *n* - A **study** based on **aggregate** or **group data** for some loosely defined **population** (eg, one defined by geographic area or by occupation) as it exists at some **point** or points in **time** and done to investigate the **relationship** of an **exposure** to a known or presumed **risk factor** for a specified **disease**. Generally, exposure is measured in the **aggregate** for the **population** and the measure of disease is by **prevalence**. Examples: An investigation of the role of sodium in hypertension in different countries of the world by relating per capita consumption of sodium to prevalence of hypertension in those countries; investigation of the change in rates of bladder cancer in the US in relation to use of saccharin. Typically, such studies are undertaken and viewed as **hypothesis** generating (as opposed to hypothesis testing). Generally, a **positive relationship**, as suggested by an increasing rate of disease with increasing exposure to the risk factor of interest, is taken as suggestive evidence of a causative role of the exposure in the disease process.

ecology *n* - [Ger *ökologie*, fr *ök-* ec- + *-logie* - logy] 1. A branch of science concerned with the interrelationship of organisms and their environment. 2. The totality or pattern of **relationships** between organisms and their environment.

edit *n* - An instance of **editing**.

edit, **editing**, **edited**, **edits** *v* - To adapt or refine to bring about uniformity or conformity with a **standard**.

edit check *n* - The process of reviewing a **data item** on a completed **data form** for deficiencies in the way it was completed, or in the values reported.

edit period *n* - A time **period** used for collecting or batching **data forms** or **records** for **editing** and for reporting counts of forms or **records** received and numbers of deficiencies noted.

edit query *n* - A **statement**, usually in the form of a question, generated from a review of a completed **data form** that draws attention to some suspected **error** or deficiency in a completed item; normally requires some action by personnel responsible for **generation** of the **data**; considered to be a **turnaround document** when the query is written and when a written response is required from the person or site being queried to resolve or close the query. rt: **data query**

editor *n* - 1. One who **edits** (eg, a desk editor, forms editor, data editor), especially one whose occupation is editing. 2. One who has overall responsibility for the content of some document or periodical, such as a **journal** or newspaper. 3. A **computer program** that permits its user to create or modify statements in other computer programs.

editorial review committee *n* - A **committee** in the organizational structure of an **investigative body** that has responsibility for reviewing **manuscripts** produced by that body, usually prior to submission for **presentation** or **publication**.

effect *n* - [ME, fr MF & L; MF, fr L *effectus*, fr *effectus*, pp of *efficere*, to bring about, fr *ex-* + *facere* to make do] 1. Something that follows from or is brought about by an antecedent **event**, action, or condition. 2. **treatment effect** 3. **difference** 4. Power to bring about a certain **outcome** or **result**. 5. Outward appearance or sign.

effect, **effected**, **effecting**, **effects** *v* - To bring about, to accomplish, or to cause to come into being.

effect modifier *n* - A **variable**, **factor**, or condition that, when present, is capable of changing or moderating a particular **result** or **outcome**, eg, the time of first exposure to wild polio virus as a modifier of the **risk** of paralysis. syn: conditioning variable, **moderator variable** rt: **interaction**

effect size *n* - 1. The **size** of a **difference** due to a **factor** (defn 2). 2. **treatment difference**

effective *adj* - 1. Producing a desired **effect**. 2. Being in effect, operative.

effective sample size *n* - **Sample size** after actual or anticipated losses due to **dropouts**, missing **data**, and **treatment noncompliance**. rt: **expected effective sample size**, **observed effective sample size**

effectiveness *n* - The state of being **effective**; efficacious.

effectiveness trial *n* - A **trial** designed to assess the usefulness of a **test treatment** under conditions approximating everyday practice conditions. syn: **pragmatic trial**, **management trial** ant: **efficacy trial** rt: **community trial**, **demonstration trial**, **field trial**, **management trial** *Usage note*: See **pragmatic trial** and **explanatory trial**.

efficacy *n* - 1. The **power** to produce an **effect**, especially a desired **beneficial effect**. 2. The extent to which a **treatment** or procedure serves to produce or is capable of producing a desired beneficial effect or **result**. syn: **effectiveness**

efficacy monitoring *v* - [trials] 1. **Monitoring** (defn 2) for **efficacy**, as performed at periodic time points over the course of a trial, to determine whether the trial should be stopped or modified; as distinct from **safety monitoring**. 2. **efficacy review** (defn 1) 3. **treatment effects monitoring** rt: **safety monitoring, treatment effects monitoring, interim look, interim result** *Usage note*: Often used in contradistinction to **safety monitoring** in settings where the user wishes to distinguish between **interim looks** performed for efficacy monitoring versus those made for safety monitoring; eg, in settings where looks for safety monitoring are not counted as looks for purposes of adjusting **p-values** for **multiple looks**. The distinction is predicated on the assumption that safety and efficacy are **independent** dimensions of **treatment** — often not the case. Use **treatment effects monitoring** when the distinction is unimportant or where the monitoring performed is for efficacy and safety. See also notes for **administrative review, safety monitoring**, and **treatment effects monitoring**.

efficacy review *n* - [trials] 1. An **interim review** (defn 2) of **results** for evidence of **efficacy** of a **test treatment**, not part of or that is considered apart from an ongoing **treatment effects monitoring** process, that is done for the sole or primary purpose of determining whether that treatment shows sufficient promise to justify continuing use of it in the trial. 2. **efficacy monitoring** (defn 1) rt: **safety review** *Usage note*: Use in the sense of defn 1 is in regard to an **interim look**, planned or **ad hoc**, made for the purpose of determining whether the **test treatment** shows sufficient promise of efficacy to warrant continued use of it in the trial. Use in the sense of defn 2 is in regard to an ongoing **treatment effects monitoring** process. Use **efficacy review** for uses in the sense of defn 1. Use **efficacy monitoring** when the interim review is part of a planned ongoing process. See note for **efficacy monitoring**.

efficacy trial *n* - A **trial** designed to assess the **efficacy** of a **test treatment** under ideal conditions and in a setting not designed or necessarily intended to approximate everyday practice conditions. syn: **explanatory trial** ant: **effectiveness trial** *Usage note*: See **explanatory trial** and **pragmatic trial**.

efficiency *n* - 1. The quality or degree of being **efficient**. 2. Efficient operation as measured in some way, eg, in terms of time, cost, or energy expended per unit of effort.

efficient *adj* - [ME, fr MF or L; MF, fr L *efficient-, efficiens*, fr prp of *efficere* to bring about] Productive of a desired **effect** with economy or without waste.

ELA *n* - **Establishment License Application**

elective *adj* - Permitting a choice or option.

elective treatment *n* - A **treatment** that is not considered essential in caring for some designated condition, but that is presumed to be **beneficial** in reducing the **risk** of subsequent **morbidity** or **mortality** in those with that condition.

electronic *adj* - 1. Of, relating to, based on, or operated by, or otherwise involving the controlled conduction of electrons or other charge carried in some conducting material. 2. Of or relating to something stored, displayed, or transmitted electronically, such as **data** in a **computer**.

electronic database *n* - A **database** in which **data** and **data files** are stored, retrieved, and manipulated electronically.

electronic dataset *n* - 1. A **dataset** residing in the **memory** of a **computer** or an associated **peripheral**. 2. A dataset in a form suitable for storage, retrieval, and processing on a computer.

electronic file *n* - A **file** (defn 2) that resides in a **computer** or some other electronic device and that can be retrieved and processed electronically.

electronic form *n* - A **form** that is or may be displayed electronically (eg, on a **video screen**), especially one that is or may be completed using such displays and associated electronic devices. ant: **paper form**

element *n* - [ME, fr OF & L; OF, fr L *elementum*] One of the parts of a compound or complex whole, generally connoting irreducible simplicity.

eligibility criteria *n* - **Criteria** used for determining **eligibility**, eg, for **enrollment** into a **trial**. In trials, usually the constellation of **inclusion criteria** and **exclusion criteria** used for determining eligibility.

eligible *adj* - [ME, fr MF & LL; MF, fr LL *eligibilis*, fr L *eligere* to choose] Qualified to be chosen.

eligible, eligibility *n* - The state or condition of being **eligible**.

emancipate, emancipated, emancipating, emancipates *v* - [L *emancipatus*, pp of *emancipare*, fr *e-* + *mancipare* to transfer ownership of, fr *mancipmanceps* purchaser, fr *manus* hand + *capere* to take] To release from parental care and responsibility.

emancipated minor *n* - 1. A self-supporting **minor**. 2. A minor considered **emancipated** in some limited legal sense, generally by virtue of action or behavior; the person has the same rights, privileges, and responsibilities as an **adult** in the area of emancipation and those rights and privileges are granted without need for parental permission or consent, eg, a sexually active teenage girl seeking care in a pregnancy clinic. syn: **mature minor**

emergency *n* - An unforeseen combination of circumstances or the resulting state that calls for immediate action or disposition.

emergency use *n* - [**medicine**; in regard to a **biologic**, **drug**, or **device** under **test** but not yet approved by the **Food and Drug Administration**] Use of a test article outside the context of a **treatment protocol** of an approved study and deemed necessary in last-ditch efforts at preservation of health or life. rt: **compassionate use** *Usage note*: Emergency use of unapproved test articles is limited as indicated above and typically to situations devoid of viable alternative treatment options. Use may occur in the absence of review or approval of that use by the **institutional review board** of the institution of use.

empirical *adj* - 1. Relying on experience or **observation** alone. 2. Operating or based on observation or experience. 3. Capable of being verified by observation or experimentation.

empirical curve *n* - 1. A **curve** fitted to **observed data** points without benefit of a mathematical **model** or documented fitting procedure. 2. A curve fitted to observed data by eye.

empirical curve fit *n* - An **empirical fit** of a **curve** to **observed data**.

empirical fit *n* - A **fit** of **data** fashioned without benefit of theory or mathematical model, usually by eye.

end *adj* - Final, ultimate, lasting.

end point *n* - 1. A **point** that marks the end of a line segment or **interval**. 2. A point marking the completion of a process or a stage of a process. 3. **Limit** or **boundary** value, as in the end point of a **range**. rt: **endpoint** *Usage note*: Also may be written as one word, but not recommended because of potential for confusion with **endpoint**; see that entry for comments.

endemic *adj* - [F *endémique*, fr *endémie* endemic disease, fr Gk *endēmia* action of dwelling, fr *endēmos* endemic, fr *en* in + *dēmos* people, populace] Constantly present; belonging to or native to some region or population. rt: **epidemic, pandemic**

endpoint *n* - 1. **Limit** or **boundary** value, as in the **end points** of a **range**. 2. **end point** (defn 2) 3. **outcome measure** 4. A **primary** or **secondary outcome measure**, especially one recorded as an **event** such as death or a nonfatal event such as a myocardial infarction, that results in termination or alteration of **treatment** or **followup** of the person on whom observed. 5. Any primary or secondary outcome measure recorded as an **event** observed during the course of treatment or followup regardless of whether it results in an alteration of treatment or followup. 6. Any outcome measure recorded as an event. 7. **early stopping** 8. **stopping rule** rt: **end point** *Usage note*: Best avoided because of misuse and potential for confusion. Use **end point** in the sense of defns 1 and 2. Use outcome, outcome measure, or event in the sense of defns 3, 4, 5, and 6. Most "endpoints" (defns 3, 4, 5, and 6) noted over the course of followup in **trials** are not indicators of "end" in regard to treatment or followup. Most **protocols** call for followup, and often treatment as well, over a defined period of time even in the presence of and following intercurrent events. As a rule, there are no endpoints in this operational sense of usage, except for death. Use of the term in protocols and **manuals** for trials can cause personnel at **clinics** to stop treatment and terminate followup on the occurrence of an "endpoint" (morbid event) if they regard the term as having operational meaning. Avoid as a generic label for **morbid** and **fatal events**, and especially in settings where such events are devoid of operational implications in regard to followup or treatment. Avoid in the sense of defns 7 and 8 and especially in contexts where the term is likely to be confused with usages in the sense of defns 4, 5, or 6.

enroll, enrolled, enrolling, enrolls *v* - [ME *enrollen*, fr MF *enroller*, fr *en-* + *rolle* roll, register] 1. To **enter**. 2. **register** 3. Enter into a list, catalog, or roll.

enrollee *n* - One who is **enrolled**.

enrollment *n* - 1. The action of **enrolling** as defined by some action or **event**. 2. The state of having been or of being **enrolled**. 3. **patient enrollment** *Usage note*: The term is subject to a fair amount of confusion in **trials**, especially when used in contexts where there is no landmark demarcating enrollment. The usual landmark is **treatment assignment** or **treatment initiation**. Persons passing the landmark are considered enrolled and are counted in the **denominator** for the trial. Use in contexts where the landmark is not specified or is otherwise unclear or varying, is likely to leave readers uncertain or confused as to the true denominator for **treatment comparisons** and with concerns as to whether the treatment groups are free of **treatment related selection biases**, especially in **unmasked trials**. See **patient enrollment** for comments.

enrollment period *n* - 1. [general] The planned or actual time period for **enrollment**. 2. [trials] **patient enrollment period** syn: recruitment period

enrollment process *n* - The process and related procedures needed or associated with **enrollment** of persons or other **observation units** into a **study**; **patient enrollment process**

enrollment suspension *n* - The **suspension** of **enrollment** due to some intercurrent concern or problem, especially such a suspension due to concerns regarding the adequacy or appropriateness of the **study**, concerns regarding the **eligibility criteria** or the **consent process**, or general concerns regarding the credibility of the study. syn: suspension of enrollment rt: **protocol suspension** *Usage note*: Distinct from **treatment protocol suspension**, where the intake of new people may be suspended, but the **data collection** and **treatment** processes for those already enrolled may continue as indicated in the **study protocol**. See also usage notes for **protocol suspension** and **treatment protocol suspension**.

enter, entered, entering, enters *v* - [ME *entren*, fr OF *entrer*, fr L *intrare*, fr *intra* within; akin to L *inter* between] 1. To come or gain admission to a **group** or activity. 2. To become a member or active **participant**, eg, a **patient** who enters a **trial**. 3. To make record of.

entry *n* - [ME *entre*, fr OF *entree*, fr fem of *entrė*, pp of *entrer* to enter] 1. The act of **entering**. 2. The act of making a **record**; something entered on a record, or a **file** or a **database**, eg, **data** recorded on a **form** or keyed to a database.

entry criteria *n* - **Criteria** used to determine **eligibility** for **entry**; **eligibility criteria**. rt: **exclusion criteria**, **inclusion criteria**

epidemic *adj* - [F *épidémique*, fr MF, fr *epidemie*, n, epidemic, fr LL *epidemia*, fr Gk *epidēmia* visit, epidemic, fr *epidēmos* visiting, epidemic, fr *epi-* + *dēmos* people] Affecting many (in **absolute** or **relative** number) at one time or in a defined **time interval** within a specified region, area, or population. rt: **endemic**, **pandemic**

epidemic *n* - An outbreak or product of rapid spread, growth, or development, eg, an epidemic of measles.

epidemiological *adj* - Of, relating to, concerned with, or having characteristics of **epidemiology** or of something used by **epidemiologists**.

epidemiological study *n* - 1. A **study** designed or intended to produce information having to do with the **epidemiology** of some **disease** or health condition afflicting human beings. 2. An **observational study** done in a medical or public health setting and intended to address some **epidemiological** question or issue. 3. A study involving epidemiological methods. 4. A study involving methods similar to those used by an **epidemiologist**.

epidemiologist *n* - One who is trained in the **discipline** of **epidemiology** or is involved in the generation or **analysis** of **data** for the purpose of characterizing the patterns or determinants of disease.

epidemiology *n* - [LL *epidemia* + ISV *-logy*] 1. A **discipline** of the health sciences concerned with characterizing, controlling, or preventing **disease** or adverse health conditions of human beings or their precursors by application of knowledge gained from **observation** of their **incidence**, **frequency**, **distribution**, and pattern and by actions taken to modify or eliminate the correlates and determinants of those conditions. 2. The sum of knowledge relating to the factors and conditions determining the cause, spread, or distribution of some **disease** or adverse health condition, as in the *epidemiology of cardiovascular disease*. rt: **experimental epidemiology**

epsilon *n* - [Gk *e pilson*, lit, simple e] The 5th letter of the **Greek alphabet**, uppercase E, lowercase ε.

equal *adj* - [ME, fr L *aequalis*, fr *aequus* level, equal] 1. Of the same measure, quantity, amount, or **number** as another. 2. Identical in mathematical value or logical denotation; equivalent.

equal allocation *n* - **equal treatment assignment**

equal assignment *n* - **equal treatment assignment**

equal ignorance *n* - A state of mind characterized by an equal degree of uncertainty regarding a set of choices or options; **equipoise**.

equal treatment assignment *n* - [**trials**] A **scheme** in which the **assignment probability** for any one **treatment** is the same as for every other treatment in a **trial**; **uniform treatment assignment**.

equality *n* - The state or quality of being **equal**. rt: **justice**

equation *n* - A mathematical statement involving two quantities, one being equal to the other and separated by an equal sign, eg, $y = a + bx$.

equipoise *n* - 1. A state of equilibrium or counterbalance. 2. A state of mind characterized by legitimate uncertainty or indecision as to choice or course of action because of a **balance** of potential gains versus losses or of **benefits** versus **risks**; state considered to be an essential prerequisite to the initiation of **treatment trials**.

equitable *adj* - Having or exhibiting **equity**; dealing fairly and equally with all concerned. rt: **just**

equity *n* - [ME *equite*, fr MF *equité*, fr L *aequitat-*, *aequitas*, fr *aequus* equal, fair] Freedom from **bias** or favoritism

equivalence *n* - The state or property of being **equivalent**. rt: **bioequivalence**

equivalent *adj* - [ME, fr MF or LL; MF, fr LL *aequivalent-*, *aequivalens*, prp of *aequivalēre* to have equal power, fr L *aequi + valēre* to be strong] **Equal** in force, amount, value, or action; like in significance or import. rt: **bioequivalent**

error *n* - [ME *errour*, fr MF, fr L *error*, fr *errare*] [general] 1. A mistake, slip, lapse, or blunder. 2. A **deviation** from truth or **accuracy**. 3. [**science**] The difference between a calculated or **observed** value and its **true** or **expected value**. 4. **Variation** in **measurement** or **observation** of a quantity due to **factors** or conditions not **controlled** or that cannot be controlled, or due to mistakes. *Usage note*: Generally the term and its synonyms, such as mistake, slip, lapse, or blunder, imply the absence of motive or intent to depart from truth or accuracy. Hence, usage in scientific writing and discourse should be reserved for instances where motive is absent or not suspected. Appropriate, non-neutral, terms, such as falsehood, untruth, lie, or fabrication, should be used when motive is presumed or present. Similarly, the term should not be used as a euphemism for departures or deviations that are the result of willful intent, such as in characterizing a departure from a **treatment protocol** as being due to error when in fact it was due to conscious wilful acts. See **random error** and **systematic error** for additional comments.

error margin *n* - A **range** about a specified value beyond which something is considered to be unlikely, eg, the set of values lying outside a 95% **confidence interval** about some **point estimate**. In opinion surveys, typically stated as the difference between the upper and lower **boundary** value for the interval, as in *the margin of error is 13 percentage points* for a survey involving 55 people and yielding a point estimate of 38% for the response of interest. syn: margin of error rt: **safety margin**

error mean square *n* - **mean square error**

error term *n* - 1. The term in a **regression model**, typically denoted by e or ε, denoting **error** associated with the **measurement** or **observation** of the **dependent variable**; generally assumed to have an **expected value** of 0 when the **model** is used in **data analysis**. 2. **error variance**

error variance *n* - **Variance** associated with the **error term** in a **model** having a **random** source of error, such as in a **regression model**.

escalate, escalated, escalating, escalates *v* - To increase in amount, extent, intensity, or number.

escalation *n* - The state of being **escalated** or the act of escalating.

establishment *n* - A place of business; a public or private **institution**.

Establishment License Application (ELA) *n* - An **application** made to the **Food and Drug Administration** for permission to manufacture a **drug** or **biologic**.

estimate *n* - 1. A numerical value or **interval**, such as a **mean**, **median**, **variance**, or **interquartile range** based on **observed data** and serving as an approximation to some true underlying **parameter**. 2. Any value or interval that is intended or used to approximate some true underlying value or interval.

estimate, estimated, estimating, estimates *v* - [L *aestimatus*, pp of *aestimare* to value, estimate, fr *aes* copper] 1. To determine the size, extent, or nature of by **calculation** or other procedures that are intended to provide an approximation of the **true** value. 2. To judge tentatively or approximately the value, worth, or significance of.

estimated sample size *n* - The **number** of **observation units** required for a **study**, as derived from a **sample size calculation** or in some other way.

estimation *n* - The act of **estimating** something; **estimate**.

estimator *n* - 1. An expression, usually mathematical in form, that **estimates** a **population parameter**. 2. The actual value of such an expression for a given set of **observed data**.

eta *n* - [ME, fr LL, fr Gk *ēta*, of Sem origin; akin to Heb *hēth* heth] The 7th letter of the **Greek alphabet**, uppercase H, lowercase η.

ethic *n* - [ME *ethik*, fr MF *ethique*, fr L *ethice*, fr Gk *ēthikē*, fr *ethikos*] 1. A **principle** stating what is right or good and that serves or is to serve as a basis for guiding behavior or conduct. 2. A system of moral principles or values; **ethics**.

ethical *adj* - [ME *etik*, fr L *ethicus*, fr Gk *ēthikos*, fr *ēthos* character] 1. Of or relating to **ethics**. 2. Conforming to accepted professional **standards** of conduct.

ethical committee *n* - **ethics committee**

ethical drug firm *n* - 1. A **firm** that develops, tests, and markets **prescription drugs** (eg, as opposed to one that markets only **generic** prescription drugs). 2. A firm that markets the **drug** products it develops. *Usage note*: Not recommended because of its pejorative tone; use implies that firms not satisfying the definition are "unethical". Term becoming archaic.

ethical principles of medical care *n* - **medical ethics, principles of**

ethicist *n* - 1. One whose specialty is the study of **ethics**. 2. Broadly, anyone professing knowledge of or understanding of ethics via formal study, profession, or activity, eg, a member of the clergy or bar responsible for guiding or counseling people with regard to moral or ethical issues. *Usage note*: In the context of **treatment effects monitoring committee** or other committees having a similar function for **trials** and for **institutional review boards**, often loosely applied; often any nonhealth professional, especially one who is a member of the clergy, a lawyer, or academician concerned with theology or philosophy.

ethics *n* - 1. A **discipline** dealing with the study of the general nature of morals and of the choices made or open to those bound or influenced by those morals. 2. The **rules** and **standards** of conduct governing or guiding a profession. See also **ethic** and **medical ethics**.

ethics committee *n* - 1. A **committee** responsible for the review of **research projects** involving **human beings** to ensure ethical **design** and **conduct** (see **involve**); variously known as **ethics review committee**, **institutional review board**, **Helsinki committee**, **human experimentation committee**, and **human volunteers committee**. 2. **treatment effects monitoring committee** (not a recommended synonym)

ethics review committee *n* - 1. **ethics committee** 2. **treatment effects monitoring committee** (not a recommended synonym)

ethnic *adj* - [ME, fr LL *ethnicus*, fr Gk *ethnikos* national, gentile, fr *ethnos* nation, people] 1. Of or relating to a racial, national, tribal, linguistic, or cultural origin or background. 2. Being a member of an ethnic group.

ethnic origin *n* - The racial, national, tribal, linguistic, or cultural **origin** or background of a person or group of persons. rt: **race**

evaluable *adj* - Capable of being evaluated for some purpose or end. *Usage note*: See comment for **evaluable study patients**.

evaluable patient *n* - **evaluable study patient**

evaluable patients *n* - **evaluable study patients**

evaluable study patient *n* - [trials] A **study patient** considered suitable for inclusion in some **tabulation** or **analysis** by virtue of having had some **event** or satisfying some condition during the course of **treatment** (eg, having a recurrence of a cancer; having received the **assigned treatment** and having taken it for a specified period of time). *Usage note*: See note for **evaluable study patients**.

evaluable study patients *n* - [**trials**] The **subgroup** of **study patients** considered to **satisfy** certain conditions and, as a result, are retained for **analysis**. *Usage note*: Generally, use of the term implies a violation of a basic **analysis principle** in that the subgroup used for making **treatment comparisons** is, itself, subject to **treatment related selection bias**. As a result, treatment comparisons are likely to be **confounded** by the **selection variable** and, hence, the **treatment difference** noted, if any, may have more to do with selection bias than with the treatment being tested. The possibility of confounding exists whenever the selection variable is observed after the initiation of treatment (as with any **treatment compliance variable** in any analysis where only those patients receiving a specified amount of the treatment are selected for analysis).

evaluate, evaluated, evaluating, evaluates *v* - 1. To determine or fix the value of something. 2. To determine the significance or worth of by appraisal or **study**.

even *adj* - [ME, fr OE *efen*; akin to OHG *eban* even] Being one of a **sequence** of natural **numbers** starting with 2 and counting by twos; a number exactly divisible by two. ant: **odd**

event *n* - [MF or L; MF, fr L *eventus*, fr *eventus*, pp of *evenire* to happen, fr *e-* + *venire* to come] 1. An occurrence, incident, or experience, especially one of importance or **significance**. 2. **clinical event** 3. **binary outcome measure** 4. The actual occurrence of a condition or feature that is defined by a **binary outcome measure**.

event rate *n* - 1. The **number** of persons or **observation units** in a defined **population** experiencing or displaying the undesired state of a **binary outcome** over a defined **time period**, divided by the number of persons or observation units in that population at **risk** of that outcome in that time period and expressed as a **rate** (done by multiplying the decimal fraction obtained by 10 raised to some power, typically, 2 or 3). 2. The number of **incident events** observed in a defined population over a specified time period,

divided by the number of persons or observation units in that population at risk of an incident event in that time period and expressed as a rate.

ex- *prefix* - [ME, fr OF & L; OF, fr L, fr *ex* out of, from; akin to Gk *ex, ex-* out of, from, OSlav *iz*] 1. out of, from 2. not 3. former

ex officio *adj* - By virtue or because of an **office** or position. *Usage note*: Used to denote members of a **committee** or **board** that serve because of the office or position held to distinguish them from elected or appointed members. Depending on circumstances, the rights and privileges of members so designated may be the same as for other members or may be restricted. Unless otherwise indicated, the rights and duties should be assumed to be the same as for other members. Indicate if positions are without vote.

exact, exacting *adj* - [L *exactus*] 1. Exhibiting or marked by strict, particular, and complete accordance with fact or procedure. 2. Marked by thorough consideration or minute **measurement** of small factual or numerical details.

exact, exacted, exacting, exacts *v* - [ME *exacten*, fr L *exactus*, pp of *exigere* to drive out, demand, measure, fr *ex-* + *agere* to drive] To demand and obtain by force or authority.

exam *n* - **examination** (defns 2, 3, and 4)

examination *n* - 1. The state or result of being examined. 2. **test** (defns 8 and 9) 3. An assessment made by medical personnel in a recognized medical facility in relation to diagnosing, assessing, treating, or caring for a person. 4. **patient examination** 5. In **trials**, often any **visit** by a person to a **study clinic**, even in the absence of any **examination** in the usual medical sense of that term (not recommended, use **visit**). rt: **visit** *Usage note*: Subject to mild forms of misuse, as in defn 5. Avoid as a synonym for **visit**.

examine, examined, examining, examines *v* - [ME *examinen*, fr MF *examiner*, fr L *examinare*, fr *examen*] 1. To make or give an **examination**. 2. To inquire into closely; to investigate.

exclude, excluded, excluding, excludes *v* - [ME *excluden*, fr L *excludere*, fr *ex-* + *claudere* to close] To **prevent** or restrict the entrance of; to ban from participation, consideration, or **inclusion**. ant: **include**

exclusion *n* - [L *exclusion-, exclusio*, fr *exclusus*, pp of *excludere*] The state of being **excluded**; something that is excluded. ant: **inclusion**

exclusion criteria *n* - [**trials**] **Criteria** set forth in the **protocol** of a trial that, when met for a **study candidate**, render that person ineligible for **enrollment**. ant: **inclusion criteria**

executive *adj* - Designed for or relating to execution or carrying into effect; having administrative or managerial responsibility.

executive committee (EC) *n* - [**multicenter trials**] A **committee** within the structure of some studies, especially **multicenter studies**, responsible for direction of the day-to-day affairs of the study. One of the **key committees** in the organizational structure of a **multicenter trial**. Usually consists of the **officers of the study** and perhaps others selected from the **steering committee** and typically headed by the **chair** or **vice-chair** of the steering committee and reporting to that committee. rt: **steering committee** *Usage note*: Sometimes used interchangeably with steering committee (not recommended). The term, **executive committee**, should be reserved for settings in which it is part of or subservient to a larger committee or body. In settings where there is only one leadership committee, use steering committee.

exempt *adj* - [ME, fr L *exemptus*, pp of *eximere* to take out] Set apart; free of responsibilities or requirements to which others are subject.

exempt research *n* - 1. **Research** falling into one or more of the categories exempted from the review and approval policies set forth in the code of federal regulations for **institutional review boards**.[117] 2. Research involving **human subjects** (see **involve**) and classified as being **exempt** from IRB review and approvals policies after review by an IRB. 3. Research considered to be in an exempt category by the performing investigator and carried out without an IRB review. *Usage note*: Note that defns 2 and 3 have different operational implications. The option implied in defn 3 may not be permissible in some settings. For example, it is not permissible when the IRB makes the determination after review of the proposed research. An investigator in those settings is obligated to submit to an IRB, regardless of the investigator's judgment as to whether or not the proposed research qualifies as being exempt. The determination is made by the IRB after review of the proposed research. Proceeding, as implied in defn 3, in such settings has the potential of placing the investigator in violation of local IRB regulations. See note for **involve** *v* for comment on the meaning of **involve**, as in *research involving human beings*, in relation to use of that term in regulations relating to IRBs.

exemption *n* - The state of being **exempt**.

expand, expanded, expanding, expands *v* - [ME *expaunden*, fr L *expandere*, fr *ex-* + *pandere* to spread] 1. To open up. 2. To increase the extent, **number**, content, volume, or reach of. 3. To subject to mathematical expansion.

expanded *adj* - To have extended reach, influence, impact, or availability.

expanded access *n* - [**medicine**] **expanded availability**

expanded availability *n* - [**medicine**] **Availability** of a **drug** outside existing limits of usage; especially such availability prior to FDA **licensure** for a given **indication** or use. syn: expanded access rt: **compassionate use**

expect, expected, expecting, expects *v* - [L *exspectare* to look forward to, fr *ex-* + *spectare* to look at, fr *spectus*, pp of *specere* to look] 1. To anticipate or look forward; to anticipate or look forward to the coming or occurrence of something. 2. To consider probable or certain.

expectancy *n* - 1. The state of being **expected**. 2. Something expected.

expectation *n* - 1. The act or state of anticipation. 2. Something **expected**. 3. **expected value**; **mathematical expectation**

expected assignment ratio *n* - The **assignment ratio** mathematically **expected** for a specified **assignment scheme**. syn: **specified assignment ratio**

expected effective sample size *n* - The **number** of **treatment assignment units** (usually people) specified when a **study** is planned, less deductions for losses due to **drop out** and, in **trials**, less reductions due to anticipated losses from treatment **noncompliance**. rt: **observed effective sample size**

expected frequency *n* - The **frequency expected** under ideal or specified theoretical conditions and assumptions, eg, the expected frequency of females in a **population** assuming a **uniform distribution** for sex. rt: **expected number**

expected number *n* - The **number** or **count expected** under ideal or theoretical conditions or assumptions. rt: **expected frequency**

expected power *n* - The **power** for detecting a specified **difference**, as determined prior to the start of a **study**, eg, in the case of a **trial**, the power expected from a given **sample size** (as set when planning the trial) for a specified **treatment difference** and for anticipated losses due to **drop out** and **noncompliance**. rt: **conditional power**, **observed power**

expected treatment assignment ratio *n* - The **assignment ratio expected** using a given set of **treatment assignment probabilities**. syn: **specified assignment ratio** rt: **observed treatment assignment ratio**

expected value *n* - The sum of the **product** of the values of a **random variable** and **probabilities** of occurrence for those values; for **continuous random variable**, the integral of the product of a **probability density function** and the random variable itself over all possible values of the variable; **mathematical expectation**. rt: **expected frequency**, **expected number**, **parameter**

expedite, expedited, expediting, expedites *v* - [L *expeditus*, pp of *expedire*] To execute promptly; to accelerate the process or progress of; speed up.

expedited review *n* - 1. A **review** performed in prompt order and more expeditiously than ordinary. 2. A review performed by the **chair** of an **institutional review board** or by a member (or members) of an IRB, as designated by the chair; as distinct from a review performed by the full board. Provisions for expedited reviews are limited, by regulation, to proposals involving no more than minimal risk and to minor changes to approved projects.[117]

experience *n* - [ME, fr MF, fr L *experientia* act of trying, fr *experient-*, *experiens*, prp of *experiri* to try, fr *ex-* + *-periri* (akin to *periculum* attempt)] Something personally encountered, undergone, or lived through; an **event** or series of events encountered, undergone, or lived through.

experiment *n* - [ME, fr MF, fr L *experimentum*, fr *experiri*] 1. A procedure or **test** (defn 6) carried out under planned **controlled** conditions in order to discover an effect or law, to **test** (defn 3) or establish a **hypothesis**, to demonstrate a known fact or law, or for evaluation of the procedure or test, as in a **clinical trial**. 2. A procedure or process extending over time (eg, the treatment of gunshot wounds as practiced by surgeons of Ambroise Paré's time) abruptly changed because of circumstances (depletion of boiling oil — the standard treatment for gunshot wound — because of the intensity of the battle to capture the castle of Villaine; 1537) thus proving a **fortuitous** opportunity to assess the effect of the change against some **outcome measure** (In the case of Ambroise Paré: *I raised myself very early to visit them, when beyond my hope I found those to whom I had applied the digestive medicament, feeling but little pain, their wounds neither swollen nor inflamed, and having slept through the night. The others to whom I had applied the boiling oil were feverish with much pain and swelling about their wounds. Then I determined never again to burn thus so cruelly the poor wounded by Arquebuses*[119]); **fortuitous experiment**; **natural experiment**. *Usage note*: Most usages of **experiment** are in settings where there is a known or implied active process involved in designing and carrying out the experiment, as implied in defn 1. The term should be preceded or followed by appropriate modifiers when that is not the case, as with usages in the sense of defn 2.

experiment, experimented, experimenting, experiments *v* - To conduct an **experiment**; to test or try.

experimental *adj* - 1. Of, relating to, or based on experimentation. 2. Serving the ends of or used as a means of experimentation; not **observational**. 3. Relating to or having the characteristics of an experiment.

experimental design *n* - Any **design** or plan for conducting an **experiment**, especially that portion related to the **test variable** and description of ways in which it is to be manipulated. In the case of **trials**, usually that portion of the design or plan specifying the **treatments** to be studied, the **treatment assignment ratio**, the plan for assigning **treatment units** to the various **study treatments**, and the **treatment protocol**. rt: **study design**

experimental drug *n* - 1. A **drug** not yet tested in human beings, or one undergoing such testing as a possible prelude to licensure. 2. The **test treatment** in a **drug trial**. rt: **clinical epidemiology**, **descriptive epidemiology** *Usage note*: Usage in the sense of defn 2 is not recommended, except in settings where the conditions for defn 1 apply, such as perhaps in a **phase I** or **phase II trials**.

experimental epidemiology *n* - A subspecialty within the discipline of **epidemiology** involving the use of designed **experiments**, such as **clinical trials** (defns 1, 2, or 3) to investigate the role of some **factor** or **agent** in the generation, amelioration, delay, or prevention of **disease**. rt: **clinical epidemiology**

experimental error *n* - The **error** or **variation** remaining after all other **sources of variation** have been accounted for; the error not accounted for by the **hypothesis** or **model**. Variously referred to as **experimental error**, **error term**, **chance variation**, **extraneous variation**, or **random variation**. *Usage note*: Note that the errors referred to in this setting are naturally occurring, not mistakes.

experimental study *n* - Any **study**, such as a **clinical trial** (defns 1, 2, or 3), in which the **investigator** manipulates one or more **variables** in order to **observe** the effect of the manipulation on some process or **outcome**.

experimental treatment *n* - 1. A **treatment** that has not been tested in human beings or that is being tested but has not yet been approved for general use. 2. [**clinical trials**] **test treatment**

experimental trial *n* - A **trial**, especially an **efficacy** or **effectiveness trial**, involving two or more **study treatments**, at least one of which is largely untested. *Usage note*: Redundant; avoid, since the term **trial** (defn 1) itself conveys the notion of experimentation.

experimental unit *n* - The **unit** in an **experimental design** that receives or is to receive the **treatment** or a level of the **factor** of interest; equivalent to **treatment assignment unit** in **trials** and usually to **observation unit**.

experimental variable *n* - A **variable** that denotes the levels of a **factor** or **treatment** to be applied or that are applied in an **experiment**. The values assumed by the variable will correspond to the number of levels represented for a factor or treatment in the **design**. It will be **binary** in form in settings where the factor or treatment appears or is used at only one level, the value 1 indicating presence or use of the factor or treatment and the value 0 denoting absence of the factor or treatment. Typically referred to as **treatment variable** in **trials**.

experimentation *n* - 1. The act or process of carrying out an **experiment**. 2. The act or process of trying something not tried before. 3.

The act or process of performing an activity or procedure to determine whether it can be performed or performed as planned.

expert *adj* - [ME, fr MF & L; MF, fr, L *expertus*, fr pp of *experiri*] Having or displaying special skills or knowledge derived from training and experience.

expert *n* - [F, fr *expert*, adj] One having special skills or knowledge derived from training or experience.

expert system *n* - A **system** of **rules**, such as contained in a **computer program**, developed using experience or knowledge of **experts** to interpret or classify conditions or results presented to it [Hand, 1984].[64] For example, presentation of symptoms to yield a list of possible **diagnoses**. A form of artificial intelligence. Also known as **knowledge-based system**.

explanatory *adj* - Serving to explain.

explanatory trial *n* - A **trial** that is or is to be designed to explain how a **treatment** works [see Sackett, 1980;[135] Sackett and Gent, 1979;[136] Schwartz and Lellouch, 1967[139]]. Often used in contradistinction to **pragmatic trial**. syn: **efficacy trial** ant: **pragmatic trial**, **management trial** *Usage note*: Not generally a useful characterization, except, perhaps, where there is a need or desire to emphasize the nature of the trial as distinct from other types, most notably management trials. The difficulty is that the distinction is often blurred in that explanatory trials provide information on management and vice versa. Further, it may not be possible to reliably classify trials as to intent vis-a-vis explanatory or management, unless the characterization is applied by the **investigators** themselves. See **pragmatic trial** for additional comments.

explanatory variable *n* - 1. A **variable** that accounts for or explains an observed **association** or **difference**. 2. **independent variable**

exploratory data analysis *n* - 1. **Data analysis** performed for the purpose of attempting to find **relationships** of importance in the **data** or **subgroups** or subsets of the data that explain observed results; usually performed without benefit of prior **hypotheses**. 2. **data dredging**

exponent *n* - [L *exponent-*, *exponens*, prp of *exponere*] A **number**, symbol, or algebraic expression written above and to the right of a mathematical expression or number to indicate its **power**, eg, *2* in the expression 10^2.

exponential *adj* - 1. Of or relating to an **exponent**. 2. Involving a **variable** in an exponent, eg, *x* in the expression e^x. 3. Capable of being expressed or approximated by an exponential function.

exponential distribution *n* - A **probability density function** of the form

$$f(x) = \frac{1}{\theta}e^{-x/\theta} \ \ for \ x > 0; \ 0 \ elsewhere$$

with **mean** θ and **variance** θ^2. The distribution has applicability in engineering and the life sciences in relation to reliability studies and queuing, eg, it characterizes the waiting time between successive **events** in a **Poisson process**; also referred to as the negative exponential distribution, a special case of the **gamma distribution**.

Exponential distribution

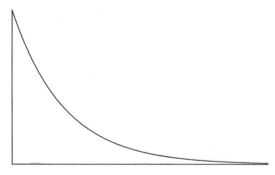

expose, exposed, exposing, exposes *v* - [ME *exposen*,fr MF *exposer*, fr L *exponere* to set forth, explain, fr *ex-* + *ponere* to put, place] Subject to **risk** from a harmful condition.

exposed *n* - [**epidemiology**] 1. A person (or group of persons) subject to **risk** of acquiring a **disease** from **contact** with or **exposure** to the infectious **agent** for that **disease**, eg, polio virus. 2. A person (or group of persons) subject to risk of acquiring some disease or adverse health condition from contact with or **exposure** to some causative or presumably causative agent, eg, development of leukemia from exposure to low levels of radiation or development of high blood pressure from a diet high in sodium. 3. A person (or group of persons) subject to risk or of deriving protection from contact or exposure to some agent. rt: **exposed group**

exposed group *n* - A **group** of persons having been or presumed to have been **exposed** to some **agent** or condition known to be or suspected of being causative of a **disease** or **adverse** health condition or of playing a role in causation.

exposure *n* - Being or having been exposed.

external study validity *n* - The extent to which study **results** provide a correct and proper basis for **generalization** to a larger **target population**; generally a matter of conjecture except in studies in which sampling procedures are used to select study members. See also **generalizability**. rt: **internal study validity, validity**

extramural *adj* - Being or occurring outside or beyond the **limits** or confines of a specified organizational **unit** or entity. ant: **intramural**

extramural funding *n* - 1. Monies awarded or provided from outside one's own **institution** or **agency**. 2. **Funding** provided by an agency or **organization** to some unit or organization external to it; in the case of **NIH**, monies provided to awardees in relation to its **extramural research program**. ant: **intramural funding**

extramural research *n* - **Research** performed outside the confines or the direct control of the **institution** funding it. In the parlance of **NIH**, research funded by **grants** or **contracts** and not part of its **intramural research program**. ant: **intramural research**

extraneous *adj* - [L *extraneus*] 1. Existing on or coming from the outside. 2. Not forming an essential or vital part; unnecessary.

extraneous source of variation *n* - In **study design** and conduct, a **source of variation** due to conditions or **factors** beyond the **control** of the **investigator**.

extraneous variation *n* - **Variation** arising from extraneous sources, eg, that due to **random** variation or **error**.

extrapolate, **extrapolated**, **extrapolating**, **extrapolates** *v* - [L *extra* outside + *E- polate*, as in *interpolate*] To infer, **predict**, extend, or project beyond something recorded, **observed** or experienced, eg, to use **data** contained in a table of heights and weights to extrapolate to heights and weights beyond the limits of the table.   ant: **interpolate**

F

F *n* - [6th letter of the English alphabet] Symbol for a **statistic** based on the **F distribution**; F for the developer of the statistic, **Ronald Fisher**.

F distribution *n* - The sampling **distribution** of the **ratio** of two **independent chi-square random variables**, each divided by its **degrees of freedom** (v_1 and v_2, for the **numerator** and **denominator** variable, respectively). The F distribution is used in **analyses of variance** to gauge the statistical likelihood of an observed value of the **F test statistic** under the **null hypothesis**. The distribution is tabled for various values of v_1 and v_2. The distribution approaches the **chi-square distribution** with v_1 degrees of freedom divided by v_1 as v_2 approaches infinity. First described by **Ronald Fisher** and named in his honor.[47] syn: variance-ratio distribution

F distribution

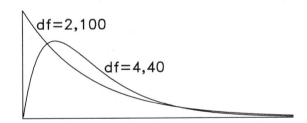

F test *n* - 1. A **test of hypothesis** based on the **F test statistic**. 2. The value of the F test statistic for a given set of **data**.

F test statistic *n* - 1. A **test statistic** of the general form:

$$\frac{U/v_1}{V/v_2}$$

where U and V are **independent random variables** having **chi-square distributions** with v_1, v_2 **degrees of freedom** for U and V, respectively; used for **analysis of variance** and calculated by taking the **ratio** of **independent variances** estimated from **observed data** and having v_1 and v_2 degrees of freedom, respectively. 2. The calculated value of the **statistic** for a given set of **data**.

fabricate, fabricated, fabricating, fabricates *v* - [ME *fabricaten*, fr L *fabricatus*, pp of *fabricari*, fr *fabrica*] Makeup for the purpose of deception; invent. rt: **dry lab, forge**

fabricated data *n* - **Data** made up for the purpose of deception. syn: **dry labbed data, falsified data, forged data** rt: **bogus data, fudged data, scientific misconduct**

fabrication *n* - 1. The act or process of **fabricating**. 2. The product of fabricating; lie; falsehood.

factor *n* - [ME, fr MF *facteur*, fr L *factor* doer, fr *factus*] 1. Something that actively contributes to the production of a result or outcome or that brings about a change; **determinant**. 2. A **variable** or condition manipulated or controlled in an **experiment**; a **categorical variable** or specific value of that variable, especially in an experimental setting. 3. A substance that functions in or promotes the function of a particular physiological process or body system. 4. A component part of a **number** or quantity, that when multiplied by its other component parts, yields that number or quantity. 5. A multiplier or divider used to express change or difference, eg, **rate** increased by a factor of 10.

factor, factoring, factored, factors *v* - To resolve into **factors**.

factor analysis *n* - A method of **multivariate analysis** in which the goal is to represent an array of **data** on individual **observation units**, each observed on a number of **variables** and involving varying degrees of **interrelationships**, by **linear combinations** of the **data**; each such combination being referred to as a **factor** or dimension of the data and used to help identify the components or **determinants** of some process, behavior, or **outcome**. For example, the analysis of responses to questions in an intelligence test to identify the different forms of intelligence represented.

factorial *adj* - Of, relating to, or being a **factor** or a **factorial**. ant: **nonfactorial**

factorial *n* - 1. The product of all **positive** integers from 1 to n; denoted as n!; 0! = 1. 2. A **factorial design** or **factorial experiment** in which some or all of the various **factors**, conditions, or **treatments** of interest are arranged or administered in combinations as in a **complete** or **incomplete factorial**.

factorial design *n* - 1. An **experimental design** in which all or some of the **factors** or **treatments** appear in combination with all or some of the other factors or treatments, as in a **complete factorial treatment design** or **incomplete factorial treatment design**. 2. **factorial treatment design** rt: **complete factorial treatment design, incomplete factorial treatment design, hierarchical experiment**

factorial experiment *n* - An **experiment** in which some or all of the levels of one **experimental variable** appear in combination with some or all of the levels of another such variable. Said to be a **complete** factorial experiment when all combinations of the one experimental variable appear in combination with all combinations of the other experimental variable and said to be **incomplete** when some but not all of the possible combinations are represented. rt: **hierarchical experiment**

factorial structure *n* - A **structure** in which the **factors**, traits, conditions, or **treatments** have a **factorial** arrangement or **design**.

factorial treatment design *n* - A type of **treatment design** in which one **treatment (factor)** is **crossed** (full or partial) with another treatment (factor). For example, a 2 x 2 factorial design in a **parallel trial** to evaluate the usefulness of counseling to reduce sodium intake and caloric intake in relation to blood pressure control; in its simplest form with just two levels for each factor (counseling or no counseling) yields four counseling regimens: AB, $\bar{A}$B, A$\bar{B}$, and $\bar{A}\bar{B}$, where A represents counseling for sodium reduction and $\bar{A}$ denotes absence of such counseling, and where B represents counseling for caloric restriction and $\bar{B}$ denotes absence of such counseling.

rt: **complete factorial treatment design, incomplete factorial treatment design**

factorial treatment structure *n* - A **structure** in which some or all of the **treatments** are arranged as a **complete** or **incomplete factorial**.

failure *n* - [alter of earlier *failer*, fr AF, fr OF *faillir* to fail] The condition or fact of not achieving the desired or expected end result or end; not a success.

fallacy *n* - [L *fallacia*, fr *fallac-*, *fallax* deceitful, fr *fallere* to deceive] 1. **False** or mistaken idea or notion. 2. Plausible argument or **relationship** using fallacious **data** or specious reasoning. rt: **ecological fallacy**

false *adj* - [ME *fals*, fr OF & L; OF, fr L *falsus*, fr pp of *fallere* to deceive] 1. Not genuine. 2. Intentionally untrue; adjusted or made so as to deceive; tending to mislead 3. Not true; inconsistent with the facts. ant: **true**

false negative *n* - [epidemiology] 1. Someone falsely classified as not having some **disease** or condition on the basis of a diagnostic test or **screening** procedure, eg, a woman who has a negative Pap smear of the cervix but has cancer of the cervix. 2. A **result** of a **test** or diagnostic procedure that leads to such a **false classification**. ant: **false positive** rt: **sensitivity, specificity**

false positive *n* - [epidemiology] 1. Someone falsely classified as having some **disease** or condition on the basis of a diagnostic test or **screening** procedure, eg, a woman who has a positive Pap smear of the cervix but does not have cancer of the cervix. 2. A result of a test or diagnostic procedure that leads to such a false classification. ant: **false negative** rt: **sensitivity, specificity**

falsified data *n* - 1. **Data** made **false** by a purposeful act; **fudged data; bogus data** (defn 1). 2. Made-up **data**; also **dry labbed data, fabricated data**, or **forged data**. rt: **scientific misconduct**

falsify, falsified, falsifying, falsifies *v* - [ME *falsifien*, fr MF *falsifier*, fr ML *falsificare*, fr L *falsus*] 1. To state untruthfully; misrepresent. 2. To make false by altering or adding to. 3. To makeup; **fabricate; forge**.

FDA *n* - **Food and Drug Administration**

feasibility study *n* - A **study** designed and performed for the purpose of determining whether it is possible to perform a **full-scale study** or a specified set of tasks or functions in relation to such a full-scale study, eg, a study aimed at testing the ability of investigators in selected **field centers** to recruit specified numbers of **patients** in a designated time period. rt: **demonstration study, pilot study**

feasibility trial *n* - A **trial** designed and performed for the purpose of determining whether it is possible to perform a larger more complicated **full-scale trial** or a specified set of tasks or functions in relation to such a full-scale trial, eg, a trial aimed at testing the feasibility of administering different dietary treatments to free-living healthy people. rt: **demonstration trial, pilot trial**

feasible *adj* - [ME *faisible*, fr MF, fr *fais-* stem of *faire* to make do, fr L *facere*] Capable of being done or carried out; capable of being used.

fee *n* - [ME, fr MF *fé*, *fief* fr OF, of Gmc origin; akin to OE *feoh* cattle, property, OHG *fihu* cattle; akin to L *pecus* cattle, *pecunia* money, *pectere* to comb] 1. A fixed charge. 2. A charge for a service rendered. 3. An amount paid or to be paid for a service rendered or activity performed.

fee-for-service *n* - 1. A **fee** paid or to be paid to a purveyor for a service rendered or activity performed. 2. **fee-for-service agreement**

fee-for-service agreement *n* - An **agreement** in which the amount paid or to be paid to a purveyor of a service is determined by the amount of service rendered.

fetal tissue *n* - Any of the products of the **fetus** during gestation, including the placental membrane.

fetus *n* - [ME, fr L, act of bearing young, offspring; akin to L *fetus* newly delivered, fruitful] 1. A developing human embryo, especially after attaining a basic embryologic structure, eg, after the 12th week of development to the moment of birth. 2. An unborn or unhatched vertebrate, especially after attaining a basic embryonic structure.

Fibonacci, Leonardo (Leonardo Pisano) - (1170 (circa) - 1250 (circa)) Italian born (Pisa) mathematician and algebraist; studied commercial arithmetic and mathematical literature of Hindu and Arabic cultures; largely responsible for introduction of the Arabic system of numbers and notation into Western culture. Responsible for **Fibonacci sequence**.

Fibonacci numbers *n* - 1. **Numbers** from a **Fibonacci sequence**. 2. **Fibonacci sequence**

Fibonacci sequence *n* - A **sequence** of **numbers**, 1, 1, 2, 3, 5, 8, 13, 21, ⋯, in which each successive number (after the first two) is the **sum** of the previous two in the sequence; named after **Leonardo Fibonacci**.

fiducial *adj* - 1. Taken as a standard of reference. 2. Founded on faith or trust.

fiducial distribution *n* - A **distribution** derived from the **distribution** of **estimators** that contains all relevant information from a **sample**. Similar in concept to **a priori probability density**, but having a different genesis and interpretation. rt: **fiducial inference, fiducial limits**

fiducial inference *n* - A type of **inference** due to **RA Fisher** based on **fiducial distributions** having to do with **populations** of **parameters**. Similar in concept, but not genesis or interpretation, to inferences based on **confidence intervals**. The object of the inference is to make probabilistic statements regarding the values of unknown **parameters**. "Fiducial" because the inference relates, in effect, to the trust one has in inferences based on confidence intervals. rt: **fiducial distribution, fiducial limits**

fiducial limits *n* - **Limits** between which a **parameter** is assumed to lie. Not to be confused with **confidence limits** even if the two sets of limits are the same, as they may be in special cases. rt: **fiducial distribution, fiducial inference, confidence interval, confidence limits**

field *adj* - 1. Made, conducted, or used in the **field** (defn 1). 2. Operating or active in a general setting, especially in contradistinction to the usual setting of a factory, **office**, **clinic**, or **laboratory**.

field *n* - [ME, fr OE *feld*; akin to OHG *feld* field, OE *flōr* floor] 1. An area of activity or operation that exists or is performed in a general setting, such as a **community**; as distinct from a specialized setting such as a factory, **office**, **clinic**, or **laboratory**. 2. A set of one or more characters (**bytes**) treated as a whole in a **record** or a **file**; a set of one or more columns on a punch card or spaces on a **data form** used to record a designated type of information. rt: **community**

field center *n* - A **center** that operates or exists outside a designated factory, **office**, or **laboratory**.

field clinic *n* - A **clinic** that operates or exists outside the traditional confines and setting for a **clinic**.

field monitor *n* - 1. One who **monitors** operations in the **field**. 2. An individual employed by the **sponsor** or a **center** of a **trial** (eg, **coordinating center**) to visit participating **clinics** to monitor data collection procedures; **study clinic monitor**. rt: **circuit rider**

field survey *n* - A systematic collection of **data**, usually through the use of **questionnaires** administered to persons in a general **population**.

field trial *n* - 1. A **trial** carried out in the **field** (defn 1); as opposed to a **clinic** or hospital. 2. **community trial** 3. **demonstration trial** *Usage note*: Subject to varying use; not informative without use of additional descriptors to make sense of meaning clear. In a technical sense, any trial not involving medical care or treatment in the usual sense of those terms is a field trial in the sense of defn 1. Often used in reference to trials done in the field with geographic region as the unit of assignment.

figure *n* - [ME, fr OF, fr L *figura*, fr *fingere*] 1. **Number** or amount. 2. A written or printed character. 3. A **graphic** representation of a set of **data**, of a geometric form, or of textual material. rt: **chart**, **diagram**, **table**

file *n* - [MF, fr *filer* to spin, fr LL *filare*, fr L *filum*] 1. A **device** by which paper **records** are kept for storing and retrieval. 2. A collection of related **records** (eg, as represented by a series of punch cards or as contained on a magnetic tape or **disk** or in the **memory** of a **computer**) that is or may be treated as a logical unit or entity.

file, filed, filing, files *v* - The act of placing or arranging something (eg, **data items**, **records**) in a **file**.

file drawer problem *n* - The tendency of or expectation for **investigators** to leave or abandon **results** of **studies** in one's file drawer unpublished, especially in relation to those that are **nil** or **negative**. Often used in relation to references to **publication bias**.

final *adj* - [ME, fr MF, fr L *finalis*, fr *finis* boundary, end] 1. Not to be altered or undone; of or relating to the last or concluding action or process. 2. Of or relating to the ultimate purpose or result of some process or action.

final data analysis *n* - 1. **Data analyses** carried out at the end or last stage of a **study**, eg, analyses performed during the **termination stage** of a **trial**. 2. Data analyses performed in relation to the final version of a **manuscript** or **report**.

final examination *n* - **final patient examination**

final patient examination *n* - 1. The last **examination** of a **patient** prior to **close-out**. 2. The last examination of a patient prior to **enrollment** (not recommended usage).

find, found, finding, finds *v* - [ME *finden*, fr OE *findan*; akin to OHG *findan* to find, L *pont-*, *pons* bridge, Gk *pontos* sea, Skt *patha* way, course] To come upon by searching or purposeful effort.

finite *adj* - [ME *finit*, fr L *finitus*, pp of *finire*] 1. Having definite or definable **limits** or **boundaries**. 2. Completely determinable in theory or in fact by counting or **measurement**; not **infinite**. ant: **infinite**

finite population *n* - A **population** having a **finite** (countable) number of elements or units.

firm *n* - [Ger *firma*, fr It, signature, deriv of L *firmare* to make firm, confirm, fr *firmus*] A **business** or enterprise.

fiscal *adj* - [L *fiscalis*, fr *fiscus* basket, treasury; akin to Gk *pithos* wine jar] Of or relating to financial matters.

fiscal year (FY) *n* - An accounting **period** of one **year** defined by the firm, agency, or corporate entity to which it applies; for the US Government starting with October 1 and ending with September 30.

Fisher, Sir Ronald Aylmer - (1890 - 1962) Born in London; died in Adelaide. English mathematical statistician responsible for numerous innovations in the field of **statistics**, most notably **maximum likelihood**, **analysis of variance**, and **randomization**. Much of his early work was done in relation to agricultural experiments at Rothamsted Experimental Station. His 11 page paper on field experiments, published in 1926, served as the basis for his widely cited book on design of experiments.[47]

Fisher's Exact Test *n* - A **nonparametric statistical test** for comparing two **proportions** from **independent samples**; **exact** because the **probability** of observing a value as extreme or more extreme than the one observed for the **test statistic** is calculated from the **hypergeometric distribution** for a 2x2 **contingency table** with **row** and **column** totals fixed.

fit *adj* - [ME; akin to ME *fitten*] Adapted to an end or state; put into a suitable state.

fit *n* - [ME, fr OE *fitt* strife] 1. The conformity or **agreement** between **observed data** and a **curve** based on a mathematical model or **empirical fit**. 2. The conformity or agreement between an **observation** and that predicted or computed using a mathematical model.

fit, fitted, fitting, fits *v* - [ME *fitten* to marshal troops, fr or akin to MD *vitten* to be suitable, akin to OHG *fizza* skein] 1. To be suitable or proper for. 2. To conform correctly or suitably close to a defined shape or profile. 3. To insert or adjust until suitably positioned or situated. 4. To be in agreement or accord with; to cause to conform or comply. 5. To adjust to a given set of points, as in **curve fitting**.

fix, fixed, fixing, fixes *v* - [ME *fixen*, fr L *fixus*, pp of *figere* to fasten] 1. To establish, definitely set, or **assign**. 2. To make an accurate determination of. 3. To set in order or **adjust**. 4. To make firm, stable, or stationary. 5. To give a final or permanent form to.

fixed assignment *n* - **fixed treatment assignment**

fixed assignment design *n* - **fixed treatment assignment design**

fixed assignment ratio *n* - **fixed treatment assignment ratio**

fixed assignment schedule *n* - **fixed treatment assignment schedule**

fixed sample size design *n* - [**trials**] 1. A **design** in which the **number** of **observation units** to be **enrolled** is fixed as determined by a **sample size calculation** prior to the start of **enrollment** or as fixed by other considerations (eg, cost or availability of patients). 2. Any **nonsequential sample size design**, even if the sample size is not fixed or determined before the start of the trial. ant: **sequential sample size design**

fixed treatment assignment *n* - [**trials**] Any method of **treatment assignment** involving a **fixed treatment assignment ratio**. ant: **adaptive treatment assignment**

fixed treatment assignment design *n* - [**trials**] A **treatment assignment design** in which the **treatment assignment ratio** is **fixed**. ant:

adaptive treatment assignment design

fixed treatment assignment ratio *n* - [**trials**] An **assignment ratio** that remains **fixed** over the course of **enrollment**.

fixed treatment assignment schedule *n* - [**trials**] A **treatment assignment schedule** in which **treatment assignment probabilities** remain **fixed** over the course of **enrollment**. ant: **adaptive treatment assignment schedule**

fixed-cost *adj* - Of or relating to a monetary cost fixed by **agreement** or statement; unlike **cost-reimbursement** and **fee-for-service**.

fixed-cost contract *n* - A **contract** in which there is an **agreement** between the **contractor** (defn 1) and purveyor of goods or services on the amount to be paid for said goods or services, regardless of actual costs incurred.

fixed-effects model *n* - A **mathematical model**, typically used in **analysis of variance**, in which the values representing **effects** are considered fixed and, hence, are represented by **parameters** in the model. ant: **random-effects model** rt: **mixed-effects model**

flat *adj* - [ME, fr ON *flatr*; akin to OHG *flaz* flat, Gk *platys*] 1. Having a smooth **continuous** horizontal surface. 2. Being or characterized by a straight horizontal **line**.

flat file *n* - Any **file** in which **data** elements are organized and arrayed as if they are unrelated and logically of equal importance (eg, an unordered sequence of **records** as contained on magnetic tape or a **diskette**). rt: **hierarchical file**

floppy *adj* - Being soft and flexible; tending to flop.

floppy disk *n* - **diskette**

flow *adj* - Of or relating to a smooth or **continuous** transition.

flow diagram *n* - **flowchart** (defn 1)

flowchart *n* - 1. A **chart** or **diagram** that provides a step-by-step progression through a procedure or system; when presented as a chart, usually a sequence of numbered written instructions; when presented as a diagram, usually displayed with a mix of text and connecting lines and symbols to display the sequence of steps; also flow diagram. 2. [**medicine**] A **spreadsheet** in two **dimensions** (**rows** and **columns**) with one of its dimensions corresponding to different **measures** (eg, laboratory tests) and with the other dimension corresponding to **time**; used to record and review data for a **patient**.

Flow diagram

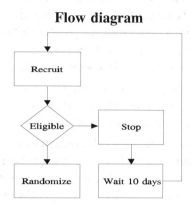

follow *n* - The act or process of **following**.

follow, followed, following, follows *v* - [ME *folwen*, fr OE *folgian*; akin to OHG *folgēn* to follow] 1. To go or come after a person or thing in place, time, or sequence. 2. To keep **track** of. 3. To result or occur as a consequence or effect. 4. To accept as authority, obey; to be or act in accordance with.

follow up, followed up, following up *v* - 1. To maintain contact with a person or some larger **observation unit** through periodic **visits**, telephone calls, or letters so as to continue **observation** or to be in a position to do so when appropriate; in the case of **trials** typically done in relation to **treatment administration** or assessment of the effects of **treatment**. 2. To pursue in an effort to take some action or step; to take appropriate action, eg, to follow up on a lead. 3. To contact periodically in **trials** and other forms of **prospective followup** for the purpose of observing or **monitoring** the effects of some procedure or **treatment** or to note the occurrence of some **outcome** or **event** for **data collection**; the process implied proceeds forward in real time and typically involves **direct contact** with **study participants** or their **surrogates**. 4. Any of various kinds of activities or processes intended to generate **prospective data** for the object of followup. The activity or process for the object of followup starts at a point in time determined by some act, **event**, or **exposure** and proceeds in time from that point. The act, event, or exposure may have occurred in the past with followup proceeding to a point in the less distant past, to

the present, or to a point in the future, or it may occur in the present with followup proceeding to a point in the future.

following *adj* - Coming next in time, order, or sequence.

followup *adj* - [also **follow-up**] 1. Done, conducted, or administered in the course of **follow up**, as in a **followup study**. 2. Of, relating to, concerned with, or being something done as a followup, especially in relation to previous actions, procedures, or **observations**.

followup *n* - [also **follow-up**] 1. The act of or an instance of **followup**. 2. Something done in or as followup, eg, reexamination of a person as part of **scheduled followup**. 3. Maintenance of contact with a person or **observation unit** for care or administration of **treatment**. 4. **patient followup**

followup cohort *n* - 1. A **group** of people (or larger **observation units**) followed forward in time. 2. A group of people **enrolled** in a **study** and followed forward in time.

followup data *n* - **Data** collected on an **observation unit** or a set of observation units after **enrollment** of that unit or units in a **study**.

followup data collection visit *n* - [**trials**] Any **data collection visit** that takes place after a person has been **assigned to treatment**.

followup examination *n* - **followup patient examination**

followup observation *n* - 1. An **observation** made at a designated point in the course of **followup**. 2. A series of observations made at various **time points** over the course of followup. 3. An item of **data** collected on a **person** (or larger **observation unit**) after **enrollment** in a **study**.

followup patient examination *n* - A **patient examination** done at a **followup visit**.

followup period *n* - 1. A **period** of **time** from **enrollment** of an **observation unit** (usually a person) in a **study** to the termination of **followup** of that unit. 2. A period of time in the course of a study defined by the start of followup of the first observation unit **enrolled** and by the end of followup of the last unit enrolled; **followup stage**.

followup stage *n* - [**trials**] 1. A **stage of trial** with **followup** as the sole objective; typically starting with the completion of **treatment administration** and ending with the start of the **termination**

stage. The stage does not exist in trials in which treatment and followup proceed concurrently, as in the **treatment and followup stage**. 2. Such a stage occurring after the **close-out stage**.

followup study *n* - 1. A **study** in which **data collection** for those **enrolled** proceeds forward in time, either from a point in the past to a more recent point in the past, from a point in the past to the present or one in the future, or from the present to a point in the future. 2. **concurrent followup study** See *study* for list. syn: **cohort study**, longitudinal study, **prospective study** ant: **cross-sectional study** *Usage note*: All **trials**, by definition, involve **followup** and in this general sense are, therefore, members of this larger class of studies. However, the term is best reserved for the subset excluding trials to avoid confusion. See **cohort study** for additional comment.

followup study design *n* - The portion of a **study design** that details methods and procedures to be used for following those **enrolled** in the **study** and for **data collection** during **followup**.

followup survey *n* - A **survey** that is done as a **followup** to one done previously. ant: **cross-sectional survey**

followup variable *n* - A **variable** observed or to be observed during **followup**. rt: **baseline variable**

followup visit *n* - [trials] Any **study clinic visit** by a person after **treatment assignment**, especially a **required followup visit**. See **required** and **non-required followup visit** for classes of visits. See also **treatment adjustment**, **interim**, **close-out**, **post close-out**, and **post-trial followup visit** for specific types of followup visits.

food *n* - [often attrib ME *fode*, fr OE *fōda*; akin to OHG *fuotar* food, fodder, L *panis* bread, *pascere* to feed] Material, usually of plant or animal origin and consisting essentially of protein, carbohydrate, and fat, used in the body of an organism to sustain growth, repair, and vital processes and to furnish energy.

Food and Drug Administration (FDA) *n* - An **agency** within the US **Department of Health and Human Services** and a part of the **United States Public Health Service** (USPHS) having broad regulatory powers relating to the content and nature of claims made in the labeling of **food** products and food additives, cosmetics, **medical devices**, and **drugs** intended for or subject to interstate commerce. The agency has authority to grant, withhold, or rescind licenses to market drugs and medical devices and to require studies establishing their **safety** and **efficacy** as conditions for approvals to market; see **Investigational New Drug Application**, **New Drug Application**, **Abbreviated New Drug Application**, and **Pre-Market Approval Application**. Major division within the FDA include:[115]

Center for Biologics Evaluation and Research (CBER)
Center for Devices and Radiological Health (CDRH)
Center for Drug Evaluation and Research (CDER)
Center for Food Safety and Applied Nutrition (CFSAN)
Center for Veterinary Medicine (CVM)
National Center for Toxicological Research (NCTR)

force *n* - [ME, fr MF, fr (assumed) VL *fortia*, fr L *fortis* strong] Strength or energy exerted or brought to bear.

force of mortality *n* - **Hazard rate** for death.

forge, forged, forging, forges *v* - [ME, fr OF, fr L *fabrica*, fr *fabr*-, *faber* smith] To make or imitate falsely with the intent to deceive.

forged data *n* - Made-up **data**. rt: **falsified data**, **scientific misconduct**

forgery *n* - Something **forged**.

form *n* - [ME *forme*, fr OF, fr L *forma* form, beauty] 1. A paper **document** consisting of a collection of **data items** and **data fields** in which the data items serve to characterize the types of information required and the fields represent blank spaces to be used for recording the requested information. 2. Any such arrangement, including those represented electronically on video screens. rt: **data form**, **data record**, **record**, **questionnaire**

formless *adj* - [general] Devoid of or wanting in form; having no delineation or form. [**data collection**] Not involving use of **paper forms**.

formless study *n* - **paperless study** *Usage note*: Not recommended; use other terminology, such as **paperless study**, to avoid risk of being jocular or pejorative.

forms inventory *n* - An **inventory** of forms completed, received, or processed.

fortuitous *adj* - [L *fortuitus*; akin to L *fort-*, *fors*] Occurring by **chance**; fortunate; lucky.

fortuitous experiment *n* - A condition imposed by **fortuitous** circumstances that provides a basis for making an **observation** or drawing a **conclusion** regarding some **test** or procedure; not an **experiment** in the usual sense; see usage note for **experiment**. rt: **natural experiment**

forward *adj* - [ME fr OE *foreweard* fr *fore-* + *-weard* -ward] Proceeding or advancing in **time** or **sequence**; proceeding or advancing in steps from simple to complex, or from one to many; done or arranged in logical order or sequence. ant: **backward**

forward stepwise regression *n* - **Stepwise regression** typically performed by proceeding from a mandated set of **regressors** (eg, the set considered to be important as based on previous work plus selected demographic variables) to a larger, but still limited, set done by adding regressors with the ultimate goal of finding an appropriately restricted set. As distinct from **simultaneous regression**. See **stepwise regression** for more details. See **backward stepwise regression** for alternative approach.

fractile *n* - [as an adj: pertaining to fraction or breakage] One of a contiguous set of **ranges** of values of a **frequency distribution**, such that each set accounts for the same number or fraction of counts represented in the distribution, eg, the fractiles of a **uniform** age distribution over the range 25 through 55 that is to be divided into 3 fractiles would have the values 25 - 35, 35 - 45, and 45 - 55; also **quantile**; see **centile**, **decile**, **quintile**, **quartile**, **percentile**, **tercile** for specific types.

frame *n* - A skeleton structure that provides a basis for future work or action, eg, a **sampling frame** or the framework of a physical structure.

fraud *n* - [ME *fraude*, fr MF, fr L *fraud-*, *fraus*; akin to Skt *dhvarati* he bends, injures] Broadly, deceit or trickery; specifically, a deception deliberately practiced to secure unfair or unlawful gain; an act of deceiving or misrepresenting; intentional perversion of the truth to induce another to part with something of value or to surrender a right. *Usage note*: Avoid as an accusation, absent supporting evidence of intent. Two identical acts, both equally injurious, may be judged to have been the result of different motivations or causes and, hence, one may be

fraudulent, given an intent on the part of the one performing the act to deceive, and the other may be simply the result of oversight or **error**. The element of intent is evident in the definitions of fraud, as given in the *Oxford English Dictionary*[109] and *Black's Law Dictionary*.[10] Even acts of omission can be fraudulent if intended to deceive. OED: *1. The quality or disposition of being deceitful; faithlessness, insincerity. 2. Criminal deception; the using of false representations to obtain an unjust advantage or to injure the rights or interests of another. 3. An act or instance of deception, an artifice by which the right or interest of another is injured, a dishonest trick or stratagem. 4. A method or means of defrauding or deceiving; a fraudulent contrivance; in modern colloquial use, a spurious or deceptive thing.* Black's Law Dictionary: *An intentional perversion of truth for the purpose of inducing another in reliance upon it to part with some valuable thing belonging to him or to surrender a legal right. A false representation of a matter of fact, whether by words or by conduct, by false or misleading allegations, or by concealment of that which should have been disclosed, which deceives and is intended to deceive another so that he shall act upon it to his legal injury. Anything calculated to deceive, whether by a single act or combination, or by suppression of truth, or suggestion of what is false, whether it be by direct falsehood or innuendo, by speech or silence, word of mouth, or look or gesture.*

fraudulent *a* - Characterized by, based on, or done by **fraud**; deceitful.

fraudulent data *n* - **fabricated data**; **falsified data**; **forged data** rt: **scientific misconduct**

free *adj* - [ME, fr OE *frēo*; akin to OHG *fri* free, Gk *prays* gentle] 1. Having the right or privilege to be unrestricted or unconstrained, as in *you are free to withdraw from a study whenever you so choose*. 2. Not obstructed or impeded; not restricted. 3. Not subject to government regulation. 4. Not costing or charging anything. rt: **win** *Usage note*: Subject to misuse in everyday usage, especially in the sense of defn 4, as in *Congratulations, you have won a free TV!* (as printed on an official looking "prize" notice from yet another sweepstakes). Typically, a careful reading of the "fine print" on the "notice of award" reveals that to receive the "free gift", one has to be prepared to invest time (eg, by traveling to a distant point to listen to or watch a detailed sales pitch) or buy something. Avoid as a disingenuous claim. See also note for **win**.

free treatment arm *n* - 1. A **treatment** that is selected by the **study physician** or **study patient**. 2. A **study group** that receives the **treatment** selected by study physicians or study patients.

freedom *n* - [ME *fredom*, fr OE *frēodōm*, fr *frēo* free + *-dōm* -dom] The absence of constraint or condition.

freeze *n* - The state of being **frozen**.

freeze, froze, frozen, freezing, freezes *v* - [ME *fresen*, fr OE *frēosan*; akin to OHG *friosan* to freeze, L *pruina* hoarfrost, OE *frost* frost] To cause to become fixed, immovable, or unalterable.

frequency *n* - 1. The **number** or **relative number** of persons, places, or things represented by a **count** or **proportion**. 2. The number or relative number of persons, places, or things in a **class** or **category**. rt: **relative frequency** *Usage note*: The term **frequency** refers to either absolute or relative counts; usually clear from context. If there is a possibility of confusion, it is wise to be explicit by using the appropriate modifiers, absolute or relative.

frequency distribution *n* - An arrangement of **data** that exhibits the **frequency** or **relative frequency** of the occurrence of the values of the **variable** represented by the distribution, eg, the frequency distribution of age gives the number or relative number of persons observed having specified ages.

frequency function *n* - 1. A **function** giving the **frequency** of variate values of a **variable** as a function of different values of the variable (**distribution function**); for **continuous variables**, the frequency in an elemental small **interval**. 2. **probability density function**

frequency histogram *n* - **histogram**

frequency matching *v* - A process in which one **group** (eg, **controls**) is purposely selected so as to have the same or approximately the same **frequency distribution** as another group (eg, **cases**) for a **variable** or combination of variables (eg, age and gender). ant: **pair matching** rt: **individual matching, category matching, group matching**

frequency polygon *n* - A **graph** of a **frequency distribution** of **grouped data** arising from a **continuous variable** involving a series of straight lines connecting points corresponding to frequencies and positioned at the midpoints of the **class intervals** represented in the distribution; the point corresponding to the lowest class is connected to the point on the **x-axis** corresponding to the lower limit of the interval for that class, and the point for the highest class is connected to the point on the x-axis corresponding to the largest value represented in the interval for that class. Similar in general form and construction to a **histogram** where the rectangles representing frequencies are replaced by a series of connected points, with the points positioned at the midpoint of the class intervals represented in the distribution.

Frequency polygon

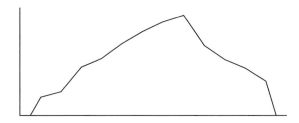

frequency table *n* - A tabular representation of a **frequency distribution** as a **table** with as many lines as **categories** or **class intervals** (plus one for the **total**) and where the **frequency** is given for each line represented.

frequentist *n* - 1. Being or relating to a school of thought in which **inferences** about a particular **dataset** depend on the **probability distribution** for particular **parameter** values based on the hypothetical notion of a **study** being repeated many times under the same conditions; also referred to as **sampling** theory approach. 2. One who performs a **frequentist analysis**. rt: **Neyman-Pearson theory**

frequentist analysis *n* - A method of **data analysis** based on the notion that a **study** can be repeated many times under the same conditions and that **inferences** should be based on the hypothetical frequencies of repeated **outcomes** under a given **hypothesis**. Analyses are expressed as verdicts regarding the acceptance or rejection of **null** or **alternative hypotheses**, **p-values** interpreted as an "observed" **type I error rate**, or **confidence intervals**. rt: **frequentist** *Usage note*: Most analyses presented are of this form and usually are referred to simply as analyses without the modifier **frequentist**. Generally the characterization **frequentist analysis** is used only in contradistinction to a method of analysis not requiring a frequentist view, as in **Bayesian analysis**.

fudge, fudged, fudging, fudges *v* - [origin unknown] 1. To exceed the proper bounds or **limits** of something. 2. To devise as a substitute without adequate basis; fake; makeup. rt: **forge**

fudged data *n* - **Data** adjusted or modified to comply with or be within a **standard** or **limit**. rt: **falsified data, forged data, scientific misconduct**

full *adj* - [ME, fr OE; akin to OHG *fol* full, L *plēnus* full, *plēre* to fill, Gk *plērēs* full, *plēthein* to be full] **Complete**; containing as many as possible or permissible; lacking restraint, check, or qualification; being at the highest degree.

full factorial *n* - **complete factorial**

full factorial treatment design *n* - **complete factorial treatment design**

full mask *n* - **complete mask**

full-scale *adj* - Of, relating to, or involving a major commitment of resources.

full-scale trial *n* - 1. A **trial** undertaken following a **pilot** or **feasibility trial**, especially one with a large **sample size** relative to that of the pilot or feasibility trial. 2. A **definitive trial**. (defn 1). rt: **feasibility trial, pilot trial** *Usage note*: See **definitive trial**.

function *n* - [L *function-*, *functio* performance, fr *functus*, pp of *fungi* to perform; prob akin to Skt *bhunkte* he enjoys] 1. A mathematical correspondence that **assigns** exactly one element of one set to each element of the same or another set. 2. A **variable** (quality, trait, or **measurement**) that depends on and varies with another, eg, height varying as a function of age.

fund *n* - [L *fundus* bottom, piece of landed property] A sum of money or other resources whose principal or interest is set apart for a specific purpose or activity.

fund, funded, funding, funds *v* - 1. To provide money for a **project** or activity. 2. To place money in an account for a specific purpose.

funding *adj* - Of or relating to the process of obtaining or providing money.

funding agency *n* - An **agency** that provides fiscal support for a specified purpose or activity. syn: **sponsoring agency**

funding agreement *n* - An **agreement** between the payer and payee concerning the nature and extent of **funding** in return for a specified product or completion of some task.

funding application *n* - **Funding proposal**, especially one prepared in relation to a **grant application**. syn: **funding request** rt: **contract proposal**

funding award *n* - A **grant** or **contract** awarded to an **institution** for a designated **project**.

funding office *n* - The **office** responsible for fiscal negotiations and disbursement of funds in relation to a **funding proposal**. rt: **grants management office, contract office**

funding officer *n* - The head of the **funding office**. rt: **grants management officer, contract officer**

funding proposal *n* - A **proposal** from an **applicant, offerer,** or **proposer** for **funding** a specified activity. syn: **funding application, funding request** rt: **contract proposal, grant proposal**

funding request *n* - A **request** for **funding** in relation to some **project** or activity; **funding proposal**.

G

Galton, Francis - (1822 - 1911) Englishman, educated at Cambridge in medicine but, after receiving an inheritance giving him the freedom to travel and for a life of leisure, abandoned medicine in favor of work in meteorology, genetics, and statistics. His contributions to **statistics** include approaches to **analysis** and the development and use of **regression** procedures.

gamma *n* - [ME, fr LL, fr Gk, of Sem origin; akin to Heb *gimel* gimel] The 3rd letter of the **Greek alphabet**, uppercase Γ, lowercase γ.

gamma distribution *n* - A **probability density function** of the form:

$$f(x) = \frac{\lambda}{\Gamma(n)}(\lambda x)^{(n-1)}e^{-\lambda x}$$

for x > 0 and where Γ is the **gamma function**. The **distribution** has **mean** n/λ and **variance** n/λ^2. Includes, as special cases, the **chi-square distribution** and the **exponential distribution**.

gamma function *n* - A mathematical **function** of the form:

$$\Gamma(x) = \int_0^\infty t^{x-1}e^{-t}dt$$

for x > 0, or the real part of x > 0 if x is complex.

Gauss, Carl Friedrich - (1777 - 1855) Renowned German mathematician and astronomer noted for major contributions to **statistics**. His work includes development of a theory of **estimation** based on **least squares**.

Gaussian *adj* - Of or relating to a **variable** or **function** having a **normal** or normal-like **distribution**.

Gaussian distribution *n* - **normal distribution**

gender *n* - [ME *gendre*, fr MF *genre*, *gendre*, fr L *gener-*, *genus* birth, race, kind, gender] 1. Characterization of **sex** (defn 2) based on observed functions, anatomy, behaviors, or affectations. 2. The sex of assignment by oneself or someone else. rt: **sex** *Usage note*: Not to be used interchangeably with **sex**; see sex for reasons.

generalizability *n* - The state or quality of being **generalizable**. *Usage note*: That state or quality in the case of a **sample** derives from use of defined sampling procedures and **populations**, thereby providing a scientific basis for the generalizations or **inferences** made. However, that formal basis is usually absent in trials and generalizations, as a rule, must therefore be made on a judgmental, nonstatistical, grounds. One's willingness to apply the conclusions of a trial to the broader setting of general medical care and to a more **heterogeneous** set of patients then those studied is a matter of judgment. The notions of generalizability and **validity** in the context of trials are different and should not be confused. Generalizability relates to the extent to which the conclusions derived from a trial can be generalized beyond the setting of the trial and the particular people studied in the trial. Validity relates to comparisons within a trial and to the extent to which the **treatment differences** can be legitimately attributed to the **treatment variable**. See usage note for **validity**.

generalizable *adj* - Having generality; being able to **generalize** or to **infer** from.

generalize, generalized, generalizing, generalizes *v* - To draw a general **conclusion** from; to give general applicability to; to give a general form to; to derive or induce.

generalized *adj* - Made general.

generally recognized as safe and effective (GRASE) *n* - A designation accorded a **drug** already in use for a specified indication by a panel of experts convened by the **Food and Drug Administration** that, when made, removes the drug from the testing and licensing requirements of a **new drug** for that indication.[49, 52, 116] rt: **Drug Efficacy Study**

generate, generated, generating, generates *v* - [L *generatus*, pp of *generare*, fr *gener-*, *genus* birth] To bring into existence; produce; procreate; beget.

generation *n* - 1. The act or process of bringing into being. 2. The **average** span of time from **birth** of **parents** to birth of offspring. 3. A **group** of persons constituting a single step in the line of descent from an ancestor. 4. A group of persons born over a **time period** corresponding to a generation (defn 2); such a group living contemporaneously.

generation effect *n* - [epidemiology] **Variation** or **change** in the health or well-being of successive **generations** due to changes in environment, life style, and health practice; such variation or change seen in successive **birth cohorts**. rt: **cohort effect**

generator *n* - One or something that **generates**.

generic *adj* - [F *générique*, fr L *gener-*, *genus*, birth, kind, class] Being or having a nonproprietary name.

generic drug *n* - A **drug** marketed under a nonproprietary name after patent protection for an approved **proprietary drug** has expired; drug similar in function and action to a specified proprietary drug or to another FDA-approved drug and having the same active ingredients as that drug. Marketing requests subject to review and approval by the **Food and Drug Administration**; see **Abbreviated New Drug Application**. syn: me-too drug rt: **pioneer drug**

geometric *adj* - 1. Of, relating to, or according to the methods or principles of geometry; increasing in a **geometric progression**. 2. Utilizing rectilinear or simple curvilinear motifs or outlines in design; of or relating to art based on simple geometric shapes.

geometric distribution *n* - A **probability distribution function** of the form:

$$f(x) = pq^x, \quad x = 0, 1, 2, \cdots$$

where x is the **trial** in which the first success is observed in a series of **independent Bernoulli trials**, each having a **probability** of success of p and with q = 1 - p. The distribution has **mean** 1/p and **variance** q/p^2; referred to as a geometric distribution because successive terms form a **geometric progression**.

geometric mean *n* - The nth **root** of the product of n **positive numbers**; eg, 4 for the numbers 2, 4, and 8; 5 for the numbers 1, 5, 5, and 25; 5.3835633 for the numbers 4, 5, 6, and 7. The geometric mean is always less than the **arithmetic mean** except where all the numbers are the same. Used to "average" rates of change; calculation facilitated by the fact that the **logarithm** of the geometric mean is the **arithmetic mean** of the **logarithms** of the individual values. See **mean** for list.

geometric progression *n* - A **sequence** of terms such that the **ratio** of one term to the one preceding it is the same as for any other two adjoining terms, eg, the sequence: 1, 1/2, 1/4, 1/8, 1/16, 1/32, etc.

giga- *prefix* - [ISV, fr Gk *gigas* giant] One billion, denoted by the symbol g or G.

gigabyte (gB, GB) *n* - 1,073,741,824 (ie, 2^{30}) **bytes**, denoted by the symbol gB or GB; roughly one billion bytes. rt: **kilobyte**

glossary *n* - A list of terms, abbreviations, and letter and symbol designations used in a written work and their meanings; typically appearing as front or back matter to such work.

goal *n* - [ME *gol* boundary, limit] The **objective** or end toward which an effort is devoted; **objective**. rt: **aim, objective, purpose**

gold *n* - [often attrib ME, fr OE; akin to OHG *gold* gold; OE *geolu* yellow] Something having or regarded as having high value or quality.

gold standard *n* - [According to *Webster*,[159] a monetary standard under which the basic unit of currency is defined by a stated quantity of gold and which is usually characterized by the coinage and circulation of gold, unrestricted convertibility of other money into gold, and the free export and import of gold for the settlement of international obligations.] A **measure, method**, or **procedure** widely regarded as being the best available or being of the highest quality possible; often used to express confidence in the answer or result provided by such a measure, method or procedure or in the desirability of such a measure, method, or procedure, as in *the clinical trial is the gold standard for treatment evaluation*. *Usage note*: Limit use to settings where there is a recognized hierarchy of value or quality on some dimension or scale. Presumptive when used in reference to one's own methods or procedures.

golden *adj* - 1. Of greatest value or importance; precious. 2. Of a high degree of excellence; superb.

golden rule *n* - 1. A guiding principle. 2. Golden Rule: a rule of ethical conduct based on biblical teaching admonishing one to do onto others as they would have them do onto oneself; Matthew (7:30) *Therefore all things whatsoever ye would that men should do to you, do ye even so to them: for this is the law and the prophets*; Luke (6:31) *And as ye would that men should do to you, do ye also to them likewise.*

Gompertz, Benjamin - (1799 - 1865) English actuary and astronomer responsible for the mathematical relationships described by a **curve** named in his honor, **Gompertz's curve** and an approximation regarding the risk of dying with increasing age, **Gompertz's law**.

Gompertz's curve *n* - A **curve**,[61] named for its originator, **Benjamin Gompertz**, of the form:

$$y = ka^{b^x}$$

or log y = log k + (log a) b^x, where 0 < a < 1 and 0 < b < 1; a type of **growth curve**; a modified exponential curve.

Gompertz's law *n* - A **relationship** between age and the **risk** of death, noted by **Gompertz**, in which risk increases as a **geometric** function of age.

good *adj* - [ME, fr OE *gōd*; akin to OHG *guot* good, Skt *gadh* to hold fast] Of favorable character or tendency; suitable.

goodness *n* - The state or quality of being **good**.

goodness of fit *n* - 1. The extent to which **observed** and **expected frequencies** agree, as in a **goodness of fit test**. 2. The extent to which **observed data** are fitted by a **curve**.

goodness of fit test *n* - A **statistical test** designed to assess the extent of **agreement** between **observed data** and those **expected** under some theoretical **model** or observed under some other circumstance, eg, the **chi-square goodness of fit test**.

Gosset, William S - (1876 - 1937) English industrial statistician noted for his work regarding exact **error probabilities** of **statistics** and in essence derived the **t-distribution**. Published under the pseudonym of **Student** as a condition of employment at the Guinness Brewery in Dublin, Ireland.

grand *adj* - [MF, large, great, grand, fr L *grandis*] 1. Having more importance than others; having higher **rank** than others bearing the same general designation. 2. Being inclusive or comprehensive.

grand mean *n* - The **mean** based on the **grand total**.

grand total *n* - The **total** for the entire collection of **data** or values; the total overall.

grandfather *n* - The father of one's mother or father; forefather.

grandfather drug *n* - A **drug** exempted from requirements contained in the Food, Drug, and Cosmetic Act of 1938. The Act set forth standards for licensure of **new drugs**, including the requirements for **New Drug Applications** (NDAs). Drugs in use prior to the Act were exempted from the requirement of NDAs. *Usage note*: The term, **grandfather**, derives from clauses contained in the voting laws of various southern states exempting descendants of men voting prior to 1867 from new and more stringent voting eligibility requirements; the clauses had the effect of disenfranchising black people.

grant *n* - [general] Something given or granted; the act of granting; **grant-in-aid**; **grant application**. [research] 1. An **award** of monies from a federal agency to a state or local governmental unit, or to a private or public **agency**, **institution**, or foundation, to support specified **research** as described in a **grant application**. 2. An award of monies made in response to any research grant application (defn 2). 3. Materials or goods provided in lieu of money for the conduct of specified research, eg, drugs supplied by a drug company for use in a **trial**. 4. **research grant application** rt: **contract, cooperative agreement** *Usage note*: The term carries the connotation of gift or giving and, hence, is best reserved for awards providing a wide degree of control of the research by the recipient of the award. A grant, as opposed to a **cooperative agreement** or **contract**, is generally made in anticipation of relatively little involvement in the work by the sponsor. Medical **research**, at least in the US, is funded via both grants and contracts. Hence, the two terms should not be used interchangeably. They have different operational implications, especially in relation to review and administration in the NIH setting [Department of Health and Human Services, 1982;[34] Department of Health, Education, and Welfare, 1977[35]]. In a broad sense, an NIH grant is a gift made to an investigator's **institution** to allow that **investigator** to perform research specified by the investigator. An NIH contract is a legal written agreement between the NIH and the investigator's institution to perform designated services or work under the general direction of the NIH. Normally, the grant mode of support is reserved for **investigator-initiated proposals** and for **sponsor-initiated proposals** as outlined in **requests for applications** (RFAs). The contract mode of funding is usually reserved for activities coming about via **requests for proposals** (RFPs). Normally, the mode of funding, once established, remains unchanged over the course of an activity, with notable exceptions. Institutes of the NIH do convert traditional RO 1 grants to **cooperative agreements** in some **multicenter trial** settings (eg, as happened in the Glaucoma Laser Trial). Similarly, they can change from grant to contract or contract to grant support during the life of an activity. For example, a switch from grant to contract took place during the Diabetic Retinopathy Study in relation to funding for the coordinating center for that study. In addition, the initiator role can change for activities that proceed from a feasibility phase to a full-scale phase. A case in point is the Systolic Hypertension in the Elderly Program (SHEP). The initial feasibility trial grew out of investigator initiative and was funded via grants. The full-scale phase was initiated via an RFP from the NIH and was funded via the contract mode of support. Usually the NIH will use the same type of funding vehicle for all sites in a multicenter study, but there are exceptions here as well. For example, some institutes have used grants to fund clinics in such settings and contracts for core units, such as coordinating centers. There are differences between the two modes of funding, at least as practiced by the NIH, in the amount of control and direction that is or can be exercised by the NIH. In general, use of the contract mode signals a more active hand in the design, organization, execution, and analysis of the research by the NIH than is typically the case with grant support.

grant application *n* - 1. An **application** submitted to a federal governmental agency for a **grant-in-aid**. 2. **research grant application** 3. **grant proposal** rt: **contract proposal**

grant proposal *n* - A **funding proposal** that, if awarded, involves or is to involve funding via a **grant**. rt: **contract proposal**

grant-in-aid *n* - 1. A federal **grant** of **funds** to a state or local governmental unit or to some **agency**, **institution**, or foundation to subsidize or support some designated activity or project. 2. **grant** (defn 2)

grantee *n* - One who has a **grant** in return for which the person or party intends to perform certain activities or functions. rt: **contractor**, **subcontractor** *Usage note*: See **contract** and **grant**.

grants management office *n* - 1. The **office** in the **sponsoring agency** whose members are responsible for awarding, funding, and administration of **grants**. 2. That office in a **lead center**, serving as a **surrogate** for the **sponsoring agency**, under the **consortium mode of funding** and involving use of grants for dispersal of funds to the other centers. 3. **business office** (defn 3) rt: **contract office** *Usage note*: Care should be taken to distinguish between usage in the sense of defn 2 as opposed to that in the sense of defn 1. Use in the sense of defn 3 is not recommended in that such offices typically have responsibilities for administering **contracts** as well as grants.

grants management officer *n* - 1. The individual in the **sponsoring agency** who is responsible for awarding and funding **grants** for specified **projects**. 2. Such a person in a **lead center** under the **consortium mode of funding** and involving the use of grants for dispersal of funds to the other centers. rt: **contract officer** *Usage note*: Care should be taken to distinguish between usage in the sense of defn 2 as opposed to that in the sense of defn 1.

grantsmanship *n* - The "art" or practice of applying for **grants**, especially where not directly related to the scope or nature of work proposed and that are considered by the **applicant** to increase the prospect of **funding**; generally having to do with the organization or presentation of material and documentation related to budget and cost projections; **contractsmanship** when applying for **contracts**.

graph *n* - A visual display (**diagram**), typically two dimensional, consisting of a series of points, **lines**, line segments, **curves**, or areas, intended to represent or depict the way in which one **vari-**

able or **factor** is related to another variable or factor.

graph, **graphed**, **graphing**, **graphs** *v* - 1. To represent with a **graph**. 2. To plot **data** or a **variable** as a graph.

graphic *adj* - [L **graphicus**, fr Gk **graphikos**, fr **graphein** to write] 1. Formed, by writing, drawing, or engraving. 2. Of, relating to, or concerned with a **graph**. 3. Of, relating to, or concerned with written or printed words or symbols or devices used in writing or printing or to represent sound or to convey meaning.

graphic *n* - 1. A **graphic** representation; **graph**. 2. A display generated by a **computer** and displayed on a **computer screen** or by some other imaging device, especially one that can be manipulated by the user.

graphic display *n* - 1. **graph** 2. A display on a **video screen**, especially one designed to provide a depiction corresponding to the print version of the display.

GRASE *n* - **generally recognized as safe and effective**

Greco-, **Graeco-** *prefix* - [L *Graeco-*, fr *Graecus*] Pertaining to **Greek** or Greece.

Greco-Latin square *n* - An **n** by **n** array of Roman and Greek letters arranged such that each Roman and Greek letter appears once and only once in each **row** and **column** of the array, eg, as depicted below (4 by 4 Greco-Latin square):

Cβ	Dγ	Aα	Bδ
Aδ	Cα	Bβ	Dγ
Dα	Bδ	Cγ	Aβ
Bγ	Aβ	Dδ	Cα

rt: **Latin square**

Greco-Latin square treatment design *n* - [**trials**] A **design** involving combinations of **treatments** arranged in the form of a **Greco-Latin square**. The design represents an extension of the **complete block treatment design** and is used to control **variation** associated with rows as well as **columns**. **Permutations** of such arrangements, when rows are viewed as corresponding to **patients** and columns to time or order of **treatment**, represent forms of **complete treatment crossover designs** involving the simultaneous use of two treatment modalities, one represented by Roman letters and the other by Greek letters. Use of such arrays in **crossover trials** has the

advantage of eliminating the effect of treatment order as a source of **variation** since each patient represented in an array receives each of the treatments and each treatment follows every other treatment once and only once in any given array. rt: **Latin square treatment design**

Greek *n* - [ME *Greke*, fr OE *Grēca*, fr L *Graecus*, fr Gk *Graikos*] The Indo-European language of the Greek people.

Greek alphabet *n* - An alphabet consisting of 24 characters:
ΑΒΓΔΕΖΗΘΙΚΛΜΝΞΟΠΡΣΤΥΦΧΨΩ
αβγδεζηθικλμνξοπρστυφχψω
alpha (Αα), beta (Ββ), gamma (Γγ), delta (Δδ), epsilon (Εε), zeta (Ζζ), eta (Ηη), theta (Θθ), iota (Ιι), kappa (Κκ), lambda (Λλ), mu (Μμ), ni (Νν), xi (Ξξ), omicron (Οο), pi (Ππ), rho (Ρρ), sigma (Σσ), tau (Ττ), upsilon (Υυ), phi (Φφ), chi (Χχ), psi (Ψψ), omega (Ωω).

group *n* - [often attributed to F *groupe*, fr It *gruppo*, of Gmc origin; akin to OHG *kropf* craw] 1. A collection of individuals with a common characteristic, relationship, or aim; eg, a collection of people working together on a specific **research project**; **study group**; **research group**. 2. A collection of objects regarded as a **unit**. rt: **aggregate**

group data *n* - **Data** characterizing a **group**; especially in the absence of **data** for individual units or elements comprising the group, such as that used in **ecological studies** for measuring **exposure** to some known or presumed **risk factor**; **aggregate data**. rt: **grouped data** *Usage note*: Not to be confused with **grouped data**.

group matching *v* - 1. **frequency matching** 2. **category matching** rt: **individual matching**, **pair matching**

group randomization *n* - [**trials**] Treatment assignment via **randomization** in which the **randomization unit** is an aggregate of **treatment units**, such as members of a household, members of a hospital ward, or members of a **community**. rt: **group treatment assignment**, **unit randomization**

group sequential *adj* - 1. Of, relating to, or concerned with a **sequential** process in which the **unit** defining the **sequence** is an **aggregate** of **observations** or **treatment units**. ant: **unit sequential** 2. Relating to or based on a method of **hypothesis testing** involving use of accumulating data, augmented before each new **test** by an added set of **observation** (as in **group sequential interim data analysis**); the testing process continues until the **null hypothesis** is rejected, or some other **boundary** condition is encountered or crossed.

group sequential analysis *n* - **group sequential interim data analysis**

group sequential design *n* - [trials] A **sequential design** (**open** or **closed**) in which **treatment comparisons** are made only at designated time points or intervals (eg, every 6 months), after **enrollment** of specified numbers of **patients** (eg, after every 50 **randomizations**), or after occurrence of specified numbers of **events** (eg, after every 10 deaths) and the results of which are used to decide whether or not to continue the trial. *Usage note*: See **sequential design data analysis**.

group sequential interim data analysis *n* - [trials] A method of **interim data analysis** that is carried out after **enrollment** of specified numbers of **observation units** (usually persons), eg, for the first time when enrollment reaches 50 and again when it reaches 100, 150, etc. See DeMets and Ware [1980][32] and Pocock [1977].[125] *Usage note*: See **interim data analysis**.

group treatment assignment *n* - [trials] **Treatment assignment** in which the **assignment unit** is an aggregate of **treatment units**, eg, a **design** with household as the assignment unit and individual household members as the treatment unit. rt: **unit treatment assignment, group randomization**

grouped data *n* - 1. A collection of **data elements** (eg, the recorded ages of the **population enrolled** into a **trial**) that relate to individual members or units of a **population** and that are combined to provide some summary **measure** or **statistic** for that population. 2. A set of **data** defined by a **class** or **class interval**. *Usage note*: Not to be confused with **group data** or **aggregate data**.

growth *n* - A stage in the process of development; progressive development; progression; increase.

growth curve *n* - 1. A **curve** describing **growth**, eg, one showing the **expected** weights and heights of children by age. 2. Any of a series of curves, such as **Gompertz's curve** and the **logistic curve**, having the general form of ar

elongated s due to a **rate** that is progressively changing over the time course of the process; changes proceeding from slow to rapid and back again to slow.

guardian *n* - 1. One who is responsible for the care or protection of another. 2. One who has legal responsibility for the care of another and for management of that person's affairs, eg, guardian of a **child**.

guess *n* - An act or instance of **guessing**; a conjecture arrived at by guessing; surmise.

guess, guessed, guessing, guesses *v* - [ME *gessen*, prob of Scand origin; akin to ON *geta* to get, guess] To **predict** a **result** without adequate **information** or knowledge; to assume or presume without adequate information or knowledge; to arrive at a correct **conclusion** by conjecture or supposition.

guesstimate *n* - [blend of **guess** and **estimate**] An **estimate** that is little more than a guess because of inadequate information or knowledge.

guideline *n* - A statement of policy or procedure issued to serve as a guide in a specified setting or application. rt: **rule, principle** *Usage note*: Generally, a guideline is constructed as an aid, hence it may be ignored without penalty. Use **rule**, requirement, regulation, or some other appropriate term when the policy or procedure is to be followed without fail.

guinea pig *n* - 1. Any of variously colored, stout-bodied, short-eared, nearly tailless, South American burrowing rodents of the genus Cavia cobaya widely domesticated as pets and for **research**. 2. A person needlessly or frivolously experimented upon. 3. A person subjected to untested procedures. 4. A person exposed to procedures having no intrinsic **benefit**. 5. A person exposed to procedures considered to entail more **risks** than benefits. 6. A person enrolled into a **trial** considered to violate existing **ethics** or **norms** or **standards** for care. *Usage note*: (In regard to people) Use with caution, especially in relation to implied claims or assertions of wrong doing. Usually evocative and emotion-laden and intended to suggest needless experimentation, experimentation so poorly done so as to have no benefit, or use of persons as objects of experimentation in settings involving undo risk or sacrifice. In the context of **trials**, often used in regard to a subset of persons considered to have been denied adequate **treatment** or to have been needlessly exposed to risk without the prospect of offsetting benefit; often in references to the subset receiving the **control treatment** in a **placebo-controlled** trial. Most uses in the context of trials, whether or not intentional, have the effect of impugning the judgment of **sponsors** of the trial for having funded it and of **institutional review boards** and **ethics committees** for having approved the trial.

H

half *n* - [ME, fr OE *healf*; akin to L *scalpere* to cut, OE *sciel* shell] One of two equal or approximately equal parts into which something is divided.

halo *n* - [L *halos*, fr Gk *halōs* threshing floor, disk, halo] The aura of sentiment, glory, or veneration surrounding or associated with an idealized person, thing, or activity.

halo effect *n* - 1. An **effect** (usually **positive** or **beneficial**) due to the attention one receives; an effect having more to do with being the focus of attention (eg, as received by virtue of being in a **study** aimed at effecting some change or improvement) than with the reason for the attention; **Hawthorne effect**. 2. A **positive** coloring of **observations** of a person due to a positive aura of the observer; the effect produced by such coloring in an observation or **report**. 3. A tendency to recall past **events** and **experiences** in a **positive** light; such a tendency involving the more likely recall and reporting of positive events or experiences than **negative** events or experiences; a tendency in which positive events or experiences are emphasized and negative events and experiences are de-emphasized. syn: **Hawthorne effect** rt: **bias, Heisenberg effect, placebo effect, placebo reactor** *Usage note*: The term is typically reserved for instances in which the effect is positive or beneficial, as suggested by the modifier **halo**. The term, especially when used in the sense of defn 1, has connotations similar to **placebo effect**. Placebo effect is due to suggestion and supposition, whereas halo effect is due to attention. Hence, the two terms should not be used interchangeably.

handbook *n* - 1. A **book** capable of ready transport and serving as a concise reference for a specific area or activity organized for ease of use; **study handbook**. 2. **manual** *Usage note*: See **study manual of operations** for difference between handbook and manual in study settings.

haphazard *adj* - Occurring without any apparent order or pattern. syn: **random** (not recommended) *Usage note*: Use when characterizing a process that is unordered but not meeting the **scientific** definition of random, or where there is uncertainty as to whether that definition is satisfied. Do not equate haphazard with random in scientific writing or discourse. Distinct from **random**, in that there is no mathematical basis for characterizing a haphazard process.

haphazard treatment assignment *n* - A **treatment assignment** that is made in a **nonrandom**, arbitrary fashion not according to any apparent plan or **design**.

haphazardization *n* - 1. An act of assigning or ordering that is the result of a **haphazard** process. 2. An **order** or **sequence** that is the result of a process considered to be akin to **randomization** but lacking in scientific base (as detailed for **random** *adj, scientific*). rt: **randomization** *Usage note*: Not to be confused or used interchangeably with randomization. See note for randomization.

hard *adj* - [ME, fr OE *heard*; akin to OHG *hart* hard, Gk *kratos* strength] 1. Not speculative or conjectural; specific. 2. Free of weakness or defect. 3. Rigid; not flexible. 4. permanent ant: **soft**

hard disk *n* - [computers] A magnetic storage medium, involving a **disk** or series of disks, permanently affixed to a piece of **hardware** capable of storing and providing access to large quantities of **data**.

hard endpoint *n* - **hard outcome**

hard outcome *n* - [trials] Any **outcome measure** not subject to major **errors** of interpretation or **measurement**, eg, death or some other serious explicit **clinical event**. ant: **soft outcome**

hardware *n* - 1. Fittings, tools, utensils, or parts of machines made of metal. 2. The actual **electronic** and electrical **devices** contained in a vehicle, such as a spacecraft, or in an apparatus, such as a **computer**.

harmonic *adj* - [L *harmonicus*, fr Gk *harmonikos*, fr *harmonia* harmony] 1. Being characterized by periodicity or **frequency**. 2. Characterized by a component frequency of a harmonic motion (as of an electromagnetic wave) that is a whole number multiple of the fundamental frequency.

harmonic mean *n* - The reciprocal of the **arithmetic mean** of the reciprocals of the individual numbers, eg, the harmonic mean for the values 3, 6, and 8 is $[(1/3 + 1/6 + 1/8)/3]^{-1} = 4.8$. See *mean* for list.

Hawthorne effect *n* - An effect on the person under study (usually **positive** or **beneficial**) by being under study; behavior influenced by knowledge of the fact that one is being studied. The name arises from the site of the study at which the phenomenon was observed — a Western Electric plant located in Hawthorne, Illinois. That plant was the site of a series of studies starting in the late 1920s. Collected works contained in a monograph entitled *Management and the Worker* and published in 1964.[132] syn: **halo effect** (defn 1)

hazard *n* - [ME, fr MF *hasard*, fr Ar *az-zahr* the die] 1. A possible source of danger; **risk**. 2. Chance **event**; accident. 3. The **probability** of a failure in a specified interval of time; **hazard rate**. 4. **hazard function**

hazard function *n* - 1. A **function** describing the **hazard** (defn 3) as a function of time. 2. The **hazard rate** at various points in time.

hazard rate *n* - 1. An idealized or theoretical **rate** for an infinitesimally small **time interval** (**instantaneous rate**); the **probability** of the **event** in time interval t + Δt, as Δt approaches 0. Synonymous with **force of mortality** when the hazard is death. 2. The number of new **events** that occur in a period of time per **person-time** of **observation** during the period, eg, **person-years**.

hazard ratio *n* - The **ratio** of two **hazard rates**.

head *n* - [ME *hed*, fr OE *hēafod*; akin to OHG *houbit* head, L *caput*] person; person count

head fee *n* - A **fee** based on person count, eg, a fee in the amount of $2,500 paid by a drug company to an **investigator** for each person **enrolled** into a **trial** and followed for 8 weeks.

health *n* - [often attrib ME *helthe*, fr OE *hǣlth*, fr *hāl*] 1. The general condition or state of one's body. 2. The condition of being sound in body, mind, or spirit; freedom from physical **disease** or pain.

health scientist administrator *n* - An individual at the **National Institutes of Health** who is responsible for providing technical and scientific

assistance to investigators under the **grant** mode of **funding**.

Heisenberg effect *n* - An **effect** in which the act of **measuring** one of two related **variables** has an effect on the other variable. Named after Warner K Heisenberg (1901 - 1976), German atomic physicist, for a **principle** in quantum mechanics. Also referred to as the uncertainty principle. rt: **halo effect**

Helsinki committee *n* - **ethics review committee**; as referred to in some parts of the world, eg, in Israel. See also **institutional review board**.

Helsinki Declaration *n* - **World Medical Association Declaration of Helsinki**

Helsinki Resolution *n* - **World Medical Association Declaration of Helsinki**

Henle-Koch's postulates *n* - A series of **postulates** that if satisfied are considered **sufficient** to support the **inference** that a particular living organism causes a specified **disease**. Formulated by Friedrich Gustav Jakob Henle (1809 - 1885; German physician and professor of anatomy) and put forward in an essay published in 1840; refined by Robert Koch (German; 1843 - 1910; student of Henle's; discover of tubercle bacillus; Nobel prize for medicine 1905) and first presented in lectures delivered in 1884 and 1890. The three basic requirements for the inference are that the organism in question 1) is always found with the disease it is postulated to cause; 2) is not found with any other disease; 3) after isolation and culture, is capable of producing the disease in experimental settings. As summarized by Last [1988][84] the postulates or conditions are: 1) The agent must be shown to be present in every case of the disease by isolation in pure culture; 2) The agent must not be found in cases of other diseases; 3) Once isolated, the agent must be capable of reproducing the disease in experimental animals; 4) The agent must be recovered from the experimental disease produced. rt: **causal relationship**

hetero-, heter- *prefix* - [comb fr MF or LL; MF, fr LL, fr Gk, fr *heteros*; akin to Gk *heis* one] Other; different; other than usual. ant: **homo-**

heterogeneous *adj* - [ML *heterogeneus*, *heterogenus*, fr Gk *heterogenēs*, fr *heter-* + *genos* kind] Varied, mixed, not the same; consisting of dissimilar parts or constituents. ant: **homogeneous**

heteroscedastic *adj* - Having unequal **variances** or **scatters**; not **homoscedastic**. Displaying marked variability.

hexadecimal *adj* - Of, relating to, or being a **number system** with base 16.

hexadecimal number system *n* - A **number system** with base 16 in which numbers are represented as sequences of **digits**, 0 through 9, and letters A through F (corresponding to numeric values 10 through 15, respectively) and are processed as corresponding to a sum of products in which each product is a number, 0 through 15, multiplied by 16 raised to the power corresponding to the position of the number in the sequence. For example, the hexadecimal number, 47, corresponds to $4 \times 16^1 + 7 \times 16^0$, and equals 71 decimal. A single character or digit (**byte**) is represented by 2 hexadecimal numbers, eg, $(3B)_{\text{base 16}} = (0011\ 1011)_{\text{base 2}} = (;)_{\text{ASCII}}$ rt: **binary number system, decimal number system**

hierarch *n* - [MF or ML; MF *hierarche*, fr ML *hierarcha*, fr Gk *hierarchēs*, fr *hier-* + *-archēs* -arch] A person high in a **hierarchy**.

hierarchical *adj* - Of, relating to, or arranged in a **hierarchy**.

hierarchical database *n* - A **database** in which each **data record** is broken into logically related segments and the segments are connected by pointers in an ordered tree-like arrangement. Viewed from the perspective of "ownership", a single record in such a database may "own" many other records, but any given record may be "owned" by just one other record.

hierarchical experiment *n* - An **experiment** involving a **hierarchical experimental design**. syn: **nested experiment**

hierarchical experimental design *n* - A class of **experimental designs** in which **treatments** (**factors**) are **nested**. For example, in the context of **trials**, consider a design involving use of three different treatment modalities, (eg, public service advertising (A), group counseling (B), and drug treatment (C)) in which drug treatment is administered to individuals within groups, counseling is performed on groups from defined communities, and defined communities are exposed to public service ads.

A_1				A_2			
B_1		B_2		B_1		B_2	
C_1	C_2	C_1	C_2	C_1	C_2	C_1	C_2

rt: **factorial experiment, hierarchical experiment, split-plot design**

hierarchical file *n* - A **file** (defn 2) in which **records** are ordered or accessed in some ordered **hierarchical** fashion.

hierarchy *n* - An ordered or ranked series or **classification**.

Hill, Sir Austin Bradford - (1897 - 1991) British medical statistician of the London School of Hygiene, considered by many as the modern day father of clinical trials; known for his writings in relation to the need for trials and on the design, implementation, and conduct of trials.

histogram *n* - [Gk *histos* mast, web + E *-gram*] A graphic representation of a **frequency distribution** of **grouped data** for a **continuous variable** formed using a series of contiguous rectangles (except where separated by groups having zero frequency) with widths (as displayed on the **x-axis**) corresponding to the intervals covered in the grouping and having areas proportional to the frequencies in the intervals per unit of interval length. rt: **frequency polygon**

Histogram

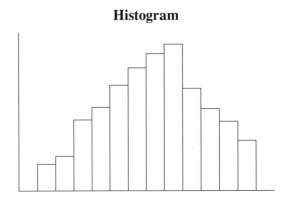

historical *adj* - Of or relating to the past.

historical control *n* - 1. A **control** based on past experience. 2. A **control** (defn 1) based on **data** collected or **observations** in a period of time previous to that pertaining to the group being studied. 3. A hypothetical person having a specified disease and subject to the expected course of that disease prior to a change in the diagnosis or treatment of that disease. 4. **histori-cal control group** syn: **nonconcurrent control**, **nonparallel control** ant: **concurrent control** *Usage note*: Subject to varying usage. Normally, usage pertains to **data** obtained or provided from an **observational study** done in the past and having defined diagnostic, **data collection**, and followup procedures. However, the term may also be used with much less implied rigor, as with definition 3 in references to the **natural history** of a disease prior to the advent of a new treatment. The careful user and writer will take care to distinguish between usages supported with a defined, rigorously collected, **dataset** versus those lacking in this regard, as in defn 3. The nature of the usage should be made clear by specifying the data source (or lack thereof) in relation to the use. Most usages are in contexts involving a new treatment in the absence of **controlled trials** and in relation to claims based on outcomes observed with the new treatment in contrast to those observed prior to introduction of the new treatment in similar kinds of patients.

historical control group *n* - A **control group** observed in a period of time previous to that pertaining to the **study group**. In the setting of **trials**, generally not a valid alternative to a **concurrent control group**. Use of this method of **control** should be limited to settings in which the **disease** or condition was reliably diagnosed using accepted diagnostic procedures, where **treatment** was uniform over the time in which the controls were identified and is different from the treatment being studied, in which the disease or condition has a predictable course or **out-come**, and in which it is impractical or unethical to carry out a **controlled trial**. ant: **concurrent control group**

historical controls *n* - A collection of **patients** used as a **comparison group** who were diag-nosed and treated for the **disease** or condition of interest in the past and in a time frame predating that pertaining to the **study group**(s).

history *n* - [L *historia*, fr Gk inquiry, history, fr *histōr*, *istōr* knowing, learned; akin to Gk *eidenai* to know] 1. An account of a person's previous experience, eg, an account of a person's previous illnesses and medical conditions and **treatment** as recorded in a **medical record**. 2. An assem-bly of facts relating to some event or condition, eg, as provided by a patient in taking a medical history. 3. An assembly of facts or **data** relating

to the natural course of a disease, eg, as for a group of patients in relation to a **natural history study**.

home *adj* - Operating or occurring in a **home**.

home *n* - [ME *hom*, fr OE *hām* villege, home; akin to Gk *kōmē* villege, L *civis* citizen, Gk *koiman* to put to sleep] One's place of residence; domicile.

home visit *n* - 1. A **visit** that take place in one's home. 2. **study home visit**, **patient home visit**

homeo-, home- *prefix* - [L & Gk; L *homoeo-*, fr Gk *homoi-*, *homoio-*, fr *homoios*, fr *homos* same] Like or similar.

homeopathic *adj* - Of or relating to **homeopathy**; of a diluted or ineffective nature, as in **homeo-pathic dose**.

homeopathic dose *n* - A **dose** of a **substance** or **drug** at **homeopathic** level. In **trials**, eg, some **vaccine trials**, a **control treatment** consisting of minute quantities of the same substance or drug given as the **test treatment**.

homeopathy *n* - [Ger *homöopathie*, fr *homöo-* home- + *pathie* -pathy] A **system** of **medical treatment** based on the use of minute quantities or **doses** of remedies that in massive quantities or doses produces **effects** similar to those of the **disease** or condition being treated.

homo-, hom- *prefix* - [L, fr Gk, fr *homos*] One and the same; alike. ant: **hetero-**

homogeneity *n* - 1. The quality or state of being **homogeneous**. 2. The state of being similar or having similar values.

homogeneity of variance *n* - A condition in which the **variances** of two or more **popula-tions**, **distributions**, or **variables** are the same or not dissimilar enough to be considered different.

homogeneous *adj* - [ML *homogeneus*, *homogenus*, fr Gk *homogenēs*, fr hom- + *genos* kind] Of the same or similar kind, uniform, not mixed. ant: **heterogeneous**

homogenous *adj* - Of, relating to, or exhibiting homogeny; **homogeneous**

homoscedastic *adj* - [*hom-* + Gk *skedastikos* able to scatter, fr *skedannynai* to scatter] Having equal **variances** or **scatters**; not **heteroscedastic**.

hour *n* - [ME, fr OF *heure*, fr LL & L; LL *hora* canonical hour, fr L, hour of the day, fr Gk *hōra*] 1. The 24th part of day (defn 2); 60 minutes. 2. The time of day reckoned with a 12-

hour clock and designated am or pm, eg, 1:30 am meaning one hour and 30 minutes after midnight. 3. The time of day reckoned with a 24-hour clock and recorded as a four-digit number with 0000 being midnight, eg, 0130 for one hour and 30 minutes after midnight. 4. A customary or particular time. *Usage note*: See **time measure**.

hourly *adj* - 1. Occurring **hour** by hour. 2. Computed or determined in terms of an hour. *Usage note*: See **time measure**.

house *n* - [often attrib ME *hous*, fr OE *hūs*; akin to OHG *hūs* house] 1. A building that serves as living quarters for one or a few families. 2. A commercial firm.

human *adj* - [ME *humain*, fr MF, fr L *humanus*; akin to L *homo* man] 1. Of, relating to, or characteristic of man. 2. Consisting of human beings.

human experimentation committee (HEX committee) *n* - **institutional review board**

human subject *n* - **subject** (defn 1) *Usage note*: Usually redundant. Subjects are understood to be human in most usages in the context of **clinical trials**. Limit use of **human** as a modifier to settings where there is a need to distinguish use from that of defn 2 for subject. See usage note for **subject** for additional comments.

human volunteers committee *n* - **institutional review board**

hyper- *prefix* - [ME *iper-*, fr L *hyper-*, fr Gk, fr *hyper*] 1. above; beyond; **super** 2. excessive 3. That which is or exists in a space of more than 3 dimensions.

hypergeometric distribution *n* - A **probability distribution** of the form:

$$f(k) = \frac{\binom{M}{k}\binom{N-M}{n-k}}{\binom{N}{n}} \text{ for } k = 0, 1, 2, 3, \cdots, n$$

that gives the **probability** of obtaining exactly **k** elements of one kind and **n** - **k** elements of another if **n** elements are chosen at **random** without replacement from a **finite population** having **N** elements, **M** of which are of the first kind and **N** - **M** are of the second kind. When **N** is large compared to **n**, the distribution is approximated by the **binomial distribution**.

hypothesis *n* - [Gk, fr *hypotithenai* to put under, suppose, fr *hypo-* + *tithenai* to put] 1. An assumption or statement, not yet proven by **experiment** or **observation**, adopted for the sake of testing its soundness or to facilitate investigation of a class of phenomena. 2. An assumption or concession made for the sake of argument; an interpretation of a particular situation or condition taken as the ground for action. 3. A theory or speculation put forward as a possible explanation of some phenomenon or process. rt: **alternative hypothesis**, **null hypothesis**, **research hypothesis**, **treatment hypothesis**

hypothesis test *n* - **test of hypothesis**

I

iatrogenic *adj* - [Gk *iatros* physician + E *-genic*] Inadvertently induced by physician action or word.

Id, ID *n* - identification

Id check digit *n* - A **check digit** that is part of an **identification number** that is used as a check for transcription errors in that number.

IDE *n* - **Investigational Device Exemption**

IDEA *n* - **Investigational Device Exemption Application**

identification *n* - An act of **identifying**; the state of being identified; evidence of identity.

identification number, Id number *n* - 1. A unique **number**, combination of numbers, or combination of numbers and letters or other **symbols**, used to identify or designate, especially one used for record storage and retrieval. 2. **patient identification number; study identification number** *Usage note*: Note that **number** in this usage is as defined by defn 3 for **number**.

identifier *n* - 1. One or something that identifies or labels. 2. A symbol that serves to **identify**, indicate, or denote some **variable, record, file**, or **dataset**.

identify, identified, identifying, identifies *v* - 1. To establish the **identity** of. 2. To ascertain the nature, origin, or characteristics of. 3. To consider as identical or equal to.

identity *n* - [MF *identité*, fr LL *identitat-*, *identitas*, irreg fr L *idem* same, fr is that] 1. The quality or condition of being the same as something else. 2. The collective aspect of the set of characteristics by which someone or something is known or identified. 3. An **equation** that is satisfied for all values of the **variables** represented.

ignorance *n* - The state or fact of being **ignorant**.

ignorant *adj* - Lacking knowledge or understanding.

illusory *adj* - Deceptive, not real, **spurious**.

illusory correlation *n* - A **correlation** between two **variables** that arises from something other than a **causal relationship**. rt: **nonsense corre-** lation, spurious correlation

imbalance *n* - [general] The state of being out of **balance**; not in equilibrium; out of **proportion**. [**trials**] 1. A difference in the **distribution** of a **baseline characteristic** among the **treatment groups**, especially one considered to be large and unlikely. 2. An observed **assignment ratio** that differs from the one expected, especially a departure considered to be beyond the **range** of **chance**.

imbalance minimization treatment assignment *n* - [**trials**] An **adaptive treatment assignment scheme** in which **assignment probabilities** change as a function of the **observed** departure from the desired or **expected assignment ratio** (eg, decreasing the assignment probability for a **treatment** for which the number of previous **assignments** exceeds the desired ratio and increasing the probability for a treatment for which the number of previous assignments is less than the desired assignment ratio). See **urn model treatment assignment, biased coin treatment assignment**, and **minimum likelihood treatment assignment** for types.

immune *adj* - [L *immunis*, fr *in-* + *munia* services, obligation; akin to L *munus* service] 1. Free or exempt from. 2. Marked by protection; not **susceptible**. 3. Having or producing antibodies or lymphocytes capable of reacting with a specific antigen.

implement, implemented, implementing, implements *v* - To put in place; to carry out.

implementation *n* - The act or process of **implementing** something; the state resulting from being implemented.

important *adj* - [MF, fr OIt *importante*, fr L *important-, importans*, prp of *importare*] Marked by or indicative of **significant** worth or consequence; valuable in content or **relationship**.

imputation *n* - The act of imputing; something imputed.

impute, imputed, imputing, imputes *v* - [MF *inputen*, fr L *imputare*, fr *in-* + *putare* to consider] To ascribe or attribute.

in-, il-, im-, ir- *prefix* - [ME, fr MF, fr L; akin to OE *un-*; ME, fr MF, fr L, fr *in* in, into] 1. not, non-, un 2. in, within; into 3. toward

in vitro *adj, adv* - [NL, lit, in glass] Outside the living body and in an artificial environment.

in vivo *adj, adv* - [NL, lit, in the living] In the living body of a plant or animal.

inactive *adj* - Not **active**; quiescent; chemically or biologically inert. ant: **active**

inactive control *adj* - [trials] Of or relating to a **control** that is or is intended to be **inactive**. ant: **active control** rt: **negative control**

inactive control treatment *n* - [trials] A **control treatment**, such as a **placebo** or **sham treatment** or **nontreatment**, not capable of producing an **effect**, except perhaps a **placebo effect**. ant: **active control treatment** rt: **negative control treatment**

inactive dose *n* - **inactive treatment dose**

inactive substance *n* - A **substance** that does not have biological activity, such as a **placebo**, and is incapable of producing a **treatment effect**, other than perhaps a **placebo effect**. ant: **active substance**

inactive treatment *n* - A **treatment** not capable of producing an **effect**, other than a **placebo effect**; includes **placebo treatment**, **sham treatment**, and **nontreatment**. ant: **active treatment** rt: **inactive control treatment**

inactive treatment dose *n* - A **treatment dose** that is below the level capable of producing noticeable **effects**. ant: **active treatment dose** rt: **treatment dose**

incidence *n* - [epidemiology] 1. The **number** of occurrences, within a specified **time period**, of a **disease**, condition, or **event** in a defined **population** assumed or known to be **free** of that disease, condition, or event at the start of that time period. 2. **incidence rate**

incidence rate *n* - [epidemiology] Incidence (defn 1) divided by **number** at **risk** (ie, that portion of a defined **population** known or assumed to be **free** of the **disease**, condition, or **event** of interest at the start of the **time period** used for the calculation); often expressed per 100, 1,000, or 10,000 (or some other multiple of 10) population at risk.

incident *adj* - Something related to or **dependent** on another thing or condition.

incident case *n* - 1. A **case** (defn 2) occurring in a specified **time period** in persons at **risk** of being identified as a case within a defined **population**. 2. **incident event**

incident event *n* - 1. The occurrence of an **event** for a person or **observation unit** at **risk** of the event over a specified time period and in a defined **population**. 2. **binary outcome** (defns 2 and 4)

include, included, including, includes *v* - [ME *incuden*, fr L *includere*, fr *in-* + *claudere* to close] 1. To take in or comprise as part of a whole. 2. To contain within or between. ant: **exclude** (defn 1)

inclusion *n* - [L *inclusion-, inclusio*, fr *inclusus*, pp of *includere*] The state of being **included**; something that is included. ant: **exclusion**

inclusion criteria *n* - [trials] The set of **criteria** used for determining **eligibility** for **enrollment** into a trial; **entry criteria**. ant: **exclusion criteria**

incomplete *adj* - [ME *incompleet*, fr LL *incompletus*, fr L *in-* + *completus* complete] Not **complete**; not finished; not **full**.

incomplete block *n* - 1. A **block** that includes or is to include only some of the **treatments** or levels of a **factor** or **variable** represented in a **design**. 2. A **block** in which a **treatment** is not to be used, or one in which a treatment is not represented the number of times specified in the **treatment design**. ant: **complete block**

incomplete block design *n* - An **experimental design** with **blocks** that are not **complete**, ie, blocks in which one or more **treatments** (or levels of a **factor** or **variable**) are not represented, or in which treatments are not represented in the **ratio** specified in the **treatment design**. ant: **complete block**

incomplete block treatment design *n* - [trials] A **treatment design** with **blocks** in which only certain of the **study treatments** are represented, eg, a design involving three treatments, but only two per block. ant: **complete block treatment design**

incomplete crossover *n* - Not a **complete crossover**.

incomplete crossover treatment design *n* - 1. A **crossover treatment design** that provides for **administration** of some, but not all, of the **study treatments** to the **experimental units** (eg, patients) in the **trial**. 2. A crossover treatment design in which each of the individual experimental units receive some, but not all, of the treatments represented in the design. rt: **complete crossover treatment design**

incomplete factorial *n* - 1. A **factorial design** or **factorial experiment** in which only some of the combinations of **factors**, conditions, or **treatments** possible in a **complete factorial** appear, are used, or are administered; eg, the combinations $A\bar{B}$, AB, and $\bar{A}B$ in a **trial** involving the treatments A and B and **matching placebos**, $\bar{A}$ and $\bar{B}$, respectively. 2. Any factorial arrangement that is **incomplete**, even if complete for a defined subset of the factors, conditions, or treatments represented, eg, an arrangement in which the combinations $A\bar{B}$, AB, $\bar{A}B$, and $\bar{A}\bar{B}$ are represented but in a trial involving a third treatment, C, not used in combination with A, $\bar{A}$, B, or $\bar{B}$. syn: partial factorial ant: **complete factorial**

incomplete factorial treatment design *n* - [trials] A type of **parallel treatment design** involving some, but not all, combinations of the **treatments** used in the trial, eg, a **double-masked placebo-controlled** design involving **drugs** A and B and three **treatment groups**: $A\bar{B}$, $\bar{A}B$, and AB, in which $\bar{A}$ and $\bar{B}$ correspond to **placebo treatments** matching drugs A and B, respectively. syn: partial factorial treatment design, **incomplete factorial** ant: **complete factorial treatment design**

incomplete Latin square *n* - [trials] 1. A **Latin square** not having all possible **permutations** of the **treatments** represented. 2. A Latin square in which one or more of the treatments are not represented in one or more of the possible permutations for the square.

incomplete treatment assignment block *n* - [trials] A **treatment assignment block** that is **incomplete**, ie, one not including one or more of the **study treatments** or one that is only partially filled.

incomplete treatment assignment block design *n* - [trials] A **treatment design** in which only certain **study treatments** are represented in a **block**, eg, a design involving three treatments, A, B, and C, in which only two of the three treatments are represented in any given block. ant: **complete treatment assignment block design** rt: **balanced incomplete treatment assignment**

block design

increment *n* - [ME, fr L *incrementum*, fr *increscere* to increase] One of a series of regular additions or progressive **steps**.

incremental funding *n* - **Funding** provided at specified times (eg, once a year) or after completion of specified tasks over the course of a **project**.

IND *n* - **Investigational New Drug**

IND cross-reference *n* - A **reference**, typically by **IND number**, in one **Investigational New Drug Application**, to information contained in another INDA; done to allow the FDA to consider information contained in the referenced application when reviewing the application containing the cross-reference.

IND number *n* - A **number** assigned by the **Food and Drug Administration** for identifying an **Investigational New Drug Application**.

IND safety report *n* - **investigational new drug safety report**

IND trial *n* - 1. A **trial** done under an **INDA**. 2. A trial requiring an INDA. 3. A trial involving one or more **new drugs** (defn 1). rt: **Investigational New Drug Application** *Usage note*: Subject to confusion when a trial involves a mix of **new drugs** (defn 1) and **approved drugs** (defn 1).

INDA *n* - **Investigational New Drug Application**

independence *n* - The quality or state of being **independent**. ant: **dependence**

independent *adj* - [general] 1. Not **dependent**; not subject to control by something or someone else. 2. Not affiliated with a larger controlling unit. [statistics] 1. The property in which the **joint probability** of some composite **event** or condition is given by the **product** of the **probabilities** of the individual events or conditions comprising that composite event or condition. 2. A **variable** that is not subject to influence or to being dictated or determined by others. 3. Numbers or expressions not capable of being deduced, derived, or determined from or expressed in terms of the set of numbers or expressions under consideration, eg, **independent contrast**. ant: **dependent** *Usage note*: The term should not be used in scientific writing and discourse in the absence of a basis for its use. Typically, that basis derives from mathematical considerations, operational considerations, or from actual maneuvers to ensure independence (such as those done in the **randomization** process to ensure that assignments issued are independent of patient and physician preferences). See **correlation coefficient** for additional comments.

independent contrast *n* - A **contrast** (defn 5) that is not capable of being derived or expressed by any other **linear** combination of contrasts; **orthogonal contrast**.

independent double data entry *n* - **Data entry** in which data are entered (keyed) by two different people working independently of one another; as distinct from **dependent double data entry**. rt: **quasi-independent double data entry**

independent event *n* - An **event** that is not **dependent** on other events or conditions for occurrence. In a probabilistic sense, events are said to be independent if and only if the **joint probability** of those events is the product of the probabilities of the individual events.

independent random variable *n* - A **random variable** that is not **dependent** on other variables or conditions for the value it assumes. In a probabilistic sense, variables are said to be **independent** if and only if the values of the **joint probability density functions** of all the variables together is the **product** of the **probability density functions** of the individual variables. ant: **dependent random variable**

independent sample *n* - A **sample** that is not **dependent** on other samples for the values it assumes, ie, one that is in no way influenced or capable of being influenced by any other sample that may be selected.

independent variable *n* - 1. A **variable** that is not **dependent**; **independent random variable**; **treatment variable**. 2. The **variable** manipulated in an **experiment**; **treatment variable**; **experimental variable**; **input variable**. 3. In equations involving variables, usually the variable(s) to the right of the equation sign and whose value(s) determine the value(s) to the left of the equation sign, for example see **regression equation**; often designated by the letter x or X with a unique subscript to distinguish it from other such variables if more than one. 4. A variable used as if it were an independent variable even if not, in a strict sense, independent of others, as with **regressors** in **multiple regression analysis**. 5. A characteristic or measure being observed or made, especially one that is hypothe-

sized to influence some event or manifestation. ant: **dependent variable** rt: **independent random variable**

index *n* - [L *indic-*, *index*, fr *indicare* to indicate] 1. A value associated with a **variable**, **record**, **data item**, or **file** used to indicate position, location, or order of the variable, record, data item, or file in some ordered arrangement. 2. A list of entries, typically appearing at the end of a **document**, used to locate materials contained in the corpus of the **document**; typically consisting of a series of topics, terms, or subject headings each followed by one or more page numbers corresponding to pages in the document containing the listed term or having information pertinent to the topic or subject listed. 3. A value or **score** derived from a collection of **items** or **measures**. 4. An **electronic file** or paper document that is used to aid in locating information or documents contained in different documents or locations, eg, **MEDLINE** and Index Medicus for locating papers in the medical literature. 5. A device, such as the pointer on a gauge, used to indicate value or quantity.

index case *n* - The first **case** in a defined **group** (eg, family or group of **patients**) to come to attention or to be affected by some **disease** or condition. rt: **proband**, **propositus**

index group *n* - The **group** of **primary** interest in a **comparative study**; usually the **test treated group** in a **controlled trial**, **cases** in a **case-control study**, and the **exposed group** in a comparative **cohort study**. rt: **comparison group**, **reference group**

indexed file *n* - [computers] A **file** in which the user has direct access to any **record** through a directory that indicates the location of every record in the file; the directory may be used for any of a variety of functions involving the retrieval, insertion, deletion, or modification of records.

indexed journal *n* - A **journal** whose contents are indexed in a paper or electronic file, such as Index Medicus or **MEDLINE**.

indexed literature *n* - **Literature** that is indexed in some paper or electronic file, such as Index Medicus and **MEDLINE** for medical **journals** and NLM Current Catalog and CATLINE for medical books.

indexed sequential access method (ISAM) *n* - [computers] A method of accessing **records** in an **electronic file** by locating those records via an index file that contains, for each record in the file, the value of the index variable and the location of the record in the master file. The indexed file is ordered on the index variable and searched using values of the index variable supplied by the user.

indicate, indicated, indicating, indicates *v* - [L *indicatus*, pp of *indicare*, fr *in-* + *dicare* to proclaim, dedicate] 1. To point out or point to; to be a **sign**, **symptom**, or **index** of or for; to demonstrate or suggest the need, necessity, or advisability of or for. 2. To state or express.

indication *n* - 1. Something that **indicates**; **sign** (defn 2). 2. Something indicated as necessary or expedient. 3. A specific state or condition for which something is indicated, eg, the indication named in a **new drug application** or listed in a **label insert**.

indicator *n* - 1. One or something that indicates; pointer. 2. **tracer substance** 3. Something, such as litmus paper, that by change in color or some other change shows the state, condition, or concentration of a solution.

indicator variable *n* - A **binary variable** used to indicate presence or absence of some condition or factor, usually in some **regression model**; **dummy variable**.

indirect *adj* - [ME, fr ML *indirectus*, fr L *in-* + *directus* direct] 1. Not **direct**; deviating from a direct line or course. 2. In mathematics, being or involving proof of a proposition or **theorem** by demonstration that its negation leads to absurdity or contradiction. ant: **direct**

indirect contact *n* - 1. A **contact** of one person or party with another person or party through a third person or party. 2. A contact of one person or party with another person or party that is through or the result of a third person or party. 3. A contact of one person or party with another person or party arising from use of intermediary vehicles, agents, or parties, eg, such a contact arising in response to a mass mailing or to ads in newspapers or on radio or TV. ant: **direct contact** rt: **indirect patient contact**

indirect cost *n* - A **cost**, usually expressed as a **percentage** of **direct costs**, that is not identifiable with a specific product, activity, or function, but is nonetheless considered to be an associated cost. rt: **direct cost, total cost**

indirect data entry *n* - 1. **Data entry** performed using code sheets or other **documents** produced from the original **study forms** and documents. 2. Data entry not performed at the **data generation site**. ant: **direct data entry**

indirect distribution of funds *n* - Any system of **funding** in which **funds** flowing to a **site** from a **sponsor** are via a party other than the sponsor, as in **consortium funding**. ant: **direct distribution of funds**

indirect funding award *n* - A **funding award** made to a **site** by another site with funds from a **sponsor**, as in a **consortium award**. ant: **direct funding award**

indirect patient contact *n* - [trials] **Contact** of a **patient** with a **study clinic** that is the result of actions of intermediaries or **surrogates** of the clinic, eg, referring physicians, or that is the result of a general publicity, advertising, or mailing campaign designed to encourage interested patients to contact the clinic. ant: **direct patient contact**

indirect patient recruitment *n* - Any method of **patient recruitment** that involves **indirect patient contact**. ant: **direct patient recruitment**

indirect rate adjustment *n* - A method of **rate adjustment** in which the **crude rate** observed in a **study population** is compared to a **standardized rate**, as obtained from a **standard population** by deriving a **weighted mean** rate using the observed distribution of the study population as weights. The crude rate, divided by the resulting weighted mean rate, is referred to as the **standardized mortality** (or **morbidity**) **ratio** (abbreviated SMR); a ratio of less than 1 indicates an experience in the study population that is better than that of a standard population having the same distribution as the study population and a ratio greater than 1 indicates the experience is worse than that of such a standard population. The method is used for small study populations (because of unreliable rate estimates for **subgroups** formed using the **adjustment variable**). See **direct rate adjustment** for alternative method. rt: **standardization**

indirect research cost *n* - **Indirect costs** incurred by the **institution** housing a **research project**; typically those arising from providing for general administrative support and for providing space, heat, light, and the like in connection with the project. rt: **direct research cost, total research cost**

indirect standardization *n* - **indirect rate adjustment**

individual *adj* - [ML *individualis*, fr L *individuus* indivisible, fr *in-* + *dividuus* divided, fr *dividere* to divide] Of or relating to, or distinctly associated with an **individual**; being an individual or existing as an indivisible whole; existing as a distinct entity.

individual *n* - A particular being or organism as distinct from others; a human being; a particular person.

individual matching *v* - A process in which an **observation unit**, usually a person (eg, a **control**), is selected to **match** another (eg, **case**) on a **variable** or combination of variables (eg, gender and age). rt: **frequency matching, pair matching**

induce, inducing, induced, induces *v* - [ME *inducen*, fr L *inducere*, fr *in-* + *ducere* to lead] 1. To move by persuasion or influence; to call forth or bring about by influence or stimulation. 2. To determine by **induction**; to **infer** from particulars.

induct, inducted, inducting, inducts *v* - [ME *inducten*, fr ML *inductus*, pp of *inducere*, fr L] 1. To put in formal possession; to admit as a member. 2. To introduce, initiate or **enroll**.

induction *n* - 1. **Inference** of a general **conclusion** or **principle** from particulars. 2. A conclusion arrived at by induction. 3. In **mathematics**: a **method** of demonstration or proof of a proposition consisting of proving the first case and the case immediately following an arbitrary case for which the proposition is assumed to hold. 4. The act or process of **inducting**. rt: **deduction**

industry *n* - [ME *industrie* skill, employment involving skill, fr MF, fr L *industria* diligence, fr *industrius* diligent, fr OL *indostruus*, fr *indu* in + *-struus* (akin to L *struere* to build)] 1. Systematic labor, especially for some useful purpose or stated end in relation to the production of something of value; the commercial production and sale of goods or services. 2. A specific branch of manufacture and trade, such as the **drug industry**. rt: **drug industry, company**

inequality *n* - [ME *inequaltié*, fr L *inaequalitat-*, *inaequalitas*, fr *inaequalis* unequal, fr *in-* + *aequalis* equal] The quality of being unequal or uneven; a formal statement of inequality, as in **Bonferroni's inequality**.

infant *n* - [ME *enfaunt*, fr MF *enfant*, fr L *infant-*, *infans*, fr *infant-*, *infans*, adj, incapable of speech, young, fr *in-* + *fant-*, *fans* prp of *fari* to speak] A person in the first stage of life following birth; a person in the first year or two of life following birth.

infectious *adj* - Capable of causing infection; communicable by infection.

infectious dose *n* - 1. A **dose** of an infectious agent or organism that causes or is capable of causing infection. 2. A dose of an anti-infectious **drug**, agent, or substance that fails to prevent infection. rt: **infectious median dose, lethal dose**

infectious median dose *n* - 1. The **dose** that causes or is estimated to cause infection in 50% of the organisms, experimental animals, or persons receiving the dose. 2. The dose of an anti-infectious agent that fails to prevent infection in 50% of those to which or whom it is administered. Referred to as the ID_{50} in **bioassays** and in analyses involving **logit** or **probit transformations**. rt: **infectious dose, lethal median dose**

infer, inferred, inferring, infers *v* - [MF or L; MF *inferer*, fr L *inferre*, lit, to carry or bring into, fr *in-* + *ferre* to carry] To **conclude** from facts, **observations**, or premises; to surmise or arrive at a **conclusion**.

inference *n* - 1. The act or process of **inferring**, eg, in relation to generalizations or **conclusions** derived from a **sample** or set of **observations**, to a larger set or universe. 2. Something inferred; a proposition arrived at by inference; the premises and conclusions of a process of inferring.

infinite *adj* - [ME *infinit*, fr MF or L; MF, fr L *infinitus*, fr *in-* + *finitus* finite] [general] Extending indefinitely, endless; immeasurably, or inconceivably great or extensive; inexhaustible. [scientific] Extending beyond, lying beyond, or being greater than any preassigned finite value however large; characterized by an infinite number of elements or terms. ant: **finite**

infinite population *n* - 1. A **population** whose value or **distribution** is not effected by **sampling** without replacement; a population that is not **finite**. 2. The set of values that can be assumed by a **continuous variable**.

inform, informed, informing, informs *v* - [ME *informen*, fr MF enformer, fr L informare, fr in- + *forma*, from] To impart information or knowledge. *Usage note*: See notes for **informed** *adj* and for **informed consent**.

information *n* - 1. Knowledge obtained from investigation or study. 2. **Data** or facts.

informed *adj* - 1. Having information; based on possession of information. 2. Having information conveyed in an intelligible fashion. 3. Being in possession of information and understanding it; knowledgeable. *Usage note*: Most uses as a modifier of **consent** are in the sense of defns 1 or 2. Those uses are different from that implied for defn 3. Defn 3 implies evidence (**data**) or use of an active process intended to ensure that the information conveyed is understood by the recipient. Uses in the sense of defns 1 or 2 imply a passive process with regard to understanding. Use should be assumed to be in the passive sense, unless accompanied with details of the process or evidence supporting use in the sense of defn 3. See **informed consent** for added comments.

informed consent *n* - A decision by a person (or that person's **parent, spouse, guardian**, or representative) to submit (or to be submitted) to some procedure or to be **enrolled** into some **research project**, after being informed of its purpose, procedures, possible **risks** and **benefits**, and of the consequences of refusing to consent, if any. For trials, generally a **preassignment consent**, given after being informed of the purpose of the trial, why the person is eligible for **enrollment**, the **test** and **control treatments** being evaluated and of associated potential risks and benefits, the method of **treatment assignment**, the level of **treatment masking**, and the options for treatment and care if consent is not given. rt: **deferred consent, documented consent, post-assignment consent, signed consent, oral consent, written consent** *Usage note*: Often, the modifier *informed* is more an expression of wishful thinking on the part of the user rather than of documented fact and, hence, is usually best dropped. Its use is best reserved for settings in which there are steps built into the **consent process** to ensure an informed decision based on evidence of comprehension of what is involved, or for settings in which the decision can be demonstrated to have been informed. See **informed** *adj* for added comments.

informed consent *v* - 1. The giving or obtaining of an **informed consent**. 2. The process of obtaining **consent**. For **trials**, normally a process involving a dialogue between a representative of the trial and a **study candidate** (or surrogate) prior to **enrollment** that entails presentation of information (usually presented orally and in writing) detailing the purpose of the trial, why the person is eligible for **enrollment**, the **test** and **control treatments** being evaluated and the potential **risks** and **benefits** associated with use of each, the method of **treatment assignment**, the level of **treatment masking**, and the options for treatment and care if consent is not given. The process may involve several dialogues over a period of time. Consent may be given by a surrogate, such as a **parent, spouse**, or **guardian**, for the candidate in cases in which the candidate is a **minor** or is otherwise unable to engage in the consent process. The fact of consent is normally documented by the signature of the candidate or surrogate on a **consent statement**. syn: **preassignment consent** rt: **consent process, deferred consent, documented consent, post-assignment consent, signed consent, oral consent, written consent**

infraction *n* - [L *infractus*, pp of *infringere* to break off] Violation, **protocol departure**.

initial *adj* - [MF & L; MF, fr L *initialis*, fr *initium* beginning, fr *initus*, pp of *inire* to go into, fr in- + *ire* to go] 1. Of or relating to the beginning; placed at the beginning; first.

initial, initials *n* - The first letter of a name; the first letter of the first, middle, and last name of a person.

initial, initialed, initialing, initials *v* - To acknowledge, authenticate, or give approval by affixing the **initials** of the authorizing or responsible person or agent.

initial design stage *n* - The first stage of a **trial**; concerned with design and planning. See **stage of trial** for list of stages.

initiate, initiated, initiating, initiates *v* - [LL *initiatus*, pp of *initiare*, fr L, to induct, fr *initium*] To cause or facilitate the beginning of.

initiation *n* - The act or instance of beginning.

innovate, innovated, innovating, innovates *v* - [L *innovatus*, pp of *innovare*, fr in- + *novus* new] To introduce as or as if new; to invent or improvise, especially in an imaginative manner.

innovation *n* - The introduction of something new; a new method, device, or idea, especially one that is imaginative or **unique**.

innovative *adj* - Of or relating to **innovation**. *Usage note*: Best avoided in most writing detailing design, methods, and procedures, especially in relation to one's own work. The emphasis should be on description, not characterization.

innovator drug *n* - The first marketed use of a **drug** for a given **indication**, according to a specified **dosage** and route of administration.

input *n* - 1. Something put in, eg, **data** into a **computer** for **analysis**. 2. The act or process of putting in. 3. **independent variable** ant: **output**

input device *n* - [**computer**] A **device**, such as a keyboard on a **computer terminal**, used for **input** of **data** or commands. rt: **output device**

input/output device *n* - [**computer**] A **device** on a computer, such as disk drive, that may be used for **input** or **output**. rt: **input device**, **output device**

input variable *n* - 1. A **variable** supplied by an operator of a **computer program** to perform an operation, eg, any one of the variables needed to calculate a **sample size** for a **trial**. 2. **independent variable** (defn 2)

insert *n* - 1. Something added or extra that is inserted or is for insertion. 2. **label insert**

insert, inserted, inserting, inserts *v* - [L *insertus*, pp of *inserere*, fr *in-* + *serere* to join] To put or trust in.

instantaneous rate *n* - The idealized or theoretical **rate** as the interval to which the rate pertains approaches zero; **hazard rate** when the interval is a time measure.

institution *n* - An established organization, corporation, or agency, especially one that has a public character.

institutional *adj* - Of or relating to an **institution**.

institutional review board (IRB) *n* - A **committee** or **board**, as set forth in guidelines and regulations emanating from the **United States Public Health Service** concerning research involving human beings,[88] appointed by authorities within a research **institution** and constituted to review and approve studies to be carried out on human beings by **investigators** from that institution. The review focuses on the **ethics** and legitimacy of the proposed research from the perspective of **risk-benefit** and on the adequacy

of the proposed safeguards for would-be volunteers or individuals put at **risk** in or by the research. The risk may be a **direct** consequence of procedures performed or may be an **indirect** consequence of the work (eg, invasion of privacy or breaches of confidentiality). The review deals with, but is not restricted to, the nature and adequacy of the **consent process** and related **consent statement** when there is to be **contact** with individuals, and in all cases, whether or not there is contact, to a review of the adequacy of procedures to preserve individual anonymity and confidentiality of the information provided or obtained. Technically, the guidelines and regulations apply only to projects funded or to be funded by the federal government, but most institutions require IRB review and approval of all research involving human beings before it may be undertaken, regardless of funding source. The name arises from the regulations issued by the US Public Health Service and is, in one sense, unfortunate in that it is not suggestive of the functions actually performed. See also note for **involve**. syn: **ethics committee**, **Helsinki committee**, human experimentation committee, human volunteers committee

instrument *n* - [ME, fr L *instrumentum*, fr *instruere* to arrange, instruct] 1. **Data collection form**, especially one that is used to measure or derive some score or index, such as an intelligence test or personality profile. 2. A mechanical, electronic, or other kind of device used for determining or measuring the value of a **variable** or entity under observation. *Usage note*: Normally best avoided in the sense of defn 1 in that usage in this sense often suggests or implies a greater degree of precision and accuracy than normally possible or achieved.

integrity *n* - 1. An unimpaired condition; soundness. 2. Firm adherence to a **code** or **standard** of moral or ethical value.

intelligence *n* - [ME, fr MF, fr L *intelligentia*, fr *intelligent-*, *intelligens* intelligent] The ability to learn, understand, or comprehend or to deal with new or trying situations in a constructive manner; reason.

intelligent *adj* - [L *intelligent-*, *intelligens*, prp of *intelligere*, *intellegere* to understand, fr *inter-* + *legere* to gather, select] 1. Having or indicating **intelligence** or mental capacity; revealing or reflecting good judgment or sound thought;

skillful. 2. Possessing intelligence; guided or directed by intellect; rational. 3. Able to perform detailed instructions or functions, such as those performed by an **intelligent computer terminal**.

intelligent computer terminal *n* - A **computer terminal** containing a **microprocessor** that can be programmed to allow the user to perform tasks independent of the computer to which it is connected. syn: smart computer terminal ant: **dumb computer terminal**

intelligent terminal *n* - **intelligent computer terminal**

intention *n* - What one intends to do or bring about. *Usage note*: Intention is different from the reality of what is accomplished. Intention has to do with motivation as represented by a state of mind and may or may not lead to the desired end result. See also **intention to treat**.

intention to treat *n* - [**trials**] A philosophy or state of mind in which there is an **intent** to account for all **observation units** enrolled into a trial and to perform **analyses by assigned treatment**, regardless of observed course of **treatment**. *Usage note*: Not recommended, although in common usage. Use only in the presence of language detailing the operational implications of the intent, as in **analysis by assigned treatment**. See also usage note for **intention**.

inter- *prefix* - [ME *inter-, enter-*, fr MF & L; MF *inter-, entre-*, fr L *inter-*, fr *inter*; akin to OHG *untar* between, among, Gk *enteron* intestine, OE *in* in] Between or among (such as in *inter-patient variability* or in *inter marry*). rt: **intra-**

interacting variable *n* - 1. [**epidemiology**] A **variable** whose state or level influences the size or nature of the **effect** observed or existing between two factors of interest (eg, cigarette smoking in relation to some **disease** state and degree of **exposure** to some agent in a **case-control study**). 2. [**trials**] Any **variable** that influences the nature or size of a **treatment difference**. See *variable* for list. rt: **confounding variable** *Usage note*: It is important, in the case of trials, to distinguish variables that are known to be **independent** of **treatment assignment** and ensuing treatment processes (eg, any variable observed before treatment assignment) from those that are not (variables observed after the initiation of treatment) or from those that may not be (eg, variable observed after treatment assignment but prior to the initiation of treat-

ment). The distinction is important in **trials** when trying to understand the biological relevance of the variable in the treatment process. An **interaction effect** due to a variable known to be independent of treatment assignment, eg, sex of the patients studied, is clearly of more importance in deciding how the treatment should be used, than one in which there is uncertainty in this regard because the variable was observed after the start of treatment and where the observations are subject to a treatment related observation **bias**.

interaction *n* - [general; **Mutual** or **reciprocal** action or influence; **antagonism** or **synergism**; a **joint** effect of two or more **variables** or **factors**.] [**experiments, trials**] 1. A relationship in which changes in **response** (**dependent variable**) produced by changes in one or more **treatments** or factors (**independent variables**) depend on other treatments or factors. 2. A **relationship** in which the nature or magnitude of the **test-control treatment difference** for the **outcome** of interest in a **trial** depends on the state of those treated, as defined by one or more **baseline characteristics** or **variables** (eg, sex and age on entry). rt: **qualitative interaction**, **quantitative interaction**, **confounding**, **interacting variable** *Usage note*: To be used as an explanation of an observed **treatment effect** in trials, the variable in question should influence the size or nature of the **treatment difference** observed, and the difference should be large enough so as to be unlikely to have arisen by **chance** alone. Avoid using as a **weasel term**. Note also that interaction and **confounding** have different conceptual bases and implications and, hence, should not be confused. In both cases, for trials, the variable in question must be related to outcome. In the case of confounding, the variable has to be differentially distributed by treatment group; in the case of interaction, the variable has to influence the **treatment difference** observed. The existence of an interaction does not affect one's ability to compare among the treatment groups, the presence of a confounder does. Confounding influences one's certainty regarding the existence of a treatment effect itself since the difference can be explained either by the treatments applied or by the confounding variable. Interaction influences one's certainty as to the extent to which a result may be applied to a broader population, eg, does the treatment work for both males and females or only for males or females? See also usage notes for **interacting variable** and for **confounding variable**.

interaction effect *n* - An **effect** due to an **interaction**; **treatment interaction effect**.

intercept *n* - The **point** of **intersection** of a **line** or **curve** with an **axis** in a coordinate system, eg, the point at which a line crosses the **y-axis**. rt: **slope**

interest *n* - [ME, prob alter of earlier *interesse*, fr AF & ML; AF, fr ML, fr L, to be between, make a difference, concern, fr *inter-* + *esse* to be] 1. Involvement with or participation in something. 2. **proprietary interest**

interim *adj* - Done, made, or occurring within an **interval** or intervening time; during; within.

interim *n* - [L, adv, meanwhile, fr *inter* between] An intervening time; **interval**.

interim analysis *n* - **interim data analysis**

interim data analysis *n* - [trials] 1. **Data analysis** carried out during a **trial** for the purpose of **treatment effects monitoring**. 2. Any data analysis done before data collection is completed, for whatever reason, but usually concerned with assessments of **treatment effects**. rt: **sequential data analysis** *Usage note*: There are subtle distinctions between **interim data analysis** and **sequential data analysis** (see usage notes for **sequential** and **sequential data analysis**) that should be preserved in usage. Strictly speaking, the term, **interim data analysis**, applies to any trial, (**fixed sample size design** or a **sequential design**) in which interim analyses are done. However, the recommended convention is to reserve the term for fixed sample size designs and to use the term, **sequential data analysis**, when referring to the analyses required for sequential designs. See also note for **sequential data analysis**.

interim followup *n* - 1. **Followup** that is in addition to that required or specified in the **study protocol**; eg, added followup taking place between **scheduled followup visits**. 2. **unscheduled followup**

interim followup visit *n* - [trials] Any **followup visit** that takes place after **enrollment** of a person into a trial that is not part of the required sequence of **followup visits** and that is initiated because of some problem or concern; ordinarily

not counted as a **required followup visit** unless it takes place within the specified time period for a required visit and all the required procedures for that visit are carried out as part of the interim visit; **nonrequired followup visit**. ant: **required followup visit**

interim look *n* - [trials] 1. A **look** at the **results** of a trial while under way, especially when performed for the express purpose of determining whether the trial should be stopped or modified. 2. Any summary of **interim results** made during the course of a trial having the potential of being used to stop or modify the trial. 3. **interim result** rt: **multiple looks**, **administrative review**, **efficacy review**, **safety review**, **treatment effects monitoring**

interim result *n* - [trials] 1. Any **test-control treatment difference** observed during the **trial**. 2. A test-control treatment difference observed during the trial which results in a **protocol** change, especially a **treatment protocol** change.

interim review *n* - 1. A **review** performed during the course of an activity to determine whether the activity should be allowed to continue unaltered. 2. In the context of **trials**, a review based on observed **data** from the trial. rt: **administrative review**, **efficacy monitoring**, **interim look**, **performance monitoring**, **safety monitoring**, **treatment effects monitoring**

interim visit *n* - **interim followup visit**

intermediate *adj* - [ML *intermediatus*, fr L *intermedius*, fr *inter-* + *medius* mid, middle] Being or occurring in the middle; between.

intermediate endpoint *n* - **intermediate outcome**

intermediate outcome *n* - 1. An **outcome** considered to be **predictive** of some more important outcome. 2. An outcome considered to be on the path to some more important outcome. 3. **surrogate outcome** *Usage note*: See **surrogate outcome**.

intermediate variable *n* - A **variable** that is related to both the **independent** and **dependent variables** of a **study**. syn: contingent variable

internal *adj* - [L *internus*; akin to L *inter* between] Existing or situated within the **limits** or surface of something, such as within a study structure or within a body.

internal study validity *n* - The degree to which **differences** among the **comparison groups** in a **study** can be attributed to the **variable** of interest (eg, **treatment** in a **clinical trial**). rt: **external study validity, validity** *Usage note*: See **validity**.

interobserver agreement *n* - The extent to which an **observation** or **measurement** of some **variable** (eg, blood pressure) **agrees** with a similar observation or measurement made by a different **observer**, especially such agreement for observations or measurements made at the same time or in close temporal proximity to each other. ant: **interobserver disagreement** rt: **interobserver variation, intraobserver agreement**

interobserver disagreement *n* - The extent to which an **observation** or **measurement** of some **variable** (eg, blood pressure) **disagrees** with a similar observation or measurement made by a different **observer**, especially such disagreement for observations or measurements made at the same time or in close temporal proximity to each other. ant: **interobserver agreement** rt: **interobserver variation, intraobserver disagreement**

interobserver error *n* - **interobserver variation**

interobserver variation *n* - The extent to which an **observation** or **measurement** of some **variable** (eg, blood pressure) **varies** from a similar observation or measurement made by a different **observer**, especially such variation for observations or measurements made at the same time or in close temporal proximity to each other. rt: **interobserver agreement, interobserver disagreement, intraobserver variation**

interpolate, interpolated, interpolating, interpolates *v* - [L *interpolatus*, pp of *interpolare* to refurbish, alter, interpolate, fr *inter-* + *polare* (fr *polire* to polish)] 1. To **estimate** a **value** or **function** lying between known or **observed** values. 2. To insert between. ant: **extrapolate**

interquartile *adj* - Of or relating to that which is between **quartiles**.

interquartile range *n* - A **range**, defined by the upper **limit** (**end point**) of the 1st **quartile** and the lower limit of the 3rd quartile; accounts for 50% of the **values** or **observations** represented in the **distribution**.

interrelate, interrelated, interrelating, interrelates *v* - To bring into mutual **relation**; to have a **mutual relationship**.

interrelated *adj* - Having a **mutual** or **reciprocal relationship**.

intersect, intersected, intersecting, intersects *v* - [L *intersectus*, pp of *intersecare*, fr *inter-* + *secare* to cut] To meet and cross at a common **point**, as two **lines**; to share a common area; to overlap.

intersection *n* - 1. The act or process of **intersecting**. 2. A place or area where two or more things, such as lines, intersect. 3. The set of elements common to two or more sets. rt: **intercept**

interval *n* - [ME *intervalle*, fr MF, fr L *intervallum* space between ramparts, interval, fr *inter-* + *vallum* rampart] 1. The **time** between **events** or states; a pause. 2. A space or separation between objects, units, or states. 3. A set of real **numbers** between two numbers, including or excluding one or both of the end numbers.

interval censored *adj* - Of or relating to being **censored** within an **interval**. rt: **left censored, right censored**

interval censored observation *n* - 1. An **observation** subject to **censorship** within an **interval**. 2. Absence of observation (defn 1) because of censorship within an interval. rt: **left censored observation, right censored observation**

interval data *n* - **Data** from a **continuous variable**, such as age or family income, that are presented or used as **categorical data**.

interval estimate *n* - An **estimate** of an **interval** or **range**, eg, as defined by the **limits** of a **confidence interval** or by **fiducial limits**. rt: **point estimate**

interval estimation *n* - The act of arriving at an **interval estimate**. rt: **point estimation**

intervene, intervened, intervening, intervenes *v* - [L *intervenire* to come between, fr *inter-* + *venire* to come] 1. To occur, fall, or come between; to lie or be inserted between two things, **events**, or states. 2. To enter or appear as irrelevant or as a **nuisance**; to exert influence, such as through an **intervening variable**. 3. To interfere with, interrupt, or effect a change through action.

intervening variable *n* - 1. A **variable** that blocks or alters the effect of another variable. 2. **intermediate variable** syn: mediator variable

intervention *n* - [trials] 1. A **test treatment**, especially one in a **trial** involving nonmedical treatments and well people, such as in a diet trial involving use of different counseling procedures to assess their usefulness in effecting and sustaining changes in eating behavior. 2. Any **study treatment**; **test** or **control treatment**. *Usage note*: Not recommended as a synonym or replacement for the term **treatment** for reasons discussed in *Explanatory notes* (page xx). Use **treatment**, **study treatment**, **test treatment**, or **control treatment**, as dictated by context. Not recommended because of its ambiguous nature. In a technical sense, anything that one does to another is a form of interference, and, hence, a form of **intervening** (defn 3 of **intervene**), whether or not related to administration of a **study treatment**. The most common usages of the term are in settings where there is a desire to play down the clinical aspects of a trial or where there are no such aspects, as in studies of well people involving nonmedical study treatments, eg, in trials involving education or other nonmedical schemes for modifying the risks of developing subsequent **disease**. However, even in these settings, the term **treatment** is a more apt descriptor of what is done. See **treatment** for additional comments.

intervention study *n* - 1. A **study** in which there is an effort to change the natural course of a **disease** or health condition by attempting to alter **risk factors** or precursors associated with that disease or condition. 2. **trial** *Usage note*: not a recommended synonym for **trial**. See comments for **study** and **intervention** for reasons.

intervention trial *n* - **Trial**, especially one involving well people and nonmedical **treatments** such as use of counseling schemes designed to effect lifestyle changes. *Usage note*: Not a recommended term. See **intervention** for reason.

interventionist *n* - [trials] The person who applies the **treatment(s)** in a **trial**, especially the **test treatment**. *Usage note*: Used primarily in settings involving nonmedical treatment(s), eg, education schemes designed to modify behavior associated with increased **risk** of subsequent **disease**. Also used when there is a desire or need to de-emphasize or avoid medical connotations or responsibility. Not a recommended term. See **intervention** for reason.

interview *n* - [MF *entrevue*, fr (*s*)*entrevoir* to see one another, meet, fr *entre-* + inter *voir* to see] An interaction, face-to-face or via telephone or other forms of **electronic** hookup, involving two

or more people, for the purpose of soliciting **information** from the **interviewee**.

interview, interviewed, interviewing, interviews *v* - To solicit **information** from an **interviewee**.

interview study *n* - A **study** in which the prime source of **data collection** is by **interview**; as opposed to **record reviews** or data collected by physical **examination**.

interviewee *n* - One who is **interviewed**.

intra- *prefix* - [LL, fr L *intra*, fr (assumed) OL *interus*, adj, inward] In, within, or inside of. rt: **inter-**

intramural *adj* - Being or occurring within the **limits** or confines of a specified organizational unit or entity. ant: **extramural**

intramural funding *n* - 1. Monies provided or awarded from within one's own **institution** or **agency** for work to be done within or under the direct control of one's own institution. 2. **Funding** provided by an agency or organization to some unit or subdivision of that agency or **organization**; in the case of **NIH**, monies provided to units within the NIH for conducting its **intramural research program**. ant: **extramural funding**

intramural research *n* - **Research** performed within the confines or under the direct control of the **institution** funding it. In the parlance of **NIH**, research performed within the institution as part of the its **intramural research program**. ant: **extramural research**

intraobserver agreement *n* - The extent to which an **observation** or **measurement** of some **variable** (eg, blood pressure) **agrees** with a similar observation or measurement made by the same **observer**, especially such agreement for observations or measurements made at the same time or in close temporal proximity to each other. ant: **intraobserver disagreement** rt: **intraobserver variation, interobserver agreement**

intraobserver disagreement *n* - The extent to which an **observation** or **measurement** of some **variable** (eg, blood pressure) **disagrees** with a similar observation or measurement made by the same **observer**, especially such disagreement for observations or measurements made at the same time or in close temporal proximity to each other. ant: **intraobserver agreement** rt: **intraobserver variation, interobserver disagreement**

intraobserver error *n* - **intraobserver variation**

intraobserver variation *n* - The extent to which an **observation** or **measurement** of some **variable** (eg, blood pressure) **varies** from a similar observation or measurement made by the same **observer**, especially such variation for observations or measurements made at the same time or in close temporal proximity to each other. rt: **intraobserver agreement, intraobserver disagreement, interobserver variation**

intuition *n* - [LL *intuition-*; *intuitio* act of contemplating, fr L *intuitus*, pp of *intueri* to look at, contemplate, fr *in-* + *tueri* to look at] The act or facility of knowing without evident rational thought and **inference**; immediate cognition.

intuitive *adj* - 1. Known or perceived by **intuition**. 2. Knowing or perceiving by intuition. 3. Possessing or given to intuition.

invariant *adj* - 1. Unchanged by specific mathematical or physical operations or **transformations**. 2. **Constant**; unchanging. ant: **variant**

invasive *adj* - 1. Tending to spread; such as cancer cells invading healthy tissue. 2. Involving entry into the living body, especially in relation to surgical procedures.

invasive procedure *n* - [**medicine**] Any **procedure** that involves penetration of the skin barrier, such as for biopsy, x-ray, angiogram, or blood drawing; normally done for either **diagnostic** or **therapeutic** purposes.

inventory *n* - 1. An itemized **list** or **count** of goods, assets, or **documents** on hand, received, or on deposit. 2. **forms inventory** 3. A list or count of persons enrolled into a **study**.

inventory, inventorying, inventoried, inventories *v* - Counting or making the entries required for creating or maintaining an **inventory**.

inverse *adj* - [L *inversus*, fr pp of *invertere*] 1. Opposite in order, nature, or purpose. 2. The result of inversion. 3. An inverse function or operation; denoted by a power of -1 in mathematical expressions involving an inverse operation, eg, logarithm^{-1} denotes **inverse logarithm, antilogarithm**, or **antilog**.

inverse log *n* - **inverse logarithm**

inverse logarithm *n* - The **number** corresponding to a given **logarithm**, eg, logarithm$_{10}^{-1}(2) = 100$. syn: antilogarithm, antilog ant: **logarithm**

inverse sine *n* - The **inverse** function to the **sine**; if y is the sine of Θ, then Θ is the inverse sine

of y; also sine^{-1} or arcsine; sine$^{-1}(1/2) = 30°$. syn: arcsine ant: **sine**

inverse sine transformation *n* - A **variance** stabilizing **data transformation** of the form:

$$y = sine^{-1}\sqrt{x}$$

typically performed on **proportions** when in the **range** 0.05 to 0.20 and 0.80 to 0.95 to make them more amenable to **analyses** involving standard statistical techniques. See **square root transformation** for corresponding transformation for **Poisson variable**. syn: arcsine transformation

investigate, investigating, investigated, investigates *v* - [L *investigatus*, pp of *investigare* to track, investigate fr *in-* + *vestigium*, footprint, track] To **observe** or **study** by inquiry and by the **collection** and **analysis** of **data**.

investigation *n* - 1. That body of activities related to **investigating**. 2. **study**

investigational *adj* - Of or relating to **investigation**.

Investigational Device Exemption (IDE) *n* - An **exemption** granted by the **Food and Drug Administration** to allow use of a **medical device** prior to approval; granted in response to an **Investigational Device Exemption Application**. See **Investigational New Drug** for corresponding term for **drugs**.

Investigational Device Exemption Application (IDEA) *n* - An **application** directed to the **Food and Drug Administration** by the manufacturer or **sponsor** of a **medical device** for permission to evaluate the device in human beings [Food and Drug Administration, 1983].[50] See **Investigational New Drug Application** for corresponding term for **drugs**. rt: **Pre-Market Approval Application**

investigational drug *n* - **investigational new drug**

investigational new drug *n* - 1. A **new drug** being evaluated as a possible prelude to a submission of a **New Drug Application**. 2. A new drug being evaluated as part of an **Investigational New Drug Application**. 3. A new drug for which the **Food and Drug Administration** has issued an IND number in response to an **Investigational New Drug Application** (INDA). syn: investigational drug

Investigational New Drug (IND) *n* - 1. **Investigational New Drug Application** 2. **investigational new drug** rt: **new drug, New Drug Application**

Investigational New Drug Application (INDA) *n* - An **application** made by a **sponsor** (defn 4) to the **Food and Drug Administration** for permission to evaluate a **new drug** (defn 1) using human beings (see usage note for **new drug**); application required for use of a new drug (defn 3), use of an existing drug for a new **indication**, or an **approved drug** at a new **dosage**, strength, or new route of administration. The typical application will contain proposals for one or more trials. Trials proposed in an application may not start prior to approval of the application. The FDA has 30 days following receipt of an application to object to an application. The application is considered approved 30 days after receipt in the absence of written query or objection. See also **IND trial.** syn: Notice of Claimed Investigational Exemption for New Drug rt: **IND trial**

investigational new drug safety report *n* - A report to the **Food and Drug Administration** of an **adverse drug experience** in relation to an **investigational new drug** that is both serious and unexpected; written or telephoned. In relation to such reports, the regulations specify for written reports: *The sponsor shall notify FDA and all participating investigators in a written IND safety report of any adverse experience associated with use of the drug that is both serious and unexpected. Such notification shall be made as soon as possible and in no event later than 10 working days after the sponsor's initial receipt of the information. Each written notification shall bear prominent identification of its contents, ie, "IND Safety Report". Each written notification to FDA shall be transmitted to the FDA division of the Center for Drug Evaluation and Research or the Center for Biologics Evaluation and Research which has responsibility for review of the IND. In each written IND safety report, the sponsor shall identify all safety reports previously filed with the IND concerning a similar adverse experience, and shall analyze the significance of the adverse experience in light of the previous, similar reports. In regard to telephone reports, the regulations specify: The sponsor shall also notify FDA by telephone of any unexpected fatal*

or life-threatening experience associated with use of the drug in the clinical studies conducted under the IND no later than 3 working days after receipt of the information.[48] syn: IND safety report, **safety report** (defn 2) rt: **serious adverse drug experience, unexpected adverse drug experience**

investigative *adj* - Of or relating to **investigation.**

investigative body *n* - **investigative group**

investigative group (IG) *n* - The entire set of personnel involved in the conduct of a **study**; in **multicenter trials** includes **center directors** and support staff, representatives from the **sponsoring agency**, and **study committee** members. syn: **research group**, investigative team, **study group** (not a recommended synonym, see usage note for **study group**)

investigative team *n* - **investigative group**

investigator *n* - 1. Broadly, one who **investigates**. In the case of **research**, generally one who has a **key** role in conducting the research or some aspect of the research. 2. **study investigator** 3. **clinical investigator** *Usage note*: Use appropriate modifiers when referring to a particular subset of investigators, eg, **clinical investigator** when referring to the subset of people responsible for administration of treatment in a **clinical trial**. Avoid as a generic designation when used to the exclusion of others having investigator status, as in use as a synonym for **clinical investigator** in settings also involving nonclinical investigators. See **principal investigator** and **center** for added comments.

investigator's brochure *n* - A **brochure**, prepared and maintained by the **sponsor** (defn 5) of a **new drug** in relation to an **investigational new drug**; required by the **FDA** in relation to an **investigational new drug application**; distributed to investigators carrying out work in relation to said **IND**; contains detailed information regarding the chemical nature of the drug, its mode of action or presumed mode of action, and a summary of available animal as well as clinical data relating to the **safety** and **efficacy** of the drug; sponsor is obligated to revise and update the brochure as work proceeds and information accrues as to the nature of the drug and its safety and efficacy.

investigator-initiated research proposal *n* - 1. A **research proposal** conceived, prepared, and submitted to a prospective **sponsor**, without a formal solicitation by the sponsor. 2. An unsolicited **grant proposal** submitted to the **NIH**, such as an RO 1 **grant application**. ant: **sponsor-initiated research proposal** rt: **grant proposal** *Usage note*: The initiating force behind a proposal is not always clear, especially in the case of large scale **multicenter trials**, even for those funded by grants not solicited by **requests for applications** (**RFA**s). Typically, investigators will not undertake the task of preparing fully developed proposals for such trials, in itself is arduous and expensive, without some indication from the **sponsor** that they will be accepted for review and that the proposed work is consistent with the general charge or scope of interest of the sponsor. See note for **sponsor-initiated research proposal** for added comments.

involve, **involved**, **involving**, **involves** *v* - [ME *involven* to roll up; wrap, fr L *involvere*, fr in- + *volvere* to roll] 1. To engage or **enroll** as a **participant**. 2. entail 3. To relate closely; connect. *Usage note*: **Involve**, as in *research involving human subjects* in the Code of Federal regulations for **IRBs**,[117] has a broad meaning and is not to be read or interpreted as being restricted to uses in the sense of defn 1 where someone is actually enrolled into a **study** or is otherwise contacted or seen by an **investigator** in relation to a **research project**. **Research**, in the IRB sense of that term, is considered to involve **human beings** and, hence, is subject to review and approval prior to initiation even where there is to be no contact with persons (as in a **case-control study** based on **chart** reviews). The involvement in such cases is indirect and arises because an investigator is using something related to a person, such as a person's **medical record** or a biopsy specimen or **data** pertaining to that person.

iota *n* - [L, fr Gk *iōta*, of Sem origin; akin to Heb yōdh yod] 1. The 9th letter of the **Greek alphabet**, uppercase I, lowercase ι.

IRB *n* - **institutional review board**

item *n* - 1. One of the distinct parts of a whole, eg, a specific **question** in a **questionnaire** or a specific entry on a **data form**. 2. A particular **entry** in a listing.

iteration *n* - 1. A single **replication** of an **iterative process**. 2. **iterative process**

iterative *adj* - Involving **repetition**, as in computational **iteration**.

iterative process *n* - A computational **procedure** in which the results of each preceding **step** are used as the basis for the next step and where the results of each step represent an approximation to some **estimate**. Typically the procedure is started with some arbitrary **value** and continues for a designated number of replications or until some condition is achieved, eg, one in which the difference between the two succeeding estimates is less than some specified amount.

J and K

j, J *n* - [10th letter of the English alphabet] Something shaped like the letter J.

j-shaped *adj* - Of or relating to a shape resembling the letter j.

j-shaped curve *n* - 1. A **curve** shaped like the letter **j** or its mirror image; **asymmetrical** and rising or falling sharply to the **right**. 2. A curve with its lowest **ordinate** value at the lower **limit** of the **range** of values represented on the **x-axis** and rising monotonically to the right and at an ever increasing **rate** to its zenith at the upper limit of the range of values represented on the x-axis. 3. A curve with its largest **ordinate** value at the lower **limit** of the **range** of values represented on the **x-axis** and falling monotonically to the right and at an ever decelerating **rate** to its nadir at the upper limit of the range of values represented on the x-axis. rt: **s-shaped curve, u-shaped curve**

j-shaped curve

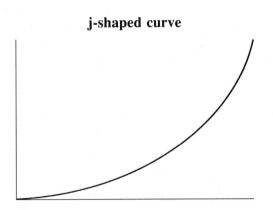

j-shaped distribution *n* - A **distribution** resembling the letter **j**; one rising sharply to the **right** and having its major **mode** at or near the **left** extreme of the distribution. rt: **u-shaped distribution**

jackknife *adj* - 1. Of or relating to something having general purpose or utility. 2. Of or relating to something **crude** or something not **exact** or **precise**.

jackknife estimate *n* - An **estimate** derived using a **jackknife method**. rt: **jackknife method, bootstrap estimate**

jackknife method *n* - A largely **nonparametric method** of gauging the accuracy of an **estimate**; done by calculating estimates of the desired estimate for each of the **n** different subsets of the **data** having **n** - 1 of the **observed data** points; notion due to Quenouille; name due to Tukey and intended to suggest something of general purpose or utility; see Miller [1974][105] and Diaconis and Efron [1983][36] for review. rt: **bootstrap estimate, bootstrap sample**

joint *adj* - [ME, fr MF, fr pp of *joindre*, fr OF] 1. combined; together 2. Common to two or more. 3. United, joined, or sharing with another. 4. Being a function of or involving two or more **variables**.

joint density function *n* - A **density function** for two or more **random variables** operating together; **bivariate density function** when involving only two variables. syn: multivariate density function rt: **bivariate density function**

joint distribution *n* - A **distribution** for two or more **random variables** operating together; **bivariate distribution** when involving only two variables. syn: multivariate distribution rt: **bivariate distribution, univariate distribution**

joint frequency distribution *n* - A **frequency distribution** for two or more **variables** operating together.

joint probability function *n* - A **probability function** for two or more **random variables** operating together.

journal *n* - [ME, service book containing the day hours, fr MF, fr *journal*, adj, daily, fr L *diurnalis*, fr *diurnus* of the day, fr *dies* day] 1. A printed **document** produced and distributed on a regular basis and containing materials of interest to intended readers, especially one for which there is a charge and that is available by subscription; newspaper, magazine, or newsletter; **scientific journal**. 2. A record of transactions or actions related to some activity, **file, dataset,** or account. 3. **log** (defn 2) 4. An account of day-to-day events or actions. 5. A record of experiences, ideas, or reflections kept regularly for private use; diary.

journaling *v* - The act of recording or creating entries in a **journal** (defn 2 or 3).

judge, judged, judging, judges *v* - [ME *juggen*, fr OF *jugier*, fr L *judicare*, fr *judic-*, *judex* judge, fr *jus* right, law + *dicere* to decide, say] 1. To form a considered opinion via thoughtful assessment of available evidence and via **testing** of premises. 2. To make an evaluation or arrive at an assessment after careful consideration.

judgment *n* - The process of forming a considered opinion or assessment by discerning **comparison** and **testing**; an opinion or assessment so formed.

just *adj* - [ME, fr MF & L; MF *juste*, fr L *justus*, fr *jus* right, law; akin to Skt *yos* welfare] Conforming to **standards** of correctness or fairness.

justice *n* - [ME, fr OF, fr L *justitia*, fr *justus*] The maintenance or administration of what is **just** and fair, especially by impartial methods and procedures.

justice, principle of *n* - A **principle** in **medical ethics** that asserts that the care and **treatment** performed or offered in a research setting involving human beings must be done in a **just** and **equitable** fashion, not to the **benefit** of a few or to the exclusion of others [Levine, 1986].[88] See also **medical ethics, principles of**.

juvenile *adj* - [F or L; F *juvénile*, fr L *juvenilis*, fr *juvenis* young person] Physiologically immature or undeveloped; not yet an **adult**; **child**.

k, K *n* - [11th letter in the English alphabet] 1. Shorthand for **kilo**, denoting thousand, eg, $30k for $30,000; 100k **bytes** for 100,000 bytes. 2. **kappa** (defn 2)

Kaplan-Meier product limit *n* - A **nonparametric method** developed by Kaplan and Meier [1958][73] for estimating cumulative **event rates** using **conditional probabilities**. The method is especially suited to situations, such as encountered in **trials**, in which persons are **enrolled** over a period of time and followed to a common calendar time point.

kappa *n* - [Gk, of Sem origin; akin to Heb *kaph*] 1. The 10th letter of the **Greek alphabet**, uppercase K, lowercase κ. 2. **kappa statistic**

kappa statistic *n* - A **statistic** used to assess the degree of **agreement** existing in the **categoriza-**tions or **classifications** by two different people assessing the same **data** or **records** or by the same person at two different times. The statistic is defined by the **ratio** of the **observed** agreement in the categorization provided by the two readings divided by that expected by **chance** alone, assuming the two readings are **independent** and unrelated. The statistic is **positive** if the agreement is greater than that predicted by chance and **negative** if less than that predicted by chance. A value of 0 indicates agreement equal to that predicted by chance, a value of 1 indicates perfect agreement, and a value of -1 indicates no agreement (perfect disagreement). The statistic has the form:

$$\kappa = (p_o - p_e)/(1 - p_e)$$

where p_o is the observed agreement between the two readings and p_e is the agreement expected by chance alone, both measured as proportions of all readings.

Kefauver-Harris Act of 1962 *n* - [After chief sponsors, Carey Estes Kefauver, D, Tennessee, Rep 1939 - 1948; D, Tenn, Senate 1948 - 1963; Oren Harris, D, Arkansas, Rep, 1941 - 1966; officially *Drug Amendments of 1962*] Amendments to the Food, Drug, and Cosmetic Act of 1938, aimed at strengthening the regulatory powers and authority of the **Food and Drug Administration** in regard to denying licensure to **drugs** judged to be ineffective or unsafe and in being able to remove such drugs from the market when found to be unfit.

Kendall's tau *n* - A measure of **correlation** involving **ranks** based on the number of rearrangements or reorderings required to make one ranking agree with another.[75] The measure is given by:

$$\tau = 1 - \frac{4Q}{n(n-1)}$$

where **Q** is the total number of reorderings required and **n** is the number of observations being ranked.

key *adj* - Of basic importance; essential; fundamental.

key *n* - 1. Something that explains, identifies, or provides answers or solutions. 2. A list of words or phrases used for explanation or for **coding** or **classification**. 3. A button on a keyboard that, when pressed or struck, causes a character to appear or to be recorded on a page or screen. The method of creation may be mechanical, as with a typewriter and paper, or **electronic**, as with a keyboard connected to a video screen or to an **electronic device** used for storage of information.

key, **keyed**, **keying**, **keys** *v* - 1. To assign or identify with a **label**, **code**, or **classification**. 2. The conversion of a **data** element to a coded or electronic format by use of a **key**, such as found on a keyboard.

key committee *n* - [**multicenter trials**] A committee essential to the operation of the trial; generally any of the following: **steering committee**, **executive committee**, **advisory-review committee**, **treatment effects monitoring committee**, and **advisory-review and treatment effects monitoring committee**. syn: major committee

keying *n* - The process of converting handwritten text, spoken words, or recorded **data** to printed or electronic form by use of **keys** on a keyboard.

kilo- *prefix* - [F, modif of Gk *chilioi*] Thousand

kilobyte (kB, KB) *n* - 1,024 (ie, 2^{10}) **bytes**.

Klimt, Christian Robert - (1918 - 1994) MD **epidemiologist** and **trialist**; received MD degree from the University of Vienna in 1944 and DrPH from The Johns Hopkins University in 1952; played a major role in the design and conduct of several large-scale **multicenter trials**, starting with the University Group Diabetes Program;[156] was a founding member of the **Society of Clinical Trials** and served as its president, 1984 - 1985.

knowledge-based system *n* - **expert system**

Koch's postulates *n* - **Henle-Koch's postulates**

kurtosis *n* - [Gk *kyrtosis* convexity, fr *kyrtos* convex; akin to L *curvus* curved] 1. The flatness or peakedness of a **unimodal distribution**, especially with respect to the concentration of values near the **mean** as contrasted with the concentration expected for a **normal distribution**. 2. **kurtosis statistic** rt: **leptokurtosis**, **platykurtosis**

kurtosis statistic *n* - A **statistic**, denoted, α_4, used to characterize or measure the **kurtosis** of a **distribution**; defined by the 4th **moment** divided by the square of the 2nd moment of the individual values comprising the distribution about their **mean**; the statistic has the value of 3 for the **normal distribution**.

L

label *n* - [ME, fr MF] 1. A slip (as of paper or cloth) inscribed and affixed to something for identification or description; written or printed matter accompanying an article to furnish identification or other information; a descriptive or identifying word or phrase 2. An isotope or other substance used for identification or tracing.

label insert *n* - A printed document containing detailed factual information concerning the **indication** for usage of a **drug**; information provided typically includes description of or information pertinent to the drug compound itself, known or presumed mode of action, method and mode of administration, recommended **doses** and **dosages**, recommended period of use, known **side effects** and potential risks and toxicities associated with use, and warnings and cautions concerning use, including an enumeration of known contraindications for use. The insert is prepared as part of a **New Drug Application** (NDA) process by the manufacturer or marketing agent of the drug. The content of and information provided in the insert are subject to the review and approval of the **Food and Drug Administration** (FDA). The drug may not be marketed for the named indication without an approved label insert. The content of the label is subject to revisions and modifications after approval of the NDA as requested by the manufacturer or marketing agent and as approved by the FDA, or as dictated by the FDA. So named because the printed document representing the label is affixed to the exterior of the package containing the drug as a detachable appendage or is placed inside the package (hence also **package insert**). The insert, as such, is not normally dispensed with prescriptions of the drug but may be available on request and can be found in the *Physicians' Desk Reference*.[122] Certain classes of drug products (eg, oral contraceptives) must be dispensed to users with written warnings and precautions. syn: package insert

laboratory *n* - [ML *laboratorium*, fr L *laboratus*, pp of *laborare* to labor, fr *labor*] 1. A facility equipped for study primarily by **experimentation** or for testing and **analysis** in some area of **study** or activity. 2. A place providing opportunity for experimentation, observation, or practice in a field of study or learning. 3. A place equipped to perform tests and analyses of bodily fluids and specimens. rt: **central laboratory**, **local laboratory**

laden *adj* - Carrying a load or burden.

lag *adj* - [prob of Scand origin; akin to Norw dial *lagga* to go slowly] 1. Being comparatively slow. 2. delayed; last.

lag *n* - 1. One that lags or is last. 2. The act or the condition of lagging. 3. Comparative slowness or retardation. 4. An amount of lagging or the **time** during which lagging exists; a space of time or **interval** between related **events** or phenomena, eg, the time between initiation of a **treatment** and achievement of its full effect, as in **treatment lag**.

lambda *n* - [Gk, of Sem origin; akin to Heb *lāmedh* lamed] The 11th letter of the **Greek alphabet**, uppercase Λ, lowercase λ.

landscape *adj* - Of or relating to an **orientation** of a **page**, photograph, or painting so as to be wider than high. ant: **portrait**

landscape *n* - [D *landschap*, fr *land* + *-schap* -ship] [general] A pictorial representation, such as a painting or photograph, of natural scenery suggesting wide expanse by **orientation** on the long **axis** of the canvas or sheet so as to be wider than high. [printed **document** or **graphic**] Visual material intended to be viewed, interpreted, or read on or along the long **axis** of the **page** on which displayed; **landscape page orientation**. rt: **portrait**

landscape page orientation *n* - A **page** layout in which the majority of the printed and visual information is arrayed on the long axis of the page. ant: **portrait page orientation** rt: **landscape**

large *adj* - [ME, fr OF, fr L *largus*] 1. extensive; broad 2. Having more than usual power, capacity, or scope; comprehensive. 3. Exceeding most other things of like kind, especially in quantity or size; big. 4. Dealing in great numbers or quantities. ant: **small** rt: **big**

large and simple trial *n* - **big and simple trial**

large trial *n* - **big trial**

Latin *adj* - [ME, fr OE, fr L *Latinus*, fr *Latium*, ancient country of Italy] 1. Of, relating to, or composed in Latin; of or relating to the Italic language of ancient Latium and Rome.

Latin square *n* - 1. An **n** by **n** array of Latin (Roman) letters arranged such that each letter appears once and only once in each **row** and **column** of the array. For example, in a 4 by 4 array:

C	D	A	B
A	C	B	D
D	B	C	A
B	A	D	C

2. **Latin square treatment design** rt: **Greco-Latin square**

Latin square treatment design *n* - A **treatment design** in which **treatments** to be assigned or the order of use is designated by the arrangement of letters in a **Latin square** array. The design represents an extension of the **randomized complete block treatment design** in that it **controls variation** associated with **columns** as well as **rows** in the array. **Random permutations** of such arrays, when rows are viewed as corresponding to **patients** and columns to time or order of **treatment**, represent forms of **complete treatment crossover designs**. Use of such arrays in **crossover trials** has the advantage of eliminating the effect of treatment order since each patient represented in an array receives each of the treatments and each treatment follows every other treatment once and only once in any given array.

law *n* - [ME, fr OE *lagu*, of Scand origin; akin to ON *log* law; akin to OE *licgan* to lie] 1. A **statement** of a **relationship** of **events** or phenomena that is known to be invariant under given conditions. 2. A general relation proved or assumed to hold between mathematical or logical expressions; **theorem**.

law of large numbers *n* - A **theorem** in **statistics** that asserts that the **probability** that the **absolute difference** between the **mean** of a **sample** drawn from a defined **population** and the true mean of that population is greater than an arbitrarily small amount approaches zero as the size of the sample approaches **infinity**.

lay *adj* - [ME, fr MF *lai*, fr LL *laicus*, fr Gk *laikos* of the people, fr *laos* people] 1. Not having a profession; not gainfully employed. 2. Not having or from a particular profession; not having or from the domain of professions typically required or represented. 3. Not ecclesiastical. rt: **nonhealth professional** *Usage note*: Subject to confusion because of implied differences in defns 1 and 2. Use in the sense of defn 1 is in reference to lack of profession or employment. Use in the sense of defn 2 is in reference to one having a different profession, as in characterizing a member of the law profession as a lay member of a **treatment and effects monitoring committee**. Preferably avoided in the sense of defn 2, except where accompanied by detail setting the usage apart from that in the sense of defn 1. See **lay committee member** for additional comments.

lay committee member *n* - [**trials**] 1. A **committee** member who does not have a profession, eg, one who is retired or who is not gainfully employed. 2. A committee member having a profession outside the biomedical field, also **nonhealth professional**; eg, a lawyer or theologian. *Usage note*: Often at least one position on the **advisory-review**, **advisory-review and treatment effects monitoring committee**, or **treatment effects monitoring committee** in **multicenter trials** will be designated to be filled with a **lay** (defn 1) person or a **nonhealth professional** or will be filled by such persons even if the positions are not so designated. The characterization **lay** should be reserved for usages in the sense of defn 1 for **lay committee member**. Use **nonhealth professional** in the sense of defn 2 for reasons indicated in comments for **lay**. Typically a **lay** (defn 1 or 2) member is chosen to balance or broaden the perspective of the committee. Often the position or the person filling the position is viewed as having to do with **patient advocacy**. That view may restrict the perspective of the person filling the position and may unwittingly suggest the lack of such advocacy from others on the committee. The designation of **advocate** should be reserved for positions designated for advocates or incumbents of positions chosen from advocacy groups.

lay representative *n* - 1. One who is considered, chosen, or designated to represent the laity, especially in relation to some cause or perspective. 2. A **lay** person selected or designated to fill some position or to perform some function within a **trial**, eg, a position on the **treatment effects monitoring committee**. 3. **nonhealth professional** rt: **patient advocate** *Usage note*: See note for **patient advocate**.

LD *n* - **lethal dose**

lead *adj* - Acting or serving as a lead or leader; being first or ahead.

lead center *n* - 1. A **center** designated in a **multicenter study** to take the **lead** in testing or performing certain procedures in a study or which is otherwise designated to assume a leadership position in a study. 2. The center responsible for disbursing funds to other centers in a study fully or partially funded under a **consortium agreement**. rt: **parent center**

lead clinic *n* - [multicenter trials] 1. A **clinic** responsible for testing proposed **patient examination** and **data collection** procedures prior to their use in other clinics. 2. The first clinic funded, especially when that clinic is responsible for developing and testing data collection procedures to be used in the trial.

lead time bias *n* - A **bias** due to **differences** in the length of **followup** of the **groups** being compared that is the result of differences in how the time point for initiation of followup is determined, eg, a **comparison** of **events rates** in two groups after **diagnosis** of some **disease** or health condition, when the diagnosis tends to be made earlier in one group than in the other because of the use of better diagnostic procedures. The bias, if present but undetected, can lead to erroneous conclusions. For example, the survival of two groups receiving different forms of therapy for a disease such as lung cancer will not be a valid indication of the usefulness of those therapies if the disease in the one group is diagnosed earlier than in the other group.

lead-in *adj* - Of, being, or relating to that which precedes or comes before, especially as a prelude or introduction. rt: **run-in** *Usage note*: See **lead-in period**.

lead-in *n* - 1. Something that precedes or comes before, especially something done or offered as a prelude or introduction to a main event or

activity. 2. **lead-in period** rt: **run-in** See note for **lead-in period**.

lead-in period *n* - [trials] 1. A **period** of **time** prior to **enrollment** and within the **baseline period** during which **study candidates** are placed on a **treatment** similar to one of those to be evaluated in the **trial** to assess their tolerance to or acceptance of a treatment, or to provide information on **treatment compliance**. The treatment administered may be similar to the **control treatment**, as in the Coronary Drug Project [Coronary Drug Project Research Group, 1973],[30] or may be a **test treatment** [CAST Investigators, 1989].[19] Typically, candidates judged to have had **adverse reactions** to the treatment or to have unsatisfactorily adhered to the prescribed **treatment schedule** are not enrolled. See Brittain and Wittes [1990][16] for a discussion of usefulness of the procedure. 2. **baseline period** syn: **run-in period** rt: **placebo lead-in period** *Usage note*: Preferred to **run-in period** because the meaning of the base term, **lead-in**, is closer to that implied for the period than for **run-in** and for reason stated in the note for **run-in period**.

least *adj* - [ME *leest*, fr OE *lǣst* superl of *lǣssa* less] 1. Lowest in importance or position. 2. Smallest in size or degree; smallest possible.

least squares *adj* - [statistics] Of or relating to the **least squares method** or to a set of squared values, the sum of which is the smallest possible as the result of using an **estimate** produced by that method.

least squares curve fit *n* - A **curve fit** that is the result of using **estimates** produced by the method of **least squares**.

least squares estimate *n* - An **estimate** that is produced by the **least squares method**.

least squares method *n* - A method of **estimation** and **curve fitting**, due to **Gauss**, in which the **estimates** produced or used have the property that the sum of squared differences of the individual **data** points from the estimate or fitted curve is the smallest possible. syn: method of least squares

left *adj* - [ME, fr OE, weak; akin to MLG *lucht* left; fr the left hand's being the weaker in most individuals] 1. Designating, belonging to, or located to the north when facing east. 2. Located in the direction of the left hand; located nearer the left hand than the right hand. 3.

[**statistics**] Points on the **x-axis** located nearer or positioned in the direction of the **origin**, as seen in the **positive** quadrant. ant: **right**

left censored *adj* - Of or relating to being **censored** on or to the **left** of some designated **point** or **event**. ant: **right censored** rt: **interval censored**

left censored observation *n* - 1. An **observation** subject to **censorship** on the **left**. 2. Absence of observation (defn 1) because of censorship on the left. 3. Inability to observe because of censorship on the left. *Usage note*: Observations on most people **enrolled** in **followup studies** are exposed to varying degrees of left censorship from the entry point backward in time. However, this form of censorship is not usually of concern in characterizing the course of a **disease** or in comparing groups over time since most such characterizations and assessments are made from a **baseline** established as part of the **enrollment** process and proceed forward in time. ant: **right censored observation** rt: **interval censored observation**

left skew *adj* - [**statistics**] Of or relating to a **frequency distribution** that is **asymmetrical** with an extended **tail** to the **left**. syn: negative skew ant: **right skew**

left skew distribution *n* - 1. A **nonsymmetrical distribution** with an extended **tail** to the **left** of the **mode**. 2. A **distribution** having a **negative** value for the **statistic** measuring **skewness** of a distribution. syn: negative skew distribution ant: **right skew distribution** rt: **skewness**

Left skewed distribution

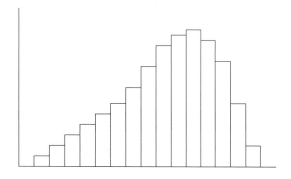

left skewness *n* - **Skewness** to the **left**. syn: negative skewness ant: **right skewness**

left tail *n* - [**statistics**] That portion of a **distribution** at the extreme **left**. ant: **right tail**

leptokurtic *adj* - Of, relating to, or concerned with a **distribution** that is more peaked and tailed than a **standard** distribution as evaluated by some **measure**, such as the **kurtosis statistic**. ant: **platykurtic** rt: **leptokurtic distribution**

leptokurtic distribution *n* - A **unimodal distribution** being more peaked and tailed than a **normal distribution**; such a **distribution** having a **kurtosis statistic** greater than 3. ant: **platykurtic distribution** rt: **leptokurtosis**

leptokurtosis *n* - A condition of being more peaked and tailed than a standard **distribution**. ant: **platykurtosis** rt: **kurtosis, leptokurtic distribution**

lethal *adj* - [L *letalis, lethalis*, fr *letum* death] Deadly; capable of causing death.

lethal dose (LD) *n* - A **dose** of radiation, **drug**, or other agent or substance that causes death or is capable of causing death. rt: **lethal median dose, infectious dose**

lethal median dose *n* - The **dose** that causes or is **estimated** to cause death in 50% of the organisms or experimental animals to which administered; referred to as the LD_{50} in **bioassay** work and in analyses involving **logit** or **probit transformations**. rt: **lethal dose, infectious median dose**

level *n* - [ME, fr MF *livel*, fr (assumed) VL *libellum*, alter of L *libella*, fr dim of *libra* weight, balance] Amount or degree.

level of masking *n* - **masking level**

level of significance *n* - **significance level**

level of treatment adherence *n* - **treatment adherence level**

liaison *adj* - [F, fr MF, fr *lier*, fr OF] 1. Of or relating to communication for establishing and maintaining cooperation and mutual understanding, eg, as conducted by a **project officer** on behalf of a **funding agency**.

license *n* - [ME, fr MF *licence*, fr L *licentia*, fr *licent-, licens*, prp of *licēre* to be permitted; akin to Latvian *līgt* to come to terms] 1. Official or legal permission to do or own a specified thing. 2. A permission granted by a competent authority to engage in a business, occupation, or activity that is not otherwise unlawful.

licensed drug *n* - 1. **approved drug** 2. A **biological product** and use proposed in a **Product License Application approved** by the **Food and Drug Administration**.

licensure *n* - The granting of a **license**.

licensure trial *n* - A **trial** designed and conducted for the purpose of **licensure**; a trial considered to be key for or in a **New Drug Application**; a **phase III drug trial**. rt: **pivotal trial**

life *n* - [ME *līf*, fr OE *lif*; akin to OE *libban* to live] 1. The property or quality manifest in functions such as metabolism, growth, respiration, response to stimuli, and reproduction that distinguishes a living organism from one that is dead. 3. The characteristic state or being of a living organism. 4. A living being, especially a human being. 5. That period of time between birth or inception and death.

life event *n* - Change or disruption in **life** due to some important **event**, usually **negative**, such as the death of a loved one or diagnosis of a serious disease that affects the view or perception of subsequent life, or that alters subsequent life patterns.

life expectancy *n* - The length of **time** a person or object is expected to survive or to continue functioning, as determined under specified assumptions and conditions; referred to as **unconditional life expectancy** or simply as **life expectancy** when the length of time is from birth or prior to use and **conditional life expectancy** when from some point after birth or use. *Usage note*: Measures of life expectancies for people to determine premiums for life insurance and pay out schedules for retirement annuities. They are also used as rough indicators of change in the "health" of a population over time or of differences in the "health" of various populations as they exist at some point in time. Estimates of life expectancies are, in effect, predictions of the future based on past experience. In reality, the actual life experience of a population is determined by the forces to which it is exposed. Past experience is useful in predicting the future only to the extent that the forces in effect in the past remain in effect for the future. Life expectancies are influenced by changes in medical practice and public health measures, as well as by the natural forces to which populations are exposed, including war and natural disasters. The life expectancies typically quoted for populations are

means, eg, for the US population, 1990, 72.7 and 79.4 for white males and females, respectively.[113] The **mean life expectancy** and **median life expectancy**, as a rule, differ. For example, the mean life expectancy for the US population (1989) was 75.3 years, compared with 78.9[112] for the median. Conditional life expectancies are predictions, in effect, of life remaining given survival to a designated age or point. For example, the 1990 mean life expectancy for a white female surviving to age 65 is 19.1; the corresponding figure for a white male is 15.2.[113] rt: **conditional life expectancy, unconditional life expectancy, lifetable**

lifetable *n* - An assembly of **data** in **table** or **graph** form that summarizes the survival (or mortality) experience of the **observational units** (eg, people or objects such as light bulbs) from some specified starting point. In the life sciences, the starting point is usually a specified age (as in most lifetables compiled by demographers), some **event** (such as **diagnosis** of **disease**), or **enrollment** into a **study** (as in a **clinical trial**).

lifetable analysis *n* - A method of **analysis** that relies on a count of the number of **events** observed and the time points at which those events occurred, relative to some zero point. The event may be death or some other event. In **clinical trials**, the time to an event for a **patient** is usually measured from the **time of enrollment**. **Treatment effects** are assessed by comparing **events rates** in the different **treatment groups**.

lifetime *n* - The duration of existence of a living being or thing.

lifetime prevalence *n* - 1. **Prevalence** over a **lifetime**. 2. Prevalence through a **point** in **life**. rt: **period prevalence**

likelihood *adj* - Of or relating to **probability** or **chance**.

likelihood *n* - **Probability** or **chance**.

likelihood function *n* - The **probability density** (or mass) **function** viewed as a function of the unknown **parameters** of the **probability distribution**, given a particular dataset. Since specific values of each parameter correspond to different hypotheses, one can calculate the "likelihood" of specific hypotheses given the data. **Likelihood** is not equivalent to **probability** and the likelihood function cannot be manipulated in the same manner as a probability density function. Usually it is more convenient to work with the **natural logarithm** of the likelihood function (called the log likelihood). The origin of the concept of likelihood is due to RA Fisher.

likelihood principle *n* - [**statistics**] A **principle** that asserts that all of the information for assessing one **hypothesis** versus an **alternative hypothesis**, given a set of **data** and an assumed **model**, is contained in the **likelihood function** of the hypotheses for the data as given.[41] In the case of **trials**, the principle implies that the interpretation of a given set of data, in regard to the amount of support provided for one **hypothesis** versus another, is independent of the reason for the **analysis**, ie, is not influenced by the number of **interim looks** performed in the past or by whether or not the trial was subject to a **stopping rule** [Dupont, 1983;[40] Cornfield, 1966[29]].

likelihood ratio *n* - The **ratio** of the **likelihood function** evaluated at two particular **parameter** values (corresponding to two particular **hypotheses**). The ratio (or its **logarithm**) can be interpreted as the strength of evidence in favor of one hypothesis versus the other.

likelihood ratio test statistic *n* - A **test statistic** based on a **likelihood ratio**.

limit *n* - [ME, fr MF *limite*, fr L *limit-*, *limes* boundary] 1. A place or area enclosed by a **boundary** or bounds. 2. Something that bounds, restrains, or confines. 3. A prescribed **maximum** or **minimum** amount, quantity, or number. 4. A number that for an infinite sequence of numbers is such that ultimately each of the remaining terms of the sequence differs from this number by less than any given **positive** amount. rt: **alert limit, normal limit**

limits of prediction *n* - **prediction limits**

Lind, James - (1716 - 1794) British naval surgeon; contributed to improved hygiene aboard ships at sea. Conducted what is often cited as the first modern day **controlled trial**; 1747 at sea on 12 sailors having scurvy. The study demonstrated the value of fresh oranges and lemons in treating the disease.[91]

line *n* - [often attrib ME *linen*, fr *line* flax, fr OE *līn*] 1. A horizontal **row** of written or printed characters. 2. A **boundary limit** or **region**, eg, as implied with **baseline**. 3. Route or avenue, as in **mainline** or **on-line**. 4. A **continuous** tracing, straight or curved; generated by a moving point

and having an extension only along the path of the point.

linear *adj* - 1. Of, relating to, resembling, or having a **plot** or **graph** that is a **line**, especially a straight line. 2. Relating to, based, or depending on sequential development or steps. 3. [**mathematics**] Having a single dimension; being of the first degree with respect to one or more **variables**; of, relating to, based on, or being a **linear equation**, linear differential equation, linear function, linear transformation, or linear algebra. ant: **nonlinear**

linear combination *n* - The sum of two or more terms, each in the first **degree**, and each multiplied by a **constant**, at least one of which is not zero, eg, $5x_1 + 7x_2 + 2x_3$, or more generally, $a_1x_1 + a_2x_2 + a_3x_3$, where a_1, a_2, and a_3 are constants. rt: **contrast**

linear correlation *n* - **Correlation** involving **regression equations** that are **linear** in form.

linear equation *n* - 1. An **equation** of the first **degree** in any of its variables or **parameters**, eg, $y = \beta_0 + \beta_1 x$; **linear regression model**. 2. An equation of the first degree in relation to its parameters, even if not of the first degree in relation to all its variables, eg, $y = \beta_0 + \beta_1 x^2$ where **y** and x^2 are variables and β_0 and β_1 are parameters. ant: **nonlinear equation**

linear estimate *n* - An **estimate** that is based on a **linear combination** of the observed values of the **random variable**, eg, the **mean**.

linear model *n* - [**statistics**] A **model** equation of the first **degree** with respect to its **parameters**, ie, one in which all parameters have unit **power**; **linear regression model**. ant: **nonlinear model**

linear regression *n* - **Regression** involving a **linear regression model**. ant: **nonlinear regression**

linear regression analysis *n* - **Regression analysis** involving a **model equation** that is **linear** with respect to its **parameters**. ant: **nonlinear regression analysis**

linear regression model *n* - A **regression model** in which the **outcome variable**, y_i (value for the *i*th person or **observation unit**), is a **linear combination** of a series of **independent variables** (**observations** or **regressor variables**), x_{1i}, ⋯, x_{ki} and **parameters** (**regression coefficients**), β_0, β_1, ⋯, β_k plus an **error term**, ε, having the form $\beta_0 + \beta_1 x_{1i} + \beta_2 x_{2i} + \cdots +$

$\beta_k x_{ki} + \varepsilon$; linear because all parameters in the expression have unit power. The primary use of the model in **clinical trials** is for **adjustment** for **baseline differences** among the **treatment groups** when estimating **treatment effects**. The outcome variable is some measure observed during or after **treatment** and should be **continuous**. However, the model is fairly **robust** to departures from the assumption. As a result it is sometimes used as a rough and ready form of adjustment for **discrete** outcome measures, sometimes even for **binary outcome** measures, though the appropriate model for such measures is the **logistic regression model**. ant: **nonlinear regression model** rt: **multiple linear regression model, logistic regression model**

linear regression procedure *n* - Regression procedure involving a **linear regression model**. ant: **nonlinear regression procedure**

linear trend *n* - A **trend** characterized by a straight line.

link, linking, linked, links *v* - To couple or connect.

linkage *n* - The manner or style of being united; the quality or state of being linked.

list *n* - [F *liste*, fr It *lista*, of Gmc origin; akin to OHG *lista* edge] A series of items, such as numbers or words, arrayed in a column or columns.

literature *n* - [ME, fr L *litteratura* writing, grammar, learning, fr *litteratus*] 1. The body of published writings on a particular subject or topic. 2. A specific paper from that body. rt: **indexed literature**

literature control *n* - A **historical control** based on **data** contained in published **literature**.

loading dose *n* - A **dose**, usually given on initiation of therapy, intended to establish a target concentration that is then maintained with subsequently smaller doses.

local *adj* - [ME *localle*, fr MF *local*, fr LL *localis*, fr L *locus* place] 1. Of or relating to a particular place, especially one serving the needs of a defined area or locale. 2. Not general or widespread. 3. Involving or affecting only a restricted part or organ; topical. rt: **central**

local area network (LAN) *n* - [computers] A **network** of interconnected **computers**, **peripheral equipment**, and **software** created and maintained to allow users in a given locale to interact one with another and to use and share in the use of common **datasets** and **files**.

local laboratory *n* - 1. A **laboratory** that serves a single **center** in a **multicenter study**. 2. A laboratory located within the same geographic region as its users, eg, one located in the same city or institution as its users. 3. A laboratory set up and operated for the benefit of a specific person or set of persons in relation to some research activity or specialized function; especially one under the control of and located within one's own administrative unit and the services of which are available only to specified persons housed within that administrative unit. rt: **central laboratory**

local mode *n* - 1. Locally the **maximum** value. 2. A value in a **frequency distribution** greater than adjacent values. rt: **mode, modal class**

locate, located, locating, locates *v* - [L *locatus*, pp of *locare* to place, fr *locus*] 1. To find or fix the position of; to determine or indicate the place, site, or limits of. 2. To set or place in a particular spot or position.

location *n* - 1. The act or process of **locating**. 2. A particular place, point, or site.

location measure *n* - 1. A **measure** of a **distribution**, eg, **arithmetic mean**, **median**, or **range**, such that addition of a constant to each value of the distribution results in a shift of the measure by the same amount; **location parameter**. 2. A measure that purports to or that specifies the location of a distribution, especially one that is in some sense typical of or central to the distribution, eg, arithmetic mean, median, or **mode**. syn: measure of location rt: **scalar measure**

location parameter *n* - A **parameter** of a **distribution**, eg, **mean**, **median**, or **range**, such that addition of a constant to each value of the **variable** defining the distribution causes a shift in the location of that parameter in the distribution by an amount equal to the constant. rt: **scalar parameter**

locational *adj* - Of or relating to a particular position, point, or site.

locator *n* - One or something that locates.

locator file *n* - 1. A **file** that contains **locator information**, such as **patient** name, address, etc, that is or may be used for locating patients lost to **followup**. 2. A file that is used for locating other files.

locator information *n* - 1. **Information**, such as name, address, etc, collected as part of **baseline data** in **prospective followup studies**, used or intended for use in locating patients **lost to followup** (defn 1). 2. Information such as record number, form number, etc, used for locating **records** or **files**.

log *n* - [often attrib ME *logge*, prob of Scand origin; akin to ON *lāg* fallen tree; akin to OE *licgan* to lie] 1. **logarithm** 2. A systematic collection of entries, typically arrayed in list form and ordered by time and date, concerning transactions or steps in relation to some use, process, task, or function, eg, a computer log providing times of use.

log transformation *n* - A **transformation** in which observed values are converted to **logarithmic** values; performed to **normalize** a **frequency distribution**, to stabilize **variance** (eg, in **analysis of variance** in relation to **data** having **variances** that change as a function of the size of the values observed), or to convert a curvilinear **relationship** to a straight line relationship.[164, 5]

log-linear model *n* - A **model** in which the **expected value** of the **outcome variable** is **linear** on the **log** scale.

log-normal distribution *n* - A **normal distribution** as provided by a **log-normal random variable**.

log-normal random variable *n* - A **random variable** that, when transformed by taking its **natural logarithm**, has a **normal distribution**.

log-odds *n* - The **log** of an **odds** or **odds ratio**.

log-odds ratio *n* - The **log** of an **odds ratio**.

logarithm *n* - [NL *logarihmus*, fr *log-* + Gk *arithmos*, number] The **exponent** of a base number that is the **power** to which that base must be raised to produce a given number (eg, $100 = 10^2$ has a logarithm$_{10}$ of 2). syn: **log** ant: **inverse logarithm**

logistic, logistical *adj* - Of, represented by, or relating to a **logistic curve**

logistic curve *n* - 1. A **curve** arising from an **equation** of the form $y = (c + ab^x)^{-1}$. 2. A **growth curve** having the general form of an elongated s; **s-shaped curve**. 3. **logistic function**

logistic function *n* - 1. A **exponential function** used in mathematical **models** of **growth** and **survival** processes; **logistic regression model**.

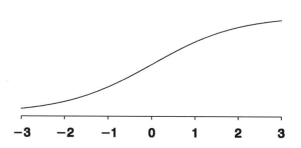

Logistic curve

2. **logistic curve**

logistic regression model *n* - A **regression model** in which the **outcome variable**, y_i (value for the *i*th person or **observation unit**), is expressed in the form $1/(1 + e^{-A}) + \varepsilon$, where **e** is the **natural constant**, $A = \beta_0 + \beta_1 x_1 + \beta_2 x_2 + \cdots + \beta_k x_k$ (a **linear combination** of a series of **independent variables** (**regressor variables**), $x_1, \cdots, x_k$, and **parameters** (**regression coefficients**), $\beta_0, \beta_1, \cdots, \beta_k$), and ε is an **error term**. The independent variables in the **clinical trial** setting are usually **baseline characteristics**. Used in settings where the outcome variable is **binary**. Values generated by the model are bounded below by 0 and above by 1 and are used to **estimate** or **predict** the **probability** (**risk**) of some **event** (eg, death) for a given value of the regressors and with the model parameters specified or estimated from observed **data**. Referred to as **multiple logistic model** when involving two or more regressors (eg, age and age^2 or age and height). rt: **linear regression model**

logit *n* - A **transformation** involving the **natural logarithm** of p/(1 - p), where **p** is given by the **logistic regression model**; arises in **bioassay** and other settings involving **binary outcomes**.

logit model *n* - **Natural log transformation** of the **logistic regression model**.

lognormal *adj* - 1. Of or relating to a **normal distribution** on the log scale. 2. Of or relating to a **random variable** that is normally distributed on the log scale.

logrank, log rank *n* - A generalization (to use with **censored data**) of the uncensored two-sample exponential scores rank test [Savage,

1956];[137] term coined by Peto and Peto [1972].[120]

logrank test statistic *n* - A **nonparametric test statistic** proposed by Mantel [1966][97] and developed by Peto and Peto [1972],[120] used in **trials** to assess the differences in the **distributions** of **events** over **time** among different **treatment groups** (usually with some **censoring**).

long *adj* - [ME *long, lang,* fr OE; akin to OHG *lang* long, L *longus,* Gk *dolichos*] Extending over a considerable length of **time** or expanse. ant: **short** *Usage note*: A relative term (as in *the board is too long*) requiring an implied or defined comparative standard. Avoid as a characterization or label without definition. That considered to be long by one may be considered to be short by another. Avoid confusion by presentation of sufficient detail to indicate sense of use. The line of demarcation between short and long is arbitrary when used as a qualitative indicator of time, as in **long-term followup** vs **short-term followup**; indicate the length of time involved or implied. See also **short**.

long-term followup *n* - **Followup** that extends over a long period of time, eg a year or longer. ant: **short-term followup**

long-term study *n* - 1. A **study** that takes a long time to complete. 2. A study involving **long-term followup**. syn: **chronic study** ant: **short-term study**

long-term treatment *n* - 1. **Treatment**, especially one involving a **drug** or other nonsurgical forms of treatment, administered over an extended period of time via multiple applications or repeated **doses** administered on a regular basis (especially such a treatment extending over a period of months or years). ant: **short-term treatment**

long-term trial *n* - A **trial** involving **long-term followup**. ant: **short-term trial**

longitudinal *adj* - 1. Dealing with the growth, change, or **observation** of an individual or group over a period of time; **followup**. 2. Of or relating to length. 3. Placed or running lengthwise. *Usage note*: Redundant as an adjective modifier of followup. All followup proceeds over time and, therefore, is longitudinal in the sense of defn 1. Avoid as a synonym for followup, as in **longitudinal study** in place of **followup study**. The term *followup* has four letters less than

longitudinal and is subject to less confusion than **longitudinal** in that context.

longitudinal study *n* - **followup study**

look *n* - 1. The act of **looking** or **examining**. 2. **interim look**

look, looking, looked, looks *v* - [ME *looken,* fr OE *lōcian*; akin to OS *lōcōn* to look] To **examine**.

lose, lost, losing, losses *v* - [ME *losen,* fr OE *losian* to perish, lose, fr *los* destruction; akin to OE *lēosan* to lose; akin to ON *losa* to loosen, L *luere* to release, atone for, Gk *lyein* to loosen, dissolve, destroy] 1. To suffer deprivation of; to be caused to part with something of value because of misfortune. 2. To miss from one's possession or from a customary or presumed place. 3. To fail to keep control of or allegiance to; to fail to keep or sustain. ant: **win**

loss *n* - [ME *los,* prob back-formation fr *lost,* pp of *losen* to lose] A person, thing, or amount that is **lost**.

loss to followup *n* - Any **loss** of **followup data** on a person (or other **observation unit**) after **enrollment** into a **study**; loss may occur because a person cannot be located for required **data collection** or because the person is unwilling or unable to submit to required data collection procedures. rt: **lost to followup** *Usage note*: The majority of losses to followup in **trials** occur because of **dropout** since most data in trials are generated via direct interview and examination of those enrolled. However, some forms of followup may continue even after a person drops out, as noted in a comment for **dropout**.

losses to followup *n* - The sum total of lost **information** because of **loss to followup**. *Usage note*: See **loss to followup** for comment.

lost *adj* - Unable to be found or located; no longer possessed; taken away or beyond reach or attainment.

lost to followup *adj* - 1. Characterized by unknown whereabouts in a **followup study**. 2. An **observation unit** in a **followup study** that cannot be followed for some **outcome** or observation of interest. rt: **losses to followup** *Usage note*: The characterization in **trials** is usually applied to a person who is unwilling or unable to return to the **clinic** for **followup examinations**. The characterization is subject to misuse, especially when used as a global characterization for a person without regard to nature or extent of information lost. In good usage, the observation or set of observations lost is specified. Specification is important when followup is possible by other means, eg, by telephone instead of by scheduled **clinic visits**. It is bad practice to use **lost to followup** interchangeably with **dropout** or **drop out**. Indeed, a person, no longer willing or able to return for **clinic visits**, is lost to followup for observations made during such visits, but not necessarily for observations that can be made in other ways, eg, by telephone interview. Even individuals who refuse any contact with study personnel may not be lost to followup for certain events, such as death.

lost to mortality followup *adj* - Characterized by **vital status** that cannot be determined because that person cannot be located or traced.

lot *n* - [ME, fr OE *hlot*; akin to OHG *hlōz*] 1. An object, such as an **urn** containing numbered balls, or a **device**, such as a pointer that can be spun, used for determining something by **chance**. 2. The use of chance for determining something.

lottery *n* - [often attrib MF *loterie*, fr MD, fr *lot* lot; akin to OE *hlot* lot] 1. A selection process, performed in public and based on **chance**, eg, as used for selection into the military or for determining the recipient of some prize or award. 2. Any selection or determination process based on **chance** such as **randomization**. *Usage note*: The most common usage of the term in **trials** is in explanations given to **candidates** for **enrollment** of the **treatment assignment** process in **randomized trials** during the **consent process** (as in, *the treatment to be administered will be determined by a random or chance process similar to that used in a lottery for choosing a winner*). The association with lotteries or the drawing of **lots** is useful in conveying the notion of chance but is not especially helpful in explaining the process implied by randomization. Lotteries are used to select one from among many, whereas all persons in a trial are "selected" and all are assigned to a treatment. Further, the notion of winning or losing, as implied with a lottery or the drawing of lots, is neither informative nor helpful in the consent process, especially in trials motivated by a true state of **equipoise**. Hence, it is perhaps more instructive to explain the process implied by randomization as being akin to making a choice by flipping a coin rather than by reference to a lottery or to the drawing of lots. See also note for **random** *adj, scientific*.

M

main *adj* - [ME, fr OE *mǣgen-*, fr *mǣgen* strength] chief, **principal**, **primary**

main effect *n* - The **effect** associated with or produced by a **treatment** or **factor** in a **factorial experiment**.

mainframe *n* - 1. The **central processing unit** of a **computer** exclusive of **peripheral** and remote **devices**. 2. A large, fast, multitask, multipurpose computer. rt: **supercomputer**

mainline *adj* - Being in or of the mainstream.

mainline paper *n* - [**trials**] A **paper** detailing the **design**, **methods**, or **baseline results** of a **trial** or containing original **results** related to the primary **objective** of a trial and written by study personnel commissioned by the **investigative group** or their representative. syn: **primary publication** rt: **secondary paper**

major *adj* - [ME *maiour*, fr L *major*, compar of *magnus* great, large] 1. Greater in importance, interest, **rank**, or stature. 2. Greater in number, quantity, or extent. 3. Having attained **majority**.

major committee *n* - **key committee**

majority *n* - 1. The greater part or number. 2. The **age** at which full civil rights are accorded to a person (age 18 in the United States).

manage, managed, managing, manages *v* - [It *maneggiare*, fr *mano* hand, fr L *manus*] To handle or direct with a degree of skill; to exercise administrative, executive, or supervisory functions.

management *n* - The act of managing; the conducting or supervision of something.

management trial *n* - A **trial** designed and conducted primarily to provide information on the value of a **treatment** in normal usage [see Sackett, 1980;[135] Sackett and Gent, 1979;[136] Schwartz and Lellouch, 1967[139]]. syn: **pragmatic trial** ant: **explanatory trial** *Usage note*: See usage notes for **explanatory trial** and **pragmatic trial**.

manager *n* - One who **manages**.

Mann-Whitney test *n* - A **nonparametric test**, extending work of Wilcoxon [1945],[165] for testing whether two **distributions** are the same; based on ranks of the individual values of the two distributions combined [Mann and Whitney, 1947].[94] See also **Wilcoxon test**.

Mantel-Haenszel test statistic *n* - A summary **chi-square test statistic**, developed by Mantel and Haenszel [1959],[98] for testing the equality of **proportions** observed in two different **groups** or **populations** after taking account of differences in the composition of the two groups or populations being compared. The approach involves a series of **2 X 2 tables** (one for each stratum of a stratification variable). The individual chi-square are combined to yield a summary chi-square.

manual *n* - 1. A **document**, typically arranged or presented in book or booklet form, intended as a reference for performing a defined set of tasks or functions; **study manual**; **study manual of operations**. 2. **handbook** 3. **protocol** (not a recommended synonym) *Usage note*: See **study manual** and **study handbook** for usage notes.

manual of operations (MoP, MOP) *n* - 1. A **document** in book or booklet form of instructional material used for performing **operations** in relation to some defined task or function. 2. **study manual of operations**

manuscript *n* - 1. A handwritten or typewritten composition, especially one prepared for submission to a **journal** or publisher. 2. Such a composition after publication in a journal, book, or magazine. rt: **paper**

manuscript masthead *n* - Identifying information displayed at the head of a **manuscript**, generally consisting of a title followed by a form of **authorship attribution**.

margin *n* - [ME, fr L *margin-*, *margo* border] 1. The part of a page or sheet at the edges; typically white space in printed documents devoid of printed material, except for headers, footers, and page numbers. 2. That which is at the edge or border of something; that which is at the **boundary** of two adjoining surfaces. 3. A spare amount, measure, or degree allowed or given for contingencies or special circumstances; a bare minimum below which or an extreme **limit**

beyond which something becomes impossible or is no longer desirable; **safety margin**. 4. A **range** about a specified value beyond which something is considered to be unlikely; **error margin**.

margin of error *n* - **error margin**   rt: **safety margin**

margin of safety *n* - **safety margin**   rt: **error margin**

marginal *adj* - [ML *marginalis*, fr L *margin-*, *margo*] Being of or relating to the summation or integration of two or more **variables** over all possible values of those variables.

marginal distribution *n* - The **distribution** resulting from summation or integration over two or more dimensions of a **joint distribution**.

marker *n* - 1. **biological marker**; genetic marker 2. Something that marks or denotes, eg, a symbol used to indicate the beginning or end of a set of **data**, a **record**, **field**, or **file**.

market *n* - [ME, fr ONF, fr L *mercatus* trade, marketplace, fr *mercatus*, pp of *mercari* to trade, fr *merc-*, *merx* merchandise] A public place where goods are sold at wholesale or retail.

marketing application *n* - An **application** for a **new drug** submitted under section 505 (b) of the Food, Drug, and Cosmetic Act; a request for certification of an antibiotic submitted under section 507 of the Act, or a **product license application** for a **biological product** submitted under provisions of the Public Health Service Act.

mask, masked *adj* - Of, relating to, or being a procedure in a **study**, especially an **experiment** or **trial**, in which a person or class of persons (eg, **patients**, **treaters**, or **readers** in a trial) is not informed of or is denied access to information known to or made available to others represented in the study or **experiment**. See **single-mask**, **double-mask**, and **triple-mask** in relation to **treatment assignment** in trials.   syn: **blind** (not recommended; see **blind** for reasons) *Usage note*: Preferred to **blind** because of negative connotations and ambiguities associated with **blind**. **Blind** carries a connotation of mindlessness or stupidity in some everyday usages, eg, *blind luck* or *blind stupidity*. The term **mask** has greater utility across a wider class of trials and settings than **blind** (eg, **blind** can be confusing in vision **trials** with **blind** treatment administration and with blindness as an

outcome measure) and is a better descriptor of the operational process implied.

mask *n* - [MF *masque*, fr OIt *maschera*] [general] Something that hides or conceals from view. [**research**] A condition imposed on an individual (or group of individuals) for the purpose of keeping that individual (or group of individuals) from knowing or learning of some condition, fact, or observation, such as **treatment assignment**, as in **single-masked**, **double-masked**, or **triple-masked trials**.   syn: **blind** (not recommended usage; see **blind** for reasons) *Usage note*: See note for **mask, masked** *adj*.

mask, masked, masking, masks *v* - To conceal by withholding, hiding, or obscuring some condition, fact, or **observation**.   rt: **censor**

masked data analysis *n* - [**trials**] 1. **Data analysis** performed by someone **masked** to **treatment assignment**. 2. Data analyses presented with the **treatment groups** masked.

masked data analyst *n* - [**trials**] A **data analyst** **masked** to **treatment assignment**.

masked data collection *n* - **Data collection** performed with the imposition of a **mask** in relation to some condition, fact, or **observation**, eg, **disease** status in a **case-control study** or **treatment assignment** in a **clinical trial**.   rt: **masked data collector**

masked data collector *n* - A **data collector** **masked** to some condition, fact, or **observation**.   rt: **masked data collection**

masked experiment *n* - 1. An **experiment** in which one or more persons or categories of persons (eg, **patients**, **treaters**, **data collectors**, the **committee** that monitors the **study** for **treatment effects**) are denied access to information concerning aspects of the experiment during its conduct. 2. **masked trial**

masked patient *n* - [**trials**] A **patient masked** to **treatment assignment**.

masked randomization *n* - 1. **Randomization** in which **treatment assignments** remain **masked** until issued. 2. **single-**, **double-**, or **triple-masked** randomization.   syn: blind randomization (not recommended; see **masked randomization** for reasons)   ant: **unmasked randomization**, open randomization   rt: **masked treatment assignment** *Usage note*: Masked randomization (defn 1) is a property of any assignment scheme in which assignments cannot be predicted and where they are not issued or released until a **patient** has been judged **eligible** and has **consented** to **enrollment**, as with assignments generated on demand by **computer**, assignments used in **sequence** as contained in sealed envelopes or in a locked **electronic file**. The actual treatment to be administered will be revealed to clinic personnel and patients when assignments are issued in **unmasked trials** and only to clinic personnel (not patients) in **single-masked trials**. The treatment is not revealed to either clinic personnel or patients in **double-** or **triple-masked trials**; the assignments themselves in such cases will be coded in some way to mask the identities of the treatments called for by the assignments.

masked reader *n* - A **reader masked** to some fact or condition, eg, **treatment assignment**, disease state or condition of the **patient**, information concerning previous **readings**.

masked reading *n* - A **reading** performed or made under **masked** conditions. The masking may relate to **treatment assignment**, disease state or condition of the **patient**, or to information concerning previous **readings**.

masked treater *n* - 1. A **treater** masked to **treatment assignment**. 2. A treater masked to some condition or fact regarding the **patient**.

masked treatment *n* - A **treatment** that is administered in a **masked** fashion; **single-masked treatment**; **double-masked treatment**; **triple-masked treatment**.

masked treatment assignment *n* - 1. Any **assignment scheme** in which **treatment assignments** remain **masked** until issued, especially any such scheme in regard to the person to be assigned and to those requesting the assignment. 2. **single-**, **double-**, or **triple-masked** treatment assignment. syn: blind treatment assignment (not recommended) ant: **unmasked treatment assignment**, **open treatment assignment** rt: **masked randomization** *Usage note*: As noted in the usage note for **masked randomization**, masked treatment assignment (defn 1) is a property of any scheme in which **treatment assignments** remain **masked** until **patients** (**treatment units**) have been judged **eligible** for **enrollment** and ready to be started on the assigned treatments, such as with the **randomization** schemes implied for **masked randomization**, as well as with **nonrandom adaptive**

schemes that are effectively masked (eg, one in which assignments are derived by a **minimization** scheme involving an algorithm that can only be reliably evaluated using a **computer**). The actual treatment to be administered will be revealed to clinic personnel when the assignment is issued in **unmasked trials** but only to selected people in **single-masked trials** and not to any one in the clinic in **double-** or **triple-masked trials**. The assignments themselves in such cases will be coded in some way so as to mask the identities of the treatments called for by the assignments.

masked treatment assignment schedule *n* - 1. A **treatment assignment schedule** that is **masked** to clinic personnel. 2. Such a schedule masked to all personnel, including those responsible for administering it. ant: **open treatment assignment schedule** *Usage note*: Note that a schedule can be masked but that assignments obtained from the schedule may not be masked, as in the case of a **trial** not involving **masked treatment administration**. Most schemes administered by **coordinating centers** in **multicenter trials** are masked in the sense of defn 1 and some in the sense of defn 2 (eg, those in which assignments are sealed or those in which assignments are generated via **computer** as needed). Most self-administered envelope schemes meet the test for being masked, except where assignments can be determined without opening the envelope (eg, where assignments can be seen by transillumination of envelopes) or where the system is perverted (eg, by opening envelopes before patients are ready to be enrolled). See also **open treatment assignment schedule**.

masked treatment effects monitor *n* - A person responsible for **treatment effects monitoring** masked to **treatment assignment**. rt: **masked treatment effects monitoring committee**

masked treatment effects monitoring *n* - [trials] **Treatment effects monitoring** in which **results** used for **monitoring** are **masked** as to **treatment assignment**.

masked treatment effects monitoring committee *n* - A **treatment effects monitoring committee masked** to **treatment assignment**, eg, as achieved by presenting such a committee with a **treatment effects monitoring report** with **treatment groups** being denoted by arbitrary letter codes obscuring treatment identity.

masked trial *n* - 1. **Single-, double-, or triple-masked trial**. 2. A **trial** in which one or more persons or categories of persons (eg, **patients**, **treaters**, **data collectors**, the **committee monitoring** the trial) are denied access to information concerning aspects of the trial during its conduct, especially in relation to **treatment assignment**. ant: **nonmasked trial**

masking level *n* - [**trials**] The degree of **masking** employed in a trial in relation to **treatment assignment** for a designated class or category of people (eg, **patients**, **treaters**, **data collectors**, **readers**, **monitors**) associated with the trial; **complete**, **partial**, or **none**. syn: level of masking *Usage note*: The level may range from complete to none, for different classes or categories of people, depending on the design and operating features of the trial. For example, it is by definition complete for patients, treaters, and monitors in a triple-masked trial and usually complete for data collectors and readers. It may be complete for one class and partial or none for other classes of people, eg, as would be the case in a nonmasked trial involving masking of some of the data collectors and masked **treatment effects monitoring**.

mass *adj* - Having a large-scale or broad character.

mass *n* - [ME *masse*, fr MF, fr L *massa*, fr Gk *maza*; akin to Gk *massein* to knead] 1. A quantity or aggregate of matter. 2. A quantity, amount, or number.

mass screening *n* - 1. **Screening** of an entire **population**. 2. Screening on a large and unrestricted basis.

mass storage device *n* - [**computers**] Large capacity secondary storage **device** (ie, not part of the main computing system), primarily used for **data** backup and off-line storage. Typically, tapes, disks, cartridges, or other exterior memory devices, that are directly addressable by the **central processing unit**.

masthead *n* - 1. The printed matter in a newspaper or periodical that gives the name of the publication, details of ownership, advertising rates, and subscription rates. 2. The name of a publication as displayed on the front cover or first page. 3. **manuscript masthead**

match *n* - [ME *macche*, fr OE *mǣcca*; akin to OE *macian* to make] 1. A person or thing similar to another; a pair suitably associated. 2. The state or condition of being **matched**.

match, matched, matching, matches *v* - [general] To cause to suit or correspond. [epidemiology] To cause sets of **observation units** (eg, pairs of persons or two groups) to be identical or similar with regard to some **characteristic** or **variable** by purposeful selection. Typically done as a means of **variance control** in nonexperimental **comparative study** settings. The matching may be done with varying degrees of exactness, eg, within a defined interval or within a **class** or **category**. rt: **category matching**, **individual matching**, **frequency matching**, **pair matching**, **pairwise matching**, **overmatching**

matched control *n* - [epidemiology] A **control** (defn 3) selected to be suitably similar to the focus of **study**, eg, a **control** in a **case-control study**; typically matching **factors** are **gender**, **race**, or **age**. Types include **category matching**, **individual matching**, **frequency matching**, and **pair matching**.

matched pair *n* - A **match** of one person (or **observation unit**) to another person (or observation unit), eg, a **control** matched to a **case** in a **case-control study**. rt: **match**

matching placebo *n* - 1. A **placebo** that is designed and intended to **match** an **active substance** in shape, form, size, color, texture, smell, taste, etc. 2. A pill (capsule or tablet) that is designed and intended to match or resemble in shape, form, size, color, texture, smell or taste a corresponding pill containing a therapeutically **active drug**; **control treatment** in **placebo-controlled trials**. *Usage note*: In general, it is difficult to prepare a perfectly matching placebo. Even under the best circumstances there may be subtle differences in color, sheen, or texture. Hence, it is usually not sufficient to indicate that a matching placebo was used; details should be provided as to the nature of the similarity.

mathematical *adj* - [L *mathematicus*, fr Gk *mathēmatikos*, fr *mathēmat-*, *mathēma* mathematics, fr *manthanien* to learn; akin to Goth *mundon* to pay attention Skt *medhā* intelligence] Of or relating to **mathematics**; precise, exact.

mathematical expectation *n* - The **expected value** of a **random variable**; the **mean** of its **distribution**.

mathematical model *n* - A **model** for some process, procedure, or **data** relationship expressed in mathematical terms. 2. **model equation**

mathematics *n* - A science dealing with numbers, forms, arrangements, and associated relationships using rigorously defined numerical and operational notation.

matrix *n* - [L womb, fr *matr-*, *mater*] A rectangular array of mathematical **elements** (eg, **coefficients** of a set of **simultaneous linear equations**) that can be manipulated mathematically and that can be combined with similar arrays of the same dimension to form sums or products; square matrix when the number of **rows** equals the number of **columns**.

mature *adj* - [ME, fr L *maturs* ripe; akin to L *mane* in the morning, *manus* good] 1. Having completed natural growth or development; **adult**. 2. Characteristic of or suitable to one who has achieved full growth or development; having undergone maturation. rt: **adult**

mature minor *n* - A **minor** who, by virtue of deed, action, or need, is regarded as an **adult** in some legal, operational, or social sense and, to that extent, is accorded the same rights and privileges as an adult, eg, a sexually active teenager receiving counseling in a school clinic regarding safe sex practices without parental consent or knowledge. syn: **emancipated minor**

maximum *n* - [L neut of *maximus*] The greatest value or quantity attained or attainable; the upper allowable or attainable **limit**. ant: **minimum**

maximum likelihood *n* - 1. **maximum likelihood method** 2. **maximum likelihood estimate**

maximum likelihood estimate (MLE) *n* - An **estimate** of a **population parameter** derived using **maximum likelihood**.

maximum likelihood method *n* - A procedure for estimating **population parameters** (eg, **means** or **variances**) from **observed data** in which the **estimates** are derived, such that they maximize the **likelihood function**.

maximum tolerable dose (MTD) *n* - The highest **dose** of a **drug** considered to be **safe** and tolerable; term arises in **phase I** and **II trials** of chemoprophylaxis drugs where increased levels of a drug are associated with increased **probability** of desired effects and increased probability of serious **side effects**. See Carter (1977) for review.[20]

me-too *adj* - Broadly, similar to or the same as; in regard to a product (such as a **drug**), similar to or identical to that product with no significant advantage over it.

me-too drug *n* - **Generic drug**, especially one designed to mimic a proprietary drug.

mean *n* - 1. **arithmetic mean** 2. **average**

mean absolute deviation *n* - **Deviation from mean**, ignoring sign.

mean deviation *n* - A **measure** of **variation** of **data**, given by the **arithmetic mean** of the **absolute deviations** from the arithmetic mean. rt: **mean square error**

mean life expectancy *n* - The **mean** length of life of a specified **population**. See usage note for **life expectancy**. rt: **median life expectancy**

mean priority score *n* - The **mean** of **priority scores** (defn 1) assigned by individual members of a **review group**. For **NIH grant reviews**, the mean of the individual priority scores multiplied by 100; number ranges from 100 (best) to 500 (worst); number subject to **adjustment** to remove effects of different scoring behaviors of various review groups.

mean square *n* - The **mean** (arithmetic) of a **sum of squares**. rt: **mean deviation**

mean square error *n* - 1. The **expected value** of the squared **difference** of an **estimator** from its true value (**parameter**); for **unbiased** estimators equal to the **variance** of the estimator. 2. The **mean** (arithmetic) of the squared differences of individual values of a **dataset** from its **estimator** of central tendency. rt: **mean deviation, root-mean square error, standard deviation**

meaningful *adj* - Having meaning or purpose.

meaningful difference *n* - 1. An **observed difference** that is considered to be beyond the **range** of **chance**. 2. **clinically meaningful difference**

measure *n* - [ME *mesure*, fr OF, fr L *mensura*, fr *mensus*, pp of *metiri* to measure; akin to OE *mǣth* measure, Gk *metron*] 1. An **estimate** of what is **expected**. 2. Amount, degree, or extent. 3. A standard amount. 4. An **instrument** or utensil for measuring. 5. The act or process of measuring; **measurement**.

measure, measured, measuring, measures *v* - 1. To ascertain by **measurement**. 2. To choose to control or regulate with caution or restraint. 3. To regulate by a **standard** or **norm**.

measure of central tendency *n* - **central tendency measure**

measure of dispersion *n* - **variation measure**

measure of location *n* - **location measure**

measure of variation *n* - **variation measure**

measurement *n* - The act or process of **measuring**; a figure, extent, or amount obtained by measuring.

measurement bias *n* - A **bias** related to a **measurement** process, eg, one that favors the recording of even numbers over odd numbers, as in some methods of measuring blood pressure.

measurement error *n* - 1. **Error** or **variability** associated with the **measurement** device or process itself; as opposed to **observer error**, **rounding error**, or **digit preference**. 2. **observer error**

measurement validity *n* - The extent to which a **measurement** actually reflects what it purports to **measure**.

median *n* - The **midpoint** value in an ordered sequence of **observations** (ie, the value having as many observations below as above it for distributions with odd numbers of observations and the **arithmetic mean** of the two middle values in distributions with even numbers of observations); one of several **measures of central tendency**. rt: **average**, **mean**, **mode**

median dose *n* - The **dose** that produces or is **estimated** to produce a **response** in 50% of those to which or whom administered. See **lethal median dose** (LD_{50}) and **infectious median dose** (ID_{50}).

median life expectancy *n* - The **median** length of life of a specified **population**. See **life expectancy**. rt: **mean life expectancy**

mediate, mediated, mediating, mediates *v* - [ML *mediatus*, pp of *mediare*, fr LL, to be in the middle, fr L *medius* middle] To effect by action as an intermediary. 3. To act as an intermediary agent in bringing about or effecting something.

mediator *n* - [LL, fr mediatus, pp] 1. One or something that **mediates**. 2. An agent, compound, **factor,** or **variable** that mediates.

mediator variable *n* - **intervening variable**

medical *adj* - [F or LL; F *médical*, fr LL *medicalis*, fr L *medicus* physician, fr *mederi* to heal; akin to Av *vī-mad-* healer, L *meditari* to meditate] Of, relating to, or concerned with physicians or the practice of **medicine**; requiring or devoted to **medical treatment**.

medical care *n* - **Care** administered by or under the supervision of a physician; especially care involving **medicines** and nonsurgical procedures.

medical chart *n* - **medical record**, **patient chart**, **patient record**

medical device *n* - An instrument, apparatus, implement, machine, contrivance, implant, **in vitro** reagent, or other similar or related article intended for use in the **diagnosis** of **disease** or other health conditions, the cure, mitigation, **treatment**, or **prevention** of disease, or intended to affect the structure or function of the human body, and that exerts its effect via some means other than through chemical action within or on the human body or by being metabolized; includes diagnostic tests, kits, pacemakers, arterial grafts, intraocular lenses, and orthopedic pins [Food and Drug Administration, 1983].[50]

medical ethics *n* - 1. A branch of **ethics** dealing with **medicine**; such a branch devoted primarily to a study of the ethics of **research** on human beings as performed in medical settings. 2. The **rules** and **standards** of conduct governing or guiding the medical profession.

medical ethics, principles of *n* - Standards set forth in the **Nuremberg Code** and subsequently enunciated in the form of principles having to do with the need for **beneficence**, **competence**, **justice**, and **respect** for persons when caring for **patients** and that serve as standards to be met in **clinical trials** or other forms of experimentation on human beings. See **beneficence, principle of; competence, principle of; justice, principle of; respect for persons, principle of**.

medical judgment *n* - A **judgment** made by a **physician** in regard to the care of a **patient** after careful consideration of available information and consideration of alternative explanations or courses of action. rt: **best medical judgment**

medical liaison office *n* - **project office**

medical liaison officer *n* - **project officer**

Medical Literature Analysis Retrieval System (MEDLARS) *n* - Electronic user-based literature retrieval system consisting of a series of databases (40+) containing about 16 million **references** (as of January 1993); databases include CATLINE, **MEDLINE**, PDQ, TOXLINE, and TOXNET; maintained by the **National Library of Medicine**.

medical record *n* - A collection of written and tabular information and related **documents**, such as reports of laboratory tests, x-ray films, and ECG tracings, concerning a specific person and related to that person's **diagnosis** or care in a specified setting. syn: medical chart, **patient record, patient chart**

medical research associate *n* - **clinical research associate**

medical treatment *n* - 1. Any **treatment** administered by or under the supervision of a physician. 2. Any treatment, other than surgery, administered by or under the supervision of a physician for treatment or **prevention** of a **disease** or adverse health condition, especially one involving use of **medicines**. ant: **surgical treatment**

medical trial *n* - 1. A **trial** in which each of the **study treatments** involve **medical treatments** (defn 2). 2. A trial in which the **test treatments** involve use of medical treatments. 3. A trial in which the primary mode of treatment is medical. ant: **surgical trial** rt: **medicine**

medically important difference *n* - An **observed difference** that is considered to be of medical importance. syn: medically meaningful difference

medically meaningful difference *n* - **medically important difference**

medicine *n* - [ME, fr OF, fr L *medicina*, fr fem of *medicinus* of a physician, fr *medicus*] 1. A preparation or substance, such as a **drug**, used in treating or preventing a **disease** or adverse health condition. 2. A discipline concerned with preservation of health or the prevention, alleviation, and cure of disease. 3. A nonsurgical **medical treatment** administered for **prevention**, amelioration, or cure of a disease or **adverse** health condition.

MEDLARS *n* - **Medical Literature Analysis Retrieval System**

MEDLINE *n* - One of the **electronic databases** of **MEDLARS**; name derived from MEDLARS online; contains **reference citations** for papers contained in some 3,600 medical journals published worldwide; files contain abstracts of cited papers (when they have one) and associated medical subject headings as applied by indexers at the NLM; files include publications starting with 1966 and have about 7.2 million entries; annual increment in excess of 360,000 (as of January 1993).

mega-, meg- *prefix* - [Gk, fr *megas* large] One million; multiplied by one million.

megabyte (mB, MB) *n* - 1,048,576 (ie, 2^{20}) **bytes**.

memory *n* - [ME *memorie*, fr MF *memoire*, fr L *memoria*, fr *memor* mindful; akin to OE *mimorian* to remember, L *memoria*, fr *memor* mindful; akin to OE *mimorian* to remember, L *mora* delay, Gk *mermēra* care, Skt *smarati* he remembers] [**computer**] A device used for storing and retrieving information within a **computer**.

meta-, met- *prefix* - [NL & ML, fr L or Gk; L change, fr Gk among, with, after, change, fr *meta* among, with, after; akin to OE *mid*, *mith* with, OHG *mit*] 1. Occurring later than or in succession to; situated behind or beyond; more comprehensive; transcending. 2. Situated to extend a discipline or activity.

meta-analysis *n* - An **analysis** performed on **data** from two or more **studies** considered to bear on an issue or question of importance (eg, the role of a **risk factor** in the **etiology** of a **disease** or the usefulness of a **treatment** for a given health condition) for the purpose of drawing a conclusion regarding that issue or question. Introduced by Glass (1976).[59] See also **ad hoc meta-analysis** and **designed meta-analysis**. syn: **overview** (not recommended) *Usage note*: The term is most often applied in settings involving the analysis of results from similar **experiments**, such as **clinical trials**. Preferred to **overview** because of wider acceptance and usage and less risk of ambiguity in usage. See **overview** for added comments.

metadata *n* - **Data** about data, especially data relating to specific **fields** in a **dataset** used to characterize the state or quality of data contained in those fields, eg, a status flag for a data field in an **electronic dataset** to inform users that a data element is aberrant or is under query via an **edit query**.

method *n* - [MF or L; MF *methode*, fr L *methodus*, fr Gk *methodos*, fr *meta-* + *hodos* way] A manner or mode of procedure, especially an orderly, logical, or systematic way of instruction, inquiry, operation, or presentation, related to some task or function.

method of least squares *n* - **least squares method**

method of moments *n* - **moments, method of**

methodologist *n* - 1. One who works on a set or system of **methods**, **principles**, or **rules** for application to some defined setting. 2. One who seeks to derive general principles and standards from a study of existing practices and procedures. 3. One who is methodical. rt: **trialist**

methodology *n* - [NL *methodologia*, fr L *methodus* + *-logia* -logy] 1. A body of **methods**, **rules**, postulates, and procedures employed in a particular discipline, subspecialty, or practice; a particular set of procedures. 2. The **study** and development of methods.

metric, **metrical** *adj* - 1. Of or relating to **measurement** or to a process of measurement. 2. Of or relating to something quantitative or measured. 3. Based on the meter; of or relating to the metric system. ant: **nonmetric**

metric data *n* - **Data** that arise from and can be arrayed on a **measurement scale** and, hence, are amenable to ordinary arithmetic operations, such as addition, subtraction, multiplication, and division. syn: **quantitative data** ant: **nonmetric data**

metric variable *n* - 1. A **variable** that is **metric**, especially one that is **continuous**. 2. A variable that is quantitative, **discrete**, or **continuous**; not qualitative or **ordinal**.

micro-, **micr-** *prefix* - [ME *micro-*, fr L, fr Gk *mikr-*, *mikro-*, fr *mikros*, *smikros* small, short; akin to OE *smēalīc* careful, exquisite] small

microcomputer *n* - 1. A small **computer** with its computing capabilities residing in a circuit board. 2. A computer having a **microprocessor**, **memory**, and **input/output** capabilities and used by a single user or a few related users; **personal computer**. rt: **minicomputer**

microprocessor *n* - A **computer** processing unit that is contained in a single chip.

mid *adj* - [ME, fr OE *midde*; akin to OHG *mitti* middle, L *medius* Gk *mesos*] Being the part in the middle; occupying a middle position.

mid-quartile *n* - The **mean** of the 1st and 3rd **quartile**; sometimes used as an **estimate** of the mean of a **distribution** if the distribution is reasonably **symmetrical**.

mid-range *n* - The **arithmetic mean** of the two values defining the **range**; a quick and dirty **estimate** of the mean if the **distribution** is **symmetrical** or reasonably so.

midpoint *n* - A point at or near the center.

mini- *prefix* - miniature; very small

minicomputer *n* - Any **computer** larger than a **microcomputer** but smaller than a **mainframe**; generally having a smaller **word size** (32 **bits** or less) and less memory (64**K** or less) than a **mainframe**, but has a faster processor and can support more input/output **devices** than a microcomputer. rt: **superminicomputer**

minimization *n* - [**trials**] A method of **adaptive treatment assignment** [introduced by Taves, 1974;[150] see also pages 84-7 of Pocock, 1983[126]] in which assignments are generated to minimize some difference function, based on counts of previous assignments among the various **treatment assignment strata**. **Randomization** is not normally used with minimization, except for making assignments when the difference function is zero. However, the method can be modified to include randomization with probabilistic assignments according to a set **treatment assignment ratio** when the difference is not zero as well to render the process nondeterministic, thereby reducing the chances of study personnel predicting future assignments. rt: **minimum likelihood treatment assignment**

minimum *n* - [L, neut of *minimus* smallest; akin to L *minor* smaller] The least value or quantity attained or attainable; the lower allowable or attainable **limit**. ant: **maximum**

minimum likelihood treatment assignment *n* - A form of **baseline adaptive treatment assignment** in which each assignment is made in such a way as to minimize the **imbalance** (measured against a desired degree of **balance**) among the **treatment groups** with regard to the **distribution** of a specified set of **baseline characteristics** [Aickin, 1982].[1] rt: **minimization**

minor *n* - A person not yet having reached the **age of majority**. rt: **emancipated minor**

minority *n* - 1. The lesser part or number. 2. The smaller of two group forming a whole. 3. A racial, religious, political, national, or other group regarded as different from a larger group of which it is a part; a member of such a group. 4. The state or period of time prior to reaching the **age of majority**.

misconduct *n* - 1. Intentional wrongdoing. 2. Deliberate **violation** of a **law** or **standard** of conduct. 3. misbehavior rt: **scientific misconduct**

mixed *adj* - [ME *mixte*] 1. Combining characteristics or features of different kinds; not **homogeneous**. 2. Made up of or involving persons, elements, or things of more than one kind; **heterogeneous**.

mixed-effects model *n* - A **model** involving both **fixed** and **random effects**. rt: **fixed-effects model, random-effects model**

MLE *n* - **maximum likelihood estimate**

mock *adj* - Of, relating to, or having the character of an imitation or of something simulated.

mock table *n* - 1. **table shell** 2. **dummy table**

modal *adj* - [ML *modalis*, fr L *modus*] Of or relating to a **mode**.

modal class *n* - 1. The **class interval** of a **frequency distribution** that has the highest **frequency**. 2. Locally, a class interval that has a higher frequency than adjacent class intervals. rt: **mode**

modality *n* - 1. The quality or state of being **modal**; a modal quality or quantity. 2. A method of **treatment**; an apparatus for administration of treatment. rt: **regimen**

mode *n* - [ME *moede*, fr L *modus* measure, manner, musical mode] 1. The most frequently occurring value in a set of **data**; one of several different **measures of central tendency**. 2. **local mode** rt: **modal class**

model *n* - [MF *modelle*, fr OIt *modello*, fr (assumed) VL *modellus* fr L *modulus* small measure, fr *modus*] 1. A collection of postulates, **parameters**, and **data** presented as a mathematical description of some process, system, or state of affairs. 2. **model equation**

model equation *n* - [statistics] In **data analysis**, an **equation** of the general form y = **A** + e, where y is the **dependent variable** observed for a given **observation unit**, **A** corresponds to some function of **observations** of **independent variables** and corresponding **parameters**, and e is an **error term** corresponding to the observation unit (generally assumed to have an **expected value** of zero). In engineering terms, the model can be viewed as being comprised of a component due to signal (A) plus one due to **error** or **noise** (e). In the case of **regression models**, as used for **analyses** of data from **clinical trials**, the observation unit is typically a person (**patient**), the independent or **regressor variables** correspond to observations of **baseline variables**

for the person, and the dependent variable is typically an **outcome measure** observed during or after **treatment** of the person. The form of **A** depends on the nature of the outcome measure; see **linear regression model, log-linear model, logistic regression model**.

moderate, moderated, moderating, moderates *v* - 1. To lessen the intensity or effect of. 2. To preside over. 3. To act as a moderator.

moderator *adj* - One or something that **moderates**.

moderator variable *n* - A **variable** that **moderates** or is capable of moderating some **result** or **outcome**; eg, the variable age of first exposure, moderates the **risk** of paralysis from infection with wild polio virus. syn: conditioning variable, **effect modifier**

modified conventional author citation *n* - 1. A form of **conventional author citation** in which, in addition to individuals, the **corporate** entity (or entities) under which the work was done is named in the **masthead** or title of a work (eg, Nancy Jones and Harry Brown for the XYZ Research Group). 2. Such a citation in a **bibliography** or **reference list**. ant: **modified corporate author citation** rt: **conventional author citation**

modified conventional authorship *n* - A form of **authorship** involving named **authors** and a **corporate** entity in the **masthead** listing of authors; see **modified conventional author citation** for example. rt: **modified corporate authorship**

modified corporate author citation *n* - 1. A form of **corporate author citation** in which the names of the individuals responsible for writing the work on behalf of the **corporate** entity appear in a footnote to the title page or in the **credits** or **acknowledgements** section of the work. 2. A citation in a **bibliography** or **reference list** in which individual names appear in relation to a corporate work. ant: **modified conventional author citation** rt: **corporate author citation**

modified corporate authorship *n* - A form of **authorship** in which the **masthead attribution** is to a **corporate** entity (eg, the XYZ Research Group), but where **authors** are listed elsewhere in the work (in the **credits** or **acknowledgements** section or in a footnote to the title page). rt: **modified conventional authorship**

modified Fibonacci sequence dosage design *n* - A **group sequential** (defn 1) **dosage design** (defn 3) for **drug** testing involving doses d, 2d, 3.333d, 5d, 7d, 9d, 12d, 16d, 21d, etc (increments of 100%, 67%, 50%, 40%, 29%, 33%, 33%, and 31%) where d is chosen to be well below the **maximum tolerable dose**. In the design the 1st **group** of **patients** tested receive dose d, the 2nd group of patients tested receive dose 2d, etc, until the maximum tolerable dose is reached. The scheme derives its name from the fact that the 2nd through 5th increments (2, 3.3, 5, and 7) are similar to **Fibonacci numbers** (2, 3, 5, and 8).

modifier *n* - One or something that **modifies**.

modify, **modified**, **modifying**, **monitors** *v* - [ME *modifen*, fr MF *modifier*, fr L *modificare* to measure, moderate, fr *modus*] To change or alter; to make less extreme; to limit or restrict the meaning of; to qualify.

moment *n* - [ME, fr MF; fr *momentum*, movement, particle sufficient to turn the scales, moment, fr *movēre* to move] 1. The **mean** of a specified power (the **n**th power for the **n**th moment) of a **variable**. 2. The **expected value** of a specified power of the **deviations** of a **random variable** from a fixed value such as the **population mean**.

moments, method of *n* - A **method** of estimating **parameters** of a **distribution** by relating **parameters** to **moments**. For example, if **k** parameters are to be estimated, the method requires equations expressing the first **k** moments in terms of the **k** parameters. Estimates are obtained from the equations using observed values for the moments.

monitor *n* - [L One that warns, overseer, fr *monitus*, pp of *monēre* to warn] 1. One or something that **monitors**. 2. A person, group of persons, **center**, or **agency** having responsibility for monitoring an aspect of an activity or process, eg, one who monitors for **treatment effects**. rt: **auditor** *Usage note*: See notes for **monitor** *v*, **record auditor**, and **record monitor**.

monitor, **monitored**, **monitoring**, **monitors** *v* - 1. To watch, observe, check, regulate, or **control** for some purpose or end. 2. An ongoing evaluation of some process or procedure for determining when and if changes in that process or procedure are required (as in **treatment effects monitoring** or **performance monitoring**). 3.

record auditing *Usage note*: In the **trial** setting, use should be limited to settings denoting or implying an ongoing process; avoid as a synonym for **audit** *v* (as in the sense of defn 3 above); see note for **audit** *v*. See also notes for **record auditing** and **record monitoring**.

monitoring committee *n* - 1. A **committee** that has **monitoring** responsibilities. 2. **treatment effects monitoring committee**

monitoring design *n* - [trials] The plans for **monitoring** a trial, including those for **performance** and **treatment effects monitoring** and the rules and guidelines to be used for decision making in relation to those monitoring processes.

monitoring limit *n* - 1. A **limit**, established before or during a **trial**, that indicates the size of the **difference** or degree of departure from some **standard** or **norm** that must be exceeded before some action is taken, eg, a limit established for **treatment effects differences** which, when exceeded, leads to a recommended change in the **treatment protocol** or to an increased state of awareness as to the need for such a change. 2. **alert limit** (defn 1); **stopping boundary**

Monte Carlo *adj* - [fr *Monte Carlo*, Monaco; resort city famous for its gambling casinos] Of or relating to the use of **random sampling** or **simulation** techniques, especially in relation to **computer** based procedures performed for the purpose of obtaining an approximate solution to a complex mathematical, physical, or operational problem; **Monte Carlo method**, **Monte Carlo simulation**.

Monte Carlo method *n* - A **method** involving **Monte Carlo simulation**, especially one where **simulation** is the primary tool for solving a complex mathematical or operational problem.

Monte Carlo simulation *n* - A **method** of **simulating** some **stochastic process** or procedure using **random** or **pseudo-random numbers**. Generally involving the repetition (usually a large number of times) of some process and done to mimic some real world process or situation in order to observe its underlying behavior or to provide an empirical solution to a complex mathematical problem.

Monte Carlo trial *n* - A **trial** (defn 3) produced by a **Monte Carlo simulation** procedure.

month *n* - [ME, fr OE *mōnath*; akin to OHG *mānōd* month, OE *mōna* noon] 1. One of the 12 divisions of a **year** in the Gregorian calendar. 2.

A period of time extending from a designated **day** in one calendar month to the corresponding day in the following month; such a period as determined by date position, eg, the first Tuesday of a month or the last day of a month. 3. A period of 30 days. 4. A period of 4 weeks (28 days). 5. The time required for the moon to complete one cycle, eg, the time from one full moon to the next. 6. The average period of time required for the moon to make one revolution of the earth; equal to 27 days, 7 hours; 43 minutes. rt: **monthly, day, week, year** *Usage note*: Subject to confusion when used as an interval time measure as seen from comparison of defns 2, 3, and 4. **Month**, as defined by defn 2; not recommended as a timing interval for **followup visit schedules** because of **variation** in periods covered from month to month. Avoid use in different definitional senses within a specific setting, and especially in study documents such as **protocol**, **manual**, or **handbook**. Be explicit as to the definition underlying the term, especially when specifying or describing the **followup visit schedules** in **trials** or **followup studies**. Note that a **visit schedule** of twice monthly implies a total of 24 or 26 followup visits over a 12 month period, depending on whether defn 2 or 4 is used. See also **bimonthly** and **time measure** for additional comments.

monthly *adj* - 1. Of or relating to a **month**. 2. Reckoned by the month. 3. Lasting a month. 4. Occurring or appearing every month; occurring or appearing once a month. rt: **month, daily, weekly, yearly** *Usage note*: See **month** and **time measure**.

MoP, MOP *n* - **manual of operations**

morbid *adj* - [L *morbidus* diseased, fr *morbus* disease; akin to Gk *marainein* to waste away] Of, relating to, associated with, or characteristic of **disease**; affected with or caused by disease. rt: **mortal**

morbid event *n* - 1. An occurrence of **disease** in a person. 2. An **event** (defn 1) deemed indicative of disease or illness in a person, eg, an episode of fever or a period of hospitalization.

morbidity *n* - 1. The state or quality of being **morbid**; the state or quality of being ill or having **disease**. 2. The **relative incidence** of disease. rt: **mortality**

morbidity curve *n* - A **curve** plotted in **Cartesian coordinates**, having an **x-axis** corresponding to

time **measured** from a designated zero point (eg, the initiation of **treatment** in a **clinical trial**) and a **y-axis** corresponding to number of people having a designated morbid condition (**disease**) or **morbidity rate**, that starts from the **origin** and that increases (as a smooth line or in a series of **discrete** steps) as new cases of the designated condition occur over time. rt: **mortality curve**

morbidity rate *n* - A quantity in which the **numerator** is the number of a defined **population** who have or are considered to have or have had a specific morbid condition (**disease**) in a specified time **period** divided by the number at **risk** of acquiring that condition in that time period; usually expressed per 100 population at risk or some larger multiple of 100. The rate may be **unadjusted (crude morbidity rate)** or **adjusted (adjusted morbidity rate)** and may correspond to **incidence** or **prevalence rate** depending on whether the numerator represents a count of **incident** or **prevalent cases**. rt: **mortality rate**

mortal *adj* - [ME, fr MF, fr L *mortalis*, fr *mort-*, *mors* death] Having caused or being about to cause death. rt: **morbid**

mortality *n* - The quality or state of being mortal; death. rt: **morbidity**

mortality curve *n* - A **curve** plotted in **Cartesian coordinates**, having an **x-axis** corresponding to time measured from a designated zero point (eg, the initiation of **treatment** in a **clinical trial**) and a **y-axis** corresponding to number of deaths or **death rate**, that starts from the **origin** and that increases (as a smooth line or in a series of **discrete** steps) as deaths occur over time (also **cumulative mortality curve**); the complement of a **survival curve**. rt: **morbidity curve**

mortality rate *n* - A quantity in which the **numerator** is the number of a defined **population** who have died in a specified time **period** divided by the number at **risk** of dying in that time period, usually expressed per 100 population at risk or some larger multiple of 100. The rate may be for a specific cause of death (**cause specific mortality rate**) or for all causes of death, and may be **unadjusted (crude mortality rate)** or **adjusted (adjusted mortality rate)**. syn: death rate rt: **morbidity rate**

moving average *n* - A type of **transformation**, typically performed in **time series analysis**, in which each value in the series is replaced by the **mean** of the values at that point and one or more of the values immediately preceding and following that point; done to smooth the observed series.

MTD *n* - **maximum tolerable dose**

mu *n* - [Gk *my*] The 12th letter of the **Greek alphabet**, uppercase M, lowercase µ.

multi- *prefix* - [ME, fr MF or L; MF, fr L, fr *mulus* much, many] 1. More than one. 2. More than two. 3. many

multi-institutional *adj* - Involving more than one institution; **multicenter**.

multi-period crossover treatment design *n* - A **treatment design** that provides for the administration of three or more of the **study treatments**, one after another in a specified or **random** order, to **experimental units** in a **trial**; each administration may be followed by a **washout period**. rt: **crossover treatment design**

multi-stage design *n* - A **design** involving two or more distinct **stages**, all part of the overall **study plan**, eg, a design involving testing of various candidate **treatments** using **crossover designs** followed by a second stage in which promising treatments are tested using a **parallel treatment design**. rt: **two-stage design**

multi-study *adj* - Of, relating to, or consisting of multiple **studies**. ant: **single-study** rt: **multi-trial** *Usage note*: Use **multi-trial** if all studies are **trials**. See note for **study** *n*.

multi-study design *n* - A **design** involving two or more **studies**; performed on the same or different **study populations**. ant: **single-study design** rt: **multi-trial design**, **multi-study structure** *Usage note*: See **multi-study**.

multi-study structure *n* - An organizational **structure** created or maintained to initiate and carry out a series of related **studies** involving the same or different **study populations**. ant: **single-study structure** *Usage note*: Use **multi-trial** instead of **multi-study** if all studies are trials. See **multi-trial structure** and **study** *n* for added comments.

multi-trial *adj* - Of, relating to, or consisting of multiple **trials**. ant: **single-trial** rt: **multi-study**

multi-trial design *n* - A **design** involving two or more **trials** performed on the same or different people and involving different **treatment protocols**. ant: **single-trial design** *Usage note*: See **multi-trial structure**.

multi-trial structure *n* - An organizational **structure** created or maintained to initiate and carry out a series of related **trials** involving the same or different **study populations**. ant: **single-trial structure** *Usage note*: Most useful when characterizing past or existing structures as to observed function or planned intent. Note that a structure created as a **single-trial structure** may ultimately be classified as a **multi-trial structure** if it serves the purpose of directing two or more trials, even if not originally created for that purpose, as in the case of the Macular Photocoagulation Studies.[92, 93]

multicenter *adj* - Having more than one **center**. ant: **single-center** *Usage note*: Preferred modifier for **trials** and **studies** involving multiple centers; preferred to **collaborative** or **cooperative** for reasons indicated in usage notes for those terms. Often used in opposition to **single-center**, especially when characterizing a set of trials as to whether single-center or multicenter. An advantage of the term is that it has an appropriate antonym, whereas there is none for **collaborative** or **cooperative**, except noncollaborative and noncooperative — both inappropriate as characterizations or labels. See **single-center** for additional comments.

multicenter study *n* - 1. A **study** involving two or more **data collection** sites, a common **study protocol**, and a **data center**, **data coordinating center**, or **coordinating center** to receive, process, and analyze **study data**. 2. A study involving at least one data collection site and one or more **resource centers**. 3. A study involving two or more data collection sites. 4. **multicenter trial** syn: **collaborative study** (not recommended), **cooperative study** (not recommended) ant: **single-center study** *Usage note*: Preferred to **collaborative study** or **cooperative study** for reasons indicated in usage notes for those two terms.

multicenter trial *n* - 1. A **trial** involving two or more **clinical centers**, a common **study protocol**, and a **data center**, **data coordinating center**, or **coordinating center** to receive, process, and analyze **study data**. 2. A trial involving at least one clinical center or **data collection site** and one or more **resource centers**. 3. A trial involving two or more **clinics** or **data collection sites**. syn: **collaborative trial** (not recommended), **cooperative trial** (not recommended) ant: **single-center trial** *Usage* *note*: Preferred to **collaborative trial** or **cooperative trial** for reasons indicated in usage notes for those two terms. See **single-center trial** for comments on line of demarcation between single and multicenter trials.

multidisciplinary *adj* - Involving or consisting of two or more **disciplines**.

multidisciplinary trial *n* - 1. A **trial** requiring the combined skills of two or more **disciplines** for the administration of one or more of the **study treatments** (eg, a trial involving use of dietary counseling and medical treatment). 2. A trial involving or requiring the combination of different disciplines for its design, operation, and analysis. *Usage note*: Virtually every trial is multidisciplinary in the sense of defn 2. Hence, the term, should be reserved for uses in the sense of defn 1, if used at all.

multimodal *adj* - Of, relating to, or having more than one **mode**, as in the sense of defn 2 for **mode** or defn 2 for **modal class**. rt: **mode, unimodal**

multimodal distribution *n* - A **distribution** having more than one **mode**, as in the sense of defn 2 for **mode** or for **modal class**.

multiphasic *adj* - Of, relating to, or having multiple **phases** or aspects.

multiphasic screening *n* - **Screening** for multiple conditions or **factors** using a series of different tests or procedures, especially such screening as performed on a person in a single **visit** to the **site** of screening for the detection of **risk factors** or **disease**. rt: **mass screening**

multiple *adj* - [F, fr L *multiplex*, fr *multi-* + *plex* -fold] Consisting of or involving more than one; many.

multiple comparisons *n* - [**statistics**, in regard to two or more **comparisons** (defn 3) involving the same **dataset**] 1. Two or more comparisons involving the same **measure**; such comparison at the same point in time (as in the Coronary Drug Project[30] involving comparison of **pairs** of treatments for a designated outcome at a single point in time); such comparison at different points in time (as in a particular **test-control treatment comparison** for a particular **outcome measure** at different points in time). 2. Two or more comparisons involving different measures; such comparisons at the same point in time (as in the Coronary Drug Project[30] involving comparison of pairs of treatments for different

outcomes at different points in time, or for **treatment group comparisons** for different **baseline characteristics**); such comparisons at different points in time (as in a particular **test-control treatment comparison** for different **outcome measures** at different points in time). 3. A comparison having an associated **p-value** or **confidence interval** that is **adjusted** to take account of the fact that it is one of several comparisons made or to be made. rt: **multiple looks, multiple outcomes** *Usage note*: Virtually every **controlled trial** involves multiple comparisons in the sense of defns 1 and 2, even those involving just two **study treatments**. Any trial involving three or more study treatments and the need for two or more **pairwise comparisons** (as in the Coronary Drug Project in the comparison of each of 5 different test treatments with a **placebo control**[30]) will involve multiple comparisons anytime the treatments are compared. Broadly inclusive of **multiple looks** and **multiple outcomes**.

multiple correlation coefficient *n* - **Correlation coefficient** produced from a **multiple linear regression model**; measures the degree of relationship between the **dependent variable** and a **linear combination** of the **independent variables**. rt: **partial correlation coefficient**

multiple linear regression *n* - **Linear regression** involving two or more **independent variables**. rt: **multiple logistic regression**

multiple linear regression analysis *n* - [**statistics**] **Data analysis** based on a **multiple linear regression model**; often used in **trials** to **adjust** for differences in the **baseline** composition of the **treatment groups** when carrying out **treatment comparisons**. rt: **multiple logistic regression analysis**

multiple linear regression model *n* - [**statistics**] A **linear regression model** involving two or more **regressor variables**.

multiple logistic regression *n* - **Logistic regression** involving a **multiple logistic regression model**.

multiple logistic regression analysis *n* - [**statistics**] **Data analysis** based on a **multiple logistic regression model**; often used in **trials** to **adjust** for differences in the **baseline** composition of the **treatment groups** when carrying out **treatment comparisons**. rt: **multiple linear regression analysis**

multiple logistic regression model *n* - [**statistics**] A **logistic regression model** involving two or more **regressor variables**. rt: **multiple linear regression model**

multiple looks *n* - [**trials**] **Treatment comparisons** made at two or more time points over the course of a **trial**; especially when done in relation to **treatment effects monitoring** and where they may lead to alteration of the **treatment protocol**. rt: **multiple comparisons** *Usage note*: Not to be confused with **multiple comparisons** as discussed in a usage note for that term.

multiple outcomes *n* - [**trials**] 1. The state or condition of having or being capable of yielding two or more **outcomes** (defn 1). 2. The state or condition of having or being capable of having two or more **outcome measures** for use in making **treatment comparisons**, as in a trial providing treatment comparisons for the **primary outcome measure** and for one or more **secondary outcome measures**. rt: **composite outcome**

multiple placebo *n* - [**trials**] A **placebo** that has two or more forms or shapes in a given trial, eg, as required for **masking** in a trial involving two or more **test treatments** having different forms or routes of administration. rt: **single placebo**, **double placebo**

multiple placebo treatment design *n* - A **treatment design** that involves two or more **placebos**, eg, as needed in a **drug trial** having two or more **test treatments**, each requiring its own **matching placebo**, eg, as used in the University Group Diabetes Program[156] for masking tolbutamide and phenformin. rt: **multiple placebo**, **single placebo treatment design**

multiple regression *n* - The **regression** of a **dependent variable** on two or more **independent variables** (defn 3).

multiple regression analysis *n* - **Data analysis** using a **multiple regression model**.

multiple stratification *n* - **Stratification** using two or more **variables** separately or together.

multiplication *n* - [ME *multiplicacioun*, fr MF *multiplication*, fr L *multiplication-*, *multiplicatio*, fr *multiplicatus*, pp of *multiplicare* to multiply] 1. The result of **multiplying**. 2. The act or process of multiplying; in its simplest term analogous to adding a quantity to itself a specified number of times. ant: **division** rt: **addition**

multiply, multiplied, multiplying, multiplies *v* - [ME *multiplien*, fr OF *multiplier*, fr L *multiplicare*, fr *multiplic-*, *multiplex* multiple] 1. To increase in number. 2. To find the **product** of by **multiplication**. 3. To perform multiplication. ant: **divide** rt: **addition**

multiprotocol *adj* - Of, relating to, or having more than one **protocol**, as in a **multi-trial study**.

multiprotocol study *n* - A **study** involving two or more **protocols** administered to the same or different people; **multi-trial study**.

multivariate *adj* - Having or involving two or more **independent variables**. ant: **univariate** rt: **bivariate**

multivariate analysis *n* - 1. **Analysis** of two or more **outcome variables** at once. 2. Analysis involving the study of two or more **independent variables** at once, as in **multiple regression analysis**. 3. Any of a variety of methods of analysis including **analysis of principal components**, **analysis of variance**, **analysis of covariance**, **components of variance analysis**, correlation analysis, **factor analysis**, linear discriminant analysis, and **regression analysis**.

multivariate density function *n* - **joint density function**

multivariate distribution *n* - **joint distribution**

mutual *adj* - [ME, fr, MF *mutuel*, fr L *mutuus* lent, borrowed, mutual; akin to L *mutare* to change] **joint**; shared in common

mutually exclusive *adj* - Being related such that each excludes or precludes the other.

mutually exclusive events *n* - **Events**, eg, birth and death or those that are the result of a **binary variable**, that are **mutually exclusive**.

N

n *n* - [14th letter of the English alphabet] 1. Symbol denoting a constant integer value; a **variable** taking on integer values. 2. Symbol denoting **sample size** or **count**; also N.

n of 1 trial *n* - A class of **trial** in which **treatments** or **doses** of a treatment are applied or administered to a person in some systematic way with the intent of arriving at a proper treatment or **dosage** for the person being treated; the person, in effect, serving as his own **control** for the evaluations.[63, 141] syn: single patient trial

n-period crossover design *n* - [**trials**] A **crossover treatment design** that involves administration of **n treatments** to each person in a **crossover trial**, one after the other in some specified or **random** order, and usually having n - 1 **washout periods**, one such period following each treatment administration.

n-way *adj* - Have **n** dimensions or directions. rt: **one-way**, **two-way**

n-way classification *n* - A **classification** made on the basis of **n** different **variables** or conditions; eg, classification on the basis of age and gender — **two-way classification**.

National Cancer Institute (NCI) *n* - See **National Institutes of Health**.

National Center for Health Statistics (NCHS) *n* - A **center** within the **USPHS** with facilities in Hyattsville, Maryland, Research Triangle Park, North Carolina, and Atlanta, Georgia; responsible for collecting, analyzing, and disseminating **data** related to the health of peoples of the US; responsible for the National Health Interview Survey (NHIS) and the National Health and Nutrition Examination Survey (NHANES); produces and disseminates a number of reports and **datasets** related to birth and death.

National Center for Human Genome Research (NCHGR) *n* - See **National Institutes of Health**.

National Center for Toxicological Research (NCTR) *n* - See **Food and Drug Administration**.

National Center of Research Resources (NCRR) *n* - See **National Institutes of Health**.

National Death Index (NDI) *n* - A central electronic registry of deaths occurring in the United States starting with 1979; operated by the **National Center for Health Statistics** [1981][111] for users interested in determining **vital status** of identified persons.

National Eye Institute (NEI) *n* - See **National Institutes of Health**.

National Heart, Lung, and Blood Institute (NHLBI) *n* - See **National Institutes of Health**.

National Institute of Allergy and Infectious Diseases (NIAID) *n* - See **National Institutes of Health**.

National Institute of Arthritis and Musculoskeletal and Skin Diseases (NIAMS) *n* - See **National Institutes of Health**.

National Institute of Child Health and Human Development (NICHD) *n* - See **National Institutes of Health**.

National Institute of Dental Research (NIDR) *n* - See **National Institutes of Health**.

National Institute of Diabetes and Digestive and Kidney Diseases (NIDDK) *n* - See **National Institutes of Health**.

National Institute of Environmental Health Sciences (NIEHS) *n* - See **National Institutes of Health**.

National Institute of General Medical Sciences (NIGMS) *n* - See **National Institutes of Health**.

National Institute of Mental Health (NIMH) *n* - See **National Institutes of Health**.

National Institute of Neurological Disorders and Stroke (NINDS) *n* - See **National Institutes of Health**.

National Institute of Nursing Research (NINR) *n* - See **National Institutes of Health**.

National Institute on Aging (NIA) *n* - See **National Institutes of Health**.

National Institute on Alcohol Abuse and Alcoholism (NIAAA) *n* - See **National Institutes of Health**.

National Institute on Deafness and Other Communication Disorders (NIDCD) *n* - See **National Institutes of Health**.

National Institute on Drug Abuse (NIDA) *n* - See **National Institutes of Health**.

National Institutes of Health (NIH) *n* - A series of institutes, divisions, and related support structures, located in Bethesda, Maryland and part of the **United States Public Health Service** (USPHS); responsible for performing and funding basic and applied research in the health field. Institutes, centers, and divisions of the NIH include:[115]

> **Division of Computer Research Technology**
> **Division of Research Grants** (DRG)
> **Fogarty International Center**
> **National Cancer Institute** (NCI)
> **National Center for Human Genome Research** (NCHGR)
> **National Center of Research Resources** (NCRR)
> **National Eye Institute** (NEI)
> **National Heart, Lung, and Blood Institute** (NHLBI)
> **National Institute of Allergy and Infectious Diseases** (NIAID)
> **National Institute of Arthritis and Musculoskeletal and Skin Diseases** (NIAMS)
> **National Institute of Child Health and Human Development** (NICHD)
> **National Institute of Dental Research** (NIDR)
> **National Institute of Diabetes and Digestive and Kidney Diseases** (NIDDK)
> **National Institute of Environmental Health Sciences** (NIEHS)
> **National Institute of General Medical Sciences** (NIGMS)
> **National Institute of Mental Health** (NIMH)
> **National Institute of Neurological Disorders and Stroke** (NINDS)
> **National Institute of Nursing Research** (NINR)
> **National Institute on Aging** (NIA)
> **National Institute on Alcohol Abuse and Alcoholism** (NIAAA)
> **National Institute on Deafness and Other Communication Disorders** (NIDCD)
> **National Institute on Drug Abuse** (NIDA)
> **National Library of Medicine** (NLM)
> **Warren Grant Magnuson Clinical Center**

National Institutes of Health Revitalization Act of 1993 *n* - An Act of the US Congress, signed into law 10 June 1993, by President Clinton, containing provisions related to the design and conduct of **trials** aimed at ensuring **valid analyses** for detecting gender and ethnic origin by **treatment interactions**. The Act requires: *In the case of any clinical trial in which women or members of minority groups will under subsection (a) be included as subjects, the Director of the NIH shall ensure that the trial is designed and carried out in a manner sufficient to provide for a valid analysis of whether the variables being studied in the trial affect women or members of minority groups, as the case may be, differently than other subjects in the trial.*[154]

National Library of Medicine (NLM) *n* - See **National Institutes of Health**.

National Technical Information Service (NTIS) *n* - A service facility of the United States Department of Commerce, located in Springfield, Virginia, that operates a public repository for documents prepared by and placed on deposit by federal agencies or their grantees or contractors. Documents for **clinical trials** may include forms, manuals, **data** listings, data tapes, etc.

natural *adj* - [ME, fr MF, fr L *naturalis* of nature, fr *natura* nature] Occurring in conformity with the ordinary course of nature or life; not modified or adulterated by human beings. ant: **unnatural** *Usage note*: Often misused, especially in everyday vernacular in relation to characterizations and claims regarding food products, as in *all natural*. Avoid in relation to admixtures consisting only in part of natural ingredients and as a claim, except in the strict sense of the term.

natural constant *n* - The quantity **e**, equal to 2.71828 (approximate to 5 places). See **natural logarithm**.

natural experiment *n* - An **observation** that is the result of conditions similar to those that might be imposed in an experimental setting, but that are the result of natural consequences or events; **natural trial**. rt: **before and after study**

natural history *n* - The course of **events observed** under **natural** conditions; especially such a history observed without **intervention**.

natural history of disease *n* - **disease natural history**

natural history study *n* - A **prospective followup study** designed to yield or that yields information on the natural course of a **disease** or health condition, especially one having minimal exclusions. Such a study within a **clinical trial** generally focuses on the **control-treated group** (especially when the **control treatment** is a **placebo** or standard medical care). However, the clinical trial setting is of limited value for such a study because of the select nature of the population **enrolled**.

natural log *n* - **natural logarithm**

natural logarithm *n* - The **power** to which **e** (natural constant) is raised to produce a given number, eg, 2 is the natural logarithm of 7.38905 since $e^2 = 2.71828^2 = 7.38905$).

natural trial *n* - A **comparison** of different **treatment** procedures produced or made possible as a result of some fortuitous circumstance (such as depletion of the supply of boiling oil for the treatment of battle field wounds, as described by Ambrose Paré during the battle to capture the Castle of Villaine in 1537) or legislative or regulatory action. rt: **before and after study** *Usage note*: Not a **trial**, except in the observational sense of that term (defn 5); use should be limited to settings where a change in a procedure occurs as a result of events or actions beyond the control of those performing the procedure.

NCHGR *n* - **National Center for Human Genome Research**

NCHS *n* - **National Center for Health Statistics**

NCI *n* - **National Cancer Institute**

NCRR *n* - **National Center of Research Resources**

NCTR *n* - **National Center for Toxicological Research**

NDA *n* - **New Drug Application**

NDI *n* - **National Death Index**

necessary *adj* - [ME *necessarie*, fr L *necessaritus*, fr *necesse* necessary, fr *ne-* not + *cedere* to withdraw] Absolutely needed, required; logically unavoidable. rt: **sufficient**

necessary and sufficient *adj* - Of or related to being required and adequate to achieve or produce some end.

necessary and sufficient condition *n* - 1. A **condition** that is required and that is adequate for achieving or producing some end or for establishing the truth of some statement. 2. [**mathematics**] A **condition** (defn 4) that must

prevail and that is adequate for showing or proving the truth of a statement or relationship. rt: **necessary condition**, **sufficient condition**

necessary condition *n* - 1. A **condition** that is required for something to be true or false. 2. A condition needed for something to work; prerequisite. 3. A condition that is a logical consequence of a given statement or fact.rt: **sufficient condition**, **necessary and sufficient condition**

negative *adj* - 1. Less than **zero** and opposite in sign to a **positive number**. 2. Denoting the absence of something; **nil**. 3. Denoting the opposite or contradictory nature of something. 4. Not affirming the presence of the organism or condition in question. 5. **adverse** ant: **positive** *Usage note*: Often used in the sense of defns 2 or 3 when characterizing a **result**; meaning the result is either **nil** or opposite or contradictory in nature. As a consequence, the mere characterization of a result as being **negative** can leave a reader or member of an audience in a quandary as to the nature of the result implied — a serious quandary in **trials**, since the medical implications of a **treatment effect** that is nil are quite different from those of one that is negative in the sense of defns 3 or 5. Confusion can be avoided by making the meaning clear in the context of usage or by adopting the convention of reserving the term for characterizations of the type implied in defn 3; use **nil** for characterizations implied by defn 2.

negative *n* - 1. Having a numerical value less than zero. 2. A reply or response that indicates refusal or the withholding of **assent**; negation or denial. 3. Something that is the opposite (complementary) of or that is a negation of something else. 4. A proposition that denies or contradicts another. 5. Being in the direction of numerical values less than zero, as in **negative skew**. ant: **positive**

negative control *adj* - 1. Of or relating to an **active control** producing or capable of producing a **negative effect** (defn 2). 2. Of or relating to a control that has no effect or that is **nil**. ant: **positive control** rt: **inactive control** *Usage note*: Not recommended in the sense of defn 2 in **trials**; use **inactive control** instead.

negative control treatment *n* - 1. A **control treatment** that is intended to produce or that produces a **negative treatment effect**. 2. An **active control treatment** that has or is intended to have an effect that is opposite to the one produced or intended to be produced by the **test treatment**, eg, a **trial** (done for the purpose of assessing the role of dietary sodium in elevating blood pressure) involving blood pressure as the **outcome measure** having a control treatment providing for diets high in sodium contrasted with a test treatment providing for diets low in sodium. 3. A control treatment that has or is intended to have an effect that is opposite to the one produced by a **positive control treatment**. ant: **positive control treatment** rt: **inactive control treatment**

negative correlation *n* - 1. A **correlation coefficient** with a **negative** sign. 2. A **relationship** between two **variables** in which the higher values of one variable are associated with the lower values of the other variable. ant: **positive correlation**

negative effect *n* - 1. An **effect** that is **adverse**. 2. An effect that is opposite in direction from that desired. 3. An effect that is not **beneficial**. 4. **nil effect** ant: **positive effect** *Usage note*: See **negative** *adj* for note.

negative predictive value of a test *n* - The **probability** of not having a **disease** given a **negative test result** for a **screening** or **diagnostic test**. rt: **positive predictive value of a test, predictive value of a test**

negative result *n* - 1. A **result** that fails to confirm a prior hypothesis or finding. 2. A **result** that is opposite in nature or direction to that postulated or desired. 3. **nil result** ant: **positive result** *Usage note*: See **negative** *adj* for note.

negative skew *adj* - **left skew**

negative skew distribution *n* - **left skew distribution**

negative skewness *n* - **left skewness**

negative study *n* - 1. A **study** that produces results that fail to confirm a prior **hypothesis** or finding. 2. A study that produces a **result** that is opposite in nature or direction to that postulated or desired. 3. A study that produces a **nil result**. ant: **positive study** *Usage note*: See **negative** *adj* for note.

negative treatment effect *n* - 1. A **treatment effect** that is **adverse**. 2. A treatment effect that is not **beneficial**; a treatment effect that is not **positive**. 3. **nil treatment effect** ant: **positive**

treatment effect *Usage note*: See **negative** *adj* for note.

NEI *n* - **National Eye Institute**

nested *adj* - Forming a sequence or hierarchy with each member contained in or containing the next; contained within.

nested case-control study *n* - 1. A **case-control study** done within a **cohort study**; one in which **cases** and **controls** are selected from that cohort. 2. An **analysis** carried out using existing **data** from a larger **cohort study** similar in concept to that done in a case-control study; in effect, a type of **subgroup analysis** of existing data in which cases and controls are defined using data collected in a cohort study and then analyzed for differences in **exposure**.

nested experiment *n* - 1. **hierarchical experiment** 2. An **experiment** within an experiment.

net *adj* - Remaining after removal of all legitimate deductions.

net change *n* - 1. **net difference** (defn 1). 2. The **difference** of two **net differences** (defn 1), eg, the weight change from **baseline** to a specified point in **followup** observed in a **trial** for the **control-treated group** subtracted from the net change observed for the **test-treated group**. rt: **net treatment effect**

net difference *n* - 1. The **difference** of a **variable** for a given object, person, or group observed at two points in time, eg, the difference in a person's body weight at one year of **followup** compared to **baseline**, as measured by the difference of the two values. 2. The difference of a variable for a given set of objects, persons, or groups observed at the same point in time, eg, the difference in mean body weights of the **test-** and **control-assigned groups** upon **enrollment** into a **trial**. 3. **net change** (defn 2).

net treatment effect *n* - [trials] 1. The **net difference** (defns 1 or 2) for a specified **outcome measure** and period of **followup** observed for a **test treatment** and **control treatment** or two different test treatments. 2. The **effect** of one treatment **relative** to another after a specified period of followup, for a designated outcome measure, eg, as measured by a **net difference** (defn 2) for the two treatment groups of interest and presented as a **ratio** of the one difference to the other (**relative risk**). rt: **net change**

network *n* - 1. An interconnected or interrelated structure or system. 2. A system of **computers**, **terminals**, **programs**, and **databases**, interconnected by hard wired connections, communication lines, or other means, created and maintained for the purpose of allowing users to communicate with one another and to interact with and share common **datasets** and **files**.

new *adj* - [ME, fr OE *nīwe*; akin to OHG *niuwi* new, L *novus*, Gk *neos*] Having come into existence or having been proposed, introduced, or made recently; not old.

new drug *n* - 1. A **new** or existing **drug** being evaluated as an **Investigational New Drug**. 2. A **drug** not classified as **GRASE** by the **Food and Drug Administration** and not in use in the way proposed prior to 1938. 3. A compound or agent of recent creation or identification being proposed for use as a drug. rt: **Investigational New Drug** *Usage note*: In the parlance of the Food and Drug Administration, **new** refers to the application or use being proposed for a drug rather than to the drug itself. Hence, a drug that has been in use for years in relation to some established indication is nevertheless **new** when proposed for a new indication. See also usage note for **drug**.

New Drug Application (NDA) *n* - An application for a license to market a **drug** for a specified **indication**; application submitted to the **Food and Drug Administration** by the manufacturer of the drug or its marketing agent; application must be approved for the drug to be marketed for the indication specified in the **application** (see **Product License Application** and **Pre-Market Approval Application** for corresponding terms for **biologics** and **medical devices**, respectively). The application contains results of the specific **phase I, II,** and **III trials** conducted in relation to the indication and submitted (generally) after completion of required phase II or III trials. rt: **new drug, Investigational New Drug Application, Abbreviated New Drug Application, approved drug** *Usage note*: As noted in the usage note for **new drug**, the reference to *new* is in regard to the indication, not to the drug itself.

Neyman, Jerzy - (1894 - 1981) Mathematician and probabilist; born in Bendrey, Monrovia (Russia); studied physics and mathematics at the University of Kharkov; held a position at Univer-

sity College in London in the 1930s where he worked with Egon Pearson; accepted a position at the University of California in 1938, where he remained; contributions include **Neyman-Pearson theory**.

Neyman-Pearson theory *n* - A **theory** of **hypothesis testing** based on the concepts of **type I** and **type II errors** and **power functions**. rt: **frequentist**

NHANES *n* - **National Health and Nutrition Examination Survey**

NHIS *n* - **National Health Interview Survey**

NHLBI *n* - **National Heart, Lung, and Blood Institute**

NIA *n* - **National Institute on Aging**

NIAAA *n* - **National Institute on Alcohol Abuse and Alcoholism**

NIAID *n* - **National Institute of Allergy and Infectious Diseases**

NIAMS *n* - **National Institute of Arthritis and Musculoskeletal and Skin Disorders**

NICHD *n* - **National Institute of Child Health and Human Development**

NIDA *n* - **National Institute on Drug Abuse**

NIDCD *n* - **National Institute on Deafness and Other Communication Disorders**

NIDDK *n* - **National Institute of Diabetes and Digestive and Kidney Diseases**

NIDR *n* - **National Institute of Dental Research**

NIEHS *n* - **National Institute of Environmental Health Sciences**

NIGMS *n* - **National Institute of General Medical Sciences**

NIH *n* - **National Institutes of Health**

nil *adj* - [L, nothing, contr of *nihil*, fr OL *nihilum*, fr *ne-* not + *hilum* trifle] Of, relating to, or being zero or nothing. *Usage note*: Preferred to **negative** in usages in the sense of defn 2 for **negative** *adj* for reasons indicated in the usage note for that term.

nil control treatment *n* - A **control treatment** consisting of **observation** only. Not to be confused with **placebo-control treatment**.

nil effect *n* - An **effect** measured as zero or near zero; a negligible effect. rt: **negative effect, positive effect** *Usage note*: See **nil** for usage note.

nil result *n* - A **result** of zero or near zero; an inconsequential result. rt: **negative result, positive result** *Usage note*: See **nil** for usage note.

nil treatment *n* - No administered **treatment**; observation only; **nil control treatment**.

nil treatment effect *n* - 1. A **treatment effect** of zero or near zero. 2. A treatment effect that is not statistically different from zero. 3. A treatment effect of inconsequential size or importance. *Usage note*: See **nil** for comment.

NIMH *n* - **National Institute of Mental Health**

NINDS *n* - **National Institute of Neurological Disorders and Stroke**

NINR *n* - **National Institutes of Nursing Research**

NLM *n* - **National Library of Medicine**

noise *n* - [ME, fr OF, strife, quarrel, noise, fr L *nausea* nausea] 1. An unwanted signal or disturbance. 2. **Variation** in recorded **data** due to **observational**, recording, or other kinds of **errors**.

noisy *adj* - Characterized by **noise**.

noisy data *n* - **Data** having **variation** due to observational, recording, or other kinds of **errors**.

nominal data *n* - Qualitative **data**, such as gender, membership in an organization, or area of residence (rural vs. urban); data not amenable to ordering.

nomogram *n* - [Gk *nomos* law + ISV -gram] A graphic representation of a mathematical **function** used for determining its value over a defined range of **input** values (eg, DuBois' nomogram [DuBois and DuBois, 1916][39]); typically consisting of calibrated scales for two input **variables** positioned such that, when a point on one scale is joined by a straight line connecting a point on the other scale, the point of intersection on a third scale corresponds to the value of the function for the designated input values.

non- *prefix* - [ME, fr ME, fr L *non* not, fr OL *noenum* fr *ne*- not + *oinom*, neut of *oinos* one] 1. Not; other than; reverse of; absence of. 2. Of little or no consequence; unimportant.

noncompliance *n* - The act or process of failing to **comply** with or to a procedure or routine; lack of conformity to rules or regulations. ant: **compliance** rt: **nonrespondent**

noncompliant *adj* - Not being in a **compliant** state; having an unwillingness to **comply**. ant: **compliant**

noncompliant person *n* - A person who is unwilling or unable to **comply** with a specified request, procedure, or routine; eg, in relation to accepting the **assigned treatment** regimen in a **trial**. ant: **compliant person**

nonconcurrent *adj* - 1. Not running **parallel**. 2. Not simultaneous in time. ant: **concurrent**

nonconcurrent cohort study *n* - 1. A **followup study** of a **cohort** from one point in the past to a more recent point in the past or to the present using existing **data**, eg, as contained in the **medical records** of members of the cohort. 2. A followup study of a cohort from a point in the past to a point in the future (followup from the point in the past to the present is based on existing data, followup from the present to a point in the future is based on **real time** observation and **data collection**). syn: retrospective cohort study

nonconcurrent control *n* - A **control** (defn 1) constructed or formulated from **observations** or **data** of the past as opposed to the more recent past or present for the object of **comparison**; eg, a **historical control** as used in assessing a new **treatment** in the absence of a **concurrent control**. syn: **nonparallel control** ant: **concurrent control**

nonconcurrent enrollment *n* - [followup studies] 1. **Enrollment** (defn 2) taking place in the past, as in a **nonconcurrent cohort study**. 2. **Enrollment** of one or more of the **study groups** over a time period different from that over which one or more of the other study groups were or are to be enrolled (eg, in studies involving multiple **study groups**). 3. Enrollment that is not **concurrent**. ant: **concurrent enrollment**

nonconcurrent followup study *n* - 1. A **followup study** having two or more **study groups** and **nonconcurrent followup** of at least one of those groups in relation to another. 2. **nonconcurrent cohort study** 3. **nonconcurrent prospective study** See *study* for list. ant: **concurrent followup study**

nonconcurrent prospective study *n* - 1. A **prospective study** in which the starting point for **followup** is in the past (eg, the occurrence of some **event** as identified from a review of hospital **records** or some other existing **data**

source) and followup proceeds forward to some more recent time in the past, to the present, or to some point in the future. The followup may not involve any contact with study members if the data desired can be obtained from existing records. 2. A followup study in which the starting point for followup of one of the **study groups** precedes that of one or more of the other study groups; **nonconcurrent followup study**. 3. **nonconcurrent-concurrent prospective study** ant: **concurrent followup study**, concurrent prospective study rt: **nonconcurrent enrollment**

nonconcurrent-concurrent prospective study *n* - 1. A **concurrent followup study** in which entry is defined by some **event**, action, **condition**, or **exposure** that occurred in the past. 2. **nonconcurrent cohort study** (defn 2)

noncrossover treatment design *n* - [trials] A **treatment design** not involving a **crossover treatment design**; **parallel treatment design**. ant: **crossover treatment design**

nonexperimental study *n* - A **study** not involving an investigator-specified **test variable**; **observational study**.

nonfactorial *adj* - Of, relating to, or concerned with something that does not have a **factorial design** or **structure**. ant: **factorial**

nonfactorial treatment design *n* - A **treatment design** not involving any **factorial** structuring of the **treatments**.

nonhealth professional *n* - [general] A person having a **profession** not related to health. [trials] Such a person selected or designated to fill some position or to perform some function within a trial, eg, such a person designated to sit as a member of the **treatment effects monitoring committee** of a trial. rt: **lay representative, patient advocate** *Usage note*: See notes for **patient advocate** and **lay committee member**.

nonlinear *adj* - 1. Of, relating to, resembling, or having a **plot** or **graph** that is not a straight line; of, relating to, resembling or having a plot or graph that is the result of a **nonlinear equation**. 2. [mathematics] Having more than one dimension; being of more than the first degree with respect to one or more **variables**; of, relating to, based on, or being a **nonlinear equation**. ant: **linear**

nonlinear equation *n* - 1. An **equation** of the second **degree** or higher in any of its variables or **parameters**, eg, $y = \beta_0 + \beta_1 x^2$; **nonlinear**

regression model. 2. An equation not of the first degree in relation to one or more of its parameters, eg, $y = \beta_0 + \beta_1{}^2 x$, where y and x are variables and β_0 and β_1 are parameters. ant: **linear equation**

nonlinear model *n* - A **model equation** not of the first **degree** with respect to one or more of its **parameters**, ie, at least one of its **parameters** exists in a form raised to a **power** other than unity; see **nonlinear regression model** for example. Used in **data analyses** for **adjustment**, **prediction**, and **hypothesis testing** in which **effects** represented by the parameters are not additive. ant: **linear model**

nonlinear regression *n* - **Regression** involving a **nonlinear model**. ant: **linear regression**

nonlinear regression analysis *n* - **Regression analysis** involving a **model equation** that is **nonlinear** with respect to one or more of its **parameters**. ant: **linear regression analysis**

nonlinear regression model *n* - A **regression model** in which the **outcome variable**, y_i (value for the *i*th person or **observation unit**) is written as some function of a series of **independent variables** (observations or **regressor variables**), $x_{1i}, \cdots, x_{ki}$ and **parameters (regression coefficients)**, $\beta_0, \beta_1, \cdots, \beta_k$ plus an **error term**, ε, and that is **nonlinear** with respect to one or more of its parameters, as in a **logistic regression model**. The primary use of regression models in **clinical trials** is in **adjustment** for **baseline differences** among the **treatment groups** when estimating **treatment effects**. See also **model equation** and **linear regression model**. ant: **linear regression model** rt: **logistic regression model, multiple logistic regression model**

nonlinear regression procedure *n* - **Regression procedure** involving a **nonlinear regression model**. ant: **linear regression procedure**

nonmask, nonmasked *adj* - Of or relating to the absence of a **mask**. rt: **masked, partially masked**

nonmask *n* - [trials] 1. A condition in which neither the person being **enrolled** in a trial or the person administering the **treatment** is **masked** to **treatment assignment**. 2. A condition in which no one involved in a trial is masked to treatment assignment. ant: **complete mask** rt: **partial mask, masking level**

nonmasked treatment assignment *n* - 1. **unmasked treatment assignment** (defns 2, 3, 4) 2. **unmasked treatment assignment** (defn 1) *Usage note*: Use only with adequate accompanying detail to make sense of usage clear. Note that the meaning of defn 1 is different from that for defn 2. See also **open treatment assignment** and **open trial**.

nonmasked trial *n* - 1. A **trial** not **single-, double-,** or **triple-masked**; a trial not involving masked administration of **treatment**. 2. A trial not involving any masking. ant: **masked trial** *Usage note*: Subject to confusion because defn 2 relates to all aspects of a trial, whereas defn 1 relates primarily to **treatment administration**. Hence, a trial nonmasked in the sense of defn 1 may, nevertheless, be masked in other regards, eg, masked readings for measurement of a specified **outcome measure**. Make nature of usage clear by providing sufficient detail to indicate sense of usage.

nonmetric, nonmetrical *adj* - Of or relating to something **qualitative**; not **metric** in the sense of defn 2 or 3. ant: **metric**

nonmetric data *n* - **Data** not based on a **measurement scale** and hence not subject to ordinary arithmetic operations; **categorical data, qualitative data**. See *data type* for list. ant: **metric data**

nonparallel control *n* - A **control** (defn 1) having a time base different from that for **cases** or a **tested treated group** of interest; **historical control**. syn: **nonconcurrent control** ant: **parallel control**

nonparametric *adj* - [**statistics**] Of or relating to a **measure** not requiring specification of assumptions regarding its underlying **distribution**; **distribution-free**; not requiring specification of **parameters**. ant: **parametric** *Usage note*: Use with caution, especially in contexts implying a sharp line of demarcation between parametric and nonparametric. Statisticians disagree as to the demarcation. Often used interchangeably with **distribution-free** though not always interchangeable. Generally applied to methods of **inference** based on **statistical tests** designed for use on **nominal** or **ordinal data**.

nonparametric method *n* - [**statistics**] A **nonparametric** method or procedure; eg, a method based on a **nonparametric test**. rt: **parametric method**

nonparametric test *n* - [**statistics**] A **test of hypothesis** that does not require specification of **parameters** for carrying it out; a **test of hypothesis** that is **distribution-free**. rt: **parametric test**

nonrandom *adj* - Of, relating to, or the result of being not **random** or something that does not conform to or satisfy the scientific definition of **random**. ant: **random** *Usage note*: In **trials**, used primarily in contexts where there is a need or desire to emphasize the nonrandom nature of a **haphazard** or systematic process, or to emphasize the failure to have **randomized**.

nonrandom trial *n* - **nonrandomized trial**

nonrandomized *v* - To have arranged, ordered, mixed, or **assigned** by use of some procedure or system other than one involving **randomization**. ant: **randomized** *Usage note*: In **trials**, used primarily in references to the **treatment assignment** process where there is a need or desire to underscore the absence of randomization in that process. See **random** *adj, scientific* for added comments.

nonrandomized trial *n* - A **trial** in which **treatment assignments** are made in some way other than via **randomization**. ant: **randomized trial** *Usage note*: Often used in contexts where there is a need or desire to emphasize the absence of randomization or the failure to have randomized. Avoid as a pejorative term, as in uses implying that only **randomized trials** are free of **treatment assignment bias**.

nonrequired followup visit *n* - [**trials**] A **followup visit** (after the **treatment assignment visit**) that is not part of the required sequence of **followup visits**, eg, one initiated by a **study patient** because of some acute problem. syn: **interim followup visit, unscheduled followup visit**

nonrespondent *n* - One who does not **respond**. ant: **respondent** rt: **noncompliance**

nonresponse *n* - Absence of a **response**. ant: **response** rt: **noncompliance**

nonresponse bias *n* - **response bias**

nonsense *n* - Something of little importance, significance, or meaning.

nonsense correlation *n* - A **correlation** between two **variables** that has little or no biological, medical, or operational importance. rt: **illusory correlation, spurious correlation**

nonsequential sample size design *n* - **fixed sample size design**

nonsequential trial *n* - 1. A **trial** involving a **fixed sample size design**. 2. A trial not having a **sequential sample size design**.

nontreatment *n* - A **null** form of **inactive treatment** not involving **treatment** of any sort or administration or use of procedures or routines intended to simulate treatment, as with **placebo** medications or **sham procedures**. *Usage note*: Used primarily in relation to characterizations of **control treatments** in **trials** where there is a need or desire to make it clear that, though the label carries the connotation of treatment, none was administered; in effect, those so assigned are subject to observation only.

nonuniform *adj* - Having varying form, manner, or degree; not the same; not constant. ant: **uniform**

nonuniform assignment ratio *n* - **nonuniform treatment assignment ratio**

nonuniform treatment assignment *n* - A **treatment assignment** scheme where the **assignment probabilities** for the various **study treatments** differ.

nonuniform treatment assignment ratio *n* - A **treatment assignment ratio** that is not **uniform**. ant: **uniform treatment assignment ratio**

norm *n* - [L *norma*, lit, carpenter's square] 1. A **standard**, **guideline**, or **principle** that serves to guide, control, regulate, or encourage proper behavior, conduct, or performance. 2. **average** (defn 3)

normal *adj* - [L *normalis*, fr *norma*] 1. Relating to, involving, or being a **normal distribution** or **curve**. 2. Perpendicular, especially perpendicular to a tangent at a point of tangency. 3. Conforming to a given type, standard, or pattern. 4. Of or relating to **average**; being usual or not deviant from expected.

normal *n* - 1. One that is normal (defn 4 **normal** *adj*). 2. Something that conforms to a **norm** or **standard** (defn 3 **normal** *adj*). 3. **normal distribution** 4. A **normal** (defn 2 of **normal** *adj*) **line** (defn 4).

normal curve *n* - A **curve** based on the **normal distribution**.

normal deviate *n* - The value of a **deviate** of the **normal distribution**; **standardized normal deviate**.

normal distribution *n* - A **symmetrical bell-shaped probability density function** of the form:

$$f(x) = \frac{1}{\sigma\sqrt{2\pi}}e^{-\frac{(x-\mu)^2}{2\sigma^2}}$$

where the **variable** x has **mean** μ and **standard deviation** σ (**variance** σ^2). Approximately 68% of the **distribution** lies within 1 standard deviation of the mean, 95% lies within 2 standard deviations, and nearly all the distribution (99.7%) lies within 3 standard deviations of the mean. A large number of **test statistics** have or are approximated by normal distributions, and hence have **critical values** based on the normal distribution.

Normal distribution

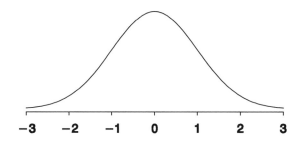

normal limit *n* - A value or **boundary** separating that which is considered **normal** from that which is not so considered. rt: **alert limit**

normal random variable *n* - A **random variable** having a **normal distribution** with a specified **mean** and **variance**; **normal variable**.

normal variable *n* - **normal random variable**

normalize, normalized, normalizing, normalizes *v* - 1. To make conform to or to reduce to a **norm** or **standard**. 2. The process of **transforming** a **variable** so as to cause it to have a **frequency function** that is **normal** or approximately so.

normalized standard score *n* - A **score** resulting from a **transformation** in which the transformed scores have a **distribution** approximating a **normal distribution**; used for **standardization**

of test scores. rt: **data transformation**, **T-score**, **Z-score**

normally distributed *adj* - Relating to, concerned with, or having a **normal distribution**.

Notice of Claimed Investigational Exemption for New Drug *n* - **Investigational New Drug Application**

NTIS *n* - **National Technical Information Service**

nu *n* - [Gk *ny*, of Sem origin; akin to Heb *nūn* nun] The 13th letter of the **Greek alphabet**, uppercase N, lowercase ν.

nuisance *adj* - [ME *nusaunce*, fr AF, fr OF *nuisir* to harm, fr L *nocēre*] Of or relating to something that is annoying, troublesome, or bothersome.

nuisance parameter *n* - A **parameter**, not directly relevant to an **estimation** process, that arises in the **sampling distribution** for the **statistic** being estimated.

null *adj* - [MF *nul*, lit, not any, fr L *nullus*, fr *ne-* not + *ullus* any; akin to L *unus* one] 1. Amounting to nothing; having no value; having no elements. 2. Having the value of zero or that value in the limit.

null hypothesis *n* - 1. In **statistics**, a **hypothesis** that asserts that there is no underlying difference in the **populations** or groups being compared with regard to the **factor**, **trait**, **characteristic**, or **condition** of interest.   2. **null treatment hypothesis** rt: **alternative hypothesis**

null treatment *n* - 1. Absence of **treatment** of any form, including that represented by **placebos**. 2. **nontreatment**

null treatment hypothesis *n* - [**trials**] A **hypothesis** that asserts that the **test treatment** has no effect or that its effect is no different from that of the **control** or **comparison treatment** with regard to a specified **outcome measure**.   ant: **alternative treatment hypothesis**

number *n* - [ME *nombre*, fr OF, fr L *numerus*; abbreviated No., no., and num. (sometimes without periods when there is little or no risk of confusion with other words or abbreviations) and denoted by the symbol #, **N**, or **n**] 1. A **count** or **total**.   2. A member of a set of **positive integers**; one of a series of symbols of unique meaning in a fixed order that may be derived by counting.   3. Any numeral, combination of numerals, combination of numerals and letters or other symbols, letters alone, or combination of

letters and other symbols used for **identification** or designation; **identification number**.

number adaptive randomization *n* - **Adaptive randomization** using the difference in the number assigned to the various **treatment groups** as the basis for **adapting**. See **adaptive treatment assignment** for other types.

number adaptive treatment assignment *n* - **Adaptive treatment assignment** using the **difference** in the number **assigned** to the various **treatment groups** as the basis for **adapting**. See **adaptive treatment assignment** for other types.

numerator *n* - The term above the line in a fraction; a number divided by a **denominator**.

Nuremberg *n* - City in the SE portion of Germany; site of World War II war crimes trials.

Nuremberg Code *n* - A set of **principles** and **standards**, enunciated during World War II war crimes trials in Nuremberg, that together are considered to represent essential prerequisites for and standards of conduct for experimentation on human beings; violation of or failure to comply with the code are considered to represent instances of inhumane treatment of human beings in the research setting. Voluntary consent is one of the essential elements of the code. The code forms the basis for the International Code of Medical Ethics as promulgated by the Assembly of the World Medical Association, London, 1949; subsequently expanded to form the basis for the **Helsinki Declaration**.[88]

O

objective *n* - Something toward which effort is or is to be directed. rt: **aim, goal, purpose**

observation *n* - [MF, fr L *observation-, observatio,* fr *observatus,* pp of *observare*] 1. An act or instance of viewing or noting a fact or occurrence. 2. **data item** (defn 2) 3. **data collection** 4. A judgment or inference from that observed; **conclusion** (defn 1).

observation unit *n* - The **unit** that forms the basis for **data collection** and **analyses** in a **study**; usually a person (**patient**) in the case of **trials**, but may be a smaller (eg, eye) or larger (eg, members of a household) unit. In trials, usually synonymous with **treatment assignment unit**.

observation variable *n* - A **variable** associated with the **observation unit** of a **study** and that is to be or has been observed at one or more points in time in the study, eg, gender as recorded upon **enrollment** or blood pressure as measured upon entry and at specified points in time during **followup**.

observational *adj* - 1. Of, relating to, or based on **observation**; especially as distinct from observation deriving from experimentation. 2. Serving the ends of or used as a means of observation; not **experimental**.

observational study *n* - A **study** (such as a **survey** or **followup study**) that has as its aim **observation** without altering or influencing that which is being observed; **nonexperimental study**; examples include **before and after study, case-history study, case-control study,** and **natural history study**. rt: **epidemiological study**

observe, observed, observing, observes *v* - [ME *observen,* fr MF *observer,* fr L *observare* to guard, watch, observe, fr *ob-* in the way, toward + *servare* to keep] To take note of; to make **observations**; to carefully watch and record as in a **research project**.

observed change *n* - **Change reported, recorded,** or **observed** for a **variable** or **function** over a specified time; **observed difference** (defn 2).

observed data *n* - **Data** noted, **collected,** or recorded in regard to some **measurement** or **assessment**. rt: **raw data**

observed difference *n* - 1. The **difference** of one value from another **reported, recorded,** or **observed** at a specified point in time, eg, the difference in **mean** body weight between two **groups** of people at entry into a **trial**. 2. The difference of a **variable** or **function** at two points in time, eg, the difference in one's body weight as measured now and one year ago.

observed distribution *n* - The **distribution** observed at or after some point in time or at or after some designated action or procedure.

observed effective sample size *n* - The **effective sample size** taking account of **observed losses** due to **drop out, missed visits,** and **noncompliance**. rt: **expected effective sample size**

observed frequency *n* - The number of values for a given **cell** of a **contingency table** or in a **category, class,** or **interval** of a **frequency distribution**.

observed frequency distribution *n* - A **distribution** of counts or numbers observed or assembled in relation to some **study** or **data collection** activity.

observed mean *n* - The **arithmetic mean** as determined for an **observed** set of **data** and a specified **variable**.

observed outcome *n* - An **outcome** recorded or observed for an **observation** or **treatment unit**.

observed power *n* - The **power** for detecting a **difference** of a specified size based on **observed results**; for **trials**, the power for a specified **treatment difference**, given an **observed sample size**, observed **data** for a specified **outcome measure**, and observed **losses to followup** due to **drop out, missed visits,** and **noncompliance**. rt: **conditional power, expected power**

observed rate *n* - **Rate** as observed or recorded. syn: **crude rate**

observed result *n* - 1. **result** (defn 4) 2. **observed treatment difference** 3. The observed value for a **measure** or **variable**. 4. **observation** (defn 4)

observed sample size *n* - The **number** of **observation units enrolled** in a **study** upon completion of **enrollment** or at some designated point during enrollment. rt: **calculated sample size**

observed treatment assignment ratio *n* - The **treatment assignment ratio** observed during or upon completion of **enrollment**. rt: **expected treatment assignment ratio**

observed treatment difference *n* - [trials] The **treatment difference** estimated or derived from **observed data** for a given **outcome variable**, especially the **primary** or a **secondary outcome variable**, as it exists at some point in the course of **followup** for the **test treatment** versus the **control treatment** or for one test treatment versus another test treatment.

observed treatment effect *n* - 1. A **treatment effect** produced by the use or administration of a **treatment**. 2. Treatment effect as **estimated** from **observed data**.

observed value *n* - A **value** (such as a count or the value of a **variable**) observed or recorded.

observed variable *n* - The value of a **variable** as determined by **observation** or as recorded.

observer *n* - One who **observes** and **records** for the purpose of documentation, as in relation to **data collection**; **reader**

observer bias *n* - **Bias** (defn 2) on the part of an **observer** that influences or is considered to influence the way in which **observations** are made or recorded, eg, **digit preference**.

observer error *n* - **Error** in a **measurement** or **observation** that is due to the one making the measurement or observation. rt: **measurement error, observer bias, observer variation**

observer variation *n* - 1. **Variation** in a **measurement** or **observation** that is due to **observer error** or differences in the way the observer makes or records the measurement or observation. 2. Variation from observer to observer making the same kind of measurement or observation; **inter observer variation**.

odd *adj* - [ME odde, fr ON oddi point of land, triangle, odd number; akin to OE *ord* point of a weapon] Being one of a sequence of natural numbers counting by twos starting with 1, ie, 1, 3, 5, 7, etc; a number not exactly divisible by two. ant: **even**

odd-even method of treatment assignment *n* - An **alternation method of treatment assign-**ment based on the order in which **observation units** are **enrolled**, eg, one in which **patients** with odd **ID numbers** are assigned to the **test treatment** and those with even ID numbers are assigned to the **control treatment** of a **trial**, or a scheme in which patients seen on **odd** numbered days are **assigned** to the **test treatment** and those seen on even-numbered days are assigned to the **control treatment** of a trial, or a scheme in which every other person seen is given the test treatment of a trial.

odds *n* - 1. A **ratio** of two numbers that indicate the **chance**, or one's belief regarding the chance, that some **event** or **outcome** will occur versus some other event or outcome; the two numbers may be **probability measures** ($3/5 \div 2/5$ or $0.60 \div 0.40$) or may be the **numerators** of two numbers having the same **denominator** (3/2 or 3:2). 2. The differential in the amount of money required from one party relative to the other in making a wager, eg, a 3:2 wager by A versus B that the Dallas Cowboys will beat the Detroit Lions the next time they meet requires A to put up 3 dollars to every 2 dollars wagered by B; A will collect 2 dollars for every 3 dollars wagered if the Cowboys win and will lose 3 dollars for every two wagered by B if the Cowboys lose. 3. The observed odds, eg, as derived from a **case-control study**. rt: **relative betting odds**

odds ratio *n* - [epidemiology] A **relative** measure of **risk** in the form of the **ratio** of two **odds**, especially as arising from **observational studies**; variously expressed depending on setting and assumptions.[84, 72] For example, the odds ratio for exposure as provided from a **case-control study** is *a/b* to *c/d* or *ad/bc* (the ratio of cross-products), where *a*, *b*, *c*, and *d* correspond to counts of independently sampled people with (**cases**) and without (**controls**) a given **disease** as represented in a **two-by-two table** of the form:

	Exposed	Not exposed
Cases	*a*	*b*
Controls	*c*	*d*

In a **prospective study** with unbiased subject selection where individuals are classified on exposure and then observed for development of **disease**, the **relative risk** is given by $a/(a + c) \div b/(b + d)$; approximated by $a/c \div b/d$ or ad/bc for rare diseases. syn: relative odds rt: **relative**

risk, risk ratio *Usage note*: See note for **relative risk**.

off *prep* - Used as a function word to indicate the **suspension** of an activity or condition. ant: **on**

off study *adj* - [**trials**] 1. Of or relating to a person not receiving the **assigned study treatment** in a **trial**. 2. Of or relating to a person in a trial for whom use of the **assigned treatment** has been **suspended** or **terminated** for medical or other reasons, eg, intolerable **side effects** or the development of some other disease conditions requiring other forms of treatment. 3. Of or relating to a person who is no longer willing or able to remain under **followup** in a trial; of or being a **dropout**. 4. Of or relating to something done or to be done that is not part of a specified **study protocol**. ant: **on study** rt: **off treatment** *Usage note*: Not recommended because of associated ambiguities. A person can be **off treatment** and still **on study** (defn 2). To avoid confusion, use **off treatment** for uses relating to defns 1 and 2, and **dropout** for uses in the sense of defn 3. See **on study** for additional comments.

off treatment *adj* - 1. Of or relating to a person not receiving the **assigned study treatment** in a **trial**. 2. Of or relating to a person in a trial for whom use of the **assigned treatment** has been **suspended** or **terminated** for medical or other reasons, eg, intolerable **side effects** or the development of some other disease conditions requiring other forms of treatment. syn: **off study** (not recommended) ant: **on treatment** *Usage note*: see usage notes for **off study** and **on study**)

off-site *adj* - Of, relating to, or being away from the **site** at which a given activity or function is performed. ant: **on-site**

off-site audit *n* - 1. An **audit** performed away from the **site** of origin or of performance of the activity or function being audited; **desk audit**. 2. **off-site record audit** ant: **on-site audit**

off-site record audit *n* - An **audit** of **records** from a **site** at a remote location, eg, an **audit** of records received from a **clinic** at a **coordinating center**. ant: **on-site record audit**

offerer *n* - [**research**] 1. A person or party offering or proposing to carry out a designated **research project** according to specifications contained in a formal proposal submitted to the **sponsoring agency**. 2. One responding to a **request for proposal** issued from the **National**

Institutes of Health. syn: **applicant, proposer**

office *n* - [ME, fr MF, fr L *officium* service, duty, office, fr *opus* work + *facere* to make, do] 1. A position of responsibility or of executive authority. 2. A place where a particular kind of business is conducted or service rendered.

Office for Protection from Research Risks (OPRR) *n* - An **office** within the **National Institutes of Health** responsible for the promulgation and administration of regulations regarding **institutional review boards**.[117]

Office of Management and Budget (OMB) *n* - An **office** in the executive arm of the United States government; general duties include those related to review and approval of **research** initiated by **requests for proposals** and documents, such as **data forms**, to be used for conduct of such research.

Office of Research Integrity (ORI) *n* - An **office** within the **National institutes of Health** responsible for protecting the **integrity** of the **extramural** and **intramural research programs** of the **USPHS**. The office has its origins in the Health Extension Act of 1985. Responsibilities include conducting investigations and rendering judgments regarding alleged **scientific misconduct** in federally funded research. The Office conducts investigations of alleged **misconduct** at applicant or awardee institutions and in the **intramural research program** of the USPHS and presents findings in administrative hearings before the **Health and Human Services** Departmental Appeal Board. The Office was established as part of the NIH Revitalization Act of 1993;[154] prior to that responsibilities of the Office were vested in the Office of Scientific Integrity (OSI) in the Office of the Director of the NIH and in the Office of Scientific Integrity Review (OSIR) in the Office of the Assistant Secretary for Health.

Office of Research on Women's Health (ORWH) *n* - An **office** within the **National Institutes of Health**, established in 1990, having a threefold mandate: (1) To strengthen and enhance research related to diseases, disorders, and conditions that affect women and to ensure that **research** conducted by or supported by the **NIH** adequately addresses issues regarding women's health; (2) To ensure that women are appropriately represented in biomedical and behavioral research studies supported by the

NIH; and (3) To develop opportunities and support for recruitment, retention, re-entry, and advancement of women in biomedical careers.

officer *n* - [ME, fr MF *officier*, fr ML *officiarius*, fr L *officium*] One who holds an **office** of trust, authority, or command.

officers of the study *n* - Those persons within a study structure elected to designated offices or who otherwise fill or head such offices; in **multicenter** structures, such as **multicenter trials**, generally taken as the **study chair** and **vice-chair** and the heads or **directors** of key **centers** or **offices** represented in the structure, such as the **data center**, **data coordinating center**, or **coordinating center**, and **project office**.

ogive *n* - A **graph** of the **cumulative frequency** for a **continuous variable** measured, recorded, or plotted over a **range** of **class intervals** for a **frequency distribution**, consisting of a series of connected line segments formed by joining the **points** represented. The first line segment is one for the class interval having the lowest value and a nonzero **frequency** (defined by x- and y-**coordinates**, corresponding to the lower **endpoint** of that interval and 0 and the upper endpoint of that interval and the observed frequency for that interval); the last line segment is one for the class interval having the highest value and a nonzero frequency (defined by x- and y-coordinates corresponding the lower endpoint of that interval and the cumulative frequency at that point and the upper endpoint of the interval and the total frequency represented in the distribution). rt: **histogram**

OMB *n* - **Office of Management and Budget**

omega *n* - [Gk *ō mega*, lit, large o] The 24th and last letter of the **Greek alphabet**, uppercase Ω, lowercase ω.

omicron *n* - [Gk *o mikron*, lit small o] The 15th letter of the **Greek alphabet**, uppercase O, lowercase o.

on *prep* - [ME, *an*, *on*, prep & adv, fr OE; akin to OHG *ana* on, Gk *ana* up, on] A function word used to indicate active involvement in some activity, function, or process. ant: **off**

on study *n* - [trials] 1. Of or relating to a person receiving the **assigned study treatment** in a **trial**. 2. Of or relating to a person in a trial under active **followup**, regardless of whether or not **on treatment**; of or relating to one that has

not dropped out. 3. Of or relating to something done or to be done that is part of the **study protocol**. ant: **off study** rt: **on treatment** *Usage note*: Not recommended because of the difference in implication for use in the sense of defn 1 versus defn 2. A person can be **on study** in the sense of defn 2 and **off study** in the sense of defns 1 or 2 for **off study**. Avoid confusion by use of explicit terminology, such as **on treatment** for uses in the sense of defn 1 above. See **off study** for additional comments.

on treatment *adj* - Of or relating to a person receiving the **assigned study treatment** in a **trial**. syn: **on study** (not recommended) ant: **off treatment** *Usage note*: See notes for **on study** and **off study**.

on-line *adj* - [computers] Being done under the control of a computer, eg, **on-line data entry**.

on-line data acquisition *n* - 1. **Acquisition** of **data** as they are generated, usually by direct **electronic** linkage to the **generation site**. 2. **direct data entry** (defn 1)

on-line data entry *n* - **Data entry** performed as **data** are generated by use of **computer**-driven **video screens** and displayed prompts. rt: **on-line data acquisition**

on-site *adj* - Of, relating to, or being at the **site** at which a given activity or function is performed. ant: **off-site**

on-site audit *n* - 1. An **audit** performed at the **site** of origin or performance of the activity or function being audited. 2. **on-site record audit** ant: **off-site audit**

on-site record audit *n* - An **audit** of **records** from a **site** at that site, eg, an **audit** of records generated at a **clinic** during a **study site visit**. ant: **off-site record audit**

one *adj* - [ME *on*, *an*, fr OE *ān*; akin to OHG *ein* one, L *unus* (OL *oios*) Skt *eka*] Being or comprised of a single unit, entity, or object.

one-armed bandit *adj* - Of, relating to, or concerned with a single **stochastic process**. rt: **bandit, two-armed bandit**

one-armed bandit *n* - Slot machine; a machine for gambling in which each round of play starts with the player inserting a specified number of coins, often one, into a slot on the machine; the player then pulls a lever (arm) to spin a set of dials, the positions of which after spinning determine the **outcome** of the game, ie, loss of the coins inserted or return of a number of coins equal to or in excess of the number inserted depending on the configuration of the dials. So named because of the lever used for spinning the dials and because of the expected monetary loss when playing. Used in **statistics** in relation to **chance** or **stochastic processes**, as in relation to games of chance or **randomization**. rt: **bandit, two-armed bandit**

one-sided *adj* - **one-tailed**

one-sided alternative *n* - **one-tailed alternative hypothesis**

one-sided test *n* - **one-tailed test**

one-tailed *adj* - [**statistics**] Being, having, or characterized by one **tail**, as in a **one-tailed alternative hypothesis**; also **one-sided**. ant: **two-tailed**

one-tailed alternative hypothesis *n* - A **composite hypothesis** serving as an **alternative** to the **null hypothesis** that specifies a **range** of permissible values of a **parameter**, all of which lie to one side of the **null** value (eg, H_o: $\mu_1 = \mu_2$ versus H_a: $\mu_1 > \mu_2$). rt: **two-tailed alternative hypothesis**

one-tailed confidence interval *n* - A **confidence interval** with just a **lower** or **upper end point**, dictated by a **type I error** associated exclusively with one of the two **tails** of the **distribution** for the **estimate**.

one-tailed test *n* - [**statistics**] A **test of significance** based on the **null hypothesis** versus a **one-tailed alternative hypothesis**. ant: **two-tailed test**

one-way *adj* - Being or related to movement or progression in one direction; having one dimension or direction. rt: **two-way**

one-way classification *n* - A **classification** based on a single **characteristic**, **factor**, or **variable**, eg, classification of individuals by gender. rt: **two-way classification**

open *adj* - [ME, fr OE; akin to OHG *affan* open, OE *ūp* up] [general] 1. Freedom of choice or option. 2. Free from concealment. 3. Having no enclosing or confining barrier; not **closed**. [**trials**] 1. Of or relating to **treatments** assigned or administered as chosen or dictated by the treating physician or **patient**. 2. Of or relating to a system of **treatment assignments** in which assignments are known or can be determined by those responsible for administration of the

treatments, eg, a scheme in which the assignments to be made are posted in a **clinic** for all to see or an **odd-even** method of treatment assignment involving **unmasked treatments**. 3. Not **masked**. 4. Of or relating to a trial still **enrolling** patients. *Usage note*: The most common usage is as a euphemism for **treatment designs** in which the **treatment** to be administered is selected by the **study physician** or **patient**. Avoid in such contexts by using more informative terms, as noted in comments for **open trial**.

open class interval *n* - A **class interval** not having a specified upper or lower **end point**.

open label *adj* - [**trials**] Of or relating to a **trial** in which **study treatments** are administered in **unmasked** fashion; characterization used primarily in relation to **drug trials**. *Usage note*: Avoid; use **unmasked**. See also notes for **open** and **open trial**.

open label trial *n* - 1. **nonmasked drug trial** 2. Any **nonmasked trial**. *Usage note*: Not recommended because of potential for confusion with **open trial** (defns 1, 2, or 3). Use **nonmasked trial**.

open randomization *n* - **unmasked randomization**

open sequential design *n* - [**trials**] A **sequential design** with an **open** region of indecision; design does not provide for an upper limit on the number of **patients** that may be **enrolled** because the **observed treatment difference** may never enter a **region** of decision; differs from **closed sequential design** in that the region of uncertainty is circumscribed for closed designs. An observed difference that lies outside the region of indecision favors an **alternative treatment hypothesis** in which the **test treatment** is superior or inferior (depending on the **boundary** crossed) to the **control** or **comparison treatment**.

open sequential trial *n* - A **trial** with an **open sequential design**.

open treatment assignment *n* - 1. **Treatment assignment** resulting from an **open treatment assignment schedule**, eg, as from a schedule posted in the **clinic** giving the order of assignment. 2. **uncontrolled treatment assignment** (defn 2) *Usage note*: Not a recommended term; if used at all, use with caution for reasons stated in usage note for **open trial**.

open treatment assignment schedule *n* - A **treatment assignment schedule** that is not

Open sequential design

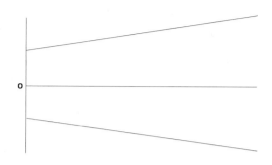

masked ant: **masked treatment assignment schedule** *Usage note*: Note that a treatment assignment schedule is considered to be open even if the treatments are not identified by name, as in the case of a schedule for a **double-masked trial** in which assignments correspond to numbers of bottles containing **placebo** or **test** medications. See also **masked treatment assignment schedule**.

open trial *n* - 1. A **trial** in which the treating physician (or some other person in a **clinic**) or the **patient** selects the **treatment** to be administered. 2. A trial in which **treatment assignments** are known in advance of being made, eg, schemes where assignments are posted or in systematic schemes, such as **odd-even methods of treatment assignment**, where the scheme is known. 3. A trial in which treatments are not **masked**; **nonmasked trial**. 4. A trial still **enrolling**. 5. A trial involving an **open sequential design**. *Usage note*: Generally used as a euphemism for a trial not involving adequate safeguards against **treatment assignment bias** (defns 1 or 2). Avoid by use of appropriate descriptors such as **uncontrolled treatment assignment** in the sense of defn 1 and **unmasked treatment assignment** in the sense of defn 2. Use **nonmasked trial** in the sense of defn 3. If used in the sense of defns 4 or 5 make certain that the term is not taken to denote conditions described in defns 1, 2, or 3.

operate, operated, operating, operates *v* - [L *operatus*, pp of *operari* to work, fr *oper-*, *opus* work; akin to OE *efan* to perform, Skt *apas* work] 1. To perform a function. 2. To perform an **operation** or series of operations. 3. To produce an appropriate **effect**.

operation *n* - [ME, *operacioun*, fr MF *operation*, fr L *operation-*, *operatio*, fr *operatus*, pp] 1. The act of performing a practical work or something involving the application of principles or process. 2. The quality or state of being functional or operative. 3. An **invasive** procedure carried out on a living body, especially one involving surgery. 4. Any of various mathematical or logical processes (such as those represented by **addition** or **multiplication**) of deriving one entity from others according to specified **rules**.

operations committee *n* - [**trials**] 1. A **committee** concerned with overall **operation** within a **trial**. 2. A committee concerned with some aspect of operations within a trial. 3. A standing committee that performs the functions of the **treatment effects monitoring committee** or those functions and others (such as those of an **advisory-review committee**); such a committee in a **multicenter trial** sponsored by the **Veterans Administration**.

operations office *n* - 1. The unit or agency of an **organization** charged with oversight or with planning and direction. 2. **data coordinating center; coordinating center**

OPRR *n* - **Office for Protection from Research Risks**

oral *adj* - [L *or-*, *os* mouth; akin to OE *ōra*, border, L *ora*] 1. Uttered by mouth or in words; spoken. 2. By mouth. *Usage note*: See usage note for **verbal**.

oral assent *n* - 1. **Assent** obtained on the basis of an **oral** exchange between the requestor and assenting party; especially one not written or signed. 2. Assent based on a written statement read to the assenting party, as in a telephone **interview** or in the case of a direct contact with a person unable to read. 3. **Documented assent** based on an oral exchange between the requestor and assenting party. syn: **verbal assent** (not recommended; see note for **verbal**) rt: **documented assent, signed assent, written assent**

oral consent *n* - 1. **Consent** obtained on the basis of an **oral** exchange between the requestor and consenting party; especially one not written or signed. 2. Consent based on a written statement read to the consenting party, as in a telephone **interview** or in the case of a direct contact with a person unable to read. 3. **Documented consent** based on an oral exchange between the requestor and the consenting party. syn: **verbal**

consent (not recommended, see note for **verbal**) rt: **documented consent, signed consent, written consent**

order, ordered *adj* - 1. Of or relating to ordered arrangement of objects or elements. 2. Having elements arranged or identified according to a plan or rule. 3. Having elements labeled by **ordinal numbers**.

order *n* - [MF *ordre*, fr ML & L; ML *ordin-*, *ordo* ecclesiastical order, fr L arrangement, group, class; akin to L *ordiri* to lay the warp, begin] 1. An arrangement of objects or elements according to some rule or system. 2. An ordering based on the numerical value of some identifier (eg, an arrangement of **records** by **ID number**) or **variable** (eg, age in an ordering of individuals from youngest to oldest). 3. An arrangement of **data elements** having numerical values, from smallest to largest or largest to smallest. rt: **rank, rank order**

order, ordered, ordering, orders *v* - To place or arrange in **order**.

order statistic *n* - A **statistic** based on numerical **order** of **data elements**; eg, the rth order statistic is the rth value in a numerical ordering of **data elements** from smallest to largest; other order statistics include **median, mid-range,** and **range**.

ordinal *adj* - [LL *ordinalis*, fr L *ordin-*, *ordo*] Of a specified **order** or **rank**.

ordinal data *n* - **Nonmetric data** that provide a **measure** of **rank** or **order** but that are not amenable to ordinary arithmetic operations, eg, a measure of socioeconomic class.

ordinal number *n* - 1. A **number** designating the place or position of a **data element** represented in an ordering or ranking. 2. A number assigned to an ordered set that designates both **order** and **count**. rt: **cardinal number**

ordinate *n* - [NL (*linea*) ordinate (*applicata*), lit, line applied in an orderly manner] 1. **y-coordinate** 2. **y-axis** rt: **abscissa**

ordinate axis *n* - **y-axis**

organization *n* - 1. An administrative and functional structure of **business** or activity; the personnel of such a structure. 2. The act or process of organizing or of being organized. 3. A collection of people engaged in a business or activity.

ORI *n* - **Office of Research Integrity**

orient, oriented, orienting, orients *v* - [F *orienter*, fr MF, fr *orient*] To set or arrange in any determinate position or direction.

orientation *n* - The state of being **oriented**; arrangement, alignment, or positioning, as in **landscape** or **portrait page orientation**.

origin *n* - [ME *origine*, prob fr MF, fr L *origin-*, *origo*, fr *oriri* to rise] 1. The point or place at which something begins, starts, or derives from. 2. The **xy-coordinate** of (0,0) in a plane **Cartesian coordinate** system.

original *adj* - Being the first instance in which something is used or proposed; not secondary, derived from something else, or imitative. rt: **unique** *Usage note*: Use with caution in relation to work or methods, especially in the absence of a literature search to establish or support a claim of primacy. Usually best avoided in characterizations of one's own work or methods used. See also **unique**.

original *n* - 1. An authentic work; a firsthand work. 2. That from which a copy, reproduction, transcription, or translation is made.

original data *n* - 1. **Data** not previously seen or reported. 2. Data seen or reported for the first time. 3. Data that are the product of an **original investigation** or **study**. 4. Data generated or collected in relation to a study. 5. Data analyzed and reported by the same **agency, group,** or persons generating or collecting them.

original document *n* - 1. **source document** 2. The **original** (defn 2) of a **document**. rt: **primary document**

original record *n* - 1. **source record** 2. The **original** (defn 2) of a **record**. rt: **primary record**

orphan *adj* - [LL *orphanus*, fr Gk *orphanos*; akin to OHG *erbi* inheritance, L *orbus* orphaned] Of or relating to being an orphan; of or being odd, alone, or isolated, eg, **orphan drug**.

orphan drug *n* - A **drug** that has limited marketing potential because of the rarity of the **disease** or condition for which it is intended. Legislation enacted in 1983 in the US provides tax incentives and a seven-year period of exclusive marketing rights to companies involved in developing and marketing such drugs. To qualify as an orphan drug under the legislation, the disease or condition for which the drug is intended must afflict fewer than 200,000 people in the US.

orthogonal *adj* - [MF, fr L *orthogonius*, fr Gk *orthogōnois*, fr *orth-* + *gōnia* angle] 1. **Intersecting** or lying at right angles; having perpendicular slopes or tangents at the point of intersection. 2. Having a sum of products that is zero (or 1 in certain instances) under specified conditions. 3. Of or related to being statistically **independent**.

orthogonal contrast *n* - A **contrast**, such that in relation to another, the sum of the **pairwise** products of the **coefficients** of the contrasts is zero.

ORWH *n* - **Office of Research on Women's Health**

other *n* - One that remains of two or more; a different person or thing; another person or thing.

outcome *n* - [general] Something that follows as a consequence of some antecedent action or **event**. [trials] 1. An **event** or **measure** observed or recorded for a particular person or **treatment unit** in a trial during or following **treatment** and that is used to assess the **safety** or **efficacy** of a **study treatment**. 2. **Primary** or **secondary outcome measure**, especially one measured or recorded as an **event**; **outcome variable**. syn: **endpoint** (not recommended) *Usage note*: Preferred to **endpoint**; see **endpoint** for reasons.

outcome adaptive random treatment assignment *n* - **Adaptive random treatment assignment** based on observed **outcomes**, eg, **play-the-winner treatment assignment** schemes.

outcome adaptive randomization *n* - A **treatment assignment process** using **outcome adaptive random treatment assignment**.

outcome adaptive treatment assignment *n* - **Adaptive treatment assignment** based on observed **outcomes**, with or without **randomization**.

outcome event *n* - [trials] 1. An **outcome measure** that is **binary** (especially the positive (defn 2) state of such a measure, eg, death or a **morbid event**). 2. The **event** of **primary** interest in a **trial** with events as **outcome measures**; usually the event used for **sample size calculations** or the one receiving the most attention in **data analyses**.

outcome measure *n* - 1. [trials] An **observation variable** recorded for a **treatment unit** (obser-

vation unit) at one or more time points after **enrollment** for the purpose of assessing the effect of a **study treatment**. 2. A **measurement** or observation used to measure the **effect** of an **experimental variable** in a defined experiment. syn: **outcome variable**

outcome research *n* - **Research** in the health care field aimed at the evaluation of **treatment** and care procedures based on the **outcomes** produced or observed; typically morbidity or mortality or other indicators of outcome, such as observed or reported **side effects** associated with a treatment or care procedure, change in symptomatology, change in functional status, or change in indicators of **quality of life**. *Usage note*: Although technically **trials** are forms of outcome research, the term is typically reserved for research of a nonexperimental, observational nature.

outcome variable *n* - [trials] An **observation variable** recorded for persons (**observation units**) at one or more time points after **enrollment** for the purpose of assessing effects of the **study treatments**. syn: **outcome measure**

outlier *n* - 1. Any value, reading, or **measurement** outside specified **limits**, especially one that is so far removed from other values that the appropriateness of its use in **analyses** is in question. 2. An extreme value considered to be in **error** or where such is considered to be a distinct possibility.

output *n* - **Data** or information flowing from a **computer** as a result of **input** or calculations and manipulations performed by the computer. ant: **input**

output device *n* - [computers] A **device**, such as a printer or **video display terminal**, used for **output**. rt: **input device**

over *adj* - external; outer

over-the-counter drug *n* - A **drug** that may be purchased without a **prescription** such as aspirin or a cold remedy; nonprescription drug.

overmatch *n* - A state or condition in which **matching** done for **variance control** in a **comparative observational study** obscures or is thought to obscure a true **causal relationship** between an **independent variable** and the **dependent variable**; occurs when a variable used for matching is related to the independent variable and influences the way in which it exerts its effect on the dependent variable. *Usage note*: Use of the term relates to variables used in matching, not to the closeness of the match achieved for any given variable. Often used as a **weasel term** to "explain" the failure to show an expected relationship or causal relationship. Avoid as an explanation of such failures except where accompanied with **data** and arguments supporting the claim. See also notes for **vacuous term** and **weasel term**.

overmatch, overmatched, overmatching, overmatches *v* - To **match** to a greater degree or amount than desired or required. rt: **undermatch** *Usage note*: See **overmatch** *n* for note; see also **vacuous term** and **weasel term** for notes.

overrepresent, overrepresented, overrepresenting, overrepresents *v* - To **represent** in larger or higher amount or degree than desired or required. ant: **underrepresent** rt: **overstudy** *Usage note*: See note for **underrepresent**.

overstudy, overstudied, overstudying, overstudies *v* - To **study** more than desired or required. ant: **understudy** rt: **overrepresent** *Usage note*: See note for **understudy**.

overview *n* - 1. A general **survey** or summary. 2. **meta-analysis** *Usage note*: Not a recommended synonym for **meta-analysis** for reasons indicated in the usage note for **meta-analysis**. Technically, the dictionary definition of overview is as given in defn 1 and, hence, the term may be confused with a survey or summary not involving any meta-analysis. The possibility of confusion is avoided with **meta-analysis**, since it has only one definition. Usage as a synonym for **meta-analysis** due to Richard Peto and coworkers; first referred to as **pooling** and subsequently as **overview**.[168, 169, 121] See **meta-analysis** for additional usage notes.

overview analysis *n* - **meta-analysis**

P

p, P *n* - [16th letter of the English alphabet] Symbol denoting a **probability** value; value usually denoted by **p**, but may also be denoted by **P**.

p-value *n* - [statistics] **Probability value** associated with an **observed test statistic** that corresponds to the **proportion** of times one would expect to observe a value as extreme or more extreme than the one observed if the **null hypothesis** were true, eg, a p-value of 0.05 for an **observed result** means that on **average** 1 in 20 replications of the study would be expected to yield a result as extreme as or more extreme than the one observed if the null hypothesis were true. Sometimes also P-value. rt: **significance level**, **statistical significance** *Usage note*: Traditionally, a p-value of 0.05 or smaller has been taken as evidence of **statistical significance**. However, it is prudent to avoid that tradition, especially in settings where the observed result and associated test statistic is just one among many of interest. It is better in that case to treat the p-values as additional descriptors of the observed **data** rather than **quantitative** indicators of statistical significance.

package *n* - 1. A commodity or product that is uniformly wrapped or boxed. 2. A **computer program** and related documentation that are designed for performing a specified function or activity.

package insert *n* - **label insert**

page *n* - [MF, fr L *pagina*; akin to L *pangere* to fix, fasten] 1. One side or face of a leaf of document, eg, a numbered page in a **book** having text or other displays on both sides or faces of all or most of its leaves. 2. Both sides or faces of a leaf of a document together, eg, a page in a **manuscript** having text or displays on only one side or face of its individual leaves.

page orientation *n* - The **orientation** or positioning of a **page** for use or reading; **landscape** or **portrait page orientation** when the two dimensions of the page are different.

pair *n* - [ME *paire*, fr OF, fr L *paria* equal things, fr neut pl of *par* equal] 1. Two similar or associated things. 2. Two corresponding things designed for use together. 3. Two or more corresponding things of a defined set (eg, brothers and sisters), each of which is or can be viewed as being paired with any other member of the set. rt: **match**

pair, paired, pairing, pairs *v* - 1. To arrange into **pairs** or to cause to become a **pair**; to make into a pair. 2. To arrange into sets involving one or more pairs. rt: **matching**

pair matching *v* - **Matching** one person, thing, or object to another such person, thing, or object, as in a **design** involving **matched pairs**; **pairwise matching**. rt: **category matching, frequency matching, group matching, individual matching**

paired comparisons *n* - 1. A method of **ranking** based on a series of **comparisons** in which an evaluator or judge indicates the member of any given **pair** preferred; eg, the ordering BCA resulting from the paired comparisons: AvsB, AvsC, and BvsC, in which the preferences were B, C, and B. 2. Comparisons involving each of several different **test treatments** with the same **control treatment**, eg, the Coronary Drug Project,[30] involving five different test treatments, each compared with the same control treatment.

paired observations *n* - **Observations** or **measurements** made on **paired observation units**, eg, education level of husband and wife or intraocular pressure of the right eye contrasted with the left eye. rt: **correlated observations**

paired sample *n* - A **sample** comprised of paired **observation units** or **treatment units**, eg, pairings of siblings, husbands and wives, or of matching anatomical parts such as eyes or hands. The pairing may be established before sampling by natural conditions or consequences, eg, as a result of birth, marriage, anatomy, or other physiological, geographic, or social conditions, or it may be established on an arbitrary basis simply for purposes of the study, eg, by **pairing** or **matching** individuals before **enrollment** on the basis of **disease** characteristics or other demographic or prognostic characteristics, or simply on the basis of order of arrival at a **study site**. rt: **paired treatment design**

paired treatment design *n* - A **parallel treatment design** in which **treatment units** are paired and assigned to treatment as members of a **block** (defn 2). The pairing may be a part of the design, as in some **sequential designs**, or may be imposed simply as a means of **variance control**. The pairing may be arbitrary (eg, **patients** paired on the basis of their arrival at a **clinic**) or natural (eg, the use of twins or paired body parts, such as hands or eyes; see the Glaucoma Laser Trial [Glaucoma Laser Trial Research Group, 1991][60] for an example based on eyes). rt: **paired sample**

pairwise *adj* - Relating to or being arranged or considered together, as a **pair** or pairs.

pairwise comparison *n* - 1. **Comparison** of different **pairs**. 2. Comparison of each **test-treated group** with the **control-treated group** in a **trial** involving two or more **test treatments** and a **control treatment**.

pairwise matching *v* - A process in which the second element of what is to be regarded as a **pair** when **matched** is selected to match the first element on one or more features or characteristics. ant: **frequency matching**, **group matching** rt: **individual matching**

pandemic *adj* - [LL *pandemus*, fr Gk *pandēmos* of all the people, fr *pan-* + *dēmos* people] 1. Occurring over a wide geographic area. 2. Occurring over a wide geographic area and effecting a large number of people. rt: **endemic**, **epidemic**

paper *n* - [ME *papir*, fr MF *papier*, fr L *papyrus* papyrus, paper, fr Gk *papyros* papyrus] 1. **manuscript** 2. Thin smooth sheets of fibrous material used for writing and printing; a single sheet of such material.

paper form *n* - A **form** printed or completed on **paper**; as opposed to an **electronic form**. ant: **electronic form**

paper-writing committee *n* - A **committee** charged with or having responsibility for writing a designated **paper**, especially one being prepared for submission to a **journal** for possible **publication**; publication committee (defn 2).

paperless *adj* - Not involving the use of **paper**; not comprised of or consisting of **paper**.

paperless data entry *n* - 1. **on-line data entry** 2. **direct data entry**

paperless form *n* - **electronic form**

paperless study *n* - A **study** that has no **paper forms**, especially one in which **data** are recorded electronically as they are collected using **video display terminals**. syn: formless study

parallel *adj* - [L *parallelus*, fr Gk *parallēlos*, fr *para* beside + *allēlōn* of one another, fr *allos* ... *allos* one ... another, fr *allos* other] 1. Similar, analogous, or interdependent in development. 2. Readily compared; companion. 3. Running or occurring at the same time; **concurrent**.

parallel control *n* - A **control** (defn 1) **parallel** (defn 3) to that to which **compared**, eg, **control-assigned patients** in a **trial** involving a **parallel treatment design**. syn: **concurrent control** ant: **nonparallel control**

parallel design *n* - **parallel treatment design**

parallel experiment *n* - 1. An **experiment** that is similar to another or that may be readily compared with another. 2. An experiment related to and carried out at the same time as another.

parallel group design *n* - [trials] A **treatment design** involving two or more **treatment groups**, **concurrent enrollment** of **observation units** to those groups, and **assignment** of observation units to one and only one of those treatment groups. **Treatment comparisons** involve different but (presumably) comparable observation units. ant: **crossover treatment design** rt: **between-person trial**

parallel group trial *n* - A **trial** having a **parallel treatment design**. syn: **between-person trial**

parallel patient *n* - A **patient** with the same general disease, demographic, and health characteristics as those **enrolled** into a **trial** and who is **treated** and **followed** in a fashion similar to those enrolled. rt: **parallel track**

parallel study *n* - 1. A **study** that is similar to another or that may be readily compared with another. 2. A study related to and carried out at the same time as another.

parallel time design *n* - 1. **parallel treatment design** 2. Any **design** providing for **concurrent enrollment** of **observation units** to the different **study groups**.

parallel track *n* - 1. A policy of the **Food and Drug Administration** (1992)[33] designed to provide **expanded availability** of promising **drugs** for the desperately ill prior to approval of an **NDA**. Requests for expanded availability are subject to review and approval of the **FDA** and are required to include provisions for organized **data collection** and assessment pertaining to use. The policy provides for use of promising drugs outside the context of **IND trials**. The policy was developed as a result of pressure from AIDS activists, in particular those associated with the AIDS Coalition to Unleash Power (ACTUP). 2. A course of activities running **parallel** to those of a **trial** (or set of trials) and designed to provide **treatment** and **followup** for persons not qualifying for **enrollment** into the trial or who are otherwise unwilling or unable to enroll. rt: **compassionate use, expanded availability, parallel patient, parallel study, treatment IND**

parallel treatment design *n* - A **treatment design** in which **treatment units** (usually persons) are **assigned** to receive only one of the **study treatments** and, hence, one in which the **treatment groups** are comprised of different treatment units; **noncrossover design** syn: **noncrossover treatment design** ant: **crossover treatment design**

parallel treatments *n* - **Treatments** arranged and administered in a **parallel treatment design**.

parallel trial *n* - 1. A **trial** having a **parallel treatment design**. 2. A **trial** carried out in relation to another, usually at the same time.

parameter *n* - [NL, fr *para-* + Gk *metron* measure] 1. A **constant** in a mathematical expression that characterizes some **population**, process, or the like and whose true value is generally unknown but can be **estimated**. 2. **observation variable** *Usage note*: Uses in the sense of defn 1 are incompatible with those in the sense of defn 2. The incompatibility should be avoided by restricting use to the sense of defn 1 and by using **variable** in the sense of defn 2. Most of the confusion arises in clinical medicine in which "parameter" is commonly used as a synonym for variable.

parametric *adj* - 1. Of or relating to a **parameter**. 2. Of or relating to assumptions required in relation to a statistical **analysis** of **data**. ant: **nonparametric** *Usage note*: See **nonparametric**.

parametric method *n* - A statistical method or procedure (eg, **hypothesis testing**) that is derived from or based on some process, function, or **distribution** that is defined by or dependent on a **parameter** or set of parameters. rt: **nonpara-**

metric method

parametric test *n* - [statistics] A **test of hypothesis** that requires specification of a **parameter** or set of parameters for carrying it out; a **test of hypothesis** that is not **distribution-free**. rt: **nonparametric test**

parent *n* - [ME, fr MF, fr L *parent-*, *parens* fr prp of *parere* to give birth to] One that brings forth offspring; one that rears or nurtures.

parent center *n* - 1. A **center** that gives rise to or nurtures other similar centers. 2. A center that has administrative or operational primacy over others. 3. A center having an **affiliate, associate,** or **satellite center**. rt: **lead center**

parent clinic *n* - 1. A **clinic** with one or more **affiliate, associate,** or **satellite clinics**. 2. **lead clinic**

parent institution *n* - 1. The **institution** having administrative responsibilities for a specified **study center** and associated investigators. 2. The **center** responsible for disbursing funds to other centers in a study funded under a **consortium agreement**; the institution housing such a center.

parent study *n* - A **study** having one or more **ancillary** or sub studies.

partial *adj* - [ME *parcial*, fr MF *partial*, fr ML *partialis*, fr LL, of a part, fr L *part-*, *pars* part] 1. Of or relating to part as opposed to the whole. 2. Not general.

partial correlation *n* - In **multivariate** settings, the **correlation** of one **variable** with another, with the values of others held fixed.

partial correlation coefficient *n* - The **coefficient** describing the **association** between two **variables** in a setting involving multiple variables (three or more) in which the values of those other variables are held fixed.

partial factorial *n* - **incomplete factorial**

partial factorial treatment design *n* - **incomplete factorial treatment design**

partial mask *n* - [trials] 1. A condition in which only some members of a designated class or category of people associated with a trial (eg, **patients, treaters, data collectors, readers,** or **monitors**) are **masked** to **treatment assignment** and **administration**. 2. The state of being **partially masked**. 3. A **mask** that is not **complete** in the sense of defns 1 or 2 of **complete mask**. 4. A **double mask** in which a specified subset of people are not masked, eg, the subset responsible for changing **dosages** of the assigned treatment over the course of the trial. 5. A double mask that is complete from one perspective but not from another; a mask in a trial with two or more pairs of **test** and **control treatments** in which the treatments represented in a given pair are masked one to the other, but not with respect to all other pairs, eg, an asthma trial with a **parallel treatment design** involving two or more test-control pairs of treatments in which all test and control treatments are to be administered via nasal inhalation and in which the two treatments represented by any given pair are to be dispensed from identical canisters, but in which the shape, form, or size of such canisters (and perhaps the required number of inhalations from them) for one such pair of treatments is different from that for another such pair. rt: **complete mask, nonmask, masking level**

partially balanced block *n* - 1. A **block** that is **balanced** from one perspective but not from another. 2. A **treatment assignment block** in which the **assignment ratio** is satisfied for some, but not all, of the treatments.

partially confounded *n* - [**research**] 1. A state in which an **effect** produced by one **variable** (eg, **treatment** in a **trial**) is partially obscured or accentuated because of another variable that also exerts an influence on the effect of interest; treatment in a trial is said to be partially confounded by a variable if the **distribution** of that variable is quantitatively, but not qualitatively, different by **treatment group** and the effect produced by the different **study treatments** differs as a function of that variable; eg, a situation in which the observed **treatment effect** differs by gender and where both gender groups are represented in the various treatment groups but in differing proportions. 2. A state of **complete confounding** in some, but not all, subsets of a **dataset**, eg, **treatment assignment** in a **multicenter trial** is said to be partially confounded with **clinic** if the treatment assignments issued for some clinics fail to include all study treatments represented in the trial. rt: **confounded, completely confounded** *Usage note*: There should be documented evidence of confounding, as demonstrated by the **joint distribution** of the variables considered to be confounded, when used as an explanation for an observed **result**. Avoid using as **weasel** clause.

partially masked *adj* - [**trials**] Of, relating to, or being a **partial mask**.

partially masked randomization *n* - **Partially masked treatment assignment** in which assignments are generated using **randomization** procedures. rt: **completely masked randomization** *Usage note*: See note for **completely masked treatment assignment**.

partially masked treatment assignment *n* - Any scheme in which the **treatment assignments** made or to be made in a **trial** are **masked** to some, but not to all, personnel who receive or are to receive them; not **completely masked treatment assignment**. rt: **completely masked treatment assignment** *Usage note*: See note for **completely masked treatment assignment**

partially masked trial *n* - 1. A **trial** in which some, but not all, of the **study treatments** are administered in a **single-** or **double-masked** fashion. 2. A trial in which some, but not all, of the staff in a **clinic** are masked to **treatment assignment**. rt: **completely masked trial, unmasked trial**

participant *n* - 1. One who **participates**. 2. **study participant**

participate, participated, participating, participates *v* - [L *participatus*, pp of *participare*, fr *particip-*, *particeps* participant, fr *parti-*, *pars* part + *capere* to take] To take part in; to have a part or share in something.

patient *n* - [ME *pacient*, fr MF, L *patient-*, *patiens*, fr prp of *pati* to suffer; akin to L *paene* almost, *penuria* need, Gk *pēma* suffering] 1. A person who is under medical or surgical care for some **disease** or medical condition. 2. **study patient**

patient accrual *n* - 1. The number of **patients enrolled** into a **trial**; the incremental change in the number enrolled. 2. The **rate** at which patients are being enrolled.

patient advocate *n* - 1. One who pleads the cause of a **patient** or a class of patients, especially as defined by some **disease** or health condition, in relation to some issue, principle, or process. 2. One who represents a class of patients, as defined by a designated disease or health condition, in some forum or setting. 3. One who is selected or appointed to serve in some group or body associated with a **trial** ostensibly as a representative of or advocate for patients **enrolled** or to be enrolled into a trial, eg, such a person serving on the **treatment effects monitoring committee**; **lay representative**; **nonhealth professional**. *Usage note*: Not generally recommended in the sense of defn 3, except perhaps in circumstances in which the person has been designated by or chosen from a bona fide patient advocacy group and in which advocacy, in the true sense of the term, is expected. Otherwise use other terms, such as **lay representative** or **nonhealth professional** to avoid the label of advocacy when not appropriate or when the implication is that only the person carrying the label is an **advocate** of patients.

patient brochure *n* - **patient information booklet**

patient chart *n* - 1. A collection of **data** and written notes pertaining to the care or **treatment** of a **patient**, especially in relation to a current episode of **disease** and treatment. 2. **patient record**

patient clinic visit *n* - 1. A **visit** made to a **clinic** by a **patient** for care or **treatment**. 2. A visit of a **study patient** to a clinic for evaluation, **treatment**, or **followup** in relation to a **study**. rt: **study clinic visit**

patient close-out *n* - [**trials**] 1. The separation of a **patient** from a **trial**, especially a planned separation such as occurs at the close of **followup**. 2. The process of separating **patients** from a **trial** at the end of the **treatment and followup stage**; typically marked by termination of **scheduled followup**, cessation of **treatment** as practiced under the **treatment protocol**, and, where applicable and appropriate, transfer of care responsibilities to some other person or facility.

patient close-out examination *n* - [**trials**] The **final patient examination** or series of such examinations performed in relation to **patient close-out**.

patient close-out followup visit *n* - A **followup visit** made by a **patient** to a **study clinic** for **data collection** and for completion of specified procedures related to **patient close-out**. rt: **patient close-out examination**

patient close-out stage *n* - 1. The close of **followup** for a **patient**. 2. The **stage** of a **trial** involving **close-out** of followup, **patient close-out stage of trial**.

patient close-out stage of trial *n* - The **stage of trial** characterized by **patient close-out**, especial-

ly that stage in a trial with a **common closing date**.

patient compliance *n* - The degree to which a **patient** follows a prescribed set of procedures or routines; synonymous with **treatment adherence** when the procedures or routines in question are those concerned with administration of a **patient's assigned treatment**. rt: **adherence**

patient contact *n* - [**trials**] **Direct** or **indirect contact** of a **patient** by personnel involved in conducting a **trial**, usually those of a **clinic**; **direct patient contact**, **indirect patient contact**.

patient enrollment *n* - The act of **enrolling** a **patient** (**treatment unit**) into a **study** as defined by some action or event. Typically, enrollment in a **trial** is considered to occur on completion of a designated **baseline visit** or on some act, eg, opening an envelope containing treatment assignment, receipt of the treatment assignment from a **coordinating center**, or on initiation of treatment.

patient enrollment period *n* - The **time period** planned for or the actual period required for **enrollment** of **patients** into a **study**. syn: patient recruitment period

patient enrollment process *n* - The process and related procedures needed for or associated with **enrollment** of **patients**; in **randomized trials** includes all **examinations** and **data collection** procedures associated with **prerandomization** and **randomization visits**.

patient examination *n* - 1. An **examination** of a **patient** performed by a physician or related personnel in relation to a **clinic visit** or hospitalization for the purpose of assessing the condition of the patient or diagnosing **disease**, or for the treatment or care of the patient. 2. [**trials**] Any such examination performed in relation to the **study protocol**, including those performed for determining **eligibility** for **enrollment**, for assigning or administering **study treatments**, and for generating **baseline** and **followup data**; **study examination**. rt: **examination**, **patient clinic visit**

patient followup *n* - [**trials**] A process involving periodic **contact** with **patients enrolled** in a **trial** for the purpose of administering the **assigned treatment**(s), observing the effects of treatment(s), modifying the course of treatment(s), or for collecting required **followup data**. rt: **followup**

patient home visit *n* - [**trials**] A **visit** to the home of a **patient** by **clinic** personnel or their agents for the purpose of care or **treatment** of the **patient** or for **data collection**.

patient identification number *n* - A unique sequence of numbers or numbers and letters used to identify a **patient**; **study identification number**

patient information booklet *n* - A **booklet** prepared for **distribution** to **patients** in relation to some **event** (eg, on **diagnosis** of a **disease**) or as a prelude to some possible action (eg, **enrollment** in a **study**). Such booklets, as used in **trials** as a prelude to enrollment, are used primarily to help ensure **informed consents**. Content, when used in that context, includes details on the nature of the trial and its underlying rationale, on the **treatments** being tested and their respective potential **risks** and **benefits**, on procedures to be performed and reasons for them, and on the **frequency** of **data collection visits** and time required for such visits. syn: patient brochure

patient mask *n* - [**trials**] A **mask** imposed on **patients** to keep them from learning the **treatment** to which they are **assigned**. rt: **physician mask**

patient monitoring *v* - **Monitoring** for changes in the health status of a **patient**, eg, monitoring for evidence of **adverse effects** of a **treatment** administered; **patient safety monitoring**.

patient population *n* - 1. The **population** of **patients enrolled** into a **study**; **study population**. 2. The general population of patients, similar to the one studied, and to which inferences and generalizations are made.

patient record *n* - 1. The cumulative collection of documents and reports relating to the **diagnosis**, care, and **treatment** of a **patient** by a physician or care facility. 2. **patient chart**

patient recruitment *n* - The process of identifying suitable patients for **enrollment** into a **study**.

patient recruitment goal *n* - The number of **patients** to be **enrolled** into a **study** as set prior to the start of the study or during **recruitment** by a **sample size calculation** or pragmatic considerations; not to be confused with **patient recruitment quota**.

patient recruitment period *n* - **patient enrollment period**

patient recruitment quota *n* - A specification, usually set before or shortly after the start of **patient recruitment** for a **study** or **trial**, that indicates the proportionate mix of patients to be enrolled with regard to some characteristic, trait, or condition (eg, the number of males versus females). *Usage note*: See **recruitment quota**.

patient recruitment stage *n* - [**trials**] The **stage** concerned primarily with **patient recruitment**. See **stage of trial** for the various stages of a trial.

patient safety monitoring *n* - [**trials**] 1. Any ongoing process of reviewing accumulated **outcome data** for groups of **patients** in a **trial** to determine if a designated **treatment** procedure should be altered or stopped; **treatment effects monitoring**. 2. The process of watching for treatment effects in an individual patient. *Usage note*: Usage in the sense of defn 2 not recommended; use **patient monitoring** instead.

pay *adj* - Leading to **pay**.

pay *n* - Something paid for a service rendered or for some other reason.

payline *n* - A term used in connection with National Institutes of Health **grants** to indicate the **priority score** required on an approved **application** to permit payment; a function of the number of approved applications received by an institute, the distribution of priority scores across applications for that institute, and the amount of money available for new research initiatives by that institute.

PC *n* - **personal computer**

Pearson, Egon Sharpe - (1895 - 1980) English-born and educated mathematician and statistician; son of Karl Pearson; responsible for what came to be known as **Neyman-Pearson theory** (not regarded by Pearson as a theory; seen by him more as a collection of principles for addressing statistical and, more broadly, scientific problems) developed through interaction with Jerzy Neyman, many over long distances via letter and occasional meetings.

Pearson, Karl - (1857 - 1936) English scientist who made numerous contributions to statistics through his work on Darwinian theory of evolution and genetics; founder and editor of Biometrika and director of Francis Galton Laboratory.

Pearson product-moment correlation coefficient
n - A **measure** of the **linear relationship** between two **metric variables**, typically denoted by the letter r when **estimated** from **observed data** and by ρ when expressed as a **parameter**. A **correlation** is said to be **positive** if the value for the one variable (or member of a pair of **observations**) increases as the other increases and is said to be **negative** if the value for the one variable increases as the other decreases. The two variables (or pairs of observations) are said to have a perfect correlation if the value for the one variable can be predicted without error from the other. The variables are said to be uncorrelated (ie, ρ or r is zero or near zero) if the value of one variable is of no value in predicting the other. rt: **association**, **dependence**, **relationship**

peer *n* - [ME, fr MF *per*, fr *per*, adj, equal, fr L *par*] One that is of equal standing with another; **compeer**

peer review *n* - 1. A **review** performed by one's **peers**, especially such a review as performed at the request of a third party to judge the adequacy of the work. 2. A critical review of one's **manuscript** performed by a person or persons selected by an editor of a **journal** to assess suitability for **publication** in that journal. 3. A critical review of a **funding application** by peers of the applicant, as requested by a **funding agency**, to provide advice to the funding agency as to suitability for funding.

peer review journal *n* - A **journal** that practices **peer review** (defn 3) in relation to the **manuscripts** it receives for possible **publication**; typically, manuscripts accepted for consideration are sent to one or more reviewers selected by editors of the journal, reviews are returned in writing to the **author**(s) along with advice as to suitability for publication; written reviews used by the editors to reach a decision about publication and as a basis for communication with the author(s) about suggested and required changes necessary for acceptance if the manuscript is not rejected.

percent *n* - One part of a whole expressed in hundredths; **percentage**. *Usage note*: Subject to considerable misuse in everyday vernacular. Baseball batting averages are thought of as percentages, but in fact are **proportions** multiplied by 1,000. The most flagrant abuses arise in advertising and merchandising (*20% off, buy now and save 30%*). The notion of **percent** or **percentage** is meaningful only in relation to a defined base. Still worse is the practice of presenting, in effect, the ratio of two numbers, both having a vague or ill-defined base, as a percentage, as in *more than a 200% savings*.

percentage *n* - 1. A **proportion** expressed per one hundred units. 2. The result obtained by multiplying a proportion by 100. *Usage note*: See **percent**.

percentage distribution *n* - A **frequency distribution** in which counts for the various **class intervals** represented in the distribution are expressed as **percentages** of the total count. rt: **relative number**, **relative frequency**

percentile *n* - [prob fr *percent* + *-ile* (as in *quartile*)] A value designating the **percent** of a **frequency distribution** equal to or below that value, eg, someone scoring in the 95th percentile of a test has a score equal to or exceeding that of 95% of those taking the test.

performance *n* - The execution of an action; the ability to perform.

performance monitoring *n* - The act of or an instance of reviewing **performance** of an ongoing activity to determine if corrective action is necessary. syn (not recommended): **data monitoring**, **safety monitoring**, **data and safety monitoring** rt: **administrative review**, **efficacy monitoring**, **multiple looks**, **safety monitoring**, **treatment effects monitoring**

performance monitoring *v* - 1. **Monitoring** (defn 2) of **performance** of some activity (or set of activities) at periodic time points over the course of the activity to determine whether the activity should be allowed to continue unaltered; in the context of **trials**, such monitoring as summarized in a **performance monitoring report**; such monitoring as part of ongoing **quality assurance**; in the context of **multicenter trials**, monitoring relating to the performance of the various **centers** in the trials. 2. **performance review** (defn 1) rt: **administrative review**, **treatment effects monitoring** *Usage note*: Not to be confused with forms of monitoring involving evaluations of **treatment results** as in **treatment effects monitoring**, **safety monitoring**, or **efficacy monitoring**. Note also that defns 1 and 2 have different operational meanings and should not be used interchangeably.

Use **performance monitoring** when the interim review is part of a planned ongoing process; use **performance review** when it is not. See also note for **administrative review**.

performance monitoring committee *n* - 1. A **committee** charged with **performance monitoring**. 2. A committee that reviews **performance monitoring reports** and takes or recommends appropriate corrective actions when indicated to deal with identified performance problems. rt: **treatment effects and performance monitoring committee**

performance monitoring report *n* - A **report** summarizing **performance** of a **center** or centers and used for **performance monitoring**. In the case of **multicenter trials**, typically prepared by the **data coordinating center** and reviewed by the full **research group**, **steering committee**, or some other body or **committee** having responsibility for performance monitoring. rt: **treatment effects monitoring report**

performance review *n* - [**trials**] 1. An **ad hoc interim review** (defn 2) of **performance** of activities or functions to determine whether the trial should be stopped or allowed to continue unaltered; eg, one done to determine whether the **rate** of **enrollment** is adequate to justify continuation of the trial. 2. **performance monitoring** (defn 1) 3. **administrative review** (defn 1) *Usage note*: Not to be confused with reviews involving **treatment results**. Note also that defns 1 and 3 have different operational meanings than defn 2. Use **performance monitoring** when the interim review is part of a planned ongoing process. See also note for **administrative review**.

period *n* - [ME *pariode*, fr MF *periode*, fr ML, L & Gk; ML *periodus* period of time, punctuation mark, fr L & Gk; L, rhetorical period, fr Gk *periodos* circuit, period of time, rhetorical period, fr *peri* + *hodos* way] 1. The span of time needed for completion of a cycle, a series of events, or an activity. 2. A portion of time demarcated by some recurring event or phenomenon, as a **circadian rhythm**.

period prevalence *n* - **Prevalence** over a defined **period** of **time**. rt: **lifetime prevalence**, **point prevalence**

peripheral *adj* - Auxiliary or supplemental to.

peripheral *n* - A **device** connected to a **computer** for **input** or **output** or for performing other auxiliary functions.

peripheral equipment *n* - Any **device** or piece of equipment connected to a **computer** used for **input** or **output** or for performing other auxiliary functions.

permutation *n* - [ME *permutacioun* exchange, transformation, fr MF *permutation*, fr L *permutation-*, *permutatio*, fr *permutatus*, pp of *permutare*] An ordered arrangement of a set of numbers, alphabetic characters, or objects.

permute, permuted, permuting, permutes *v* - [ME *permuten* to exchange, fr MF or L; MF *permuter*, fr L *permutare*, fr *per-* + *mutare* to change] 1. To change the order or arrangement of. 2. To arrange in all possible ways. 3. The act or process of changing the ordering of a set of numbers, alphabetic characters, or objects.

permuted block *n* - A **block** of **treatment assignments** representing one of the possible **permutations** of the assignments. The **number** of different arrangements of blocks of **n** assignments involving **t** different treatments and r_1 assignments to trt_1, r_2 assignments to trt_2, ⋯, r_{t-1} assignments to trt_{t-1}, and r_t assignments to trt_t is $n!/[r_1!r_2! \cdots r_{t-1}!r_t!]$, eg, $4!/(2!2!) = 6$ for a trial involving two **study treatments** arranged in blocks of size 4 (ie, ABAB, ABBA, AABB, BABA, BAAB, and BBAA).

permuted block treatment design *n* - A **design** involving permuted **blocks** of **treatment assignments**; orderings within blocks determined in some **systematic** or **random** fashion. For example, a **trial** involving three **treatments** A, B, and C, an **assignment ratio** of 1:1:1, six blocks each of size 3, and random ordering of the assignments within blocks might have the following blocks: Block 1: BCA; Block 2: ACB; Block 3: CBA; Block 4: BCA; Block 5: CAB; Block 6: CBA.

person *n* - [ME, fr OF *persone*, fr L *persona* actor's mask, character in a play, person, prob fr Etruscan *phersu* mask] human being; individual

person-time *n* - 1. The amount of **time** a person is **observed** for a designated **event** or **outcome measure**; time expressed in a **unit** consistent with the observation schedule; typically hour, day, week, or year (**person-year**). 2. The total elapsed time for a person starting from a designated point (eg, entry into a **study**) to occurrence of some **event** or **outcome** or to the present or to the end of the study in the absence of such an event or outcome. 3. [**followup studies**] The sum of times (defn 2) for the aggregate of persons represented in a defined **followup cohort**; referred to as **person-time experience**; summing based on the assumption that times are additive, ie, that a person observed for two units of time (eg, 2 years) provides the same amount of information as two persons each observed for one unit of time (eg, 1 year each).

person-time experience *n* - The sum of individual **person-times** for all persons at **risk** for the **event** or **observation** of interest.

person-year *n* - **Person-time** expressed in years; as opposed to some smaller or larger time unit. rt: **person-time experience**

personal *adj* - [ME, fr MF, fr LL *personalis*, fr L *persona*] Of or relating to a **person**; intended for exclusive use of a person; private.

personal computer (PC) *n* - 1. A small **computer** having a **microprocessor**; **microcomputer** (defn 2). 2. A desktop or portable computer.

personnel *n* - [F, fr G *personale*, *personal*, fr ML *personale*, fr LL, neut of *personalis* personal] A body of persons employed by or active in an organization, business, or service.

phase *n* - [NL *phasis*, fr Gk appearance of a star, phase of the moon, fr *phainein* to show (middle voice, to appear)] A distinguished part in a course, development, or cycle.

phase I drug trial *n* - 1. Typically the first stage in testing a **new drug** in human beings. Performed as part of an approved **Investigational New Drug Application** under **Food and Drug Administration** guidelines [Pines, 1980;[124] Food and Drug Administration, 1977[51]]; done to provide information on metabolism, pharmacologic action, and **safety** of the drug, as in a **dose escalation design**; usually not **controlled** (defn 2), ie, done without benefit of a **concurrently enrolled comparison group**. 2. **phase I trial** *Usage note*: See **phase of trial** for comment.

phase I/II drug trial *n* - A **trial** of a **new drug** designed or considered to provide preliminary information on **safety** and **efficacy**. *Usage note*: See **phase of trial** for comment.

phase I/II trial *n* - 1. **phase I/II drug trial** 2. Broadly, a **trial** involving application of a new **treatment** to human beings and conducted to

generate preliminary information on **safety** and **efficacy**. *Usage note*: See **phase of trial** for comment.

phase I trial *n* - 1. **phase I drug trial** 2. Broadly, a **trial** involving the first applications of a new **treatment** to human beings and conducted to generate preliminary information on **safety**. *Usage note*: See **phase of trial** for comment.

phase II drug trial *n* - Usually the second stage in testing a **new drug** in human beings. Performed as part of an approved **Investigational New Drug Application** under **Food and Drug Administration** guidelines [Pines, 1980;[124] Food and Drug Administration, 1977[51]]. Generally carried out on persons having the **disease** or condition of interest. The main purpose is to provide preliminary information on **efficacy** of the **drug** and to provide additional information on **safety** and associated **side effects**. May be designed to include a **control treatment** and **random assignment** of patients to **treatment**. *Usage note*: See **phase of trial** for comment.

phase II trial *n* - 1. **phase II drug trial** 2. Broadly, a **trial** involving a second stage of testing of a new **treatment** in human beings and done to generate preliminary information on **efficacy** and added information on **safety**. *Usage note*: See **phase of trial** for comment.

phase III drug trial *n* - Usually the third and final stage in testing a **new drug** in human beings in relation to a **New Drug Application**. Performed as part of an approved **Investigational New Drug Application** under **Food and Drug Administration** guidelines [Pines, 1980;[124] Food and Drug Administration, 1977[51]]. Concerned with assessment of **dosage** effects, **efficacy**, and **safety** and aimed at providing information for **labeling** in relation to use in the **clinical** setting. Usually designed to include a **control treatment** and **random assignment** to treatment. Once this phase is completed (or nearly completed) the drug manufacturer or **sponsor** (defn 5) may request permission to market the drug for the indication covered in the testing by submission of a **New Drug Application** to the Food and Drug Administration. *Usage note*: See **phase of trial** for comment.

phase III trial *n* - 1. **phase III drug trial** 2. Broadly, any **controlled trial** of a largely heretofore untested **treatment** intended primarily to generate information on **efficacy** measured against a **control treatment**. *Usage note*: See **phase of trial** for comment.

phase IV drug trial *n* - A **controlled trial** of a **drug** for a given indication performed after approval of the **New Drug Application** for that indication; typically done under circumstances approximating real-world conditions and usually with a **clinical event** as a basis for **sample size calculation** and providing for extended treatment (when appropriate) and **long-term followup** with **efficacy** and **safety** of the drug being measured against a designated **control treatment**; done with **Food and Drug Administration** approval [Pines, 1980;[124] Food and Drug Administration, 1977[51]]. rt: **post-marketing surveillance** *Usage note*: Not to be confused with **post-marketing surveillance**. Such surveillance is usually performed by observational procedures devoid of designed **concurrent comparison groups**, whereas the phase IV drug trial usually has such a comparison group, as formed by **randomization** or some other **assignment scheme**. See **phase of trial** for additional comments.

phase IV trial *n* - 1. **phase IV drug trial** 2. Broadly, any **controlled trial** involving a **clinical event** as the **primary outcome measure** and providing for extended treatment (when appropriate) and **long-term followup** with **efficacy** and **safety** of the **treatment** being measured against a designated **control treatment**. *Usage note*: See notes for **phase IV drug trial** and **phase of trial**.

phase of trial *n* - The **phase** of a **trial** from the perspective of the **sequence** of trials necessary for bringing a **treatment** into use; phase denoted by numerals indicative of order, usually I, II, and III; **classification** typically applied by **sponsors** (defn 4) or **investigators** in relation to trials done under an **IND** and based on **purpose** and **design**. *Usage note*: The classification is most commonly used in regard to **drug trials** done under an **IND** for a possible **NDA**, but sometimes used more broadly, eg, in uses in the NIH Guideline on the Inclusion of Women and Minorities as Subjects in Clinical Research[114] generated for implementing the Congressional mandate regarding **valid analysis**. The lines of demarcation separating phases are ill-defined, a fact made more evident by use, in recent years, of crossed phase descriptors (I/II and II/III). Hence, two trials, largely similar in purpose and

design can carry different phase labels. The phase characterization in relation to drug development implies order. Hence, there is the expectation that phase I trials are carried out first, followed by phase II trials and those followed by phase III trials. However in reality, the cross section of trials underway at a given point in time for a given drug is likely to span two, if not all three, phases. The amount of overlap will depend on the nature of the disease being treated and on the perceived promise of the drug in that regard. The overlap is likely to be greatest for drugs intended for use in life-limiting diseases with few established effective treatments, eg, AIDS. Further, use of a phase label does not imply existence of lower order phases. For example, a phase III trial may be undertaken in some cases in the absence of phase I or II trials. Also not to be confused with **stage of trial**. Stage of trial pertains to a class of activities within a trial as it proceeds from beginning to end.

phasic *adj* - Of or relating to **phase**; characterized by a variety of parts or phases.

phi *n* - [MGk, fr Gk *phei*] The 21st letter of the **Greek alphabet**, uppercase Φ, lowercase φ.

PHS *n* - **Public Health Service**

physician *n* - [ME *fisicien*, fr OF, fr *fisique* medicine] A doctor of **medicine**; a person skilled in the art of healing.

physician mask *n* - [trials] A **mask** imposed on **physicians** responsible for administering **treatments** intended to deny them knowledge of **treatment assignment**. rt: **patient mask**

pi *n* - [MGk, fr Gk *pei*, of Sem origin; akin to Heb *pē* pe] The 16th letter of the **Greek alphabet**, uppercase Π, lowercase π.

PI *n* - **principal investigator** *Usage note*: See **principal investigator**.

pictogram *n* - [ISV *picto-* (fr L *pictus*) + -gram] **pictograph**

pictograph *n* - [L *pictus* + E -o- + -*graph*] A **diagram** representing **statistical data** in pictorial form; frequently used in popular media for display; not recommended for scientific presentations or publications because of the possibility of distortion or misrepresentation.

pie *adj* - Round in shape.

pie chart *n* - **circle graph**

pilot *adj* - 1. Serving as a guiding device or procedure. 2. An operation or activity undertaken as a prelude to a more extensive operation or activity, such as a **pilot study**.

pilot *n* - [MF *pilote*, fr It *pilota*, alter of *pedota*, fr (assumed) MGk *pēdōtēs*, fr Gk *pēda* steering oars, pl of *pēdon* oar; akin to Gk *pod-*, *pous* foot] 1. Guide or leader. 2. **pilot study**; **pilot trial** 3. **pilot test**

pilot study *n* - A small preliminary **study** performed as a possible prelude to a **full-scale study** and intended to provide training and experience in carrying out such a study, if undertaken. rt: **demonstration study, feasibility study, pilot test, pilot trial**

pilot test *n* - 1. **pilot study** 2. **test run**; **pretest**; **dry run**

pilot trial *n* - A small preliminary **trial** performed as a possible prelude to a **full-scale trial** and intended to provide training and experience in carrying out such a trial, if undertaken. rt: **demonstration trial, feasibility trial**

pioneer *adj* - [MF *pionier*, fr OF *peonier* foot soldier, fr *peon* foot soldier, fr ML *pedon-*, *pedo*] original; earliest; first

pioneer drug *n* - 1. The first of a new class of **drug**. 2. An old (in the sense of time) drug, especially one predating current FDA guidelines and regulations.

pivotal *adj* - Vitally important; critical. *Usage note*: Use with caution, especially in relation to one's own work and as a label of anticipation, eg, *the trial being designed will be of pivotal importance.*

pivotal study *n* - A **study** considered of critical importance in reaching some **conclusion** or for substantiating some fact or **observation**. *Usage note*: See **pivotal**.

pivotal trial *n* - 1. A **trial** considered of critical importance in establishing or substantiating the usefulness of a **treatment**. 2. A **phase III** or **phase IV drug trial** intended to show or that shows a **drug** used for a given **indication** to be **safe** and **effective**. rt: **licensure trial**

PLA *n* - **Product License Application**

placebo *adj* - 1. Of or relating to the use or administration of a **placebo**. 2. Of or relating to something considered to be useless or ineffective. *Usage note*: Limit use to the sense of defn 1. Avoid nonsensical uses such as arise when the term serves as an adjective for patient or group, as in **placebo patient** or **placebo group**; use **placebo-assigned** or **placebo-treated** instead. See also notes for **placebo** and **placebo patient**.

placebo *n* - [ME, fr L, I shall please, fr *placēre* to please; the first word of the first antiphon of the service for the dead, I shall please the Lord in the land of the living, fr Roman Catholic vespers] 1. A pharmacologically **inactive substance** given as a substitute for an **active substance**, especially when the person taking or receiving it is not informed whether it is an **active** or **inactive substance**. 2. **placebo treatment** (defn 1) 3. A sugar-coated pill made of lactose or some other pharmacologically inert substance. 4. Any medication considered to be useless, especially one administered in pill form. 5. **nil treatment** 6. An ineffective treatment. rt: **double placebo, homeopathic dose, multiple placebo, placebo treatment, sham, sham procedure** *Usage note*: Subject to varying use. Avoid in the sense of defns 4, 5, and 6. Not to be confused with **sham**; see note for that entry. The use of a placebo should not be construed to imply the absence of treatment, as in designs involving **null treatment**. Virtually all trials involve some care requirements. Investigators conducting them are obligated to meet care requirements, regardless of treatment assignment and whether masked or not. For example, that requirement in the case of the University Group Diabetes Program[156] obligated investigators to do their best in maintaining all patients enrolled on standard antidiabetic diets in addition to their assigned treatments. As a result, **control treatments** involving use of placebos are best thought of as **regimens** with placebos substituting for elements of the regimens. Labels, such as **placebo patient** or **placebo group**, obscure the true nature of the treatment process and create the erroneous impression that patients assigned to receive a placebo are left untreated when that is true of only one element of the regimen. Generic labels of this sort are wrong in the literal sense of usage (there is no such being as a placebo patient except, perhaps, for one coated with lactose) and have the potential for misleading when an assignment involving administration of a placebo also involves administration of other treatments (as in a **vaccine trial** where all infants enrolled receive vaccines for diphtheria and tetanus in addition to a pertussis vaccine or matching placebo).

placebo effect *n* - 1. The **effect** produced by a **placebo**; assessed or measured against the effect expected or observed in the absence of any **treatment**. 2. The effect produced by an **inactive control treatment**, especially one involving use of a placebo. 3. The effect produced by a **control treatment** considered to be **nil** or ineffective. 4. An effect attributed to a placebo; an effect attributable to a placebo. rt: **sham effect** *Usage note*: Limit usage to settings involving the actual use of a placebo. Avoid in the sense of defns 2 and 3 when the control treatment does not involve use of a placebo.

placebo group *n* - 1. **placebo-assigned group** 2. **placebo-treated group** 3. A group not receiving or not having received any **treatment**. *Usage note*: Avoid for the reasons stated in the usage note for **placebo patient**.

placebo lead-in period *n* - [trials] A **lead-in period** in which persons receive a **placebo treatment** (as in the Coronary Drug Project [Coronary Drug Project Research Group, 1973][30]) for a time prior to **enrollment** and **treatment assignment**; typically done to help identify **compliant** individuals. See Brittain and Wittes [1990][16] for discussion of the usefulness of such strategies. syn: **placebo run-in period** rt: **lead-in period, shakedown period**

placebo patient *n* - 1. **placebo-assigned patient** 2. **placebo-treated patient** 3. A **study patient** who does not receive any **treatment**. *Usage note*: Literally, a sugar-coated patient, ala defn 3 for **placebo**. Use **placebo-assigned patient** or **placebo-treated patient** for uses in the sense of defns 1 and 2, respectively; avoid in the sense of defn 3.

placebo period *n* - [trials] A **period** of time in which a person (**treatment unit**), to be **enrolled** or already enrolled, receives a **placebo** (usually administered either in **single-** or **double-masked** fashion); when such a period precedes **treatment assignment**, usually referred to as **placebo lead-in period** or as **placebo run-in period** and used to aid in the selection of **compliant** persons or to facilitate the assessment of **eligibility**. Periods occurring after **enrollment** may arise in relation to **washouts** or cessations of **assigned treatment** in relation to episodes of intercurrent illnesses. rt: **lead-in period, shakedown period**

placebo reactor *n* - 1. A person who reports **side effects** normally associated with the **test treatment** while receiving a **placebo**. 2. A person who reacts to a **placebo** as indicated by symptoms or complaints similar to those experienced with the **test treatment**(s).

placebo run-in period *n* - **placebo lead-in period**

placebo treatment *n* - 1. A **treatment** involving the use of a **placebo**. 2. **placebo-control treatment** (defn 1) 3. An ineffective or useless **treatment** used as a **control treatment** (not recommended usage). rt: **control treatment, sham treatment** *Usage note*: Subject to misuse when used in the sense of defn 3. Use of the adjective modifier **placebo** should be reserved for settings in which a placebo is actually used, as in the sense of defns 1 or 2 for **placebo**.

placebo treatment effect *n* - 1. The **effect** produced, or capable of being produced, by a **placebo treatment** (defn 1). 2. The effect produced, or capable of being produced, by an **inactive control treatment**; placebo treatment (defn 3). *Usage note*: Subject to misuse when used in the sense of defn 2. Use of the adjective modifier **placebo** should be reserved for settings in which a placebo is actually used, as in the sense of defns 1 or 2 for **placebo**.

placebo washout *n* - Administration of a **placebo** for a defined **period** of time following administration of a **test treatment** to allow time for re-establishment of a **baseline**. Common in **crossover trials** following each treatment and prior to administration of the next one; usually administered in **single-** or **double-masked** fashion. rt: **washout period**

placebo-assigned *adj* - 1. Of, related to, or being **assigned** to receive a **placebo treatment**. 2. Of, related to, or being assigned to receive an **inactive treatment**. rt: **placebo-treated** *Usage note*: Use only in the sense of defn 1; avoid as an adjective modifier in the sense of defn 2 except when a **placebo** (defns 1 or 2) is used. See **placebo treatment** for added comments.

placebo-assigned group *n* - [trials] 1. The **group** of persons or **treatment units** assigned to a **placebo-control treatment** (defn 1). 2. The group of persons or treatment units assigned to an **inactive control treatment**. rt: **placebo-assigned patient, placebo-treated group** *Usage note*: Use only in the sense of defn 1; avoid in the sense of defn 2 when a **placebo** (defns 1 or

2) is not used. See **placebo treatment** for added comments.

placebo-assigned patient *n* - [**trial**] 1. A **patient assigned** to receive a **placebo treatment**. 2. A patient assigned to receive an **inactive control treatment**. rt: **placebo-assigned group, placebo-treated patient** *Usage note*: Use only in the sense of defn 1; avoid in the sense of defn 2 when a **placebo** (defns 1 or 2) is not used. See **placebo treatment** for added comments.

placebo-control treatment *n* - 1. An **inactive control treatment** involving administration of a **placebo** in **single-** or **double-masked** fashion. 2. Any **inactive control treatment**, including those not involving administration of a placebo. rt: **study treatment** *Usage note*: Use in the sense of defn 1. Avoid in the sense of defn 2 when a **placebo** is not used. See **placebo treatment** for added comments.

placebo-controlled *adj* - Of, relating to, or being **controlled** by use of a **placebo**.

placebo-controlled clinical trial *n* - 1. A **clinical trial** in which the **control treatment** involves the administration of a **placebo**. 2. A clinical trial involving an **inactive control treatment**. *Usage note*: Avoid in the sense of defn 2 except when a **placebo** (defns 1 or 2) is used. See **placebo treatment** for added comments.

placebo-controlled trial *n* - 1. A **trial** in which the **control treatment** involves the administration of a **placebo**. 2. A trial involving an **inactive control treatment**. *Usage note*: Avoid in the sense of defn 1 except where a **placebo** (defns 1 or 2) is used. See **placebo treatment** for added comments.

placebo-treated *adj* - 1. **placebo-assigned** (defn 1) 2. Of, related to, or being **treated** with a **placebo**. 3. Of, related to, or being treated with an **inactive treatment**. rt: **placebo-assigned** *Usage note*: Use only in the sense of defn 2; avoid as an adjective modifier in the sense of defn 3 except where a **placebo** (defns 1 or 2) is used. Use **placebo-assigned** instead of **placebo-treated** when used in the sense of defn 1. See **placebo treatment** for added comments.

placebo-treated group *n* - [**trials**] 1. The group of persons or treatment assignment units receiving or that have received a **placebo** (defns 1 or 2). 2. The group of persons or treatment units that receive an **inactive control treatment**. 3. The **group** of persons or **treatment assignment units**

assigned to a **placebo-control treatment**; **placebo-assigned group**. 4. The group of persons or treatment units assigned to receive an inactive control treatment. rt: **placebo-treated patient, placebo-assigned group** *Usage note*: Subject to misuse. Use only in the sense of defn 1. Often used in the sense of defn 3 as a synonym for **placebo-assigned group** (defn 1); avoid by using **placebo-assigned group** (since there may not be a one-to-one correspondence between being placebo-assigned and being placebo-treated). Avoid in the sense of defn 4; use **placebo-assigned group** if the inactive treatment involves use of a **placebo** (defns 1 or 2). Avoid in the sense of defn 2 when a **placebo** (defns 1 or 2) is not used. See **placebo treatment** for added comments.

placebo-treated patient *n* - 1. A **patient** receiving a **placebo** (defns 1 or 2). 2. A patient receiving an **inactive control treatment**. 3. A **patient** assigned to a **placebo-control treatment**; **placebo-assigned patient**. 4. A patient assigned to an **inactive control treatment**. rt: **placebo-treated group, placebo-assigned patient** *Usage note*: Subject to misuse. Use only in the sense of defn 1. Often used in the sense of defn 3 as a synonym for **placebo-assigned patient** (defn 1); avoid by using **placebo-assigned patient** (since usually there is not a one-to-one correspondence between being placebo-assigned and being placebo-treated). Avoid in the sense of defn 2 when a **placebo** (defns 1 or 2) is not used. Avoid in the sense of defn 4; use **placebo-assigned patient** when a **placebo** (defns 1 or 2) is used. See **placebo treatment** for added comments.

plagiarism *n* - An act or an instance of **plagiarizing**; something plagiarized. *Usage note*: Use with caution as an implied or explicit charge or accusation, especially in the absence of specific factual information supporting the charge or accusation.

plagiarize, plagiarized, plagiarizing, plagiarizes *v* - 1. To steal and pass off the ideas or words of another as one's own. 2. Use of someone else's words or documents in such a way as to imply creation and ownership; use of such words or documents, especially verbatim uses, without crediting the source. 3. To present as new and original an idea or product known by the presenter to have been developed or derived from someone else. rt: **falsify** *Usage note*: See usage note for **plagiarism**.

plan *n* - [F plane, foundation, ground plan; partly fr L *planum* level ground, fr neut of *planus* level; partly fr F *planter* to plant, fix in place, fr LL *plantare*] A method for achieving an end; an orderly arrangement of parts in an overall **design**; **design**; **protocol**.

planned meta-analysis *n* - **designed meta-analysis** *Usage note*: A plan or approach is required for any analysis. Hence, all meta-analyses are planned but only some are designed. Use **designed meta-analysis** instead of **planned meta-analysis**.

platform *n* - [often attrib MF *plate-forme* diagram, map, lit flat form] Broadly, a place from which something is launched or started; in relation to **computers**, an operating system or **program** from which other programs or procedures are launched and operated.

platykurtic *adj* - Of, relating to, or concerned with a **distribution** that is less peaked and tailed than a **standard** distribution as evaluated by a **measure**, such as the **kurtosis statistic**. ant: **leptokurtic** rt: **platykurtic distribution**

platykurtic distribution *n* - A **unimodal distribution** being less peaked and tailed than a **normal distribution**; such a **distribution** having a **kurtosis statistic** less than 3. ant: **leptokurtic distribution** rt: **platykurtic**

platykurtosis *n* - Being less peaked and tailed than a standard **distribution**. ant: **leptokurtosis** rt: **kurtosis, platykurtic distribution**

play, played, playing, plays *v* - 1. To engage in an activity having a probabilistic or chance element. 2. To take a **chance**, as in a game chance or in an activity having a probabilistic or chance element. 3. To gamble or bet.

play-the-winner treatment assignment *n* - A form of **outcome adaptive treatment assignment** for **trials** involving two **study treatments** (as a **test** and **control treatment** or as two test treatments) and a **binary outcome** for determining the success or failure of the assigned treatments. In the approach, **treatment assignments** are functions of observed **outcomes**. A success (as indicated by the state of the observed outcome measure) observed for the last **treatment unit** enrolled, causes the next treatment unit to be assigned to the treatment assigned to the last

treatment unit. A failure causes the next treatment unit to be assigned to the other treatment. The approach is used to maximize the number of treatment units assigned to the better of the two treatments as determined by observed successes. The approach is limited to conditions where success or failure can be determined shortly after the initiation of treatment (eg, in a matter of hours or a few days). Based on work of Robbins [1956,[130] 1952[131]] and extended by Zelen [1969][171] with the introduction of a probabilistic element for assignments.

plot *n* - [ME, fr OE] 1. A graphic representation, as in a **chart** or **figure**. 2. A small, defined area of ground used or to be used for a specified purpose. 3. Any object, entity, or being that is divided into two or more subparts or that can be regarded as being so divided for purposes of **design** or **analysis** of an **experiment**, as in **split-plot designs**.

plot, plotted, plotting, plots *v* - 1. To make a **plot**. 2. To locate by means of **coordinates**. 3. To locate a **curve** by means of plotted points.

PMA *n* - **Pre-Market Approval Application**

PMR *n* - **proportionate mortality rate**; **proportionate mortality ratio**

PO *n* - **project office**; **project officer**

point *n* - [ME, partly fr OF, puncture, small spot, point in time or space, fr L *punctum*, fr neut of *punctus*, pp of *pungere* to prick; partly fr OF *pointe* sharp end, fr (assumed) VL *puncta*, fr L fem of *punctus*, pp] 1. A single item or element. 2. A designated time. 3. A specified position on a **measurement scale**; a unit of measurement. 4. decimal point

point estimate *n* - An **estimate** of a **parameter** characterized by a single value or point. rt: **interval estimate**

point estimation *n* - The act of arriving at a **point estimate**. rt: **interval estimation**

point of truncation *n* - The **point** at which something is **truncated**, as in **truncated data**.

point prevalence *n* - **Prevalence** at a specified **point** in **time**. rt: **period prevalence**

Poisson distribution *n* - A **probability distribution function** of the form:

$$f(x) = \frac{e^{-\mu}\mu^{x}}{x!}$$

with **variance** and **mean** equal to μ and where the **variable** x takes on nonnegative **integer** values; used as a mathematical model for low-frequency **random** or random-like **events** (eg, traffic accidents, disintegrations of atomic particles, occurrences of a rare disease) occurring over a defined interval or span of time or space. Used instead of the **binomial distribution** for **sample size calculations** in **trials** hypothesized to have low **event rates**.

Poisson distribution

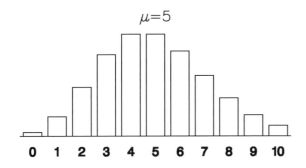

μ=5

Poisson process *n* - A **random** or random-like process producing **counts** of **events** that have a **Poisson distribution**; a process **continuous** in time or space such that the **probability** of a specified **event** during an appropriately small time interval, denoted by Δ, is approximated by αΔ, where α denotes the **event rate** and where the probability of a second event in the time interval is negligible and the probability of the event in the time interval is not dependent on what happened before.

Poisson, Simeon Denis - (1781 - 1840) French probabilist and mathematician; primary work was in the area of mathematical physics; work in **probability** was in the tradition of Laplace with emphasis on the behavior of **means** based on large numbers.

policy board *n* - **advisory-review committee**

policy committee *n* - **advisory-review committee**

policy-advisory board *n* - **advisory-review committee**.

policy-advisory committee *n* - **advisory-review committee**

poly- *prefix* - [ME, fr L, fr Gk, fr *polys*; akin to OE *full* full] 1. many; several; **multi-**; much   2. Containing an indefinite number, but more than one, of a specified substance or entity.

polychotomous variable *n* - A **discrete variable** that may assume two or more values.

polygon *n* - [LL *polygonum*, fr Gk *polygōnon*, fr neut of *polygōnos* polygonal, fr *poly-* + *gōnia* angle] A closed shape or figure defined by a series of three or more straight connecting lines, eg, a **frequency polygon**.

polynomial *n* - [*poly-* + *-nomial* (as in binomial)] 1. An algebraic expression consisting of the sum of two or more terms, each consisting of a **constant** multiplier of one or more **variables** raised, in general, to nonnegative integer powers, eg, a polynomial of **degree** n in a single real variable is of the general form: $a_0x^n + a_1x^{n-1} + a_2x^{n-2} + \cdots + a_{n-1}x^1 + a_nx^0$, where a_0, a_1, $\cdots$, a_{n-1}, and a_n are real numbers, $a_0 \neq 0$, and **n** is a positive integer.   2. A mathematical expression of two or more terms, eg, $a + bx_1 + cx_2$.

pool *n* - [F *poule*, lit, hen, fr OF, fem of *poul* cock] An aggregation (people, elements, or objects) for some common purpose or end.

pool, pooled, pooling, pools *v* - 1. [general] To combine for a common aim or end.   [**data analysis**] 2. The act or process of combining **data** collected in separate but similar studies for **analysis**, as in a **meta-analysis**.   3. The act or process of combining data from different **clinics** in a **multicenter trial**.

pooled estimate *n* - An **estimate** of a **parameter** derived by combining two or more sets of **data**.

population *n* - [LL *population-*, *populatio*, fr L *populus*] 1. A **group** or set of persons, entities, objects, or items, hypothetical or real, from which **samples** are taken or that serves as the basis for **inferences** and conclusions.   2. The total number of such persons, entities, objects, or items in a defined area or setting.

population controls *n* - **Controls** chosen from a defined **population** by **sampling** or by some other means, eg, in a **case-control study**, controls chosen from a defined community or geographic area corresponding to that from which cases were drawn.

population mean *n* - The true **arithmetic mean** of a **variable** as defined, given, or observed for an entire **population**; generally not known and, hence, a mathematical abstraction, except under circumstances in which the population is **finite** and all its values are known. Traditionally denoted by the Greek letter mu, μ, and estimated by the **sample mean**. rt: **expected value, population parameter**

population parameter *n* - A **parameter**, such as the **mean** or **variance**, of a specified **population**; generally not known and hence a mathematical abstraction, except under circumstances in which the population is **finite** and all its are known. Traditionally denoted by some Greek letter, such as μ for the **population mean** and σ for the population **standard deviation**, and estimated from observed **samples** drawn from the population. rt: **expected value, population mean, parameter**

population-based *adj* - Of, relating to, or being of a defined **population** or having a defined population base.

portrait *adj* - Of or relating to an **orientation** of a **page**, photograph, or painted material to be higher than wide. ant: **landscape**

portrait *n* - [MF, fr pp of *portraire*] [general] A pictorial representation (eg, a painting or photograph) of a person, especially of a person's face or face and upper body; usually oriented along the short **axis** of the canvas or sheet on which it is displayed so as to be higher than wide. [printed **document** or **graphic**] Visual material intended to be viewed, interpreted, or read along the short **axis** of the **page**; **portrait page orientation**. rt: **landscape**

portrait page orientation *n* - A **page** layout in which the majority of the printed and visual information is arrayed on the short axis of the page. ant: **landscape page orientation** rt: **portrait**

positive *adj* - [ME, fr ME *postif*, fr L *positivus*, fr *positus*] 1. Real and numerically greater than zero and opposite in sign to a **negative number**. 2. Denoting the presence of something; not **nil**. 3. Something real; not fictitious. 4. Affirming the presence of the organism or condition in question. 5. Something active and effective. 6. Having or expressing actual existence or quality; not speculative. ant: **negative**

positive *n* - 1. Having a numerical value greater than zero, as with a positive **difference**. 2. A reply or response that indicates **assent**, acceptance, affirmation, or acknowledgement, such as the declaratives *yes, correct, right,* or *affirmative*. 3. Having the property of being real (not fictitious or **false**) or of being active and effective, as a **positive control**. 4. Being in the direction of numerical values greater than zero, as in **positive skew**.

positive control *adj* - 1. Of or relating to an **active control** that produces or is capable of producing a **positive effect**. 2. Of or relating to a **control** that has an effect that is **positive**. ant: **negative control** rt: **active control**

positive control treatment *n* - 1. A **control treatment** that is intended to produce or that produces a **positive treatment effect**. 2. An **active control treatment** that has or is expected to have a positive treatment effect, eg, a **control treatment** involving use of suboptimal doses of the **test treatment** as in the use of a fixed dose of insulin in the University Group Diabetes Program [University Group Diabetes Program Research Group, 1970a][156] as a positive control for the test treatment involving varying doses of insulin, as required to reduce blood glucose levels to a specified limit. 3. Any form of **treatment** administered in the context of a **clinical trial** that has the potential of producing a **positive treatment effect** (defn 1), whether or not in accordance with the **study protocol**. 4. A control treatment that has or is expected to have an effect that is opposite to the one produced by a **negative control treatment**. ant: **negative control treatment** rt: **active control treatment**

positive correlation *n* - 1. A **correlation coefficient** with a **positive** sign. 2. A **relationship** between two **variables** in which the higher values of one variable are associated with the higher values of the other variable. ant: **negative correlation**

positive effect *n* - 1. An **effect** that is **beneficial** or desirable. 2. An effect measured by a **difference** that is positive. 3. A positive **treatment difference**. ant: **negative effect**

positive predictive value of a test *n* - The **probability** of having a **disease** or adverse health condition given a **positive test result** for a specified **screening** or **diagnostic test**. rt: **negative predictive value of a test, predictive**

value of a test

positive result *n* - 1. A **result** indicative of a **positive effect** (defn 2 or 3). 2. A result indicative of a **beneficial effect**. ant: **negative result**

positive skew *adj* - **right skew**

positive skew distribution *n* - **right skew distribution**

positive skewness *n* - **right skewness**

positive study *n* - 1. A **study** that produces results that confirm a prior **hypothesis** or finding. 2. A study that produces a **positive result**. ant: **negative study**

positive treatment effect *n* - 1. A **treatment effect** that is **beneficial**. 2. A **treatment difference** that is **positive** (defn 1). ant: **negative treatment effect**

post- *prefix* - [ME, fr L, fr *post*; akin to Skt *paśca* behind, after, Gk *apo* away from] **After**, subsequent to, later than, **posterior** to. ant: **pre-** *Usage note*: Generally best avoided, see page xxx (*Pre- and post- words*) in *Usage practices, cautions, and recommendations*.

post-assignment *adj* - Of or relating to that which takes place after **assignment**.

post-assignment consent *n* - [trials] A **consent** requested after **treatment assignment**; proposed by Zelen [1979].[170] Those **assigned** to receive the **test treatment** are informed of that assignment and are asked to consent (after a discussion of associated **risks** and **benefits** and treatment alternatives); those who do not consent are treated using the **control treatment**. Those assigned to the control treatment are given that treatment without discussion of alternative courses of treatment. Use of the method is usually limited to **unmasked trials** and settings involving life-threatening **diseases** in which the **control treatment** is the accepted **standard** for care and, hence, in which it is possible to justify its use without a discussion of alternative courses of treatment. ant: **preassignment consent** rt: **deferred consent, informed consent, oral consent, signed consent**

post-close-out followup visit *n* - [trials] 1. Any **followup visit** that takes place after the **close-out followup visit**. 2. Any followup visit that takes place after completion of the **close-out stage** of a trial. 3. **post-trial followup visit**

post-close-out visit *n* - **post-trial followup visit**

post-marketing surveillance *n* - Any procedure or system implemented on or after approval of a **drug, biologic,** or **device** for a given indication or use; designed to provide ongoing information on the use of the drug, biologic, or device in relation to that indication and on its **side effects**. The surveillance usually involves **survey** and **observational** techniques and is usually initiated in response to needs expressed by the **Food and Drug Administration**, the manufacturer, or some other group for added information concerning use or safety. rt: **phase IV trial**

post-randomization *adj* - Of or relating to be that occurring **after randomization**. ant: **prerandomization** *Usage note*: Avoid; use after randomization; see note for **post-**.

post-randomization examination *n* - [trials] An **examination** performed in relation to a **post-randomization followup visit** and done to satisfy **data collection** procedures in the trial.

post-randomization followup visit *n* - [trials] Any **followup visit** after the **randomization visit**. The visits may be **required** or **nonrequired**; the former class includes **treatment application and adjustment, regular, close-out,** and **post-close-out followup visits**.

post-randomization visit *n* - **post-randomization followup visit**

post-stratification *n* - 1. **Stratification** of **treatment units** or **observations** after **enrollment** or **collection** for a **subgroup analysis; stratification** (defn 3). 2. [trials] Stratification after **treatment assignment**. *Usage note*: See **stratification**.

post-stratify, post-stratified, post-stratifying, post-stratifies *v* - Broadly, to divide or arrange into **classes** or **groups** after **enrollment** or **collection**. In **trials** and **epidemiology**, to divide or arrange an assembled group of **observation units** or **treatment units** and associated **data** for a **subgroup analysis** or for some other purpose. rt: **stratify** *Usage note*: See **stratification**.

post-treatment followup *n* - [trials] 1. Any **followup** after completion of administration of the **assigned treatment**. 2. Any **followup** occurring after the first application of the **assigned treatment**. 3. **post-trial followup** *Usage note*: Best limited to use in the sense of defn 1. Subject to confusion if used in the sense of defn 2 before treatment is completed.

post-treatment followup period *n* - [**trials**] That period of **followup** defined by the period of time between cessation of **treatment** and termination of **followup**; equivalent to **followup period** (defn 1) in trials in which **study treatments** are administered in a single application or **dose** on **randomization**; period does not exist in trials in which study treatments are continuously administered over the entire course of followup.

post-treatment followup visit *n* - [**trials**] 1. **post-close-out followup visit** 2. Any **followup visit** taking place after cessation of **treatment**.

post-trial followup *n* - Any form of **followup** taking place after completion of the **close-out stage** of a **trial** or cessation of the trial.

post-trial followup stage *n* - [**trials**] A **stage of trial** occurring after the **termination stage** and intended to provide **followup data** on some **outcome measure**.

post-trial followup visit *n* - 1. Any **followup visit** that takes place after the **close of the trial**; usually to enable clinic personnel to collect **data** on a **primary** or **secondary outcome measure** for the assessment of **treatment effects**. 2. Any followup visit that takes place after the **close-out followup visit**; **post-close-out followup visit**.

posterior *adj* - [L, compar of *posterus* coming after, fr *post* after] 1. Coming after in **order**; following; later in time; subsequent. 2. Located behind a part or in the rear of a structure; situated behind.

posterior odds *n* - The **odds** that some fact is correct (eg, having a certain **disease**), given some observation or condition predicative or indicative of that fact (eg, presence of a **symptom** associated with that disease). syn: a posteriori odds

posterior probability *n* - A **probability** statement for a specified **event** conditioned by observed **data** related to that event (eg, the probability that a person has a given **disease** given the presence of some symptom associated with that disease); the quantity, P(E|C), in **Bayes' theorem**. syn: a posteriori probability rt: **a priori probability**, **conditional probability**

postulate *n* - [ML *postulatum*, fr neut of *postulatus*, pp of *postulare* to assume, fr L, to demand] A **hypothesis** advanced as an essential proposition; axiom.

potential *adj* - [ME, fr LL *potentialis*, fr *potentia* potentiality, fr L, power, fr *potent-*, *potens*] Existing as a possibility; capable of developing or of becoming a reality.

potential bias *n* - A **bias** that may arise in the future or one that is considered to exist in a speculative sense. *Usage note*: Often used in a speculative sense in relation to the role or influence that some position, **relationship**, or **association** may have or has had on one's actions or behavior, especially in relation to a real or perceived **conflict of interest**. Use with caution, especially in speculation regarding motivation for another person's behavior. Bias is easy to suggest but difficult to substantiate.

power *n* - [ME, fr OF *poeir*, fr *poeir* to be able, fr (assumed) L *potēre* to be powerful] 1. The **probability** of rejecting the **null hypothesis** when it is **false**; one minus the **type II error**. 2. **exponent** rt: **conditional power**, **expected power**, **observed power**

power function *n* - A **function** for a specified **statistical test** that gives the **power** (one minus the **type II error**; $1 - \beta$) for a **range** of values of the **parameter** of interest in the test. The function has a value corresponding to the **type I error level** of the test when the parameter has the value specified under the **null hypothesis**; elsewhere its values correspond to the power of the test for the range of **alternative hypotheses** represented by the values assumed by the parameter.

powerful *adj* - Having great **power**.

pragmatic *adj* - [L *pragmaticus* skilled in law or business, fr Gk *pragmatikos*, fr *pragmat-*, *pragma* deed, fr *prassein* to do] Relating to matters of fact or practical affairs, often to the exclusion of intellectual or artistic considerations.

pragmatic trial *n* - A **trial** done under conditions approximating those extant in everyday practice and designed and carried out for the purpose of choosing among the **treatments** tested for everyday use in ordinary settings. Often used in contradistinction to **explanatory trial**. See Sackett, 1980;[135] Sackett and Gent, 1979;[136] and Schwartz and Lellouch, 1967.[139] syn: **effectiveness trial**, **management trial** ant: **explanatory trial** *Usage note*: Of limited utility as a dimension of **classification** for reasons similar to those stated for **explanatory trials**. All trials, even if designed to mimic real-world practice, involve departures from real-world conditions. Avoid as a label; if used accompany with sufficient details to indicate the way in which the trial is **pragmatic**.

pre- *prefix* - [ME, fr OF & L; OF, fr L *prae-*, fr *prae* in front of, before] 1. Earlier than; prior to; before. 2. Preparatory or prerequisite to. 3. In advance of, beforehand. 4. In front of; anterior to. ant: **post-** *Usage note*: To be used sparingly; often unnecessary, redundant or confusing, especially when used as a prefix to an active verb conveying the notion of an act or action taking place beforehand, as in preboard, preboil, preheat, premix, prebill, preapprove, and preprint. The difficulty with most **pre-** modified verbs is that the modifications suggest acts or actions that are literally impossible or that have imaginary or mystical connotations (as in the notion of boarding a plane before it has arrived). Most **pre-** modified verbs are best used without the modifier, eg, heat instead of preheat, mix instead of premix, etc, or can be avoided with the use of some other term, such as early, as in early boarding instead of preboarding. See also *Pre- and post- words* in *Usage practices, cautions, and recommendations* (page xxx).

pre-market approval *n* - 1. **Pre-Market Approval Application** 2. Approval of a **Pre-Market Approval Application** by the **Food and Drug Administration**. rt: **investigational new drug**

Pre-Market Approval Application (PMA) *n* - An **application** to the **Food and Drug Administration**, generally based on work performed under one or more **Investigational Device Exemptions**, for permission to market a **medical device** [Food and Drug Administration, 1983].[50] See **New Drug Application** for corresponding term for **drugs** and **Product License Application** for biologics. rt: **Investigational Device Exemption Application**

preassignment *adj* - Relating to or being before **assignment** to **treatment**.

preassignment consent *n* - [**trials**] **Consent** obtained before **assignment** to **treatment**. ant: **post-assignment consent** rt: **informed consent, oral consent, signed consent**

preassignment examination *n* - [**trials**] 1. Any **examination** that is part of the evaluation process for **enrollment** into a **trial** and that is carried out prior to the **assignment examination**. 2. **baseline examination** rt: **preassignment visit, prerandomization examination, pretreatment examination**

preassignment visit *n* - [**trials**] 1. Any **visit** to a **study clinic** scheduled for or made by a **study candidate** for the purpose of evaluation for **enrollment** into a **trial** that takes place prior to the **assignment visit**. 2. **baseline visit** rt: **preassignment examination, prerandomization examination, pretreatment visit**

precise *adj* - [MF *precis*, fr L *praecisus*, pp of *praecidere* to cut off, fr *prae-* + *caedere* to cut] 1. Exactly or sharply defined or stated. 2. Strictly conforming in pattern, standard, or convention.

precision *adj* - 1. Adapted for **accurate measurement**, operation, or execution. 2. Marked by **precision**.

precision *n* - 1. The quality of being **precise** or exact. 2. The number of digits to the right of the a **decimal point** for a **continuous variable** or measure; **significant digits**. 3. The variability associated with a **variable** or **statistic** as measured by its **standard deviation** or **standard error**. rt: **accuracy**

preclinical *adj* - 1. Occurring before the **diagnosis** of **disease** is possible; of, relating to, or concerned with the period preceding manifestation of **disease**. 2. Of, relating to, or concerned with the period preceding use in human beings, eg, in reference to something done on animals or **in vitro** as a prelude to use on human beings. 3. Of, relating to, or concerned with the period preceding use in a **clinical** setting. rt: **clinical** *Usage note*: Potentially confusing because of different meanings; use sparingly and with caution. Note that the definitions refer to different periods. The reference in defn 1 is to a period of time preceding the overt onset of clinical disease in a person or persons. The reference in defn 2 is to the period preceding use of something in human beings, as in reference to studies of a compound in animals done as a prelude to possible use in human beings. The period referenced in defn 2 is extended to include the period of use in human beings in a nonclinical setting in defn 3, eg, in reference to a **phase I drug trial** involving persons free of clinical disease. See **pre-** for added comments.

predict, predicted, predicting, predicts *v* - [L *praedictus*, pp of *praedicere*, fr *prae-* pre- + *dicere* to say] To declare in advance; especially to foretell on the basis of observation, experience, **data**, or reasoning.

prediction *n* - 1. The act of **predicting**. 2. Something predicted; forecast.

prediction interval *n* - The **interval** defined by the upper and lower **prediction limits** associated with a **predicted value**; shows, on a **probability** basis, its likely **range** of **error**.

prediction limits *n* - The **limits** defining a **prediction interval**; in **regression analysis**, a **confidence interval** constructed about a future value for the **dependent variable** for a given set of values of the **independent variables**; the upper and lower values of the interval (prediction limits) are used to predict (with the **probability** used for constructing the interval) the **range** of likely future values of the **dependent variable**, given a particular set of values for the **dependent variables**. syn: limits of prediction

predictive value *n* - 1. The usefulness of some **observation**, **event**, or value in **predicting** some other event or state. 2. **predictive value of a test**

predictive value of a test *n* - [**epidemiology**] The **probability** of a given state (eg, **diseased** or not diseased) given a specified **test result** (defn 1) for a **screening** or **diagnostic test**; **negative predictive value of a test**; **positive predictive value of a test**

preference *n* - [F *préférence*, fr ML *praeferentia*, fr L *praeferent-*, *praeferens*, prp of *praeferre*] The power or opportunity to choose.

preference treatment design *n* - [**trials**] A **treatment design** that allows a person, group of persons, or institution (in the case of **multicenter trials**) choice in regard to the **treatments** used or to be used.[12, 15, 134, 139] The choice may be exercised by the person to be **enrolled** on **enrollment**, by physicians or persons responsible for administering the **assigned treatments** or by an institution on behalf of all those administering treatments at a **study clinic** in a multicenter trial. See **clinic preference treatment design**, **patient preference treatment design**, and **physician preference treatment design**.

preliminary *adj* - Coming before, especially that which is necessary to that which follows.

preliminary *n* - [F *préliminaires*, pl, fr ML *praeliminaris*, preliminary (adj), fr L *prae-* pre-

+ *limin-*, *limen* threshold] Something that precedes, is introductory, or is preparatory.

preliminary trial *n* - **feasibility trial**, **pilot trial**

premature *adj* - [L *praematurus* too early, fr *prae-* + *maturus* ripe, mature] Happening, arriving, performed, or executed before the appointed or designated time.

premature stop *n* - [general] A **stop** occurring sooner than expected; one occurring prior to the planned finish or end. [**trials**] **premature termination** syn: **early stop**

premature termination *n* - [**trials**] **Termination of a trial** before the required or specified conditions for **termination** (usually as established when the trial was designed) have been satisfied, eg, termination due to inadequate **enrollment** or because of harm due to a **study treatment**. *Usage note*: See comment for **trial stop**.

prerandomization *adj* - Of or relating to that **before randomization**. ant: **post-randomization** *Usage note*: Avoid; see note for **pre-**.

prerandomization examination *n* - [**trials**] Any **study examination** taking place before **randomization**. rt: **randomization examination**, **prerandomization visit** *Usage note*: Use **preassignment examination** when **assignment** is by means other than randomization.

prerandomization visit *n* - [**trials**] Any **study visit** taking place before **randomization**. rt: **randomization visit**, **prerandomization examination** *Usage note*: Use **preassignment visit** when **assignment** is by means other than randomization.

prescribe, prescribed, prescribing, prescribes *v* - [L *praescribere* to write at the beginning, dictate, order, fr *prae-* + *scribere* to write] 1. To write or give a medical **prescription**. 2. To lay down a rule or order.

prescribed regimen *n* - 1. **prescribed treatment regimen** 2. **regimen**

prescribed treatment *n* - 1. **treatment prescription** 2. **prescribed treatment regimen** 3. **treatment assignment** (not a recommended use)

prescribed treatment regimen *n* - 1. **Treatment regimen** prescribed for a **patient**. 2. Treatment regimen, as **prescribed** in a **study protocol**. 3. **prescribed regimen** 4. **prescribed treatment**

prescription *n* - [partly fr ME *prescripcion* establishment of a claim, fr MF *prescription*, fr LL *praescription-*, *praescriptio*, fr L act of writing at the beginning, order, limitation of subject matter, fr *praescriptus*, pp of *praescribere*; partly fr L *praescription-*, *praescriptio* order] 1. A written order by one authorized or licensed to write such orders, eg, a **physician**, for a therapeutic or corrective agent, such as a **drug**, for use on or by a designated person. 2. The execution of such a written order by one authorized or licensed to do so, such as a pharmacist. 3. The action of laying down authoritative rules or directions.

prescription drug *n* - A **drug** dispensed by **prescription**; as opposed to an **over-the-counter drug** or nonprescription drug.

presentation *n* - 1. A **manuscript** displayed (as in a poster session) or read at a professional meeting. 2. The act of presenting; something presented.

pretest *n* - A preliminary **test** of some activity, process, or procedure to determine readiness or preparedness for performing the activity, process, or procedure for real. syn: **pilot test**, **test run**, **dry run**

pretreatment examination *n* - [**trials**] Any **examination** done on or prior to the initiation of **treatment**. Synonymous with **prerandomization examination** if **randomization** and initiation of treatment take place during the same visit. rt: **pretreatment visit**, **preassignment examination**, **prerandomization examination**

pretreatment visit *n* - [**trials**] Any **visit** to a **study clinic** made by a **study candidate** for the purpose of evaluation for **enrollment** into a **trial** or for establishing a **baseline** for assessing subsequent change that takes place prior to the initiation of **treatment**. rt: **pretreatment examination**, **preassignment visit**, **prerandomization visit**

prevalence *n* - 1. The number of persons in a **population** known to have a designated **disease** or health condition at a designated **point** in **time**; **point prevalence**. 2. The number of persons in a **population** known to have a designated **disease** or health condition at anytime over a specified period of time; **period prevalence**. 3. The **proportion** of a **population** known to have a designated disease or health condition as determined at a given point in time or over a specified interval. rt: **lifetime prevalence**

prevalence rate *n* - The total number of persons in a defined **population** having a specified

disease or health condition at a specified point in time or over a defined time **interval** divided by the number in that population at **risk** of developing or acquiring that disease or health condition at that point in time or as counted at some arbitrary point within a defined interval, eg, midway into the interval; also **prevalence ratio**. rt: **prevalence**, **point prevalence**, **period prevalence**

prevalence ratio *n* - **prevalence rate**

prevalence study *n* - **cross-sectional study**

prevent, **prevented**, **preventing**, **prevents** *v* - [ME *preventen* to anticipate, fr L, *praeventus*, pp of *praevenire* to come before, anticipate, forestall, fr *prae-* + *venire* to come] To keep from happening; to hold back, forestall, or avoid.

prevention *n* - [**medicine**] 1. The avoidance of a **disease** or adverse health condition. 2. Avoiding the onset of disease or delaying the deterioration of health associated with a disease or adverse health condition by changes in lifestyle or external environment or by the administration of a preventive **treatment** (eg, immunization against the disease). rt: **primary prevention**, **secondary prevention**, **tertiary prevention**

prevention trial *n* - A **trial** that is designed to assess the **efficacy** of a **treatment** aimed at **preventing** the development or progression of a specific **disease** or health condition. syn: **prophylactic trial** ant: **therapeutic trial**, **treatment trial** rt: **primary prevention trial**, **secondary prevention trial**

preventive medicine *n* - A branch of **medicine** in which the emphasis is on **prevention** of **disease** and adverse health conditions, especially in contradistinction to the **diagnosis** and **treatment** of existent disease.

preventive, **preventative** *adj, n* - Devoted to or concerned with **prevention**.

primary *adj* - [LL *primarius* basic, primary, fr L, principal, fr *primus*] 1. First in **order**. 2. Of or being first or foremost. 3. Basic or fundamental.

primary analysis *n* - 1. [**research**] The **analysis** of greatest relevance to the **objective** of the research. [**trials**] 2. **Treatment comparisons** involving the **primary outcome**. 3. Treatment comparisons based on analyses by **treatment assigned**; **analysis by intention to treat**.

primary care *n* - [**medicine**] 1. **Care** related to the initial **diagnosis** and **treatment** of **disease** or adverse health conditions; generally rendered in response to symptoms or complaints of a **patient** presenting to a **primary care center** or in relation to routine check-ups performed at such centers. 2. Care provided to a patient at a primary care center. rt: **secondary care, tertiary care**

primary care center *n* - [**medicine**] A **center** (eg, physician office, clinic, hospital) providing **primary care**; generally the place at which **diagnosis** and care is initiated; those presenting that cannot be adequately diagnosed or cared for are referred to other facilities, such as a **secondary** or **tertiary care center**. rt: **primary care, secondary care center, tertiary care center**

primary data *n* - 1. **Data** essential to a stated end. 2. Data needed for a **primary data analysis**. 3. **original data** (defn 5) 4. **raw data** rt: **original data, secondary data**

primary data analysis *n* - 1. The **data analysis** considered of greatest importance in relation to a stated end, eg, the one of basic importance in supporting the conclusion reached from a **trial**. 2. An analysis involving the **primary outcome measure**. 3. An analysis following fundamental principles, eg, **analysis by assigned treatment**. 4. Analysis of one's own data, ie, not a **secondary data analysis** (defn 1). rt: **secondary data analysis**

primary document *n* - 1. The main or principal document in relation to some process or procedure. 2. **source document** rt: **secondary document**

primary endpoint *n* - 1. **Primary outcome variable** of **binary** form indicating presence or absence of an **event** (as opposed to a **continuous measure**). 2. The actual occurrence of such an event. *Usage note*: Avoid, for reasons indicated for **endpoint**. Use **primary outcome** or **primary outcome measure**.

primary event *n* - 1. A **primary outcome variable** that is **binary**. 2. The occurrence of an event as indicated by a primary **binary outcome measure**. 3. An event considered to be of great importance. rt: **secondary event**

primary outcome *n* - 1. [**trials**] The **event** or condition a **trial** is designed to **treat**, ameliorate, delay, or **prevent**. 2. The actual occurrence of a **primary event** in a **study participant**. 3. **primary endpoint** (not recommended; see usage note for **endpoint** for reasons).

primary outcome measure *n* - [**trials**] 1. That **measure**, among two or more, **observed** or to be observed in a trial that is considered to be of primary importance in its **design** (eg, the one used for the **sample size calculation**) or in the **analyses** performed or to be performed; may be a **continuous measure** or an **event** depending on the trial. syn: **primary outcome variable** 2. **design variable**

primary outcome variable *n* - [**trials**] The **outcome variable** designated or regarded as key in the **design** or **analysis** of a **trial**. Generally, the variable used for **sample size calculations** in the design of the trial or the one considered to be of primary importance in the analyses performed or to be performed. rt: **design variable**

primary prevention *n* - 1. The **prevention** of **disease** or an adverse health condition by the administration or implementation of preventative regimens or strategies (eg, immunization to prevent a disease or implementation of dietary changes aimed at reducing the **risk** of heart disease). 2. Efforts at the preservation of health by personal and community-wide measures; broadly, from the perspective of **epidemiology**, as given by Last[84]: The protection of health by personal and community-wide efforts, eg, preserving good nutritional status, physical fitness, and emotional well-being, immunizing against infectious diseases, and making the environment safe. rt: **secondary prevention, tertiary prevention**

primary prevention trial *n* - A prophylactic **trial** involving the use of **treatments** intended to prevent or delay the onset of **disease**, hence those **enrolled** are selected for the absence of a specified disease or adverse health condition and the **test treatment** used or to be used is one which ostensibly has the ability to prevent or delay the onset of that disease or adverse health condition. rt: **secondary prevention trial**

primary publication *n* - [**research**] 1. A **publication** containing **original data**, especially one containing a **primary result**. 2. A publication from a **study** or *investigation* considered essential in relation to the primary **purpose** or **objective** of a specific **research project**; in the case of **trials**, includes publications of primary results and on the **design**, **methods**, and **baseline results** of the trial. syn: **mainline paper** rt: **secondary publication, ancillary publication**

primary record *n* - 1. The main or principal **record** in relation to some process or procedure. 2. **source record** rt: **secondary record**

primary result *n* - [**research**] A **result** (defn 3) of direct relevance to the primary **objective** of a **study**. In **clinical trials**, a result based on the **primary outcome measure** or on the **design variable** of the trial. rt: **secondary result**, **ancillary result**

primary source *n* - 1. The origin or principle source of something, especially as identified or defined by a **source document**. 2. An **original** work, especially in relation to an idea, concept, approach, or method. 3. The creator of an idea, concept, method, or procedure, especially as documented by **publication** or in other ways. rt: **secondary source** *Usage note*: Redundant where **source** implies primacy. Limit use to settings in which there are multiple sources and a need to indicate the primacy of one of them.

principal *adj* - [ME, fr OF, fr L *principalis*, fr *princip-, princeps*] First, highest, or foremost in rank, importance, or degree; chief.

principal *n* - One who heads an office or activity by having controlling authority over that office or activity. rt: **co-principal**

principal component *n* - One of the ordered **components** identified in a **principal component analysis**. rt: **principal component analysis**

principal component analysis *n* - An **analysis** aimed at transforming a set of correlated **variables** to a new set consisting of **linear combinations** of the old set such that they are uncorrelated and ordered in terms of **variance** explained; resulting variables referred to as **components** or **principal components** in which each of the transformed variables is represented as a linear combination of the old set of variables and for which the sum of squares of the **coefficients** in the linear combination is unity; done simply to provide a more convenient way of re-expressing a set of variables. rt: **principal component**

principal investigator (PI) *n* - [**research**] 1. The person named as having responsibility for conduct of the research proposed in a **grant application** submitted to the **National Institutes of Health**; such a person named in any **funding application** submitted to the NIH, whether for **grant** or **contract** funding; such a person named on any **funding proposal**, regardless of funding

source. 2. The person in charge of a **research project**; the lead scientist on a **research project**. 3. The head of a **center** in a **multicenter study**. 4. The **chair** of a **multicenter study**. 5. The head of a **clinical center** in a **multicenter trial** rt: **co-principal investigator** *Usage note*: The term serves both as an administrative (defn 1) and leadership label (defn 2). It is a mistake to assume that an administrative role translates automatically into to a leadership role, though often the person named in the sense of defn 1 is the same person named or implied in the sense of defn 2 in the case of most investigator-initiated **single-center** research projects. Avoid use of the term, or its abbreviation, **PI**, as a leadership label in any single-center setting where more than one person is being referenced. Avoid in the sense of defn 2 in settings having multiple "principal investigators"; use **center director** and **chair of the study** to designate positions of leadership in **multicenter** settings. Avoid uses in the sense of defn 5 since those uses carry subtle connotations that those heading **resource centers** are not as "principal" to the overall effort as their clinical counterparts. See also usage notes for **co-principal investigator**, **investigator**, and **center**.

principle *n* - [ME, modif of MF *principe*, fr L *principium* beginning, fr *princip-, princeps* one taking the first part] A rule of conduct or code; a **primary source** or origin.

principle of beneficence *n* - **beneficence, principle of**

principle of competence *n* - **competence, principle of**

principle of justice *n* - **justice, principle of**

principle of respect for persons *n* - **respect for persons, principle of**

principles of medical ethics *n* - **medical ethics, principles of**

prior *adj* - [L, former, superior, compar of OL *pri* before; akin to L *priscus* ancient, prae before] Earlier in time or order; preceding. rt: **antecedent**

prior probability *n* - **a priori probability** (defn 2)

priority *adj* - Of or relating to a state of being or having precedence such as in terms of date, position, or **rank**.

priority score *n* - 1. The **score** assigned to a **research application** by an individual member of a **review group** that reflects that individual's judgment regarding the scientific merit of the proposal. In **National Institutes of Health grant** reviews, the score may range from 1 (highest scientific merit) to 5 (lowest scientific merit). 2. **mean priority score** rt: **payline**

probability *n* - 1. [statistics] The **relative frequency** with which an **event** occurs or is expected to occur. In a **finite** sampling, the number of **samples** having a specified characteristic divided by the total number of possible samples. 2. The limit of the **relative frequency** of an **event** as the number of replications of the **trial** or **experiment** giving rise to the observed frequency approaches **infinity**. [general] 3. An expression of one's belief or **confidence** in some fact or condition. 4. The **likelihood** of some **event** or condition occurring.

probability density *n* - 1. **probability density function** 2. A particular value of a probability density function. rt: **probability mass**

probability density function *n* - A **function** whose integral over a specified **interval** gives the **probability** that the value of a **continuous random variable** falls within that interval. rt: **frequency function, probability mass function**

probability distribution *n* - 1. **distribution function** (defn 2); **probability mass function** 2. **probability density function**

probability distribution function (pdf) *n* - 1. **distribution function** (defn 2) 2. **probability density function; probability mass function**

probability function *n* - **probability mass function**

probability mass *n* - 1. The **probability** associated with a given value of the **probability mass function**, eg, Pr(X = 2). 2. The probability associated with a **range** of values of a **discrete random variable**, eg, Pr(X ≤ 2). rt: **probability density**

probability mass function *n* - Probability distribution function for a **discrete variable**. rt: **probability density function**

probability sample *n* - A **sample** drawn such that every element from the underlying **population** has a known **probability** of selection. The probability may be the same for all elements (**simple random sample**) or differ depending on

some **characteristic** associated with the individual elements (as in a **stratified random sample**).

probable *adj* - [ME, fr MF, fr L, *probabilis*, fr *probare*, to test, approve, prove] Supported by evidence sufficient to establish presumption but not proof; likely but not certain.

probable error *n* - 1. A measure of **sampling variation** defined by 0.675 times the standard deviation; the multiplier derives from the fact that the lower and upper **quartiles** of a **standard normal distribution** correspond to the values -0.675 and +0.675, respectively. 2. A **confidence interval** having a **confidence level** of 0.50; for a **random variable** having a **normal distribution** defined by the interval -0.6745SD and +0.6745SD, where SD is the **standard deviation** of the variable. rt: **standard deviation, standard error**

proband *n* - [L *probandus*, gerundive of *probare*] 1. **subject** 2. **propositus**

probit *n* - [shorthand for probability unit; introduced by Bliss, 1934] A **transformation** involving the addition of 5 to a **variable** having or assumed to have a **standard normal distribution** (done to reduce the **likelihood** of **negative** values); a type of **transformation** used to estimate **dosage** in **bioassays**. The transformed value, in a **probability** sense, corresponds to the area to the left of the transformed value for a **normal distribution** with **mean** (μ) = 5 and **variance** (σ^2) = 1.

procedure *n* - [F *procédure*, fr MF, fr *proceder*] 1. A particular way of doing something or of acting. 2. A series of **steps** followed in a particular **order** or **sequence**. 3. The collective set of steps constituting a **test** or maneuver performed with or on a **patient** or **study subject** in relation to **diagnosis, treatment**, care, or **followup**.

process *n* - [ME *proces*, fr MF, fr L *processus*, fr *processus*, pp of *procedere*] A series of actions, **steps**, or **procedures** conducted toward some end.

procure, procured, procuring, procures *v* - [ME *procuren*, fr LL *procurare*, fr L, to take care of, fr *pro-* for + *cura* care] To get possession of; obtain by particular care or effort.

procurement *n* - The act of **procuring**.

procurement and distribution center *n* - [**multicenter study**] A facility in a **multicenter** structure responsible for **procuring**, packaging, and distributing a product (eg, **drugs**, laboratory supplies, forms) to selected **centers** in that structure. rt: **distribution center, procurement center**

procurement center *n* - 1. [**multicenter study**] 1. A **center** that is responsible for **procuring** materials or supplies needed by **centers** for conduct of the **study**, especially one with that as its primary or sole responsibility. 2. **procurement and distribution center**

product *n* - [ME, fr ML *productum*, fr L something produced, fr neut of *productus*, pp of *producere* in other senses, fr L *productum*] 1. The number or expression resulting from multiplication of two or more numbers or algebraic expressions. 2. Something produced or manufactured.

Product License Application (PLA) *n* - An **application** for **license** to market a **biologic** for a specified **indication**; application submitted to the **Food and Drug Administration** by the manufacturer of the biologic or its marketing agent; application must be approved for the biologic to be marketed for the indication specified in the application (see **Pre-Market Approval Application** for corresponding term for **medical devices** and **New Drug Application** for **drugs**).

product-moment *n* - A **moment** involving the **product** formed by multiplying two or more **variables**, each raised to a specified power, eg, the 1st product-moment for **deviations** of the variables x_1 and x_2 about their respective **means**, μ_1 and μ_2, is the mean of products: $(x_{11} - \mu_1)(x_{21} - \mu_2)$, $(x_{12} - \mu_1)(x_{22} - \mu_2)$, $(x_{13} - \mu_1)(x_{23} - \mu_2)$, $\cdots$, $(x_{1n} - \mu_1)(x_{2n} - \mu_2)$.

profession *n* - [ME *professioun*, fr OF *profession*, fr LL & L; LL *profession-*, *professio*, fr L public declaration, fr *professus*, pp] An area of endeavor requiring specialized knowledge and often long and intensive academic study or apprenticeship.

professional *adj* - 1. Of or relating to, or characteristic of a **profession**. 2. Engaged in one of the learned professions.

profile *n* - [It *profilo*, fr *profilare* to draw in outline, fr *pro-* forward (fr L) + *filare* to spin, fr LL] 1. A representation of something in outline. 2. A set of **data** in **table** or **graphic** form displaying the significant features of something. 3. A table or **graph** representing the extent to which one exhibits a trait or ability as determined by tests or ratings; **risk profile**.

program *n* - [F *programme* agenda, public notice, fr Gk *programma*, fr *prographein* to write before, fr *pro-* before + *graphein* to write] 1. A plan or system under which action may be taken toward an end or goal. 2. A collection of related **research** activities, as in a **program project grant**. 3. A specific research activity or **project**. 4. **computer program** rt: **project** *Usage note*: Not recommended in the sense of defn 3. Sometimes used as a substitute for the term **trial**,[156] as in University Group Diabetes Program;[156] especially as a means of de-emphasizing the experimental nature of a study. Not recommended usage. Use an appropriately informative term.

program director *n* - 1. The individual who heads a **program**. 2. The individual who heads a **research project**. 3. **principal investigator** (not recommended in the context of **multicenter studies**; see usage note for **principal investigator** for reason)

program office *n* - 1. **project office** 2. An **office** containing **project offices** for several different but related studies. 3. The office housing the headquarters of a **program**.

program officer *n* - 1. The head of a **program**. 2. One of the leaders of a program. 3. **project officer**

program project *n* - A collection of interrelated **research** activities having a common organizational structure and bearing on the same general question or issue, eg, a collection of basic and applied research projects aimed at providing a better understanding of atherosclerosis; especially such a collection funded from a single source.

program project grant *n* - 1. An NIH **grant** supporting a **program project**. 2. An **NIH grant application** for a program project.

progress *n* - [ME, fr L *progressus* advance, fr *progessus*, pp of *progredi* to go forth, fr *pro-* forward + *gradi* to go] A forward or onward movement; advance.

progress, progressed, progressing, progresses *v* - To advance or proceed; to continue unabated.

progress report *n* - 1. A **report** summarizing **progress** made in pursuing some goal or end. 2. A written report submitted to a **funding agency** near the close of a designated period of support (usually a year) containing a summary of work performed and accomplishments during the period; especially such a report submitted in relation to a request for continued support. rt: **incremental funding**

progression *n* - 1. A **sequence** of **numbers** in which each successive term may be derived from the preceding by a constant operation; a continuous and connected **series**; **sequence** 2. The action or process of **progressing**. rt: **sequence**, **series**

project *n* - [ME *proiecte*, modif of MF *pourjet*, fr *pourjeter* to throw out, spy, plan, fr *pour-* (fr L *porro* forward) + *jeter* to throw; akin to Gk *pro* forward] 1. A planned undertaking. 2. A collection of related research activities, as in a **program project**. 3. A specific research activity, such as a **study** or **trial**, having a particular goal or end. rt: **program** *Usage note*: Not recommended in the sense of defn 3. Sometimes used as a substitute for the term, **trial**, as in the Coronary Drug Project, especially as a means of de-emphasizing the experimental nature of a study.

project office (PO) *n* - 1. In the parlance of the **NIH grants** and **contracts**, the **office** located in the **sponsoring agency** within the NIH, usually staffed with one or more individuals trained in **research** or **medicine**, responsible for dealing with technical, scientific, and programmatic aspects of a **research project** funded by **grant** or **contract**; **medical liaison office**. 2. **program office**

project officer (PO) *n* - 1. The individual in the **sponsoring agency** responsible for dealing with technical, scientific, and programmatic aspects of a specified **research project**; especially one funded by the **NIH** via a **grant** or **contract**; **medical liaison officer**. 2. **Health scientist administrator** in **National Institutes of Health** grant-funded projects. 3. **program officer**

proper *adj* - [ME *propre* proper, own, fr MF, fr L *proprius* own] Characteristically belonging to the thing or being in question.

prophylactic *adj* - [Gk *prophylaktikos*, fr *prophylassein* to keep guard before, fr *pro-* before + *phylassein* to guard, fr *phylak-*, *phylax* guard] 1. Guarding against or preventing **disease**. 2. Tending to **prevent** or ward off.

prophylactic trial *n* - A **trial** that is designed to assess the **efficacy** of a **treatment** aimed at **preventing** the development or **progression** of

a specific **disease** or health condition. syn: **prevention trial** ant: **therapeutic trial** rt: **primary prevention trial**, **secondary prevention trial**

proportion *n* - [ME *proporcion*, fr MF *proportion* fr L *proportion-*, *proportio*, fr *pro* for + *portion-*, *portio* portion] 1. A part considered in relation to a whole. 2. A fraction in which the elements represented in the **numerator** are a subset of those represented in the **denominator** and hence is bounded below by 0 and above by 1 when expressed as a decimal fraction. rt: **percent**, **rate**, **ratio** *Usage note*: Not to be confused with **ratio**. The **numerator** of the two numbers forming a proportion is contained in the **denominator**. The two numbers represented in a ratio generally have different bases. Both proportions and ratios denote relationships, however, in the case of proportions the relationship is to a defined whole, whereas for ratios the relationship pertains to some variable or factor common to both numbers.

proportional *adj* - Forming a relationship with other parts or quantities; being in **proportion**.

proportional hazard *n* - A **hazard** (defn 3) **proportional** to a **baseline** hazard; in **Cox regression** a hazard assumed to be **constant** over time on the **log scale** and proportional (multiplicative) on the **antilog scale**.

proportional hazards regression model *n* - A **regression model** relating the **hazard function** to **independent (regressor) variables**, x_1, $\cdots$, x_k, and of the general form $\lambda(t,x) = \lambda_0(t) \exp(\beta_1 x_1 + \beta_2 x_2 + \cdots + \beta_k x_k)$, where $\lambda_0(t)$ is the **baseline hazard function** for an individual with all regressors equal to 0, β_1, $\cdots$, β_k are **regression coefficients**, and $\exp(\beta_k)$ is the **hazard ratio** for an individual with regressor $x_k = x^* + 1$ versus an individual with $x_k = x^*$, holding the values of the other regressors fixed.

proportionate mortality rate (PMR) *n* - Cause specific **mortality rate**; also **proportionate mortality ratio**.

proportionate mortality ratio (PMR) *n* - **proportionate mortality rate**

proposal *n* - 1. An act of putting forward or stating something for consideration. 2. Something **proposed**. 3. **funding proposal**

propose, proposed, proposing, proposes *v* - [ME *proposen*, fr MF *proposer*, fr L *proponere*] To form or put forward as a plan or intended action.

proposer *n* - The party or individual who **proposes** (normally via submission of a written proposal) to carry out a **research project**, especially in relation to a **funding proposal**; **applicant**; **offeror**.

propositus *n* - [NL, fr L, pp of *proponere*] 1. **Index case**, especially in a genetic or pedigree **study**. 2. In law, one from whom a line of descent is traced. rt: **proband**

proprietary *adj* - [LL *propietarius*, fr L *proprietas* property] 1. Of or relating to one who owns and operates some enterprise or has an exclusive right to some product. 2. Used, made, or marketed by one having the exclusive legal right. 3. Privately owned and managed and run as a for-profit organization.

proprietary drug *n* - A **drug** protected by patent or copyright against free competition as to name, product, composition, or process of manufacture.

proprietary interest *n* - An **interest** deriving from being an owner, in total or part, of a business or product.

proprietary product *n* - 1. A licensed or patented **product**. 2. A product being developed for patent, license, or copyright. 3. A product protected by patent, license, or copyright.

prospect *n* - [ME, fr L *prospectus* view, prospect, fr *prospectus*, pp of *prospicere* to look forward, exercise foresight, fr *pro-* forward + *specere* to look] 1. The act of looking forward. 2. Something awaited or that is to come. ant: **retrospect**

prospective *adj* - 1. Relating to or lying in the future. 2. Lying in the future from the perspective of a designated time point, present or past (eg, from the perspective of the date of **enrollment** into a **trial** or from that of the date of **exposure** to some agent in the past). 3. Proceeding from **cause** to **effect**. ant: **retrospective** *Usage note*: The term should be avoided when redundant or where the nature of the process or activity being referred to is clearly prospective in the real time sense, as is the case of **followup** in **clinical trials**. Trials, by definition, are prospective in real time and, hence, the term, as an adjective modifier of **trial** is unnecessary. Technically, the term is also unnecessary as a modifier of **followup** since, unless modified, as

in **retrospective followup**, it is prospective in nature by definition, whether or not performed in real time. The primary use of the term should be in opposition to **retrospective** in settings where there is a possibility for uncertainty regarding the direction of the time perspective implied. See **retrospective** for additional comments.

prospective clinical trial *n* - **clinical trial** *Usage note*: See **prospective** for note.

prospective cohort study *n* - A **cohort study** in which the **followup** is **prospective** (as opposed to **retrospective**).

prospective data *n* - 1. **Data** collected in a **prospective** fashion. 2. Data that are arrayed or used in a prospective fashion, whether or not collected in that fashion.

prospective followup *n* - **Followup** that proceeds forward in time. syn: **cohort study**, **concurrent followup study**, longitudinal study ant: **retrospective followup**

prospective followup study *n* - A **study** in which people (**observation units**) with a specific attribute or characteristic are identified and then observed for some period of time thereafter for the occurrence of the **outcome** or condition of interest, eg, development of a **disease** or occurrence of some **event**. The study may or may not involve a **comparison group** and the followup may be done in **real time** or from **records** or **data** collected and recorded in the past. **Trials** represent a special subset of followup studies with real time followup. ant: **retrospective followup study** *Usage note*: See **prospective**.

prospective registration *n* - **Registration** carried out in real time and based on current information. ant: **retrospective registration**

prospective study *n* - **prospective followup study**; **cohort study**

protocol *n* - [MF *prothocole*, fr ML *protocollum*, fr LGk *prōtokollon* first sheet of a papyrus roll bearing data of manufacture, fr Gk *prōt-* prot- + *kollon* to glue together, fr *kolla* glue; akin to MD *helen* to glue] 1. Specifications, rules, and procedures for performing some activity or function. 2. **study protocol** 3. **data collection schedule** 4. **treatment plan** *Usage note*: Subject to varying use. Often used as a synonym for **treatment**, as in *on protocol*. See usage note for **study protocol** for added comments.

protocol adherence *n* - The act of being in accord with a **protocol** as measured against rules and specifications set forth in that protocol.

protocol change *n* - A **change** made in a **protocol** as a result of thoughtful deliberation; in **trials**, usually the result of problems noted in a proposed or existing **data collection protocol** or as a result of a **treatment protocol suspension**.

protocol departure *n* - 1. A **departure** from specified **treatment, examination,** or **data collection** procedures in a **study**. 2. **treatment protocol violation** 3. **protocol change** (not recommended) syn: protocol deviation rt: **protocol infraction, protocol violation**

protocol development stage *n* - [**trials**] The second stage of a **trial**; usually undertaken after the initiation of funding and characterized by development of the **treatment** and **data collection protocols** and of procedures needed to carry out the trial. See **stage of trial** for list of other stages.

protocol deviation *n* - **protocol departure**

protocol infraction *n* - 1. **protocol violation** 2. **protocol departure, protocol deviation**

protocol monitor *n* - One who **monitors** in relation to the **protocol**, especially in relation to **compliance**.

protocol monitoring *v* - **Monitoring** aimed at detecting **departures** from the **study protocol** (defn 1) in order to take appropriate corrective actions and as a means of avoiding such departures in the future.

protocol suspension *n* - 1. **Suspension** of the **study protocol** or elements of it during the course of a **study**; such suspensions due to concerns or questions regarding the appropriateness or adequacy of the protocol or compliance to it. 2. **treatment protocol suspension** 3. Continuation of activities without the rigors of a protocol. rt: **enrollment suspension** *Usage note*: Subject to confusion. Suspension does not imply a total cessation of activities. Sometimes used simply to indicate that activities and procedures performed after the suspension were not subject to the same requirements or standards of rigor as prior to the suspension (defn 3). See also usage notes for **enrollment suspension** and **treatment protocol suspension**.

protocol violation *n* - 1. A **protocol departure** considered to be serious, eg, administration of

the wrong treatment or enrollment of an ineligible person; especially when avoidable. 2. Any **protocol departure** whether or not considered to be serious.

prove, proved, proven, proving, proves *v* - [ME *proven*, fr OF *prover*, fr L *probare* to test, approve, prove, fr *probus* good, honest, fr *profor*, in favor + *-bus* (akin to OE *bēon* to be)] 1. To **test** the truth, validity, or genuineness of. 2. To test the worth or quality of. 3. To **compare** against a **standard**. 4. To **check** the correctness or **accuracy** of. 5. To establish the existence, truth, or validity of. 6. To **demonstrate** as having a particular value or worth.

proxy *adj* - [ME *procucie*, contr of *procuracie*, fr AF, fr ML *procuratia*, alter of L *procuratio* procuration] 1. Being authorized to act or operate in place of another. 2. Being used as if a substitute for another, as with a **proxy variable**. rt: **surrogate**

proxy variable *n* - A **variable** that serves as a substitute for another variable; usually one that is easier or less expensive to **measure** or **observe** than the one it replaces. rt: **surrogate outcome variable**

pseudo *adj* - Being apparent rather than actual; **sham, spurious**.

pseudo-, pseud- *prefix* - [ME, fr LL, fr Gk fr *pseudēs*, false, fr *pseudein*, to lie] 1. Not authentic; **sham, spurious**. 2. Deceptive. 3. Apparent similarity. rt: **quasi-**

pseudorandom *adj* - Being or involving entities, such as **numbers**, that are generated, selected, or ordered by a deterministic process that can be shown to generate sequences or orders that satisfy traditional statistical tests for **randomness**. rt: **quasirandom, random** *Usage note*: Most computational schemes for generation, though usually referred to as **random number generators**, are in fact pseudorandom. Generally, they are built using deterministic computational procedures that rely on a user supplied seed to start the generation process; use of the same seed on different occasions will generate the exact same sequence of numbers.

pseudorandom number *n* - A **number** that has been generated using a deterministic process, such as those underlying most computer packages for generation, that can be shown to generate sequences of numbers that meet traditional statistical tests for **randomness** [Knuth, 1969].[81]

rt: **quasirandom number**, **random number**

pseudorandom process *n* - Any method or procedure that yields **output** that has, within the limits of detection, the mathematical properties of a **random variable** but that is known to be or believed to be **pseudorandom**. rt: **random process, quasirandom process**

pseudorandomization *n* - 1. Any **nonrandom** method of **treatment assignment** with characteristics similar to those associated with **random treatment assignment**; eg, assignments generated with most **computer** based computational schemes for **randomization**. 2. Any method of assignment assumed to have the characteristics of a **random assignment process** (such as with one based on the last digit of a patient's Social Security Number or hospital record number).

psi *n* - [LGk, fr Gk *psei*] The 23rd letter of the **Greek alphabet**, uppercase Ψ, lowercase ψ.

public *adj* - [ME *publique*, fr MF, fr L *publicus*, prob alter of *poplicus*, fr *populus* the people] Of, relating to, or affecting all the people or the area of an entire nation or state.

Public Health Service (PHS) *n* - **United States Public Health Service** (USPHS)

publication *n* - [ME *publicacioun*, fr MF *publication*, fr LL *publication-*, *publicatio*, fr L *publicatus*, pp of *publicare*, fr *publicus* public] 1. The act or process of publishing. 2. A published work.

publication bias *n* - 1. An inclination or tendency toward **publication** of results that support conclusions favoring a particular **hypothesis** or position. 2. Any influence or factor that results in a differential inclination or tendency toward publication, regardless of whether related to the nature or direction of **results** (eg, influences or factors such as gender of the investigator, source of funding for the study, or specific design and operating features of the study). *Usage note*: Most usages are in the sense of defn 1 and are offered in a speculative or cautionary sense (as opposed to a declarative sense) in that demonstration of the **bias** is often difficult or impossible. The **bias** (defn 1) operates when the decision of investigators to prepare a paper for publication is influenced by the nature or strength of the conclusion that can be drawn from the results, or when referees and editors of the journals base their decisions for acceptance or rejection on the statistical importance of the results or on the nature of the conclusions stated or implied by the results. The supposition for **trials** is that the bias is more likely to operate in trials not showing any difference (**nil result**) than for those showing a difference, and among those showing a difference the bias is assumed to be more likely for trials producing **negative results** (defn 2) than for those producing **positive results**. The bias, if operating, has serious implications for **meta-analysis**. Usages in the sense of defn 2 are quite different from those for defn 1 and should be noted as departing from the conventional definition of the bias. In the sense of defn 2, the reference is to any factor influencing publication, whether or not related to the nature or direction of results, including those fixed before or when the study is started, such as the age, gender, or rank of the investigator, or type or source of funding.

publication committee *n* - 1. A **committee** concerned with directing the development and **publication** of **manuscripts** to be or being generated from a **study**. 2. A committee designated for writing a specific manuscript; **paper writing committee**.

publish, published, publishing, publishes *v* - [ME *publishen*, modif of MF *publier*, fr L *publicare*, fr *publicus* public] 1. To make generally known by dissemination to the general public. 2. To make available to the public by deposit in a public **repository**. 3. To have one's work published.

purge *n* - An act or instance of **purging**; the removal of elements regarded as undesirable or unreliable, as in a **data purge**.

purge, purged, purging, purges *v* - [ME *pugen*, fr MF *purgier*, fr L *purigare*, *purgare* to purify, purge, fr *purus* pure + *-igare* (akin to *agere* to drive, do)] To make free of something unwanted or undesirable, as in the removal of **data** generated by a designated **clinic** from the **dataset** of a **multicenter trial** because of **fabrication** of elements of the dataset or because of major **protocol violations**.

purpose *n* - [ME *purpos*, fr OF, fr *purposer* to propose, fr L *proponere* to propose] Something set up as an object or end to be attained; intention. rt: **objective**

Q

quadratic *adj* - Of the 2nd **degree**; involving terms of the 2nd degree at most.

quadratic form *n* - A **homogeneous polynomial** of the 2nd **degree**, eg, $x^2 - 18xy + y^2$.

qualitative *adj* - 1. Pertaining to or concerned with a quality or qualities expressed as **categorizations** or in other **nonmetric** terms 2. Not amenable to **numeric analysis**. ant: **quantitative**

qualitative data *n* - **Nonmetrical data**, such as those derived from subjective assessments or from **categorizations** based on some quality or characteristic (eg, gender or marital status of a person). ant: **quantitative data** rt: **categorical data**

qualitative interaction *n* - An **interaction** in which the **sign** of the **relationship** depends on the value assumed by the **variable** of interest, eg, a treatment by gender interaction that is **positive** for one gender and **negative** for the other gender. rt: **quantitative interaction**

quality *adj* - Being of high **quality**.

quality *n* - [ME *qualite*, fr OF *qualité*, fr L *qualitat-*, *qualitas*, fr *qualis* of what kind; akin to L *qui* who] 1. A particular and essential **characteristic** or **trait**; an inherent feature. 2. A degree of excellence or superiority. 3. A distinguishing feature, trait, or characteristic.

quality assurance *n* - Any method, procedure, or approach for collecting, processing, or analyzing **data** aimed at maintaining or improving their **reliability** or **validity**; includes any or all of the following activities: **pilot testing**, **pretesting**, **repeat reading**, replicate measurement, **data editing**, **double data entry**, **performance monitoring**, aspects of **data analysis** for **treatment effects monitoring**, **site visiting** (defn 1), and **record auditing**. rt: **quality control** *Usage note*: The terms **quality assurance** and **quality control** have similar meanings and are often used interchangeably. The distinction, if any, is perhaps in relation to the extent to which the procedures or methods used for quality assurance or control are based on **sampling** and use of formal statistical procedures for **monitoring** quality. Generally, those components are more evident in quality control than in quality assurance.

quality control *n* - An aggregate of sampling and testing procedures based on statistical theory and **analysis** designed to ensure adequate **quality** in relation to a finished product. rt: **quality assurance** *Usage note*: See **quality assurance**.

quality control center *n* - A **center** concerned with **quality control**. In the case of **multicenter trials**, usually a **resource center** with responsibility for monitoring the quality of various aspects of the **data collection** or **analysis** processes employed in the trial. *Usage note*: Term not recommended except where there is a specific center with designated quality control functions over and above those normally assumed by the **data center**, **data coordinating center**, or **coordinating center**.

quality of care *n* - The degree to which **care** provided or received in some health care setting measures up to some **standard** or **norm**; typically measured in operational terms by the provider and in subjective terms by the recipient.

quality of life *n* - 1. Broadly, the quality of one's life measured against some ideal or relative **standard**. 2. An idealized **estimate** of years of life presumed to remain in which one is free of impairment, disability, or handicap. 3. **quality of life indicator** 4. **quality of life measure** rt: **quality of life indicator**, **quality of life measurement** *Usage note*: Subject to varying uses. Often used as if there are recognized standards for measurement and as if the measurement process implied is the result of an exact science when in reality there is no way of knowing or measuring the quality of one's life since that considered essential for a full life is individual and personal. Typically, measurement centers on operational indicators associated with the functions and activities of daily living. The characterization of quality is simply in terms of the extent to which those being observed are able to maintain particular functions and activities compared to a general **population** or to another **study group**.

quality of life indicator *n* - Any **measurement** or **observation** that is or that can be used as an **indicator** of **quality of life**, eg, being employed, being able to dress oneself, being able to read. rt: **quality of life**, **quality of life measure**, **quality of life measurement** *Usage note*: See **quality of life**.

quality of life measure *n* - 1. **quality of life indicator** 2. A composite measure of **quality of life** as derived from an **index** (defn 3) or as derived by combining several different indices or **quality of life indicators**. rt: **quality of life**, **quality of life indicator**, **quality of life measurement** *Usage note*: See **quality of life**.

quality of life measurement *n* - A **measurement** or a **score** derived from combining a number of different measurements or **indicators**, expressed in **relative** or **absolute** terms, used as a measure of **quality of life**. rt: **quality of life**, **quality of life indicator**, **quality of life measure** *Usage note*: See **quality of life**.

quantile *n* - One of a contiguous set of **ranges**, defined for a **frequency distribution**, such that each set accounts for the same number or fraction of counts represented in the distribution, eg, the quantiles of a **uniform** age distribution, 25 through 55, divided into 3 quantiles would be 25 - 35, 35 - 45, and 45 - 55; also **fractile**; see **centile**, **decile**, **quintile**, **quartile**, **percentile**, **tercile** for specific types.

quantitative *adj* - [ML *quantitativus*, fr L *quantitat-*, *quantitas* quantity + *ivus* -ive] Pertaining to or concerned with quantity expressed in numerical terms. ant: **qualitative**

quantitative data *n* - **Metrical data**, such as those based on counts or on some **continuous measure**, amenable to arithmetic operations. ant: **qualitative data**

quantitative interaction *n* - An **interaction** in which the direction or **sign** of the **relationship** is the same but the magnitude of the difference depends on the value assumed by the **variable** of interest; eg, a treatment by gender interaction that is of the same **sign** for both males and females but that is larger for one gender than for the other gender. rt: **qualitative interaction**

quartile *n* - [ISV, fr L quartus] One of a contiguous set of **ranges** of values that accounts for one-quarter of the total counts represented in a

frequency distribution. See also **centile**, **decile**, **percentile**, **quantile**, **quintile**, and **tercile**.

quasi- *adj* - Having a likeness to something else; resembling.

quasi- *prefix* - [L *quasi*, as if, as it were, approximately, fr *quam* as + *si* if] To some degree, almost or somewhat. rt: **pseudo**

quasi-independent double data entry *n* - **Double data entry** with both entries performed by the same person but at different times, eg, entered on one day and reentered on another day. rt: **dependent double data entry**, **independent double data entry**

quasirandom *adj* - 1. Appearing to be or resembling something **random**; random like. 2. Of, relating to, or concerned with a process considered to approximate a formal **randomization process**. 3. Being or involving entities, such as **numbers**, that are selected or ordered by some **rule** or procedure (eg, one based on the order in which people arrive at a **clinic**) that generates **sequences** that can be viewed as being like those produced or expected with a **random process** but where the rule or procedure is not amenable to testing, or if tested can be shown to yield results that do not satisfy traditional statistical tests for **randomness**. rt: **pseudorandom**, **random** *Usage note*: Not to be confused with **pseudorandom**. See notes for **random** *adj, scientific* and **pseudorandom**.

quasirandom number *n* - A **number** that has been generated by a **rule** or procedure (eg, one based on Social Security **number**) that generates **sequences** of numbers that can be viewed as being like those produced or expected with a **random process**, but where the rule or procedure is not amenable to testing, or if tested can be shown to yield results that do not satisfy traditional statistical tests for **randomness**. rt: **pseudorandom number**, **random number** *Usage note*: See note for **quasirandom**.

quasirandom process *n* - Any method or procedure claimed to be random-like or presumed to have the characteristics of a **random** or **pseudorandom process** but lacking a mathematical basis for the claim or presumption. rt: **random process**, **pseudorandom process** *Usage note*: See notes for **quasirandom** and **random** *adj, scientific*.

quasirandomization *n* - **Randomization** based on a **quasirandom** process. *Usage note*: See notes for **randomization** and **quasirandom**.

query *n* - [alter of earlier *quere*, fr L *quaere*, imper of *quaerere* to ask] 1. A question or inquiry. 2. **edit query**

query, queried, querying, queries *v* - 1. To ask questions or to make inquiries, especially in relation to resolving a doubt or question. 2. To put in the form of a question.

question *n* - [ME, fr MF, fr L *quaestion-, quaestio*, fr *quaesitus, quaestus*, pp of *quaerere* to seek, ask] 1. An interrogative expression used to test knowledge or to elicit information; **query**. 2. A subject or topic in debate or open to discussion. 3. A specific point at issue.

question, questioned, questioning, questions *v* - 1. To ask a **question** of or about. 2. To interrogate. 3. To doubt or dispute. 4. To subject to **examination** or **analysis**.

questionnaire *n* - [F, fr *questionner* to question, fr MF, fr *question*, n] 1. A document containing a series of **questions** that are to be answered by the person receiving it (as in a mailed questionnaire) or to whom administered (as in a face-to-face or telephone **interview**). 2. Any document comprised of a defined set of questions that is used to collect **data** from individuals who complete it or to whom it is administered, eg, such a document as used in a **census, survey**, or **research project; instrument, data form**. rt: **survey instrument** *Usage note*: Usage should be limited to settings where questioning is the main form of **data collection** represented in the document. Use some other term, such as **data form**, when it is only one part of the data collection process, as in most **clinical trials** involving **examination** as well as questioning.

Quetelet, Lambert Adolphe Jacques - (1796 - 1874) Belgian mathematician, statistician, anthropologist, and astronomer, whose interests included the application of mathematical methods of averages and probabilities to human beings individually and as members of groups; investigated relationship between weight and height that resulted in an **index** that bears his name.[70]

Quetelet's Index *n* - An **index** developed by **Lambert Adolphe Jacques Quetelet**[129, 70] used for relating weight to height; ie, wt/ht^2.

quintile *n* - [L *quintus* + E -*ile*] One of a contiguous set of **ranges** that accounts for one-fifth of the total counts represented in a **frequency distribution**. See also **centile, decile, percentile, quantile, quartile**, and **tercile**.

quota *n* - [ML, fr L *quota pars* how great a part] 1. A proportional part or share. 2. The number or amount representing or constituting a proportional share or limit, as in a **recruitment quota**.

quota sample *n* - A **sample** purposefully selected to satisfy specified **quotas**, expressed in **absolute** or **relative** terms, eg, a sample purposely selected to have the same proportionate mix of males and females as represented in the general **population**. *Usage note*: Not to be confused with **random sample** or **representative sample**; see those terms for usage notes.

quota sampling *n* - A method of **sampling** in which the proportionate mix of sampling elements with regard to some characteristic(s) is specified in advance and where selection is constrained to yield the desired mix. The mix specification may be arbitrarily set or may be set to match that of the **population** being sampled. rt: **representative sample** *Usage note*: Not to be confused with **random sampling**.

For the actual number of people to be enrolled into a trial, divide the number promised by 4 and multiply the time stated for getting them by 2

R

race *n* - [MF, generation, fr OIt *razza*] A division of humankind possessing transmissible genetic traits sufficient to characterize it as a distinct type. rt: **ethnic origin**

random *adj, general* - 1. Having or appearing to have no specific pattern or objective. 2. Of or designating a **chance** process in which the occurrence of previous **events** is of no value in predicting future events. 3. **haphazard** syn: **chance, haphazard, lottery** *Usage note*: Avoid; use **haphazard, chance, lottery** or **quasirandom** to avoid confusion with **random** *adj, scientific*. See also note for **lottery**.

random *adj, scientific* - 1. Of or relating to a value, **observation, assignment**, arrangement, etc, that is the result of **chance**. 2. Of or relating to a **sequence, observation, assignment**, arrangement, etc, that is the result of a **chance** process in which the **probability** is known or can be determined. 3. Of or relating to a **pseudorandom** process that has the properties of one that is random. 4. Of or relating to a single value, observation, assignment, or arrangement that is the result of **randomization**. syn: **chance, lottery** (not recommended synonyms, except in lay usage, as in **consent statements** describing the **treatment assignment process**) ant: **nonrandom** rt: **pseudorandom, quasirandom** *Usage note*: Subject to misuse. Avoid in the absence of a probability base (as in *random blood sugar* in reference to routine blood sugar determinations); use **haphazard** or some other term implying less rigor than for **random**. Misuse in the context of trials arise most commonly in relation to characterizations of treatment assignment schemes as **random** that are **systematic** or **haphazard**. See also note for **lottery**.

random *n* - [ME impetuosity, fr MF *randon*, fr OF, fr *randir*, to run, of Gmc origin, akin to OHG *rinnan* to run] A course or sequence that is the result of a **random** or **pseudorandom** **process**. *Usage note*: See notes for **random** *adj*.

random access *adj* - Permitting access in any order, especially in relation to **files** or information stored in a **computer**. ant: **sequential access** *Usage note*: This use of **random** is in the general lay sense of usage, as for **random** *adj, general*.

random access memory (RAM) *n* - [**computing**] A feature in which it is possible to access any of a defined set of **memory** locations within a **computer** in any order and where the time required for access is the same for all orders of access; achieved via use of lookup tables containing coordinates of the various memory locations. *Usage note*: See usage note for **random access**.

random allocation *n* - **random assignment**

random assignment *n* - 1. **Assignment** or designation made using **randomization**. 2. An assignment that is the result of a **random process** or **pseudorandom process**. 3. **random treatment assignment** 4. **haphazard treatment assignment** *Usage note*: Avoid in the sense of defn 4; see note for **random** *adj, scientific*.

random digit dialing *n* - A method of **random sampling** based on telephoning; typically used to select households or designated persons within households for some purpose. The sampling is done by calling a randomly ordered list of telephone numbers in the order given. The calling process continues until the required **sample size** is achieved or until all telephones numbers on the lists have been called. Those doing the sampling follow set rules regarding the number of attempts to be made to reach a working phone number before giving up and for determining whether a phone is located in a household or in some other kind of establishment (eg, a business). rt: **random sampling**

random error *n* - **Error** that is the result of a **random** or an apparently **random process**. rt: **random variable, systematic error** *Usage note*: Subject to misuse. Use should be limited to settings in which the error has no apparent explanation and has the properties of a random variable. The term should not be used to characterize variation due to **bias** or **systematic error**.

random number *n* - A **number** generated or drawn via some defined **random** or **pseudorandom process**.

random number generator *n* - A system for generating **random** or **pseudorandom numbers**, eg, a **computer program** generating such numbers.

random order *n* - 1. An ordering of a set of objects or numbers such that every possible ordering has the same **probability** of occurrence. 2. An **order** that is the result of some **randomization process**. rt: **random permutation**

random permutation *n* - 1. The act or process of changing the ordering of a specified set of items, objects, or entities by **randomization**. 2. An ordered arrangement of a set of items, objects, or entities that results from randomization. 3. One of the possible arrangements of a specified set of items, objects, or entities selected at **random**, eg, the arrangement *ACB* selected by rolling an ace with a die from among the 6 possible arrangements: (1) *ABC*, (2) *ACB*, (3) *BAC*, (4) *BCA*, (5) *CAB*, and (6) *CBA*.

random process *n* - 1. Any method or procedure that yields **output** that has the defined mathematical properties of a **random variable**. 2. **pseudorandom process** rt: **quasirandom process**

random sample *n* - A **sample** in which every **sampling unit** has a known **probability** of selection. *Usage note*: There is no guarantee that a given random sample is **representative** of the **population** from which it arises or is drawn, hence, a random sample should not be characterized as representative in the absence of methods or evidence to support the claim. See **representative sample** for additional comments.

random sampling *n* - 1. A method of **sampling** in which every member of the **population** being sampled has a known **probability** of selection. 2. A method in which every arrangement or ordering (eg, of records to be read or of **treatment assignment** in a **randomization**) has the same probability of occurrence or has a known probability of occurrence.

random start *n* - A point, determined by a **random process**, at which some process or procedure begins or is to begin, eg, the point at which one enters and begins using numbers in a table of random numbers.

random treatment assignment *n* - 1. **Treatment assignment** determined by **randomization**. 2. The **treatment assignment** for a **treatment unit** (usually a person), as determined by **randomization**. syn: **random assignment**

random variable *n* - A **variable** that may assume any one of a number of different values as determined by a **probability distribution**; the variable may be **continuous** or **discrete**. syn: chance variable, **stochastic variable**, **variable**

random variation *n* - 1. **Variation** that is **random**. 2. Variation that is due to a **random process**.

random walk *n* - A **sequence** of movements or steps, each one of which is the result of a **random process**, eg, Brownian movement.

random-effects model *n* - A **mathematical model**, eg, as used in **analysis of variance**, in which the **parameters** of a **fixed-effects model** are themselves values of **random variables**. syn: components of variance model ant: **fixed-effects model** rt: **mixed-effects model**

randomization *n* - 1. An act of assigning or ordering that is the result of a **random process** such as that represented by a sequence of numbers in a table of **random numbers** or a sequence of numbers produced by a **random number generator**, eg, the **assignment** of a **patient** to **treatment** using a **random process**. 2. The process of deriving an order or sequence of items, specimens, records, or the like using a **random process**. rt: **haphazardization**, **quasirandom** *Usage note*: Do not use as a characterization except in settings where there is an explicit or implied mathematical basis for supporting the usage, as discussed in usage notes for **random** *adj*. Use other terms implying less rigor than implied by **randomization**, such as **haphazardization**, **quasirandomization**, or **chance**, when that basis is not present or evident.

randomization breakdown *n* - A **breakdown** (defn 2) in **randomization** (defn 1) because of failure to follow the **treatment assignment schedule** as determined by a given **random process**, eg, as a result of using assignments in an order other than the one indicated. *Usage note*: A randomization process should not be characterized as having broken down without evidence of departures from the assignment schedule. It is a mistake to equate a small **p-value**, as obtained from a **randomness test**, as proof of a breakdown. Large departures (hence, small p-values) can occur by chance alone with random processes. See also **randomness test**.

randomization examination *n* - [**trials**] The **examination** at which **randomization** takes places or at which the **assignment** is revealed to the person being **enrolled**, eg, as done by opening a sealed envelope containing the assignment or by generation of the assignment from an on-site **computer**. rt: **randomization visit, treatment assignment examination**

randomization list *n* - A **list** used for making **treatment assignments** in a **randomized trial**; a list of bottle numbers or letters designating **treatment regimens** arranged in **random order** and used for making treatment assignments; a listing of **permuted blocks** arranged in random order and used for making treatment assignments.

randomization test *n* - A class of **nonparametric statistical tests** for determining the **likelihood** of some aspect of an observed **sample**; typically done by determining all possible arrangements of the sample with regard to the aspect of interest and then determining the **proportion** of the arrangements that are as extreme or more extreme (in a **probability** sense) than the one observed. Examples include **Fisher's exact test** and **Mann-Whitney test**.

randomization unit *n* - [**trials**] The **unit** to which **treatment**, as dictated by **randomization**, is or is to be applied; **treatment assignment unit**. The unit is usually a person (or a part of a person, eg, an eye) but may be an aggregate of persons, such as those occupying the same household or housed in the same hospital ward.

randomization visit *n* - [**trials**] The **visit** at which **randomization** takes place or at which the **assignment** is revealed to the person being **enrolled**, eg, as done by opening a sealed envelope containing the assignment or by generation of the assignment from an on-site **computer**. rt: **randomization examination, treatment assignment visit**

randomize, randomized, randomizing, randomizes *v* - To arrange, order, mix, or assign by use of **randomization**. ant: **nonrandomized** rt: **random** *Usage note*: See **random**.

randomized *n* - The condition of having been assigned to a **treatment** via a **random process**; normally considered to have occurred when the

treatment assignment is revealed to any member of the clinic staff, eg, when an envelope containing the treatment is opened at the **clinic**.

randomized block *n* - 1. A **block** (defn 2) of **treatment units** arranged in **random order**. 2. A **random permutation** (defn 3) of elements in a block. rt: **complete block, incomplete block**

randomized block design *n* - A **design** involving **randomized blocks**.

randomized clinical trial (RCT) *n* - A **clinical trial** in which the **treatment** to be administered to a specific **treatment unit** is selected by a **random process** from among the set of treatments considered in the trial, eg, a trial involving a single **test** and a single **control treatment** in which a coin flip determines whether a **patient** receives the test or control treatment.

randomized control *n* - [**trials**] 1. A **treatment unit** in a **trial** assigned by **randomization** to receive the **control treatment**. 2. A **control** selected by a **random process**.

randomized control trial (RCT) *n* - A **randomized trial** involving a **control treatment**. *Usage note*: Used to emphasize the fact that the trial includes a control treatment, eg, as used by Chalmers and coworkers [1981].[23] Not recommended; use **randomized controlled trial** instead (see usage note for **controlled**). If used at all, its use should be limited to trials involving a single control treatment. Strictly speaking, it is not applicable to trials involving multiple control treatments or to trials involving only test treatments. However, even if applicable, the term is not recommended because of the emphasis on the nature of the selection process for the control treatment to the exclusion of that for the test treatment or treatments. While it is true that the assignment to the control treatment is the result of a random process, the same is true for assignments to the test treatment(s). The modifier, **randomized**, used alone is sufficient to convey that notion (see **randomized controlled trial** for additional comments).

randomized controlled clinical trial *n* - 1. A **randomized controlled trial** done in a **clinical** setting. 2. A randomized controlled trial intended to have or having clinical relevance. 3. A randomized controlled trial with a **clinical event** as an **outcome measure**. *Usage note*: See **randomized controlled trial** and **randomized trial** for comments.

randomized controlled trial (RCT) *n* - 1. A **trial** involving two or more **study treatments**, **concurrent enrollment** and **followup** of the **treatment units**, and in which treatment assignments (typically **masked treatment assignments** (defn 1)) are **random** or **pseudorandom**. 2. Any trial having the features specified in defn 1, but involving **quasirandom** assignment. 3. Any trial having the features specified in defn 1 involving any assignment scheme, even one that is deterministic (eg, one involving **minimization**), in which it can be argued or in which it is reasonable to assume that the **assignment process** is not subject to influence by those being enrolled or by those responsible for enrollment (not recommended usage). 4. **randomized controlled clinical trial** *Usage note*: The modifier *randomized* should be limited to uses in the sense of defns 1 and 4. Use in the sense of defn 2 should be appropriately qualified to make readers aware of the quasirandom nature of the assignment process. The modifier should not be used for the class of trials represented in defn 3. Technically, the modifier *controlled* is not necessary in the presence of the modifier *randomized* since randomized trials are controlled by definition.

randomized response technique *n* - A **survey** technique, introduced by Warner [1965],[158] for estimating the **proportion** of a **population** engaged in an activity that is not likely to be readily reported or acknowledged (eg, homosexual behavior, drunk driving, illicit drug use, child molestation, spousal battery) because of social mores or because it is illegal. The technique involves the use of two questions, each having the same range of responses (eg, yes or no; 1, 2, or 3) in which the question to be answered is chosen by the respondent (by a coin flip or using some other randomizing device with known **probabilities**) but is not identified to the surveyor. One question is innocuous and has a known **distribution** of **responses**; the other one has to do with the behavior or activity of interest. For example, a survey designed to estimate the **frequency** of cocaine use in a population might require a respondent to answer one of the following questions (depending on whether a coin flip produces a head or a tail): *Have you ever used cocaine?* or *Were you born in December?*. The estimated frequency of cocaine use is given by the proportion of the population answering in the affirmative, minus the proportion expected to so

answer if everyone had answered the second question; in the example 0.0849, assuming an equal distribution of births over a calendar year. The technique is used to obtain a reliable **estimate** of the fraction of the population engaging in the activity by making it obvious to the respondent that the surveyor is **masked** to the question being answered; done with the intent of increasing the probability of truthful replies.

randomized trial *n* - 1. **randomized controlled trial** 2. A trial involving **random treatment assignment**. 3. A trial involving **randomization** of **treatment**. ant: **nonrandomized trial** *Usage note*: Preferred to **randomized controlled trial** for reasons indicated in the usage note for that term. Also see that comment for limitations on usage of the modifier *randomized*.

randomly selected control *n* - A **control** (defn 3) selected via some **random process** or **pseudorandom process**; not to be confused with **randomized control**.

randomness *n* - The state or quality of being **random** or random like. *Usage note*: Use with caution in assertions or statements of presumed fact regarding the "randomness" of processes such as those used for **randomization** of **treatment assignments** in **trials**. Usually, the state or quality of randomness has to be inferred. Hence, checks for "randomness", using **tests of significance** and associated **p-values**, are not, by themselves, sufficient to establish "randomness" or lack thereof.

randomness test *n* - Any of a variety of **statistical tests** applied to **data** to determine whether they are consistent with having been the product of a **random process**, eg, such a test applied to the **distribution** of **treatment assignments** across the various **treatment groups** represented in a **trial**. Most such tests are forms of **randomization tests**. Such tests, in **randomized trials**, are used primarily in relation to analyses aimed at determining whether the **observed treatment assignment ratio** is consistent with the **expected treatment assignment ratio**. The size of the resulting **p-value** is used as a guide for gauging the likelihood of a **randomization breakdown**. *Usage note*: Such tests are useful in alerting one to possible breakdowns in the randomization process, but they are not sufficient to prove the existence of breakdowns. Large departures from the expected treatment assignment ratio are possible by **chance** alone. Hence, a small p-value for the test should not be used by itself as a basis for characterizing a process as having broken down. See also **randomization breakdown**.

range *n* - [Often attrib ME, row of persons, fr MF *renge*, fr OF *rengier* to range] 1. The space or extent included. 2. The **end points** or **limits** of a series or **distribution**; such end points for a subpart of a series or distribution, eg, the end points of a **quantile**. rt: **interquartile range**, **variance**

range, ranged, ranging, ranges *v* - [ME *rangen*, fr MF *ranger*, fr OF *rengier*, fr *renc*, *reng* line, place, row] 1. To extend in a particular direction. 2. To change within **limits**.

rank *adj* - [ME, fr OE *ranc* overbearing, strong; akin to OE *riht* right] High in amount or value.

rank *n* - [MF *renc*, *reng*, of Gmc origin; akin to OHG *hring* ring] 1. **Row** or **series**, eg, as a line of soldiers arranged in close formation. 2. The numerical value affixed to a person, place, or thing corresponding to its order or position after arrangement by some process (eg, a **lottery** used conscription) or **metric variable** (eg, date of birth). 3. **Relative** standing or position. 4. The number of linearly **independent rows** in a **matrix**. 5. A social **class**.

rank, ranked, ranking, ranks *v* - 1. To arrange in **order**. 2. To take a position **relative** to others. 3. To determine the relative position of something.

rank correlation *n* - A **correlation** of **ranks** based on some **metric variable**, as in **Kendall's tau** or **Spearman's rank correlation**.

rank correlation coefficient *n* - The **correlation coefficient** derived using **ranks** based on some **metric variable**, as in **Kendall's tau** or **Spearman's rank correlation**.

rank order *n* - 1. The position of some entity, object, or person arranged according to some **metric measure** or **variable**. 2. **rank** (defn 2)

rate *n* - [ME, fr MF, fr ML *rata*, fr L (*pro*) *rata* (*parte*) according to a fixed proportion] 1. A measure of **frequency** expressed as a fraction, as in a **proportion**, or as a number expressed as a **percentage** or with some larger base divisible by 10, eg, cardiovascular deaths per 10,000 deaths. 2. A quantity, amount, or degree of something measured per unit of something else, eg, number

of neonatal deaths per 1,000 live births; number of miles traveled per unit time, as in 60 miles per hour. 3. A quantity measured with respect to another quantity, such as a monetary exchange rate. rt: **attack rate**, **crude rate**, **incidence rate**, **standardized rate** *Usage note*: Often loosely used, as in the sense of defn 1, as in **survival rate**. Strictly speaking, the term applies only for uses in the sense of defn 2.

rate, rated, rating, rates *v* - 1. allot 2. To make a determination or **estimate** of value or worth. 3. To determine or assign a **rank** or **class**.

rate adjustment *n* - **Adjustment** of a **rate**, as in **direct rate adjustment** or **indirect rate adjustment**.

ratio *n* - [L, computation, reason] A quantity that indicates the relation of one number or mathematical expression to another with respect to magnitude, quantity, or degree, as provided by the quotient of those two numbers or mathematical expressions. rt: **proportion**, **rate** *Usage note*: Not to be confused with **proportion**. The **numerator** of the two numbers forming a proportion is contained in the **denominator**. The two numbers represented in a ratio generally have different bases. Both proportions and ratios denote relationships; however, in the case of proportions the relationship is to a defined whole, whereas for ratios the relationship pertains to some variable or factor common to both numbers.

ratio estimate *n* - An **estimate** involving the **ratio** of two **variates**; in **survey sampling**, an **estimate** of a **population** total or **mean** for a designated **variable** derived by using a known population total for another variable, eg, as provided by a recent **census**, and by multiplying that total by the **ratio** of the two variates as obtained from the **sample**.

raw *adj* - [ME, fr OE *hrēaw*; akin to OHG *hrō* raw, L *crudus* raw, *cruor* blood, Gk *kreas* flesh] 1. Being in or near a natural state; not processed or refined. 2. Not **adjusted**. syn: **crude** ant: **adjusted**

raw data *n* - 1. **Measurements** and **observations** as recorded on a **data record** or **data form**. 2. Unedited data; data before any editing. 3. **Data** prior to **adjustment**. 4. **Data** contained in an electronic **data file** or a listing of the file prior to manipulation, such as those involved in **data reduction** in preparation for **data analysis**.

ray *n* - [ME, fr MF *rai*, fr L *radius* rod, ray; perhaps akin to L *radix* root] A beam of radiant energy; a stream of material particles traveling in the same line.

RC *n* - **reading center**

RCT *n* - 1. **randomized clinical trial** 2. **randomized controlled trial** *Usage note*: Not recommended notation for reasons indicated in notes for **clinical trial, randomized control trial, randomized controlled trial,** and **randomized trial.**

re- *prefix* - [ME, fr OF, fr L *re-, red-* back, again, against] 1. again; anew 2. back; backward (as in recall)

re-entry *n* - The act of entering again.

react, reacted, reacting, reacts *v* - [NL *reactus,* pp of *reagere,* fr L, *re-* + *agere* to act] 1. To exert an opposite or counterbalancing force or influence. 2. To respond to a stimulus. 3. To act in opposition to a force or influence.

reaction *n* - 1. The act or process of **reacting.** 2. Bodily response to or activity aroused by a stimulus or agent.

reactor *n* - 1. One who **reacts.** 2. Something that reacts or that produces a reaction.

read, reading, reads *v* - [ME *reden* to advise, interpret, read, fr OE *rǣdan*; akin to OHG *rātan* to advise, L *reri* to calculate] To **examine** or **observe** to determine meaning or **significance.**

reader *n* - One who **reads.**

reader mask *n* - [**trials**] A **mask** imposed on a **reader** to keep that person from learning of **treatment assignment** and course of **treatment** for those on whom readings are made or to be made. rt: **data analyst mask, data collector mask, mask, treater mask**

reading center (RC) *n* - 1. A **center** responsible for interpreting and codifying information from a specified set of materials, **records,** or documents (eg, ECGs, fundus photographs, chest x-rays, biopsy or autopsy specimens, death certificates). 2. Such a center in a **multicenter study**; see **resource center.**

real *adj* - [ME, real, relating to things (in law), fr MF, fr ML & LL; ML *realis* relating to things (in law), fr LL, real, fr L *res* thing, fact; akin to Skt *rai* property] 1. Of or relating to fixed, permanent, or immovable things (as lands or tenements). 2. Not fictional, imaginary, or artificial.

real time *n* - Present or current time; near current time (as in time critical computing).

recall *n* - Remembrance of what has been learned or experienced.

recall, recalled, recalling, recalls *v* - 1. To recollect. 2. To remind one of.

recall bias *n* - 1. A tendency to **recall** and report recent **events** more accurately than past events. 2. A tendency to **recall** and report certain facts more accurately than others. 3. Bias due to differential recall, eg, bias in a **case-control study** due to a differential in the recall of **cases** compared to **controls** in regard to past **exposures.**

receive, received, receiving, receives *v* - [ME *receiven,* fr ONF *receivre,* fr L *recipere,* fr *re-* + *capere* to take] 1. To come into possession; to acquire. 2. To serve or act as a receptacle or container.

receiver *n* - One or something that **receives.**

receiver operating characteristic (RoC) *adj* - Of, relating to, or concerned with the characteristic feature of a procedure or test under different settings or inputs.

receiver operating characteristic curve *n* - A **curve** displaying the **specificity** (on the **x-axis**) and **sensitivity** (on the **y-axis**) of a **screening test** or diagnostic procedure at different **cutpoints** of the test. Originally developed in the context of **experiments** involving the ability of a receiver to detect a signal or stimuli of differing intensities. See Begg [1991],[7] Hanley [1989],[65] and Metz [1978][103] for review.

reciprocal *adj* - [L *reciprocus* returning the same way, alternating, irreg fr *re-* + *pro-*] Inversely related; opposite.

reciprocal *n* - 1. Something in a **reciprocal** relationship to another. 2. One of a pair of numbers such that their product is one, eg, 3/4 and 4/3.

recognize, recognized, recognizing, recognizes *v* - [modif of MF *reconoisis-,* stem of *reconoistre,* fr L *recognoscere,* fr *re-* + *cognoscere* to know] To acknowledge or take notice of in some definite way; to perceive to be something or someone previously seen.

record *n* - 1. A group of related **data items** or **fields** treated as a unit, eg, a **patient chart** or completed **data collection form.** 2. A **paper** or **electronic** document that contains or is designed to contain a set of facts related to some occurrence, transaction, or the like. rt: **primary record**, **secondary record**, **source record**

record audit *n* - 1. A **comparison** of **data** recorded in one document with those recorded in another document for assessing or determining the **accuracy** or **reliability** of data; in the context of **trials**, often the comparison of data in **study records** with those in **medical charts**. 2. A comparison of information keyed from a study form with that recorded on the study form for the purpose of determining the accuracy or reliability of the keying process. 3. An **audit** of records by the **FDA** in relation to an **INDA** or **NDA**. 4. A search for external evidence that a person purported to have been **enrolled** into a **study** actually exists, eg, as done by locating the person's **medical chart** at the **site** of **enrollment**. rt: **audit**, **desk audit**, **off-site record audit**, **on-site record audit**, **record monitor** *Usage note*: Subject to varying uses and interpretations. Use with caution and with sufficient detail to make sense of usage clear. Details should include information concerning the purpose or intent of the audit and its nature, extent, and method. Usages involving the notion of comparison, as in the sense of defns 1, 2, and 3, should include details regarding the nature of the records being compared. Clearly, the number of discrepancies noted will be larger when the comparison involves records having different formats or functions (eg, study forms versus medical charts) than when records have similar formats or functions (eg, paper form versus its **electronic** counterpart as created by **data entry**). Most audits are **ad hoc** and, hence, are of little value as tools for estimating **error** or discrepancy **rates**. Rates require denominators defined by **sampling frames** or audits of all records. The absence of denominator data makes it impossible to calculate discrepancy or "error" rates. In addition, even with denominator data, resulting rates must be interpreted with caution, especially if viewed as "error" rates. Most rates are better thought of as discrepancy rates. They should not be regarded as error rates, except where one of the sources of information in the comparison is known to be correct or is regarded as being correct. Use descriptors or modifiers (such as, **random** record audit or 100% record audit) to characterize the method used for selecting records for audit or the extent of the audit. Use

on-site when the audit is performed at the site where the records were generated (eg, an audit of **clinic** records as performed by a **circuit rider** or **record monitor**). Use **off-site** when the audit is performed remote from the site of generation (as in the case of an audit of clinic records on file at the **coordinating center**). See also usage note for **audit** and **record monitoring**.

record auditing *v* - The act or process of performing a **record audit**. rt: **record monitoring** *Usage note*: May be used interchangeably with **record monitoring**, though not recommended. See notes for **record monitoring** and for **audit**, **record audit**, and **record monitor**.

record auditor *n* - 1. One who **audits records**. 2. **record monitor** *Usage note*: Use **record auditor** in relation to a person, such as one from the **FDA**, performing a **record audit** for the purpose of determining the authenticity or veracity of study records or information recorded in those records; use **record monitor** for one performing checks and **comparisons** of records during or soon after their generation as part of an ongoing **quality assurance** process in relation to **data collection** or record keeping. See also notes for **record monitor**, **record auditing**, and **record monitoring**.

record linkage *n* - A **relationship** established between **records** (eg, **baseline** and **followup forms** for a **patient** in a **trial**) in order to achieve some end or purpose (eg, assessment of changes over time as determined from data recorded on baseline and followup forms).

record monitor *n* - 1. One who **monitors** records. 2. **record auditor** 3. **circuit rider**; especially one who relies heavily on **record monitoring** as a tool for **quality assurance** of an ongoing **data collection** process. *Usage note*: May be used interchangeably with **record auditor**, though not advised. **Record monitor** should be used to designate a person having a responsibility for **quality assurance** of an ongoing data collection process via periodic checks and **comparisons** of **data forms** for the purpose of identifying and correcting errors or deficiencies noted and for the purpose of reducing similar kinds of errors or deficiencies in the future. Use **record auditor** to designate a person performing **record audits** not related to an ongoing quality assurance process, as in relation to a person performing a record audit for the **FDA** after completion of a **trial**, or for a person performing an audit during the course of a trial not employed in the trial and not having responsibility for quality assurance. See also notes for **record auditor**, **record auditing**, and **record monitoring**.

record monitoring *v* - 1. In relation to **data collection** in a **study**, an ongoing **quality assurance** process focused on record keeping and recording procedures and practices and involving periodic checks and **comparisons** of **data forms** with the aim of reducing the frequency of **errors** and discrepancies in a finished **dataset**; achieved by querying suspicious or deficient data for possible correction and by feedback procedures aimed at improving the data collection process for the remainder of the study. 2. **record auditing** *Usage note*: May be use interchangeably with **record auditing**, though not recommended. Use should be limited to that implied with defn 1. Use **record auditing** when the auditing is not related to an ongoing quality assurance process within the context of a study. See also notes for **audit**, **record auditor**, and **record monitor**.

recruit *n* - [F *recrute*, *recrue* fresh growth, new levy of soldiers, fr MF, fr *recroistre* to grow up again, fr L *recrescere*, fr re- + *crescere* to grow] A newcomer to a field or a defined activity; **enrollee**.

recruit, recruited, recruiting, recruits *v* - 1. To seek to **enroll** or fill with new members. 2. To increase or maintain the number of persons engaged or enrolled in some activity or function.

recruitment *n* - The activity or process of recruiting for **enrollment**; **patient recruitment**. rt: **screening** *Usage note*: In **trials**, usually a constellation of activities characterized by one or more **baseline examinations** performed to assess **eligibility**, to establish **baselines** for subsequent evaluations, and to carry out the **consent process**.

recruitment goal *n* - The **goal** in relation to **recruitment**, such as that for a **trial** as given by a calculated **sample size**; **patient recruitment goal**. rt: **sample size calculation** *Usage note*: Not to be confused with **recruitment quota**.

recruitment log *n* - A **log** maintained by a **recruiting study site**, such as a **clinic** in a **trial**, of persons considered for **enrollment** into a **study**. Usually maintained to provide a description of the characteristics of the **population** screened for enrollment; **screening log**.

recruitment period *n* - **enrollment period**

recruitment quota *n* - 1. The number of individuals of a specified type to be **recruited**; **patient recruitment quota**. 2. The proportionate share of a whole to be represented by a designated type or class of persons. *Usage note*: Not to be confused with **recruitment goal**. **Recruitment goal** relates to the overall number to be enrolled in a recruitment effort; **recruitment quota** relates to the mix of people to be enrolled, as specified by absolute numbers or in relative terms. The imposition of quotas in trials should be done with caution since they make achieving a stated recruitment goal more difficult in that they limit the type of people who can be considered for enrollment after individual quotas have been met. For example, a trial having a recruitment goal of 100 and a quota of 50 males and 50 females means that only males or females can be considered for enrollment once the quota is met for the other sex group, thereby prolonging the time required to achieve the stated recruitment goal of 100. Quotas should not be imposed except where there is a need or desire to carry out **subgroup analyses** within subgroups defined by the quota and where there is a need or desire to perform **comparisons** within those subgroups at a specified level of **precision**.

reduce, reduced, reducing, reduces *v* - [ME *reducen* to lead back, fr L *reducere*, fr re- + *ducere* to lead] 1. To diminish in size, amount, extent, or scope. 2. To make shorter; abridge.

reduction *n* - [ME *reduccion* restoration, fr MF *reduction*, fr LL & L; LL *reduction-*, *reductio* reduction (in a syllogism), fr L, *restoration*, fr *reductus*, pp of *reducere*] 1. The act or process of **reducing**; the state of being reduced, as in **data reduction**. 2. The amount by which something is reduced.

reduction of data *n* - **data reduction**

refer, referred, referring, refers *v* - [ME *referren*, fr L *referre* to bring back, report, refer, fr re- + *ferre* to carry] [**medicine**] To send or direct for **treatment**, aid, or information.

referee *n* - Broadly, a person to whom matters are referred for advice or resolution. In the context of a **manuscript** submitted to a **peer review scientific journal**, a person selected by an editor for the purposes of providing advice to the editor as to the suitability of the manuscript for **publication** and a written critique of the manuscript for transmission, by the editor, to the **author**(s) of the manuscript. rt: **peer review**

referee, refereed, refereeing, referees *v* - To **review** as a prelude to possible **publication** in a **peer review scientific journal** to determine whether or not a particular work should be published and, if accepted for publication, the additions, deletions, or modifications that must be made as a condition for publication. rt: **review**

reference *n* - 1. In **manuscripts** and printed documents, something that refers readers elsewhere for supporting information or material. 2. **reference citation**

reference bias *n* - A tendency or inclination to **cite** sources of information and material supporting one point of view to the exclusion of another. syn: citation bias

reference citation *n* - Information, such as contained in a **reference list** or **bibliography**, that provides **data** needed to locate information or material cited in a work, such as a **manuscript**, and presented in a standard format, eg, as required in journals. Generally, the citation includes the name of the author, title of the work, and where and by whom published. The citation may be to a **primary** or **secondary source**.

reference drug *n* - **control drug**

reference group *n* - 1. A **group** arbitrarily designated or otherwise recognized as the one to which others are to be compared, eg, the group aged 45 - 54 for **comparison of treatment differences** among **subgroups** aged 55 - 64 and ≥ 65. 2. **comparison group**

reference list *n* - **bibliography**

reference population *n* - A defined **population** used for **comparison, adjustment,** or **standardization** of results from one or more **study populations; standard population**. rt: **target population**

referent *n* - [L *referent-, referens,* prp of *referre*] One that refers or is referred to.

referral medical care center *n* - A **secondary** or **tertiary medical care center**.

referred care *n* - [**medicine**] **Care** by a person or agency provided to a **patient** on referral from a **primary** or **secondary care** source; **care** that takes place at or via a **secondary** or **tertiary care center**. rt: **secondary care, tertiary care**

regimen *n* - [MF, fr L *regimin-, regimen* rule, fr *regere* to rule] 1. A systematic plan or course of activities. 2. The plan or course of activities as specified in a **study protocol**. 3. The plan or course of activities designated for a person in a study. 4. The plan or course of activities designated for a **treatment group** in a **trial**; such a plan as contained in the treatment protocol for the trial. 5. A **prescribed** course of **treatment**. 6. A prescribed set of activities or practices for a person or persons having a specified health condition; **treatment** (defn 4).

region *n* - [ME, fr MF, fr L *region-, regio,* fr *regere* to rule] An **open** connected set of **data points**, including or excluding **boundary** points.

register *n* - [ME *registre,* fr MF, fr ML *registrum,* alter of LL *regesta,* pl, *register,* fr L, neut pl of *regestus,* pp of *regerere* to bring back, fr *re-* + *gerere* to bear] 1. A roster, ledger, list, or book in which **records** of acts, events, names, or the like are kept (eg, a register of **patients** having a particular **disease**; a register of **trials** of a particular type). 2. **registration, registry, enrollment**

register, registered, registering, registers *v* - 1. To enter into; to be **enrolled**. 2. To make an entry into a **register**. 3. To correspond exactly.

registration *n* - 1. The act of **registering**, as in entering one's name and other pertinent information into a **register**. 2. **enrollment** 3. A **document** certifying an act of registering. 4. The granting of an **application** or **license**; in regard to a **new drug**, the approval of a **new drug application** by the **Food and Drug Administration**. *Usage note*: Registration (defn 1) may or may not correspond to enrollment. Usually the act of registration (defn 1) is a necessary but not sufficient condition for enrollment. Hence, the two terms should not be used interchangeably. In the case of **trials**, registration typically takes place during the first contact with a person in relation to the **enrollment process**; signaled by the act of entering the person's name into a register or **log** or issuing an **identification number** for the person. The act of enrollment takes place when the **treatment assignment** is revealed or **treatment** is initiated and usually after **baseline** evaluations have been completed and **consent** has been obtained.

registration trial *n* - 1. A **trial** used to support a **new drug application**; a trial used to support an **application** for **license**. 2. A trial intended for support of a new drug application or application for license, if made.

registry *n* - 1. **enrollment, registration** 2. An official **data** book. 3. A specific entry in a register or data book.

regress *n* - [ME, fr L *regressus*, fr *regressus*, pp of *regredi* to go back, fr *re-* + *gradi* to go] An act or the privilege of going or coming back.

regress, regressed, regressing, regresses *v* - 1. To be subject to or exhibit **regression**. 2. To tend to approach or revert to the **mean**.

regression *n* - [Concept introduced by **Francis Galton** and used in analyses of data from **experiments** involving plant genetics[57]] 1. A functional **relationship** (postulated or **estimated**) between two or more **variables**, eg, as described in a **linear** or **logistic regression model**, and generally assessed empirically using **observed data**; sometimes used to **predict** values of one variable given the value of others. 2. An act or instance of **regression** or of **regression analysis**. rt: **regression to the mean**

regression analysis *n* - 1. **Analysis** based on a **regression model**. 2. **Estimation** of **coefficients** in a **regression model** using **observed data**; use of such coefficients in an analysis, eg, in deriving a **treatment comparison**, **adjusted** for **differences** in the **baseline** comparability of the **treatment groups**. 3. The process of finding the "best" set of **regressors** for a given model, as in **forward stepwise regression** or **backward stepwise regression**; the resulting set is typically used to describe the **dependent variable**, **y**, as a function of the chosen regressors or to predict y, given the chosen set.

regression coefficient *n* - 1. A **coefficient** in a **regression model**; see **linear regression model** and **nonlinear regression model** for examples. 2. An **estimate** of such a coefficient as obtained from a **regression analysis**.

regression curve *n* - A graphic representation of a **regression equation**, especially such a representation resulting in a **curve** (defn 3). rt: **regression line**

regression equation *n* - An **equation** expressing a postulated or observed **relationship** of one variable (**dependent variable**) to one or more **independent variables**, such as expressed in a **linear** or **nonlinear regression model**.

regression estimate *n* - An **estimate** derived from a postulated or observed **relationship** of one variable to another, eg, in a **ratio estimate**.

regression line *n* - 1. A **graphic** representation of a **regression equation** having the form of a straight **line**. 2. **regression curve** rt: **regression curve**

regression method *n* - A method of **data analysis** involving the use of a **regression model** and the **estimation** of **regression coefficients**.

regression model *n* - A **model equation** expressing a postulated or **observed** relationship between a **dependent variable** and one or more **independent variables**, eg, as a **linear** or **nonlinear regression model** or in a **proportional hazards regression model**. syn: **regression equation**

regression procedure *n* - An **analysis** procedure involving a **regression model**.

regression to the mean *n* - [Concept introduced by **Francis Galton** [1886][57] in describing the tendency of offspring generated from plant breeding experiments to be less extreme in a designated trait or characteristic than their parents] 1. The tendency or phenomenon for a characteristic, trait, or feature to be less extreme, marked, or pronounced in offspring than in parents, eg, the tendency of parents of extreme stature (tall or short) to have children less extreme in stature (ie, closer to the general mean in stature). 2. The tendency for a **variable** yielding an extreme value for a chosen **observation unit** to yield a less extreme value the next time it is observed on that particular observation unit, eg, the tendency in a study involving the selection of people with high blood pressures for the blood pressures measured after selection to be lower than those used for selection. rt: **regression** *Usage note*: Usage should be limited to settings where the determination, measurement, or variable in question is subject to the force described. Do not use simply as a means of describing a shift to less extreme values over the course of **followup** when the selection force is not operating or in settings where it is unreasonable to assume its presence.

regressor *n* - 1. Any one of the **independent variables** in a **regression model**. 2. The **independent variable**(s) in a regression **relationship**.

regular *adj* - [ME *reguler*, fr MF, fr LL *regularis* regular, fr L, of a bar, fr *regula* rule] 1. Formed, built, arranged, or ordered according to some established **rule**, **law**, **principle**, or type. 2. Recurring, attending, or functioning at fixed or **uniform** intervals.

regular followup visit *n* - Any one of a series of **visits** to be made during **followup**; also **required followup visit**. syn: **scheduled followup visit** ant: **interim followup visit, unscheduled followup visit** *Usage note*: **Regular** in this context refers to **visits** intended to take place at specified times over the course of **followup** as required for **data collection** and for carrying out procedures and assessments specified in the **study protocol**.

reimburse, reimbursed, reimbursing, reimburses *v* - [*re-* + obs E *imburse* (to put in the pocket, pay) fr ML *imburare*, fr L *in-* in- + ML *bursa* purse] To pay (money) back to someone; repay.

reimbursement *n* - The act of **reimbursing**.

reject, rejected, rejecting, rejects *v* - [ME *rejecten*, fr L *rejectus*, pp of *reicere*, fr *re-* + *jacere* to throw] To refuse to accept, consider, take, or use.

rejection *n* - The action of **rejecting**; the state of being rejected.

rejection region *n* - The **range** of values at and beyond the **critical value** of a **test statistic** that, when observed for a given set of **data**, lead to **rejection** of the **null hypothesis**. The **region** is defined by a single **critical value** for **one-tailed tests** and by an upper and lower value for **two-tailed tests**. The value(s) is (are) picked such that the region corresponds to the specified **type I error** level for the test statistic. syn: **critical region** ant: **acceptance region**

relate, related, relating, relates *v* - [L *relatus* (pp of *referre* to carry back) fr *re-* + *latus*, pp of *ferre* to carry] To show or establish a logical or **causal** connection; to have or establish a **relationship**. rt: **associate**

related *adj* - Connected by reason of an established or discoverable **relation**.

relation *n* - [ME *relacioun*, fr MF *relation*, fr L *relation-, relatio*, fr *relatus*, pp] An aspect or quality (such as structure or resemblance) that connects two or more things, parts, or beings as belonging or working together or as the same kind.

relational database *n* - **Data** elements arranged or organized in some structure or format based on **relationships** of the elements, eg, table-like structures in which the **rows** or **columns** of different **tables** can be examined, joined, or separated, based on some common relationship.

relationship *n* - The state of being **related** or **interrelated**. rt: association, correlation *Usage note*: See notes for **association** and **correlation**.

relative *adj* - 1. Being **comparative**, not **absolute** or **independent**. 2. Expressed as a **percentage** of a **total**, as in **relative frequency**, or as a **ratio**, as with a **ratio estimate** or a **coefficient of variation**.

relative betting odds *n* - **Odds** arising from a method of analysis developed by **Cornfield** [1966][29] involving the **ratio** of a **likelihood function** computed under the **null hypothesis** and under a specified **alternative hypothesis** and used to characterize the amount of support for the alternative hypothesis relative to that for the null hypothesis.

relative frequency *n* - **Frequency** represented as a **proportion** or **percentage** of **total** frequency.

relative number *n* - 1. A **number** expressed as a **proportion** or **percentage**. 2. A number expressed relative to another.

relative odds *n* - **odds ratio**

relative risk *n* - 1. A **risk** measured or stated in **relative** terms. 2. The **ratio** of **risks** for some **disease, morbid event**, or death, eg, the ratio of **incidence rates** in a group exposed to some factor to a group not exposed; approximated by the **odds ratio** for rare conditions. 3. The ratio of **hazard rates**. *Usage note*: Relative risk and odds ratio are roughly equivalent for rare conditions and may be used interchangeably in such settings; not a recommended practice since the two terms have different bases.

reliability *n* - The extent to which an **experiment, test, measurement**, or **analysis** yields the same results on **replication** under the same conditions; **repeatability, reproducibility**.

reliable *adj* - Giving the same result on **replication; repeatable, reproducible**.

repeat, repeated, repeating, repeats *v* - [ME *repeten*, fr MF *repeter*, fr L *repetere*, fr *re-* + *petere* to go to, seek] To make, do, or perform again.

repeat reading *n* - A **reading** performed again; done by a different person or by the same person at different times.

repeatability *n* - The quality of being **repeatable**; reliability, reproducibility.

repeatable *adj* - 1. Capable of being **repeated**. 2. The ability or quality of an **experiment**, **study**, **test**, **measure**, or **analysis** to yield the same **result** when repeated under similar conditions; **reliable**, **reproducible**.

repeated measures design *n* - 1. A general class of **designs** having one or more **outcome measures** amenable to repeated measurement. 2. That subset of designs defined in defn 1 in which the **primary outcome measure** is amenable to repeated measurement. *Usage note*: Note that defn 1 includes **crossover trials** and most trials having **parallel treatment designs** to the extent that the latter have at least one outcome measure amenable to repeated measurement. Defn 2 is limited to the set of designs in which the primary outcome measure (usually the **design variable**) is amenable to repeated measurement. Hence, in this sense, a trial having a parallel treatment design with mortality as the design variable is not a member of the class because the variable, death, is not amenable to repeated measurement. However, such trials, to the extent they involve other outcome measures amenable to repeated measurements (eg, a trial with mortality as the primary outcome measure and blood pressure change as a secondary outcome measure, as observed at various points over the course of treatment) are members of the class as defined by defn 1.

repetition *n* - [L *repetition-*, *repetitio*, fr *repetitus*, pp of *repetere* to repeat] The act or instance of **repeating** or of being repeated. rt: **replication**

replace, replaced, replacing, replaces *v* - To restore to a former place or position; to put something new in the place of.

replacement *n* - The action or process of **replacing**; something that replaces.

replicate *adj* - Of or relating to **replication**.

replicate *n* - One of several **experiments**, procedures, or **samples** performed or obtained under similar conditions. rt: **aliquot**

replication *n* - **Repetition** of a process, procedure, **study**, or **experiment** for the purpose of increasing the **precision** of an **estimate** or to confirm or refute some finding, **result**, or **conclusion** derived from an earlier execution of that process, procedure, study, or experiment. rt: **duplication**

Usage note: Not to be confused with **duplication**. **Replication** is an essential part of the scientific method; duplication is not. For example, replication of an experiment is necessary to establish the plausibility of a result or finding, but repetition, once a result or finding is established, is an unnecessary duplication of effort.

report *n* - [ME, fr MF, fr OF, fr *reporter* to report, fr L *reportare*, fr *re-* + *portare* to carry] A detailed accounting, especially such an accounting as contained in a written **document**.

report, reported, reporting, reports *v* - 1. To make a written record or summary. 2. To announce or relate.

repository *n* - A place, room, or container where something is deposited or stored for safekeeping and for subsequent inspection or use; **archive**. syn: **bank** *Usage note*: Usage should be reserved for settings in which the facility is established largely for collection and storage of specimens or documents, with only limited and sporadic withdrawals, as in a serum repository created primarily as a resource for pursuing questions that may arise later. If the primary function is to serve as a depot until documents or specimens are needed, as in a blood bank, use **bank**. Use **archive** if the facility is concerned with the storage and retrieval of paper or electronic records or documents.

represent, represented, representing, represents *v* - [ME *representen*, fr MF *representer*, fr L *repraesentare*, fr *re-* + *praesentare* to present] 1. To correspond in essence. 2. To serve as a sign or symbol. 3. To bring clearly to mind.

representative *adj* - Serving to **represent**.

representative sample *n* - A **sample** that is or is considered to be **representative** of some **population** (generally the one from which the sample was drawn) with regard to some characteristic(s). *Usage note*: The characterization should not be applied without supporting arguments or documentation as to why it is reasonable to expect the sample to be representative. The claim should be tied to the method of sampling used, as in **quota sampling**. Not to be used interchangeably with **random sample**. As stated in a usage note for **random sample**, there is no guarantee that a simple random sample will be representative.

reproduce, reproduced, reproducing, reproduces *v* - To produce again.

reproducibility *n* - The quality or state of being **reproducible**; **reliability**; **repeatability**.

reproducible *adj* - 1. Capable of being **reproduced**. 2. The ability or quality of an **experiment**, **study**, **test**, **measure**, or **analysis** to yield the same result when performed under similar conditions; **reliable**; **repeatable**

reproducible difference *n* - [**epidemiology**] An **observed difference** considered to be beyond the **range** of **chance** and likely to arise again if the **study** were **repeated**.

request *n* - [ME *requeste*, fr MF, fr (assumed) VL *requaesta*, fr fem of *requaestus*, pp of *requaerere* to require] The act or instance of something asked for.

request for application (RFA) *n* - A document prepared and distributed by a **sponsoring agency** to solicit **applications** pertaining to a circumscribed area of work detailed in the **request**; especially such a document prepared and distributed by an agency of the federal government, such as the **NIH**, and in which said work is to be supported by **grants**. rt: **request for proposal** *Usage note*: From the NIH perspective, both RFAs and RFPs are used as vehicles for identifying and selecting investigators and **centers** in **multicenter trials**. As a general rule (though there are exceptions), investigators have more control over the activity proposed under the NIH RFA mode of initiation and **grant** support than under the NIH RFP mode of initiation and **contract** support. The need or opportunity for NIH sponsors to assume a directive role in the activity is greater with RFPs than with RFAs. Technically, the focus in an RFP is on a defined task and on deliverables related to that task. The emphasis in an RFA is on a scientific question or issue.

request for proposal (RFP) *n* - A document prepared and distributed by a **sponsoring agency** to solicit **proposals** for execution of a specified task, especially such a document prepared and distributed by an agency of the federal government, such as the **NIH**, and in which said work is to be supported by **contracts**. rt: **request for application** *Usage note*: Not to be confused with **request for application**. See usage note for **request for application**.

require, required, requiring, requires *v* - [ME *reqeren*, fr MF *reuerre*, fr (assumed) VL *requaerere* to seek for, need, require, alter of L

requirere, fr *re-* + *quaerere* to seek, ask] To request or demand as necessary or essential.

required followup *n* - **Followup** of an **observation unit** that is a required part of the **study protocol** and that is to be done at specified times after **enrollment** of that unit.

required followup visit *n* - Any **followup visit** required as part of the **study protocol** and that is to be done at a specified time after **enrollment**; in the case of **trials**, such visits include **treatment application and adjustment followup visits**, **regular followup visits**, **close-out followup visits**, **post close-out followup visits**, and **post-trial followup visits**. ant: **nonrequired followup visit** rt: **regular followup visit**

required visit *n* - Any **visit** which is a required part of the **study protocol**; in the case of **trials**, visits include **baseline** as well as **required followup visits**. rt: **scheduled visit**

requirement *n* - Something wanted or needed; something essential to the existence or occurrence of something else.

rescue *adj* - Of or relating to something or someone to be **rescued**. rt: **salvage**

rescue, rescued, rescuing, rescues *v* - [ME *rescuen*, fr MF *rescourre*, fr OF, fr *re-* + *escourre* to shake out, fr L *excutere*, fr *ex-* + *quatere* to shake] To save or free from danger or peril. rt: **salvage**

rescue study *n* - 1. A **study** involving people with an active and uncontrolled **disease** and use of therapeutic regimens offering promise for control or amelioration of the disease, especially such studies involving people with life-threatening or life-limiting diseases. 2. **salvage study** *Usage note*: Avoid because of drama implied by **rescue** *v*, the implied promise of success, and because of connotations similar to those for **salvage study**; see also **rescue treatment** for comments.

rescue treatment *n* - A **treatment** considered necessary or prudent in the presence of indicated **signs** or **symptoms**; in the context of **trials** usually a treatment administered in addition to or in place of the **assigned treatment** in the presence of indicated signs or symptoms considered to be indicative of inadequate treatment. rt: **salvage protocol** *Usage note*: Use with caution because of implied drama. The implication is that a person to be so treated is in need of **rescue**, ie, in need of being saved or freed from a dangerous situation and that the treatment is capable of such rescue.

research *n* - [MF *recerche*, fr *recerchier* to investigate thoroughly, fr OF, fr *re-* + *cerchier*, to search] 1. [general] Careful or thorough **investigation**. 2. [**scientific**] **Systematic** investigation characterized by careful, exhaustive, and scholarly pursuits aimed at the expansion of knowledge concerning some theory, process, or procedure. *Usage note*: Subject to varying usage; often in a loose, nonrigorous sense, as in *let's research the question*. Rigorous usage should be in the sense of defn 2. The emphasis in defn 2 is on **systematic**. That emphasis is evident from the generic definition of research given in regulation of **institutional review boards**. Research therein is defined as: *...systematic investigation, including research development, testing and evaluation, designed to develop or contribute to generalizable knowledge. Activities which meet this definition constitute research for purposes of this policy, whether or not they are conducted or supported under a program which is considered research for other purposes. For example, some demonstration and service programs may include research activities.*[117]

research, researched, researching, researches *v* - To **investigate** thoroughly and exhaustively; to do or engage in **investigation**.

research application *n* - A **research proposal** in the form of an **application**; especially one submitted to a **funding agency**.

research contract proposal *n* - 1. A **contract proposal** for carrying out a designated **research** activity. 2. A **funding proposal** prepared in response to a **request for proposal**. rt: **research grant proposal**

research grant *n* - A **grant** awarded to support a designated **research** activity or **project**. *Usage note*: See **grant** for usage note.

research grant application *n* - 1. An **application** for a **research grant** submitted to an **agency** of the federal government and having a specified research plan, budget, and **principal investigator**. 2. Such an application submitted to the NIH. 3. Any application for a research grant regardless of funding source, ie, applications submitted to any federal, state, or local governmental unit, to a private or public foundation, or to some business or industrial firm.

research grant proposal *n* - 1. A **grant proposal** for carrying out **research**; **grant application**. 2. A **funding proposal** prepared in response to a **request for application**. rt: **research contract proposal**

research group *n* - The entire set of personnel involved in the conduct of a **research project** such as a **study**; in **multicenter trials** includes **center directors** and support staff, representatives from the **sponsoring agency**, and **study committee** members. syn: investigative team, **investigative group**, **study group** (not a recommended syn, see usage note for **study group**)

research hypothesis *n* - The **hypothesis** to be **investigated** in a designated **research project**; one of several hypotheses to be so investigated. syn: working hypothesis

research organization *n* - An **organization** engaged in **research**.

research program *n* - 1. **program project** 2. **research project** (defn 1)

research project *n* - 1. **Research** having a defined goal or end; a particular **study** or **trial**. 2. A collection of activities related to a designated research activity or **study**; **program project**.

research proposal *n* - A **proposal** to perform or carry out a designated **research project**; **research application**.

research subject *n* - 1. **study participant** (defn 1); **study patient** 2. One who is or is to be the object of **study**. 3. An aspect of a person that is or is to be the object of study, such as the person's medical record or a specimen collected from the person. 4. **subject** (defn 2) *Usage note*: Broadly defined in regulations for **institutional review boards** to include defns 1, 2, and 3.[117] The prerogative for IRB review and approval extends to research to be performed without any contact with those being studied, as in defn 3 with a **case-control study** based on a review of **medical records**. The review and approval requirement is independent of whether or not the persons in question are or will be aware of being studied. See also usage note for **subject**.

residual *n* - 1. That which remains; remainder. 2. The difference between results obtained by **observation** and by computation from a formula or between the **mean** of several observations and any one of them.

residual variance *n* - 1. That part of the **variance** that remains after known sources of variance are taken into account. 2. That portion of variability of the **independent variable** attributable to **experimental error**, **chance**, or **random variation**.

resolution *n* - [ME, fr MF or L; MF *resolution*, fr L *resolution-, resolutio*, fr *resolutus*, pp] A formal expression of will or intent voted by an official body or assembled group.

resource center *n* - Any **center** in a **multicenter study** involved in performing a specified set of support functions and not involved in **data collection**; in **multicenter trials** includes any of the following: **data center**, **data coordinating center**, **treatment coordinating center**, **coordinating center**, **central laboratory**, **reading center**, **quality control center**, **project office**, and **procurement and distribution center**.

respect *n* - [ME, fr L *repectus*, lit, act of looking back, fr *respectus*, pp of *respicere* to look back, regard, fr *re-* + *specere* to look] The quality or state of being esteemed or of being treated with regard and esteem.

respect for persons, principle of *n* - A **principle** in **medical ethics** that asserts that the care and **treatment** performed or offered in a research setting involving human beings must be done in a fashion denoting **respect** for those so involved [Levine, 1986].[88] See also **medical ethics, principles of**.

respond, responded, responding, responds *v* - [MF *respondre*, fr L *respondēre* to promise in return, answer, fr *re-* + *spondēre* to promise] 1. To say something in return; to reply or answer. 2. To react in **response** to. 3. To **comply**.

respondent *n* - [L *respondent-, respondens*, prp of *respondēre*] One who **responds**. ant: **nonrespondent**

responder *n* - One who **responds**.

response *n* - [ME & L; ME *respounse*, fr MF *respons*, fr L *responsum* reply, fr neut of *responus*, pp of *respondēre*] 1. The act of **responding**. 2. Something constituting a reply. ant: **nonresponse**

response bias *n* - A **bias** that arises from differences in the characteristics of people who **respond** or submit to some process or procedure as compared with those who do not. syn: nonresponse bias

response variable *n* - **outcome variable**

responsive *adj* - Giving a **response**, answering, replying.

responsiveness *n* - The state or quality of being **responsive**.

restrict, restricted, restricting, restricts *v* - [L *restrictus*, pp of *restringere*] To confine within bounds; limit; restrain.

restricted *adj* - Subject to or subjected to **restriction**; not general; limited; constrained. ant: **unrestricted**

restricted assignment scheme *n* - Any **assignment** scheme in which the **treatment assignment schedule** is designed to satisfy specified constraints or restrictions, as in **blocking** in a **fixed assignment schedule**.

restricted random assignment *n* - **Restricted assignment scheme** involving use of a **random process** to make **treatment assignments**. ant: **unrestricted random assignment**

restricted randomization *n* - **Randomization** involving restrictions, such as in **blocked randomization**; not **complete randomization**. ant: **complete randomization**, unrestricted randomization

restricted treatment assignment *n* - A **treatment assignment** that is the result of some scheme or process that is restricted in some way or other, as in **blocking**. ant: **unrestricted treatment assignment**

restricted treatment assignment schedule *n* - A **treatment assignment schedule** constructed so as to yield the **expected assignment ratio** after a specified number of **assignments**, as with **blocking** in a **fixed assignment schedule**. ant: **unrestricted treatment assignment schedule**

restriction *n* - [ME *restriccioun*, fr LL *restricition-, restricito*, fr *restrictus*, pp] Something that restricts; the act of restricting; a limitation or constraint on the use or distribution of something.

result *n* - 1. Something that arises as a logical consequence of precedent acts or events, such as a **conclusion** from a **study**. 2. **cause** 3. A finding obtained by **investigation**, **calculation**, or **analysis**. 4. **observation** (defn 4) 5. A finding that is considered meaningful or important. 6. The value or interpretation of a **test** (defn 4).

result, **resulted**, **resulting**, **results** *v* - [ME *resulten*, fr ML *resultare*, fr L to rebound, fr *re-* + *saltare* to leap] To proceed or arise as a consequence, **effect**, or **conclusion**.

retrieval *n* - The act or process of **retrieving**.

retrieve, **retrieved**, **retrieving**, **retrieves** *v* - [ME *retreven*, modif of MF *retrouver* to find again, fr *re-* + *trouver* to find, prob fr (assumed) VL *tropare* to compose] To get back again; restore; to get and bring back again, as with a file electronically stored.

retrospect *n* - [*retro-* + *-spect* (as in *prospect*)] Review of or meditation on past events. ant: **prospect**

retrospect *v* - [L *retrospectus*, pp of *retrospicere*, to look back, at, fr *retro* + *specere* to look] To review or survey past events; to look back in time.

retrospective *adj* - 1. Relating to the past; lying in the past. 2. Looking backward in time, especially in relation to some designated time point (eg, date of **exposure** to some agent in the past) or event. 3. Proceeding from **effect** to **cause**, as in an **inference** as to cause based on observed effects in a **retrospective study**. ant: **prospective** *Usage note*: While all three defns relate to the past or to things past, defn 3 refers to an inference process. Avoid where redundant, as in **retrospective case-control study**. **Case-control studies** are, by definition, retrospective in the sense of defn 3. Avoid as well where contradictory, as in **retrospective followup study** or **retrospective cohort study**. See notes for **retrospective followup study** and **prospective** for additional comments.

retrospective case-control study *n* - **case-control study**

retrospective cohort study *n* - **nonconcurrent cohort study**

retrospective followup *n* - 1. **Followup** proceeding backward in time from some designated starting time point. 2. Followup proceeding forward in time from some designated starting point in the past to a more recent time point in the past or to the present. ant: **prospective followup** *Usage note*: Not recommended because of the different meanings of the two definitions and because of the contradictory nature of **retrospective** and **followup**: The latter term implies something moving forward in time,

whereas the former term implies something moving backward in time.

retrospective followup study *n* - A **followup study** based entirely on information collected in the past, eg, one in which the progress or change in a person is tracked forward in time by a review of accumulated medical **records** for that person. ant: **prospective followup study** *Usage note*: Avoid because the term is comprised of contradictory elements since **followup** implies moving forward in time and retrospective implies moving backward in time.

retrospective registration *n* - **Registration** based on **data** collected in the past. ant: **prospective registration**

retrospective study *n* - 1. A **study** in which one moves backward in time from the present to the past or from the past to a more distant point in the past, eg, by starting with a specified **medical record** of a person having a specified **disease** and then searching backward in time to the point of diagnosis, as indicated in available records. 2. **case-control study** *Usage note*: Retrospective study is one of the synonyms for **case-control study**, though not recommended. Usage in this regard arises from the fact that the nature of the inference is retrospective, in that it proceeds from an observed effect (eg, presence of a **disease**) to a **cause** lying in the past relative to the observed effect. Technically, the term applies even if cases and controls are accumulated in a **prospective** fashion.

reverse *adj* - [ME *revers*, fr MF, fr L *reversus*, pp of *revertere* to turn back] Opposite or contrary to a previous or usual condition or procedure.

reverse site visit *n* - **reverse study site visit**

reverse study site visit *n* - 1. A **visit** having the function of a **study site visit** but performed at a site remote from the **study site**. 2. A study site visit performed at the site of the **agency** or **group** funding the visit. rt: **site visit**, **study review visit** *Usage note*: Contradictory; avoid as a label without accompanying details to make meaning clear. The modifier **reverse** is used to draw attention to the fact that the site of the visit is not at a study site and that, in this sense, it represents a departure from normal site visiting practices. The usual approach is for the visit to take place at the **study site**, or at one of the study sites in the case of a study involving multiple sites. Use of the term is not recommended because it refers to a physical impossibility, namely, visiting a site by not being there. The more general and acceptable term is **study review visit**.

review *n* - [MF *revue*, fr *revoir* to look over, fr *re-* + *voir* to see] 1. A general **survey** of previous work or materials, as in relation to preparing a review article for a **journal**. 2. The act or process of **reviewing**. 3. A critical evaluation of a work in progress for the purpose of providing constructive comments to the originator of the work. 4. A critical evaluation of previous works or events. 5. A critical evaluation of proposed work as a means of aiding in the decision as to whether to proceed with that work. 6. A critical evaluation of a **manuscript** submitted to a journal for possible **publication**; **peer review**.

review, reviewed, reviewing, reviews *v* - 1. To reexamine. 2. To look back on; to take a **retrospective** view. 3. To go over carefully and deliberately. 4. To study materials again; to make a **review**; to write a review.

review group *n* - A **group** of persons, normally recruited and appointed by the **sponsoring agency** or its representative, charged with the **review** of a **research proposal** or set of proposals for scientific merit; **study section**.

reviewer *n* - 1. One who **reviews**. 2. One who performs a critical review in relation to a **peer review**.

RFA *n* - **request for application**

RFP *n* - **request for proposal**

rho *n* - [Gk *rhō*, of Sem origin; akin to Heb *rēsh* resh] The 17th letter of the **Greek alphabet**, uppercase Ρ, lowercase ρ.

rhythm *n* - [MF & L; MF *rhy* + *hme*, fr L *rhythmus*, fr Gk *rhythmos*, fr *rhein* to flow] A regular cyclic recurrent quantitative change in a biological process or **variable**.

rider *n* - One who rides or travels. rt: **circuit rider**

right *adj* - [ME, fr OE *riht*; akin to OHG *reht* right, L *rectus* straight, right, *regere* to lead straight, direct, rule, *rogare* to ask, Gk *oregin* to stretch out] 1. Correct; conforming to the facts or truth. 2. The opposite of **left**. 3. Located in the direction of the right hand; located nearer the right hand than the left hand; of, relating to, situated on, or being on the side of the body that is furthest from the heart. 4. [**statistics**] Points

on the **x-axis** located further or positioned away from the **origin**, as seen in the **positive** quadrant. ant: **left**

right censored *adj* - Of or relating to being **censored** on or to the **right** of a designated **point** or **event**. ant: **left censored** rt: **interval censored**

right censored observation *n* - 1. An **observation** subject to **censorship** on the **right**. 2. Absence of observation (defn 1) because of censorship on the right. 3. Inability to observe because of censorship on the right; usually because of the existence or occurrence of some **event** or condition, such as death, **loss to followup**, or **withdrawal** (defn 1) precluding observation; **censored followup observation**. ant: **left censored observation** rt: **interval censored observation**

right skew *adj* - [**statistics**] Of or relating to a **frequency distribution** that is **asymmetrical** with a **tail** extended to the **right**. syn: positive skew ant: **left skew**

right skew distribution *n* - A **nonsymmetrical distribution** with a wider **range** of values to the **right** of the **mode** than to the **left**; a **distribution** with a **right skew**. syn: positive skew distribution ant: **left skew distribution**

Right skewed distribution

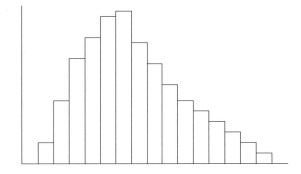

right skewness *n* - Skewness to the **right**. syn: positive skewness ant: **left skewness**

right tail *n* - [**statistics**] That portion of a **distribution** at the extreme **right**. ant: **left tail**

risk *adj* - Of or relating to **probability** or **chance** in relation to experiencing some **hazard** or adverse condition.

risk *n* - The **probability** or **chance** of some **event** or condition occurring in a defined time period, especially an adverse event or condition.

risk *v* - 1. To **expose** to **hazard** or danger. 2. To incur the risk or danger of.

risk assessment *n* - An **assessment** of **risk** associated with having some **risk factor** or accruing from exposure to some **adverse** health condition. rt: **risk profile**

risk factor *n* - 1. Any environmental **exposure**, personal **characteristic**, attribute, or **event** that affects the **probability** of developing a given **disease** or experiencing a disadvantageous change in health status [Morganstern and Bursic, 1982].[107] 2. Any environmental **exposure**, personal **characteristic**, attribute, or **event** that increases (relative to some **reference population** or **group**) the **probability** of developing a given **disease** or of experiencing an **adverse** health condition. ant: **benefit factor** 3. A **factor** or level of a factor considered or known to increase **risk** for experiencing some adverse event or health condition. 4. A factor having levels associated with increased risk and amenable to modification or amelioration via some form of **treatment** or **intervention** (eg, blood pressure levels in the hypertensive range believed amenable to reduction via dietary changes that result in reduced intake of dietary sodium). 5. A **variable** considered or known to affect the probability of experiencing some adverse event or health condition. *Usage note*: Avoid as a label without supporting evidence indicating basis for use (eg, support by giving the estimated increased risk or by citing references to the work of others establishing risk). Subject to varying use, as seen by comparison of defns 1 and 2. Note that defn 1 is broader than defn 2. Use in the sense of defn 2 is limited to instances where the probability of the event or health condition of interest is increased or assumed to be increased, whereas use in the sense of defn 1 applies so long as the probability in question is increased or decreased relative to some standard or reference. The preferred usage is in the sense of defn 2; preferred because it avoids reference to a variable or level of a variable as a "risk" factor when, in fact, the factor confers **benefit** relative to the reference population or group. Avoid mixed usages by consistency of reference (eg, by always referring to the level of a factor having increased risk as the "risk factor") or by using some other complementary term, such as **benefit factor**, when referring to the complement of a risk factor (in the sense of defn 2).

risk factor analysis *n* - [**epidemiology**] Any **analysis**, usually involving **regression** or **subgroup analyses**, that is aimed at identifying a **risk factor** for a given **disease** or health condition.

risk profile *n* - 1. A characterization of the **probability** of dying, experiencing some **morbid event**, or of developing some **adverse** health condition as a function of a **variable** influencing risk, eg, the probability of having a stroke in the next 5 years as a function of blood pressure. 2. A characterization of one's estimated risk over some defined time period of experiencing adverse health conditions; usually based on some prediction **model** involving the person's observed **demographic** and **baseline characteristics** and with risk displayed in **list**, **table**, or **graph** form.

risk profile analysis *n* - An **analysis** of one's own characteristics to derive a personal **risk profile**.

risk ratio *n* - The **ratio** of two **risks**. syn: **relative risk** rt: **odds ratio**

risk-benefit *adj* - Of or relating to the **ratio** of **risks** to **benefits**.

risk-benefit analysis *n* - [**medicine**] An assessment of the **risks** accruing to an individual **exposed** to some **treatment**, process, or procedure versus the **benefits**; **cost-benefit analysis**.

risk-benefit ratio *n* - The balance of **benefits** to **risks**; benefits measured against risks.

robust *adj* - [L *robustus* oaken, strong, fr *robor-*, *robur* oak, strength] Having or exhibiting strength; unchanging in the face of adversity. [**statistics**] Of, relating to, or concerned with a characteristic in which a procedure or **estimator** retains in some sense a specified property in the presence of departures from assumptions on which it depends.

robust estimator *n* - An **estimator** that retains its properties, such as **consistency**, in the face of departures from underlying assumptions needed to assure those properties.

robustness *n* - The state of being **robust**.

RoC, ROC *adj, n* - **receiver operating characteristic**

root *n* - [**mathematics**] 1. A **number** that when multiplied by itself an indicated number of times yields a **product** equal to a given number, eg, 2 as the 3rd root of 8, since 2x2x2 = 8. 2. A number that reduces a **polynomial equation** in one **variable** to an identity when it is substituted for that variable.

root-mean square deviation *n* - **standard deviation**

root-mean square error *n* - The **square root** of the **mean square error**. syn: root-mean square deviation, **standard deviation**

round *adj* - [ME, fr OF *roont*, fr L *rotundus*] 1. Approximately correct. 2. Exact only to a specified decimal place, eg, an observation of 14.86 to be reported to the nearest tenth would be rounded to 14.9.

round, rounded, rounding, rounds *v* - To make **round** to a specified place of **accuracy** or level of **precision**; **round off**.

round off *v* - To make **round** to a specified decimal position, as in rounding the number 67.5678 to 67.568 when reported to three places of accuracy.

round off error *n* - **Error** due to inherent limitations in the **device** used to produce or generate a **measurement** or **calculation**; **rounding error**.

rounding error *n* - 1. **round off error** 2. **Error** or **bias** introduced into some numeric **observation**, **measurement**, or **statistic** that is the result of the way in which numbers are rounded or truncated (eg, by rounding up).

routine *adj* - 1. Of commonplace or repetitious character; ordinary. 2. Of, relating to, or being in accordance with established procedure.

routine followup visit *n* - **regular followup visit**

row *n* - [ME *rawe*; akin to OE *ræw*, *rāw* row, OHG *riga* line, L *rima* slit] A number of items arranged in a horizontal line; a horizontal arrangement of items. rt: **column**

rule *n* - [ME *reule*, fr OF, fr L *regula* straight-edge, rule, fr *regere* to lead straight] 1. A prescribed guide for conduct or action, such as a **stopping rule**. 2. A regulating **principle**. 3. A mathematical formula, especially such a formula stated in words.

run *n* - 1. Something that flows or occurs in the course of a certain operation or during a certain time. 2. A continuous series, especially of things identical or similar in nature, eg, a run of 7s in a table of **random numbers**.

run, ran, running, runs *v* - [ME *ronnen*, alter of *rinnen*, vi (fr OE *iernan*, *rinnan* & ON *rinna*) & of *rennen*, vt, fr ON *renna*; akin to OHG *rinnan*, vi, to run, OE *rīsan* to rise] 1. To conduct or perform. 2. To function or proceed. 3. To extend, spread, or reach. 4. To cause to progress or move freely.

run-in *adj* - Of or relating to the start.

run-in *n* - [**trials**] 1. A **period** of **time** and set of defined activities associated with **enrollment** of an **observation unit** into a trial. 2. **lead-in period**. *Usage note*: See **run-in period**.

run-in period *n* - 1. **lead-in period** 2. **enrollment period** *Usage note*: Subject to confusion because of different meanings, depending on whether used in the sense of defn 1 or 2. Avoid by using **lead-in period** or **enrollment period**, depending on sense of usage. See also **lead-in period**.

S

s, S *n* - [19th letter of the English alphabet] Something shaped like the letter S.

s-shaped *adj* - Having or approximating the form or shape of the letter **s**.

s-shaped curve *n* - A **curve** having the shape of an elongated **s**.   rt: **j-shaped curve, u-shaped curve**

s-shaped curve

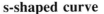
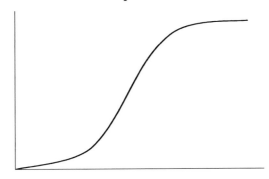

safe *adj* - [ME *sauf*, fr OF, fr L *salvus* safe, healthy; akin to L *salus* health, safety, *salubris* healthful, *solidus* solid, Gk *holos* whole, safe] Free from harm or **risk**; not threatening danger. *Usage note*: Use with caution as a claim or statement, as in *safe treatment*.

safe and effective *adj* - Producing the desired **effect** free of harm or **risk** or with an acceptable **risk-benefit ratio**.

safe and effective treatment *n* - A **treatment** considered to be **effective** and having an acceptable **risk-benefit ratio**.

safety *n* - [ME *saufte*, fr MF *sauveté*, fr OF, fr *sauve*, fem of *sauf* safe] The condition of being **safe** from undergoing or causing harm or injury.

safety committee *n* - 1. **treatment effects monitoring committee** 2. **safety monitoring committee**

safety margin *n* - An added amount, measure, or degree allowed for the purpose of avoiding something unsafe, having the potential of being

unsafe, or of reducing the likelihood of failure under extreme conditions; typically achieved by increasing the strength or robustness of something intended to withstand stresses, such as a building, or by operating well below the limit of safety as defined or known for some machine or product.   In the case of **medicine**, typically achieved by practicing or operating below the known safety limit for something, eg, in the case of a **drug** by using a lower than allowable **dose**. syn: margin of safety rt: **error margin**

safety monitoring *v* - [trials] 1. **Monitoring** (defn 2) performed at periodic time points over the course of a trial, to determine whether the trial should be stopped or modified because of safety considerations; as distinct from **efficacy monitoring**. 2. **safety review** (defn 1) 3. **treatment effects monitoring** rt: **data and safety monitoring, efficacy monitoring, treatment effects monitoring, interim look, interim result** *Usage note*: Often used in contradistinction to **efficacy monitoring** in settings where the user wishes to distinguish between **interim looks** performed for efficacy monitoring versus **safety monitoring**; eg, in settings where looks for safety monitoring are not counted as looks for purposes of adjusting **p-values** for **multiple looks**.   The distinction is predicated on the assumption that safety and efficacy are **independent** dimensions of **treatment** — often not the case. Use **treatment effects monitoring** when the distinction is unimportant or where the monitoring performed is for safety and efficacy. See also notes for **administrative review, efficacy monitoring** and **treatment effects monitoring**.

safety monitoring committee *n* - 1. **treatment effects monitoring committee** 2. A **committee** responsible for the periodic review of accumulated **data** for the purpose of determining whether the trial should be stopped or modified because of safety considerations.

safety report *n* - 1. **treatment effects monitoring report** 2. A **report** to the **Food and Drug Administration** of an **adverse drug experience** that is both serious and unexpected; written or telephoned; **investigational new drug safety report**; also **IND safety report**.

safety review *n* - [**trials**] 1. An **ad hoc interim review** (defn 2) of the **safety** of the **treatments** being used to determine whether the trial should be allowed to continue unaltered; especially one prompted by some untoward event internal or external to the trial. 2. **safety monitoring** (defn 1) rt: **efficacy review** *Usage note*: Note that defns 1 and 2 have different operational meanings and should not be used interchangeably. Use **safety monitoring** when the interim review is part of an ongoing process. See note for **safety monitoring**.

salvage *adj* - Of or relating to something to be saved or averted. rt: **rescue**

salvage *n* - [F, fr MF, fr *salver* to save] Something saved or extracted as useful or valuable.

salvage, salvaged, salvaging, salvages *v* - To **rescue** or save.

salvage protocol *n* - A **protocol** relating to a **salvage study**. rt: **rescue treatment** *Usage note*: See **salvage study** and **rescue treatment**.

salvage study *n* - In the context of **therapeutics**, a **study** designed for people considered to have been unsuccessfully treated or managed and aimed at finding an effective treatment or approach; in the context of **trials** usually one involving previously treated people who are considered to have failed to respond positively to treatment. syn: **rescue study** *Usage note*: Avoid because of negative connotations. **Salvage** in the context of **trials** has connotations of peril, wreckage, despair, and even of hopelessness. **Patients** are not likely to be consoled by being viewed as "salvage" by those to whom they look for care or by the implied peril. See **rescue treatment** for additional comments.

sample *n* - [ME, fr MF *essample*, fr L *exemplum*] 1. A **finite** part or subset of a defined **population**, selected or drawn for **study** and for deriving **estimates** and drawing **inferences** related to that population; may be drawn in some **random** fashion or may be chosen in some other way; may or may not be **representative** of the population, depending on how the sample is selected or drawn. rt: **census**, **survey** 2. A representative or typical part, item, or unit from a larger whole or group chosen for inspection or evidence of quality.

sample, sampled, sampling, samples *v* - To take a **sample** of or from.

sample distribution *n* - The **observed distribution** for a designated **variable** as provided by a **sample**. rt: **sampling distribution**

sample mean *n* - The **mean** as calculated for a **sample** and serving as an **estimate** of the **population mean**.

sample size *n* - 1. The number of **sampling units** to be drawn or selected for a **sample**; the number so selected or drawn. 2. The anticipated or actual number of elements or units constituting the **database** for a **study**, eg, the number of **patients** to be **enrolled** into a **clinical trial** or actually enrolled. rt: **recruitment goal**, **sample size calculation**

sample size calculation *n* - A mathematical **calculation**, usually carried out when a **study** is being planned, that indicates the number of **observation** or **treatment units** to be **enrolled** or studied in order to provide a specified degree of statistical **precision** for a specified level of **type I** and **type II error** protection. rt: **recruitment goal**

sample size design *n* - [**trials**] The **design** for determining **sample size**, broadly, either **fixed** or **sequential**; see **fixed sample size design** and **sequential sample size design**.

sample size requirement *n* - The **sample size** required, as indicated by a **sample size calculation** or specified **recruitment goal**.

sample survey *n* - A **survey** based on a **sampling** of the **population** of interest; as distinct from **census**.

sample variance *n* - The **variance** for a designated **variable**, as derived or calculated from a **sample** or by use of sampling.

sampling design *n* - The **design** or plan to be followed in a given instance of **sampling**, such as **cluster sampling**, **quota sampling**, **stratified sampling**, or **systematic sampling**.

sampling distribution *n* - The **observed** or **expected distribution** of a **statistic**, such as the **mean**, that is the result of **random sampling** or that is derived under the assumptions of **random sampling**.

sampling error *n* - **sampling variation**

sampling frame *n* - A structure or document that defines the **reference population** and that is used for sampling from that population; eg, a listing of the residents of a designated area used for sampling from that area.

sampling method *n* - The **method** by which **sampling** is done, eg, systematically or randomly.

sampling unit *n* - The **unit** selected or drawn in a **sampling method**, eg, ball in an urn **experiment**, person in an opinion survey, household in a study of families.

sampling variation *n* - **Variation** of results (eg, as expressed by sample **estimates**) from **sample** to sample as a consequence of differences in the **units** selected in the different samples; also referred to as **random variation**, especially in relation to **random sampling**.

sampling with replacement *n* - A system of **sampling** in which the element, object, or person drawn or selected in a **sample** is restored to the **population** (or not removed from the **sampling frame**) before the next element, object, or person is drawn or selected; eg, an **experiment** involving the sampling of balls in an **urn** in which a ball is drawn, some observation about it is made, and the ball is then replaced before the next ball is drawn; method is operational equivalent to sampling from a population of **infinite** size. rt: **sampling without replacement**

sampling without replacement *n* - A **sampling method** in which the element, object, or person drawn or selected in a **sample** is not restored to the **population** (or is removed from the **sampling frame**) after selection; eg, an **experiment** involving the drawing of 10 balls from an **urn** containing 100 balls and then observing the distribution of the 90 remaining balls with respect to some characteristic. rt: **sampling with replacement**

satellite *n* - [MF, fr L *satelit-*, *satelles* attendant] Something subordinate or **dependent**.

satellite center *n* - A **center**, subordinate to a **parent center**, organized to perform a designated set of functions at the behest of or as an agent of that parent center; **affiliate center**, **associate center**.

satellite clinic *n* - A **clinic**, subordinate to a **parent clinic**, organized and operated to **screen**, identify, **enroll**, **treat**, or **follow** a segment of the **study population** which cannot, for matters of convenience or other reasons, be seen at the **parent clinic**; **affiliate clinic**, **associate clinic**.

SC *n* - **steering committee**

scalar *adj* - [L *scalaris*, fr *scalae* stairs, ladder] 1. Having an uninterrupted series of steps or gradations; gradual. 2. Capable of being represented by a point on a **scale**.

scalar measure *n* - A **measure** or **observation** that arises from a **scale** or that can be **scaled**. syn: scale measure

scalar parameter *n* - A **parameter** of a **distribution**, such as its **standard deviation**, such that, if each value of the variable, **x**, of the distribution is replaced by the quantity, $a + b\mathbf{x}$, then the new parameter is the value of the old one multiplied by the constant, b. Generally, parameters given by powers of a scalar parameter, eg, **variance**, are also referred to as scalar parameters. Not to be confused with **location parameter**. syn: scale parameter

scale *n* - [ME, fr LL *scala* ladder, staircase, fr L *scalae*, pl, stairs, rungs, ladder; akin to L *scandere* to climb] 1. Something graduated or calibrated and used to **measure**, such as a ruler used for making linear measurements or a balance used for weighing. 2. A series of marks or points at known **intervals** used as a **measure**.

scale, scaled, scaling, scales *v* - To arrange in a graduated series; to **measure** or **observe** by or as if with a **scale**.

scale measure *n* - **scalar measure**

scale parameter *n* - **scalar parameter**

scatter *n* - The state or extent of being **scattered** or dispersed.

scatter, scattered, scattering, scatters *v* - [ME *scateren*] To distribute irregularly; to diffuse or disperse; to occur or fall irregularly in a seemingly **random** or **haphazard** pattern.

scatter diagram *n* - A two dimensional display in a plane **Cartesian coordinate** system consisting of points whose coordinates represent values of two related **variables**, eg, the 1st and 2nd blood pressure readings on people **enrolled** into a **study**. The **scatter** displayed is used as **qualitative measure** of the **correlation** of the two variables; the tendency of the points to locate along a 45 degree line with little scatter about that line represents a high degree of correlation; scatter without any apparent pattern is taken as evidence of little or no correlation.

scedastic *adj* - Denoting **dispersion** or **scatter**, especially as measured by **variance**.

Scatter diagram

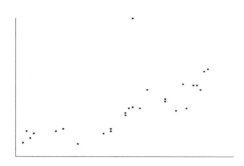

schedule *n* - [ME *cedule*, fr MF, slip of paper, note, fr LL *schedula*, slip of paper, dim of L *sceda*, *scida*, sheet of papyrus, fr (assumed) Gk *schidē*; akin to Gk *schizein*; to split] 1. A written list or sequence, as in **treatment assignment schedule**. 2. A plan for some procedure or action.

scheduled, scheduled, scheduling, schedules *v* - To place in a **schedule**; to make a schedule; to appoint or designate for a fixed time.

scheduled followup *n* - **Followup** that is planned or specified in the **study protocol**; **required followup**; not **interim followup**. syn: **required followup** ant: **unscheduled followup**

scheduled followup visit *n* - 1. **Required followup visit**; not an **interim followup visit**. syn: **required followup visit** ant: **unscheduled followup visit** 2. Any **visit** to a **study site** after **enrollment** that is **scheduled** (ie, as distinct from unscheduled, as with emergency visits), whether or not part of the sequence of followup visits specified in the **study protocol**. *Usage note*: Usage in the sense of defn 2 is not recommended when there is a potential for confusion with use in the sense of defn 1, or when used interchangeably without distinction. Whether or not a visit is scheduled, in the sense of defn 2, in studies involving specified periods of followup, such as in most **clinical trials**, is of less importance than whether or not the **data** collected and procedures performed at the visit are sufficient to satisfy the **data collection** requirements for a specified **followup period**; if so, the visit may be considered part of the required set of visits, even if it was not scheduled in advance.

scheduled visit *n* - 1. **required visit** 2. Any **visit** that is scheduled; **scheduled followup visit** (defn 2).

scheme *n* - [L *schemat-*, *schema* arrangement, figure, fr Gk *schēmat-*, *schēma*, fr *echein* to have, hold, be in (such) a condition; akin to OE *sige* victory, Skt *sahate* he prevails] A plan or program for action or carrying out some procedure.

science *n* - [ME, fr MF, fr L *scientia*, fr *scient-*, *sciens* having knowledge, fr prp of *scire* to know; akin to L *scindere* to cut] 1. The state of knowing; knowledge as distinguished from ignorance or misunderstanding. 2. An area of systematized knowledge as an object of **study**; something that may be studied or learned like systematized knowledge. 3. Knowledge covering general truths or the operation of general laws, especially as obtained and tested through the **scientific method**.

scientific *adj* - [ML *scientificus* producing knowledge, fr L *scient-*, *sciens* + *-i-* + *-ficus* -fic] Of, relating to, or exhibiting the methods and principles of **science**. *Usage note*: Subject to misuse. Often unnecessary, as in *the scientific soundness of the method*, and often used in loose lay sense, eg, *let's be scientific*. Avoid, except where needed for distinction, eg, *scientific journal* as distinct from other types of journals, or to connote real or implied rigor, as in **scientific method**. Avoid as a value term, as in *the method is not very scientific*, unless the use is supported with detail to make the basis of the judgment explicit.

scientific journal *n* - A **journal** devoted to a specific area or aspect of **science** and practicing **peer review**; see also **peer review journal**. In the area of **medicine** and related sciences, often considered to be those journals appearing in <u>Index</u> <u>Medicus</u> or **MEDLINE**.

scientific method *n* - 1. The totality of principles and processes regarded as characteristic of or necessary for pursuit of knowledge via scientific investigation, inclusive of rules for formulation of new concepts, conduct of **experiments**, **observation**, and validation of **hypotheses** by observation and experimentation. 2. A **method** of inquiry for pursuit of knowledge; characterized, in simplest terms, by identification and formulation of the problem of interest, the collection of **data** through **experiment** and **observation**, the formulation and testing of **hypotheses**, and the drawing of **conclusions**

based on those activities. *Usage note*: Avoid in loose lay sense. See note for **scientific**.

scientific misconduct *n* - 1. Willful disregard of accepted research **norms** and **standards**. 2. Any act or representation by a **scientist** that violates accepted **norms** or **standards** for **integrity**; act may relate to the **design**, conduct, **analysis**, or reporting of the project; acts include those related to **falsified** or **forged data**. 3. As defined in federal regulations (42 CFR, part 50, subpart A) for the **Office of Research Integrity**: *Fabrication, plagiarism, or other practices that seriously deviate from those that are commonly accepted within the scientific community for proposing, conducting, or reporting research. It does not include honest error or honest differences in interpretations or judgments of data.* rt: **Office of Research Integrity**

scientist *n* - [L *scientia*] One trained or learned in a **science**, especially one actively engaged in **investigations** involving **scientific method**.

score *n* - [ME *scor*, fr ON *skor* notch, tally, twenty; akin to OE *scieran* to cut] A number that expresses accomplishment or standing, expressed either in **absolute** or **relative** terms. rt: **index**

screen *n* - [ME *screne*, fr MF *escren*, fr MD *scherm*; akin to OHG *skirm* screen, L *corium* skin] 1. The process of examining and separating into different groups. rt: **triage** 2. A glass-like surface of a television or **video display terminal** used for display of images created electronically by such devices.

screen, screened, screening, screens *v* - To assess or examine in some systematic way in order to separate persons into **groups** or to identify a subset **eligible** for further evaluation or **enrollment** into some activity, eg, the process of measuring blood pressures of all persons appearing at a **clinic** for the purpose of identifying people suitable for enrollment into a **study** of high blood pressure.

screening *n* - 1. A search for persons with an identifying **marker** or characteristic, as determined by results from some **test** or **observation**, known or believed to be associated with some **disease** (or health condition presumed to have adverse health implications); see also **case detection**, **mass screening**, and **multiphasic screening**. 2. The process of evaluating **study candidates** for **enrollment** into a **study**. 3. Any of a variety of procedures applied to **data** to

identify **outlier** or questionable values. 4. A 100% inspection of items, such as in a manufacturing process, in which unacceptable items are rejected.

screening level *n* - The **cutpoint** above which (or below which) a **screening test** is considered to be diagnostic or indicative of the **disease** or condition of interest.

screening log *n* - 1. A list or **register** of people **screened** or to be screened. 2. **recruitment log**

screening test *n* - A **test** used for **screening**.

screening visit *n* - A **visit** at which **screening** is performed; eg, a **baseline visit** in relation to assessment of **eligibility** for **enrollment** into a **study**.

SD, sd *n* - **standard deviation**

SE, se *n* - **standard error**

season *n* - [ME, fr MF *saison*, fr OF, fr L *sation-*, *satio* action of sowing, fr *satus*, pp of *serere* to sow] One of the four divisions of a **year**: spring, summer, fall, and winter. A repeating time characterized by a particular feature or circumstance.

seasonal *adj* - Of, relating to, or varying in accordance with **season**.

seasonal variation *n* - **Variation** in some biological process, **measurement**, **observation**, or **reading** that is related to the **seasons** of the **year**. rt: **circadian variation**, **secular trend**, **temporal trend**, **temporal variation**

secondary *adj* - Of or being second in **order**, **stage**, or **step**. rt: **primary**, **tertiary**

secondary care *n* - [**medicine**] 1. **Care** of a **patient** at or by a **secondary care center**. 2. **Referred care** as performed by a specialist at a secondary care center. rt: **primary care**, **tertiary care**

secondary care center *n* - [**medicine**] A **center** (eg, **clinic** or hospital) that provides diagnostic services and care for **patients** referred from a **primary care center**. rt: **primary care center**, **tertiary care center**

secondary data *n* - 1. **Data** other than one's own, ie, not **primary data** (defn 3). 2. Data collected or assembled from a nonprimary source. 3. Data published by an agency or organization that were collected by some other agency, group, or persons. 4. Data of **secondary** importance in some **analysis** or presentation. rt: **primary data**

secondary data analysis *n* - 1. **Analysis** of **data** collected by someone else. 2. Analysis that is **secondary** in relation to a **primary** aim or purpose. rt: **primary data analysis**

secondary document *n* - 1. A **document** of **secondary** importance or relevance in relation to some specified use, process, or procedure. 2. A document completed from a **primary** or **source document**. rt: **primary document, source document**

secondary endpoint *n* - 1. **Secondary outcome** that is an **event** (eg, as opposed to a **continuous measure**). 2. **secondary outcome measure** *Usage note*: Use **secondary outcome** for reasons indicated in usage note for **endpoint**.

secondary event *n* - 1. A **secondary outcome variable** which is **binary**. 2. The occurrence of a **secondary outcome**, especially one that is an **event**. 3. An event triggered or caused by a **primary event**. rt: **primary event**

secondary outcome *n* - 1. An **event** or condition, generally related to the **primary outcome**, but of less clinical or medical importance than the primary outcome. 2. The actual occurrence of a **secondary event** in a **study participant**. 3. **secondary outcome measure** rt: **primary outcome**

secondary outcome measure *n* - 1. [**trials**] A **measure** related to the **primary outcome measure** considered to be of **secondary** importance in evaluation of the **study treatments**. 2. The actual occurrence of a **secondary event** in a **study participant**. 3. **secondary endpoint** (not recommended; see usage note for **endpoint** for reasons).

secondary outcome variable *n* - [**trials**] 1. An **outcome variable** related to the **primary outcome variable** considered to be of **secondary** importance in evaluation of the **study treatments** (eg, nonfatal myocardial infarctions in a trial having death as the primary outcome measure). 2. Any **outcome variable**, other than the primary outcome variable and regardless of its relationship to that variable, used for evaluation of **study treatments**.

secondary paper *n* - [**trials**] A **paper** dealing with a secondary **objective** and written by study personnel commissioned by the **investigative group** or their representative. syn: **secondary publication** rt: **mainline paper**

secondary prevention *n* - 1. **Prevention** aimed at delaying the progression of a **disease** or adverse health condition (eg, use of aspirin in **patients** who have had a myocardial infarction as a preventative measure against the occurrence of a subsequent myocardial infarction). 2. Efforts to correct departures from good health; broadly from the perspective of **epidemiology**, as given by Last:[84] *Measures available to individuals and populations for the early detection and prompt and effective intervention to correct departures from good health.* rt: **primary prevention, tertiary prevention**

secondary prevention trial *n* - A **prevention trial** involving **patients** with a history of some **disease** or condition in which the **test treatment** is administered as a possible means of preventing, or delaying further development or progression. For example, a **drug trial** involving the regular use of aspirin for the possible prevention of myocardial infarctions in patients with prior histories of myocardial infarctions. See references 151 and 30 for examples. rt: **primary prevention trial**

secondary publication *n* - [**research**] 1. A **publication** containing original **secondary results**. 2. A publication considered essential in relation to a secondary **purpose** or **objective** of a specific **research project**; in the case of **trials**, usually publications devoted exclusively to results for a **secondary outcome measure** or publications providing added information bearing on a **primary result**. syn: **secondary paper** rt: **primary publication, ancillary publication**

secondary record *n* - 1. A **record** of **secondary** importance or relevance in relation to some specified use, process, or procedure. 2. A record completed from a **primary** or **source record**. rt: **primary record, source record**

secondary result *n* - [**research**] A **result** of direct relevance to a **secondary objective** of a piece of research. In **clinical trials**, usually a result based on a **secondary outcome measure**. rt: **primary result, ancillary result**

secondary source *n* - A **source** that is not **primary**. rt: **primary source**

section *n* - [L *section-, sectio,* fr *sectus*] A distinct part or portion of a whole; **division**.

sectional *adj* - Consisting of or divided into **sections**.

secular *adj* - [ME, fr OF *seculer*, fr LL *saecularis*, fr L, coming once in an age, fr *saeculum* breed, generation; akin to L *serere* to sow] Of or relating to that which is **temporal**.

secular trend *n* - A **trend** or pattern that is time related. rt: **temporal trend** *Usage note*: Generally used to refer to a trend due to some **extraneous variable** or condition that has the possibility of influencing a time relationship of interest. For example, a trend due to learning in an ECG reading process, that in turn influences the rate of myocardial infarction observed over time for the different **treatment groups** represented in a **trial**. The existence of such a trend influences the **precision** of time related **estimates**, such as for **rates**, but does not affect the validity of **treatment comparisons** within a trial, so long as the trend is independent of **treatment assignment**.

selection bias *n* - 1. A systematic inclination or tendency for elements or units selected for **study** (usually persons in **trials**) to differ from those not selected. See **Berksonian bias** for a special type of selection bias. 2. **treatment related selection bias** (not a recommended synonym) *Usage note*: The **bias** defined by defn 1 is unavoidable in most trials because of selective factors introduced as a result of eligibility requirements for **enrollment** and because of the fact that individuals may decline enrollment (see **consent process**). The existence of the bias does not affect the **validity** of **treatment comparisons** within a trial so long as the bias is the same for all **treatment groups**, eg, as is the case when **treatment assignments** are made by **randomization**.

selection variable *n* - A **variable** used for **selection**, especially a variable used for selecting members of a defined **population** for some purpose. In **trials**, a **baseline** or **followup variable** used for selecting **treatment units** for some purpose, usually a **subgroup analysis**.

self- *prefix* - [ME, fr OE, fr *self*] By or of oneself or itself.

self-checking *adj* - Someone or something that checks oneself or itself.

self-checking digit *n* - **check digit**

semi- *prefix* - [ME, fr L; akin to OHG *sāmi-* half; Gk *hēmi-*] 1. Half or approximately half in quantity or value. 2. Occurring half way through or approximately half way through a specified

period of time, as in **semiannual**. 3. To some extent, partly, partial, incomplete. 4. Having some of the characteristics of, **quasi-**. rt: **bi-** *Usage note*: Preferred to **bi-** in relation to time designations for reasons indicated in the usage note for **bi-**. Often used to imply something that is roughly half or midway. Use more precise terminology in relation to timing when the sense of approximation conveyed via use of **semi-** is not appropriate. Note the difference in implied precision in the following phrases: *visits were performed at semiannual intervals* vs *visits were performed every 26 weeks* vs *visits were performed every 182 or 183 days*. All three expressions relate to intervals of the same length but the impressions conveyed are different.

semiannual *adj* - 1. Occurring every six **months** or approximately every six months. 2. Having a frequency of twice yearly. 3. Having a frequency of twice yearly and an occurrence cycle of every six months or approximately every six months. *Usage note*: See notes for **semi-** and **bi-**.

semimonthly *adj* - 1. Occurring every two **weeks** or approximately every two weeks. 2. Having a frequency of twice monthly. 3. Having a frequency of twice monthly and an occurrence cycle of roughly every two weeks, exactly every two weeks, or of half the number of days in a month. *Usage note*: See notes for **semi-** and **bi-**.

semiweekly *adj* - 1. Occurring every 2nd or 3rd or every 3rd or 4th **day** depending on whether reference is to a 5-day work week or to a 7-day calendar week. 2. Having a frequency of twice weekly and an occurrence cycle of every 2nd or 3rd day or every 3rd or 4th day depending on whether reference is to a 5- or 7-day week. *Usage note*: See notes for **semi-** and **bi-**.

sensitive *adj* - [ME, fr MF *sensitif*, fr ML *sensitivus*, irreg fr L *sensus*, pp] 1. Capable of detecting or discerning fine differences. 2. Of or relating to information about a person that if revealed or made known has the potential of being embarrassing or injurious. rt: **specific**

sensitive information *n* - Information pertaining to a person considered to be **sensitive**.

sensitive question *n* - A **question** used to elicit **sensitive information**.

sensitivity *n* - The quality or state of being **sensitive**. In **epidemiology** in relation to **screening tests**, the ability of a screening test to identify true **cases**, measured by the **proportion** of true cases identified by the screening test; also the **probability** that any given case will be identified by the test; also referred to as true positive rate. rt: **specificity**

sensitivity analysis *n* - [**statistics**] A type of **sensitivity testing** aimed at assessing the extent to which a finding based on some **model** can be perturbed or made to change as a result of changes in assumptions underlying the model; generally focused on those elements of the assumption not amenable to **estimation**. rt: **destructive data analysis**, **worst case analysis**

sensitivity testing *n* - Broadly, **testing** aimed at finding **limits** of **performance** or **failure**; **sensitivity analysis**.

sequence *n* - [ME, fr ML *sequentia*, fr LL, *sequel*, lit act of following, fr L *sequent-*, *sequens*, prp of *sequi*] A continuous or connected series; a set of items or elements ordered in some logical way. rt: **progression**, **series**

sequential *adj* - 1. Of, relating to, or arranged in a **sequence**; following in sequence or order. 2. Relating to or based on a method of **hypothesis testing** involving repeated use of accumulating **data**, augmented before each new test by an added **observation** or set of observations (as in **group sequential** or **unit sequential**); the testing process continues until the **null hypothesis** is rejected, or some other **boundary** condition is encountered, as in a **closed sequential design**. rt: **sequential data analysis** (defn 1)

sequential access *adj* - Permitting access in some ordered manner, as in relation to a **sequential file** (defn 2). ant: **random access**

sequential analysis *n* - **sequential data analysis**

sequential data analysis *n* - 1. Repeated **data analyses** performed in relation to a **closed** or **open sequential design**, eg, the **analysis** done after **enrollment** of a **patient**, pair of patients, or larger **block** of patients, in a **sequential trial** (defn 1), to determine whether additional patients should be enrolled; enrollment of the next patient, pair of patients, or block of patients is undertaken if the observed **treatment difference** does not exceed specified boundary limits. 2. **interim data analyses** (not a recommended synonym) *Usage note*: Ideally in the area of **trials**, the term **sequential data analysis** should be reserved for uses in relation to **unit sequential** or **group sequential designs**. Some other

term, such as **interim analysis**, should be used in reference to analysis performed for **treatment effects monitoring** in a trial having a **fixed sample size design**. While it is true that analyses performed in this context are also sequential, in the sense that they are ordered over time, they have different bases and uses than those required in relation to executing sequential designs. Hence, the two types of analyses should not be confused. See also note for **interim data analysis**.

sequential design *n* - [**trials**] 1. Any **design** with **open** or **closed** boundary **limits** where **enrollment** continues until the **observed treatment difference** for the **outcome** of interest is found to lie beyond a boundary limit. In the context of **hypothesis testing** involving a **test** and **control treatment**, differences within the boundary limits support the **null treatment hypothesis** and differences beyond a boundary limit favor the **alternative treatment hypothesis** that the test treatment is superior to the control treatment or that the control treatment is superior to the test treatment, depending on the boundary crossed. 2. **sequential dosage design** rt: **closed sequential design**, **open sequential design**, **group sequential**, **unit sequential** *Usage note*: See **sequential data analysis** for comment.

sequential dosage design *n* - Any of various schemes for choosing **dosages** of a **drug** for patients or groups of patients as they are **enrolled** into a trial; such a **scheme** as used in a **phase I/II drug trial** aimed at finding the **maximum tolerable dose**. See **modified Fibonacci sequence dosage design**, **traditional sequential dosage design**, and **up-down sequential dosage design** for examples.

sequential file *n* - 1. A **file** of **records** arranged in some logical order. 2. An **electronic file** arranged in **sequence** (as distinct from **random access**); eg, a time-ordered set of records for an individual patient.

sequential sample size design *n* - [**trials**] 1. The **sample size design** underlying a **sequential design**, ie, one in which **sample size** is a function of results observed as in an **open** or **closed sequential design**. 2. Any **scheme** in which **sample size** changes or is allowed to change as a function of observations or considerations made during the course of enrollment. ant: **fixed sample size design** *Usage note*: Best reserved for use in the sense defn 1. Not recommended in the sense of defn 2 in relation to **fixed sample size designs**, whether or not the changes are independent of observed **treatment differences**. See also **sequential data analysis**.

sequential treatment *n* - 1. An ordered **sequence** of **treatments**, eg, as administered in a **crossover trial**. 2. **stepped treatment**

sequential trial *n* - 1. A **trial** involving a **sequential design**. 2. A trial in which the decision concerning the **enrollment** of additional **treatment units** (eg, **patients**), or the continued **treatment** and **observation** of units already enrolled, is dependent on accumulated **data** in the **trial**, as in the use of **interim data analyses** to determine when it should stop. *Usage note*: The term **sequential trial** should be limited to trials having a sequential design, as in defn 1; not recommended terminology for usages in the sense of defn 2.

serial *adj* - Of, relating to, consisting of, or arranged in a **series**, **rank**, or **row**.

serial correlation *n* - The **sample correlation** between designated members of a **time series** (or space series) and those members preceding or following those members by a fixed length of time (or distance in space); eg, for a series of **observations**, $y^1, y^2, y^3, \cdots, y^{1+k}, y^{2+k}, y^{3+k}, \cdots$, the serial correlation of order k would be that for the pairs of observations defined by $(y^1, y^{1+k}), (y^2, y^{2+k}), (y^3, y^{3+k}), \cdots$; also sometimes **autocorrelation**.

serial number *n* - A **sequence** of **numbers**, or of numbers and letters, used to **identify** and indicate position in a **series**. rt: **identification number**

series *n* - [often attrib L, fr *serere* to join, link together; akin to L *sort-*, *sors* lot, Gk *eirein* to string together, *hormos* chain, necklace] A number of things or events of the same class coming one after another in spatial or temporal succession.

serious *adj* - [ME *seryows*, fr MF or LL; MF *serieux*, fr LL *seriosus*, alter of L *serius*] 1. Of or relating to a matter of importance. 2. Having important or dangerous possible consequences.

serious adverse drug experience *n* - 1. An **adverse drug experience** that is **serious**. 2. **Adverse drug reaction** that is **serious**. 3. In FDA parlance, as contained in the Code of Federal Regulations for drugs for that agency:[48] *Any*

experience that suggests a significant hazard, contraindication, side effect, or precaution. With respect to human clinical experience, a serious adverse drug experience includes any experience that is fatal or life-threatening, is permanently disabling, requires instant hospitalization, or is a congenital anomaly, cancer, or overdose. With respect to results from tests in laboratory animals, a serious adverse drug experience includes any experience suggesting a significant risk for human subjects, including any finding of mutagenicity, teratogenicity, or carcinogenicity. rt: **unexpected adverse drug experience**, **safety report**

service *n* - [ME, fr MF, fr L *servitium* condition of a slave, body of slaves, fr *servus* slave] Work done for others as an occupation.

session *n* - [ME, fr MF, fr L *session-*, *sessio*, lit, act of sitting, fr *sessus*, pp of *sedēre* to sit] A meeting or series of meetings of a group or between two individuals for the transaction of business or conducting some activity, eg, in relation to a **clinic visit**.

set *n* - A number of things of the same kind that belong together or that are used together, eg, the elements of a **dataset**.

sex *n* - [ME; fr L *sexus*] 1. The property or quality by which organisms are classified according to their reproductive functions; male and female. 2. Such a division as determined by the presence of a pair of chromosomes in the germ cells of humans, various other animal species, and some plants that, on union, combine to determine sex; XX for female and XY for male. rt: **gender** *Usage note*: Often used interchangeably with **gender**, but the two terms have different connotations, especially for uses of **sex** in relation to defn 2. Gender is the classification of sex based on observed function, anatomy, behaviors, and affectations. Generally, there is a one-to-one correspondence between the classifications made on the basis of sex (defn 2) and gender.

shakedown *n* - A process or period of testing and adjustment; a testing of something new or untried to detect faults or defects.

shakedown period *n* - 1. A period of time in the course of a **study** when **data forms** and procedures are tested prior to the official start of the study. 2. A period of time after the start of the study when procedures are still being tested and subject to change 3. The initial workup and evaluation of a person for **enrollment** into a study; especially one involving administration of **treatment**, as in a **lead-in period**, for the purpose of assessing acceptance and **compliance**. 4. The period defined by initiation of **treatment** after **enrollment**. rt: **lead-in period**

sham *n* - [perhaps fr E dial *sham* shame, alter of E *shame*] A trick that deludes; something false presented to be genuine; a spurious imitation. rt: **placebo** *Usage note*: Technically, both a **placebo** and **sham** represent a trick that deludes and, hence, share a common meaning. However, for **trials**, placebo is reserved for something taken by the person being studied, eg, a pill, whereas sham refers to something applied or done to that person by someone else, as in a sham surgical procedure.

sham effect *n* - The **effect** produced by a **sham procedure**. rt: **placebo effect**

sham procedure *n* - [trials] A bogus **procedure** designed to resemble a legitimate one and performed for the purpose of **masking** the person on whom the procedure is performed, the persons administering the procedure, or those observing the person as to whether or not the person is receiving or has received the real or bogus procedure. rt: **placebo** *Usage note*: See **sham**.

sham treatment *n* - 1. A bogus **treatment** that resembles a bona fide one; typically administered in **trials** to **mask** the person receiving a **study treatment**, those administering the study treatments, or those observing the person as to **treatment**; **sham procedure**. 2. **placebo treatment** (not a recommended synonym; see **sham** for reason)

short *adj* - [ME, fr OE *scort*] 1. Characterized by being of limited expanse or duration. 2. Characterized by being of limited stature. ant: **long** (except as a stature measure) *Usage note*: A relative term (as in *the board is short*) requiring an implied or defined comparative standard. Avoid as a characterization or label without definition. That considered "short" by one may be "long" by another. Avoid confusion by presentation of sufficient detail to indicate sense of use. The line of demarcation between short and long is arbitrary when used as a qualitative indicator of time, as in **short-term followup** vs **long-term followup**; indicate the length of time involved or implied. Similarly, the line of demarcation between short and tall is arbitrary; all such uses should be accompanied by detail indicating the implied or defined standard. See also **long**.

short-term followup *n* - **Followup** extending or to extend over a **short** period of time, eg, six months or less. ant: **long-term followup**

short-term study *n* - 1. A **study** that takes a short time to complete. 2. A study involving **short-term followup**. syn: **acute study** ant: **long-term study, chronic study**

short-term treatment *n* - 1. **Treatment**, especially one involving a **drug** or other nonsurgical forms of treatment, administered in a single or a few applications. 2. Such a treatment administered over a period of days or weeks (as opposed to months or years). ant: **long-term treatment**

short-term trial *n* - A **trial** involving **short-term followup**. ant: **long-term trial**

sib *adj* - [ME, fr OE *sibb*, fr *sibb* kinship; akin to OHG *sippa* kinship, family, L *sodais* comrade, Gk *ethos* custom, character, L *suus* one's own] 1. Kindred, related. 2. A brother or sister.

sibling *n* - 1. One of two or more individuals having at least one parent in common. 2. The issue, product, or offspring of a **parent**.

sibling center *n* - 1. A **center** that is the creation of a **parent center**. 2. A center related to another through a common **parent**. rt: **affiliate center, associate center, daughter center, satellite center, sister center**

sibling clinic *n* - 1. A **clinic** that is the creation of a **parent clinic**. 2. A clinic related to another through a common **parent**. rt: **affiliate clinic, associate clinic, daughter clinic, satellite clinic, sister clinic**

side effect *n* - A secondary by-product of an action or procedure; usually **treatment side effect** in **clinical trials**. rt: **adverse side effect, toxic side effect** *Usage note*: Use in trials should be limited to situations where there is evidence that the effect is indeed produced by a **treatment** as opposed to being merely associated with treatment. See also usage note for **drug reaction**.

sigma *n* - [Gk] The 18th letter of the **Greek alphabet**, uppercase Σ, lowercase σ.

sign *n* - [ME *signe*, fr OF, fr L *signum* mark, token, sign, image, seal; prob akin to L *secare* to cut] 1. A character indicating a mathematical operation, such as +, -, x, and ÷. 2. Something indicating presence or evidence of something; in **medicine** in relation to **disease**, any objective bodily manifestation that serves to indicate presence of **disease** or a bodily malfunction and as distinct from **symptom**. rt: **symptom**

sign test *n* - A class of **nonparametric tests of significance** in which **signed** measurements, or differences between pairs of measurements, are replaced by their signs (pluses or minuses) and then analyzed as if the signs are the result of a sample from a **binomial population**.

signed *n* - 1. Having a + or - sign. 2. Having, possessing, or bearing one's signature, as on a **signed contract**.

signed assent *n* - 1. An **assent** documented with the signature or mark of the assenting person. 2. An **assent statement** bearing the signature or mark of a person indicating that person's willingness to **assent** to that proposed. rt: **documented assent**

signed consent *n* - [**research**] 1. A **consent** documented with the signature or mark of the consenting person; such a consent indicating details regarding the nature and extent of the research, typically presented in written form (eg, as contained in a **consent form**). 2. A **consent statement** bearing the signature or mark of a person indicating that person's willingness to **consent** to that proposed in the consent statement (or explained orally in the case of illiterate persons). rt: **documented consent, disclosure statement**

signed-rank test *n* - A type of **nonparametric test of significance** based on **ranks** arising from differences of paired **observations** or measurements; see **Mann-Whitney test** and **Wilcoxon test** for examples.

significance *n* - The quality of being important or of having importance; the quality of **statistical** or **clinical significance**.

significance level *n* - [**statistics**] 1. The **probability** of rejecting the **null hypothesis** with a **test of significance** when it is **true**; **type I error**. 2. The permissible type I error level for a test of the **null hypothesis** with a specified **test statistic**. The **null hypothesis** is accepted if the test statistic yields a **p-value** which is larger than the specified level and rejected if it is equal to or less than this value. 3. **p-value**. syn: level of significance

significance test *n* - **test of significance**

significance testing *n* - [**statistics**] The act of carrying out a **test of significance** or series of such tests.

significant *adj* - [L *significant-*, *significans*, prp of *significare* to signify] Having meaning; having or likely to have influence or effect; probably caused by something other than **chance**.

significant digit *n* - 1. A **digit** position for a **continuous measure** considered to be reliable and within the **range** of **precision** of the measuring device, ie, not due to **measurement error**; eg, the first digit following the decimal point for weights recorded using a scale calibrated in tenths of a unit. 2. Any one of the digits of a **measure** beginning with the leftmost nonzero digit and extending as far to the right as necessary to include all digits considered to be within the limits of precision for the measure. 3. The rightmost digit of a measure recorded at the limit of its precision.

significant other *n* - A person of importance or meaning to an individual, especially a **peer**, such as one's spouse or mate, sister or bother, or dear friend. *Usage note*: Use should be limited to settings in which there is need or desire to be general and unrestrictive as to the persons or types of persons being referenced. Avoid as a synonym for a particular type of person, such as spouse, husband, or wife. Do not use in relation to one's parent or guardian; use parent or guardian.

simple *adj* - [ME, fr OF, plain, uncomplicated, artless, fr L *simplus*, *simplex*, lit single; L *simplus* fr *sem-*, *sim-* one + *-plus* multiplied by; L *simplic-*, *simplex* fr *sem- sim-* + *-plic-*, *plex* -fold] 1. Free from restriction; as in **simple randomization**. 2. Uncomplicated, elementary, fundamental; composed of one part. 3. Stupid; ignorant. ant: **complex** (defn 2) *Usage note*: Use with caution in the sense of defn 2. Often simplicity is in the eye of the beholder, and frequently that which is simple from one perspective is not from another. Indicate the dimension or element defining simplicity when used as a label of distinction or contrast, as in **big and simple trial**.

simple hypothesis *n* - A **hypothesis** in which the **parameter** or parameters of interest have specified values, eg, a hypothesis that the **mean** of a **distribution** is 0. ant: **composite hypothesis**

simple random sample *n* - 1. A **random sample** that arises from a sampling scheme such that every **element** or **unit** in the **population** of interest has the same **probability** of selection. 2. A random sample arising from **unrestricted randomization**. rt: **stratified random sample**

simple randomization *n* - **complete randomization**

simple treatment *n* - A **treatment** having only one **component**, eg, a treatment involving the use of a single **drug**. ant: **complex treatment**

simple treatment assignment *n* - **Treatment assignment** not involving any **restriction**, such as in **complete randomization**.

simple treatment design *n* - 1. A **treatment design** not having **factorial structured treatments**. 2. A design in which the **treatment unit** receives a **simple treatment**. ant: **complex treatment design**

simple trial *n* - 1. **data simple trial** 2. A trial easily performed; eg, one having **short followup** and an **outcome measure** easily and simply observed or measured. 3. A trial having a **simple treatment design**. 4. **big and simple trial** ant: **complex trial** *Usage note*: Avoid as a generic label; accompany with sufficient detail so as to make sense of usage clear or use additional modifiers, as with **data simple trial**. Note that use in the sense of defn 1 does not imply ease of execution; in fact, a **data simple trial** may be difficult to organize and carry out, especially if also **big**. Recognize also that people are likely to assume that simple implies low cost — an inference that may be incorrect, especially for **big and simple trials** (defn 1). The costs and efforts for such trials can be great, especially for the **coordinating center** and other core facilities having responsibilities for implementing and executing such trials. See **big and simple trial** and **simple** for added comments.

simulate, simulated, simulating, simulates *v* - [L *simulatus*, pp of *simulare* to copy, represent, feign, fr *similis* like] 1. To assume the outward appearance or qualities of; to deceive or approximate. 2. To make a **simulation** of.

simulation *n* - [ME *simulacion*, fr MF, fr L *simulation-*, *simulatio*, fr *simulare*] The act or process of **simulating**. In **statistics**, usually such an act or process in relation to representing or observing a **dynamic** process having **stochastic** elements not amenable to more exact forms of characterization, as in most **Monte Carlo simulations**.

simultaneous *adj* - [(assumed) ML *simultaneus*, fr L *simul* at the same time] 1. Existing or occurring at the same time. 2. Satisfied by the same values of a **variable**, as in **roots** of simultaneous equations.

simultaneous adjustment *n* - **Adjustment** of a **treatment effect** for one or more **covariates** using **simultaneous regression**; in distinction to **stepwise adjustment**.

simultaneous regression *n* - **Multiple regression** not involving **stepwise** selection of the **regressors** included in the **model**; as distinct from **stepwise regression**.

sine, sin *n* - [ML *sinus*, fr L, curve] A trigonometric function for an acute angle that is the **ratio** of the length of the leg opposite the angle (when considered part of a right triangle) and the hypotenuse. ant: arcsine, **inverse sine**

single *adj* - [ME, fr MF; fr L *singulus* one only; akin to L *sem-* one] Having only one relation or character; of or relating to one person. rt: **double, triple**

single blind, single blinded *n* - **single masked** See **blind** for usage note.

single masked, single mask *n* - [**trials**] 1. A condition in which those being treated are **masked** in regard to treatment but those applying the treatment are not. 2. A condition in which either those being treated or those applying the treatment (but not both) are masked in regard to treatment. 3. A condition in which only one class of people (eg, **patients**, **treaters**, or **readers**) is masked in regard to treatment. *Usage note*: See **single-mask** *adj*.

single patient trial *n* - **n of 1 trial**

single placebo *n* - A **placebo** having a single shape or form, eg, as needed in a **trial** having a **single placebo treatment design**. rt: **double placebo, multiple placebo**

single placebo treatment design *n* - A **treatment design** that involves just one **placebo**, eg, as needed in a **drug trial** having a single **test treatment**, or as needed in a drug trial with multiple test treatments, each capable of being **masked** with the same placebo. The design arises in **single-** or **double-masked trials** in which it is possible to mask all **test treatments** with a **single placebo**, as in the Coronary Drug

Project[30] (involved five test drugs and a single placebo). rt: **multiple placebo treatment design**, **single placebo**

single-blind *adj* - **single-masked** See **blind** for usage note.

single-center *adj* - Of, relating to, or comprised of one **center**. ant: **multicenter** *Usage note*: Preferred modifier for **trials** and **studies** involving a single **data collection site**. Often used in opposition to **multicenter**, especially when characterizing a set of trials as to whether single-centered or multicentered. An advantage of the term is that it has an appropriate antonym (see usage note for **multicenter**). In trials, usually used to denote a structure having a single **treatment site** (defn 1) or **data collection site**, regardless of the number of other non-data-collecting sites involved. See **single-center trial** and **multicenter trial** for additional comments.

single-center study *n* - 1. A **study** performed at a **single site**. 2. A study performed by **investigators** located at the same site or **institution**. ant: **multicenter study**

single-center trial *n* - 1. A **trial** performed at or from a single **site**: (a) Such a trial, even if performed in association with a coalition of clinics in which each clinic performs its own trial, but in which all trials focus on the same disease or condition (eg, such a coalition formed to provide preliminary information on a series of different approaches to the treatment of hypertension by stress control or reduction); (b) A trial not having any clinical centers and a single **resource center**, eg, the Physicians' Health Study.[123, 66] 2. A trial involving a single **clinic**; with or without **satellite clinics** or **resource centers**. 3. A trial involving a single clinic and a **center** to receive and process data. 4. A trial involving a single clinic and one or more resource centers. ant: **multicenter trial** *Usage note*: Note that the usual line of demarcation between single and multicenter is determined by whether or not there is more than one treatment or data collection site. Hence, a trial having multiple centers may still be classified as a single-center trial if it has only one treatment or data collection site.

single-mask, single-masked *adj* - [**experiments**] 1. Of, relating to, or being a procedure in which experimenters, but not the people being experimented upon, know the identity of the **treat-** ments being applied. 2. Of, relating to, or being a procedure in which either the experimenters or those being experimented upon, but not both, know the identity of the treatments being applied. 3. Of, relating to, or being a procedure in which one class of people (eg, **patients**, **treaters**, or **readers**) is masked to treatment identity during the course of an experiment. syn: single-blind (not recommended; see **blind** for reasons) rt: **double-mask, triple-mask** *Usage note*: Technically, the complement of the situation represented by defn 1 (ie, one in which those applying the treatments are masked and those receiving them are not, defn 2) can be characterized as single-masked. However, such masking is uncommon and, hence, the term should not be used in this sense, unless there is sufficient detail to make the sense of use explicit. Uses in the sense of defn 3 are rarer still and should be preceded or followed by sufficient detail to avoid confusion.

single-masked treatment *n* - [**trials**] 1. A **treatment** that is administered in **masked** fashion only in relation to those receiving it. 2. A treatment administered in masked fashion in relation to those receiving it or those administering it, but not in relation to both. rt: **double-masked treatment** *Usage note*: See **single-mask** *adj*.

single-masked treatment assignment *n* - [**trials**] A **treatment assignment** that is or is to be issued **single-masked**. rt: **double-masked treatment assignment, single-masked treatment** *Usage note*: See **single-mask** *adj*.

single-masked trial *n* - A **trial** that has or is to have **single-masked treatments**. rt: **double-masked trial** *Usage note*: See **single-mask** *adj*.

single-study *adj* - Of, relating to, or consisting of a single **study**. ant: **multi-study** rt: **single-trial** *Usage note*: Use **trial** if the study is a trial. See note for **study** *n*.

single-study design *n* - A **design** involving a single **study**. ant: **multi-study design** rt: **single-trial design, single-study structure** *Usage note*: See **single-study**.

single-study structure *n* - An organizational **structure** created or maintained to initiate and carry out a single **study**. ant: **multi-study structure** *Usage note*: Use **single-trial** instead of **multi-study** if the study is a trial. See **multi-trial structure** and **study** *n* for added comments.

single-tailed test *n* - **one-tailed test**

single-trial *adj* - Of, relating to, or consisting of a single **trial**. ant: **multi-trial** rt: **single-study**

single-trial design *n* - A **design** involving a single **trial**. ant: **multi-trial design** rt: **single-trial structure** *Usage note*: See **single-trial structure**.

single-trial structure *n* - An organizational **structure** created or maintained to initiate and carry out a single **trial**. ant: **multi-trial structure** *Usage note*: Used primarily in classifying structures as to intent or function in regard to whether serving one or multiple trials. See **multi-trial structure** for additional comments.

sister *n* - [ME *suster* sister, partly fr OE *sweostor* and partly of Scand origin; akin to ON *systir* sister; akin to L *soror* sister] 1. One having similar characteristics to another. 2. One having a mutual or equal relationship with another.

sister center *n* - A **center** having a relationship or association with another center, especially one performing a similar activity or function in the same or a related **study**. rt: **affiliate center**, **associate center**, **daughter center**, **satellite center**, **sibling center**

sister clinic *n* - A **clinic** having a relationship or association with another clinic, especially one performing a similar activity or function in the same or a related **study**. rt: **affiliate clinic**, **associate clinic**, **daughter clinic**, **satellite clinic**, **sibling clinic**

sister study *n* - A **study** having a relationship or association with another study, especially one involving pursuit of a similar or related issue or question. rt: **daughter study**

site *n* - [ME, place, position, fr MF or L; MF, fr L *situs*, fr *situs*, pp of *sinere* to leave, place, lay; akin to L *serere* to sow] 1. The point, place, or scene of something. 2. **study center**

site visit *n* - 1. A **visit** to a proposed or functioning **study site** by personnel not associated with the site or its **parent institution**, mandated by a **study section**, **review group**, or **sponsoring agency**, and carried out for the purpose of assessing performance potential or actual performance in order to arrive at a recommendation for **funding** or continued funding of the site. 2. **study site visit** (defn 2) rt: **reverse study site visit**

size *n* - [ME *sise* assize, fr MF, fr OF, short for *assise*] Physical magnitude, extent, or bulk; **relative** or **absolute** amount as indicated by a number, as in **sample size**.

skew *n* - A **deviation** from symmetry or true value; deviation from a straight line; slant.

skew, skewed, skewing, skews *v* - [ME *skewen* to escape, skew, fr ONF *escuer* to shun, of Gmc origin; akin to OHG *sciuhen* to frighten off] To distort from a true value or **symmetrical** form.

skew, skewed *adj* - [general] Positioned to one side; more developed on one side or in one direction than another; not **symmetrical**; running obliquely; slanting. [**statistics**] Of or relating to a **distribution** that is not symmetrical and that has a decidedly more pronounced **tail** in one direction than in the other.

skew(ed) distribution *n* - An asymmetrical **unimodal frequency distribution**. rt: **left skew distribution**, **right skew distribution**

skewness *n* - 1. Distortion or lack of straightness or **symmetry**. 2. Lack of symmetry in a **distribution**; measured by a **statistic** that has a value of 0 if the distribution is symmetrical, **positive** values if **right skewed** and **negative** values if **left skewed**.

slope *n* - 1. Upward or downward slant or inclination of a **line**, plane, or surface. 2. The **rate** of ascent or descent of a straight line per **unit** change on its **x-axis**; the tangent of the angle made by a straight line to the x-axis. rt: **intercept**

small *adj* - [ME *smal*; fr OE *smœl*; akin to OHG *smal* small, L *malus* bad] Having comparatively little size or dimension. ant: **large** *Usage note*: Use with caution as a generic label; provide accompanying detail to indicate sense of usage.

smart *adj* - Having a means of interacting; possessing intelligence. ant: **dumb**

smart computer terminal *n* - **intelligent computer terminal**

smart terminal *n* - **intelligent computer terminal**

SMR *n* - **standardized mortality ratio**

snapshot *n* - A casual (written, photographic, or electronic) recording of some event, scene, **file**, or **document** at an instant in time; made without effort to pose, arrange, or tidy. rt: **data snapshot**

society *n* - [MF *societē*, fr L *societat- societas*, fr *socius* companion] An organized group working and meeting together because of common interests or profession.

Society of Clinical Trials (SCT) *n* - A professional society formed in 1979 to promote sound design and conduct of **clinical trials** and to facilitate communications among those concerned with them.

soft *adj* - [ME, fr OE *sōfte*, alter of *sēfte*; akin to OHG *semfti* soft] 1. Lacking in strength, **robustness**, or certainty. 2. Not hard or permanent. 3. Being based on **observations** or **data** subject to varying interpretations or meanings. ant: **hard**

soft endpoint *n* - **soft outcome** *Usage note*: See **endpoint**.

soft outcome *n* - [**trials**] An **outcome measure** that is subject to **errors** of interpretation or **measurement**; usually one that depends on opinion or **observation** involving subjectivity. ant: **hard outcome**

software *n* - [**computers**] A collection of **programs**, routines, subroutines, and accompanying documentation that facilitate the programming and operation of a **computer**; as distinct from computer **hardware** (defn 2).

SoP, SOP *n* - **standard operating procedure**

source *n* - [ME *sours*, fr MF *sors*, *sourse*, fr OF, fr pp of *sourdre* to rise, spring forth, fr L *surgere*] 1. A generative force; cause. 2. A point of **origin** or procurement; beginning. 3. A **primary** or firsthand **reference**; **source document**. rt: **primary source, secondary source**

source document *n* - 1. The **original** (defn 2) of a **document**. 2. A document from which other things flow, arise, or depend. rt: **primary document, secondary document**

source of variation *n* - **Variation** due to or explained by some **procedure, process, factor**, or **variable**, as in an **analysis of variance**.

source record *n* - 1. The **original** (defn 2) of a **record**. 2. A record containing **original data**. 3. **source document** rt: **primary record, secondary record**

Spearman's rank correlation *n* - A measure of **correlation** based on **ranks** in the absence of ties; equal to the **Pearson product-moment correlation coefficient** derived using the ranked data. rt: **Kendall's tau, rank correlation**

specific *adj* - [LL *specificus*, fr L *species*] Sharing or being properties of something that allows referral to a particular **category**; exerting a distinctive influence. rt: **sensitive**

specific aim *n* - Something intended or to be pursued, such as an **aim** in a **research proposal**.

specificity *n* - The quality or state of being **specific**; the condition of being peculiar to a particular individual or group of organisms. In **epidemiology**, in relation to **screening tests**, the ability of such a test to identify **true** noncases, measured by the **proportion** of the true noncases identified by the test; also the **probability** that any given noncase will be so identified by the test, also referred to as true negative rate. rt: **sensitivity**

specified assignment ratio *n* - The particular **assignment ratio** used in constructing the **assignment schedule**. syn: **expected assignment ratio**

split *adj* - Divided or fractured.

split-half *adj* - Of or being **split** or divided into two parts of equal or unequal size.

split-half reliability *n* - The extent to which **results** obtained from a defined part of a **dataset** (eg, the first half of the dataset as divided on the basis of time) correspond to those obtained from the remaining part. rt: **reliability**

split-plot *adj* - Of, relating to, or concerned with **designs** involving subplots or their conceptual equivalent.

split-plot *n* - 1. [fr agricultural experiments] A subpart of a **plot** (defn 2), especially as demarcated for use of a particular **treatment** within a designated plot (eg, a subplot of a plot sown with a particular variety of wheat designated to receive a certain kind of fertilizer). 2. Any object, entity, or being that is split or can be regarded, in a conceptual sense, as being or having been split for purposes of **design** or **analysis** of an **experiment**, as in a **split-plot design**.

split-plot design *n* - A class of **factorial design** in which the **experimental unit** (whole **plot**) is subdivided (or can be viewed as being so divided) to allow it to receive different **treatments**; also split-unit design and sub-unit design. In the context of **crossover designs**, a **patient** may be viewed as a plot and the portions of times exposed to the different treatments defined for a given replication of the design as subplots. The effect of plot-to-plot **variation** on **treatment effect** estimated from plots diminishes as the number of plots increase.

sponsor *n* - [LL, fr L, guarantor, surety, fr *sponsus*, pp of *spondēre* to promise] 1. Broadly, one who promotes or supports. 2. A person or **agency** that is responsible for **funding** a designated function or activity; **sponsoring agency**. 3. A person or agency that plans and carries out a specified project or activity. 4. The agency or person named in an **Investigational New Drug Application** or **New Drug Application**; usually a **drug company** or person at such a company, but not always (as with an **INDA** submitted by a representative of a **research group** proposing to carry out a **phase III** or **phase IV drug trial** not sponsored by a drug company). 5. A firm or business establishment marketing a product or service.

sponsor-initiated research proposal *n* - A **research proposal** prepared in response to a request by a **sponsoring agency**, as in relation to a **request for proposal (RFP)** or **request for application (RFA)**. ant: **investigator-initiated research proposal** rt: **contract proposal** *Usage note*: The initiating forces behind **research projects** are not always clear, even when the proposals are generated in response to RFPs or RFAs or when funding is via **contracts**. Often in the case of large-scale **multicenter trials**, the initiation process is a joint one involving people at the sponsoring agency and would-be investigators, especially in the case of **NIH**-sponsored trials. For example, the Coronary Drug Project,[30] although funded by grants and ostensibly investigator-initiated, was, in fact, actively encouraged by the sponsoring institute. See note for **investigator-initiated research proposal** for added comments.

sponsoring agency *n* - The **agency**, **institution**, **organization**, or foundation that provides financial support, and often administrative and scientific support as well, for a given **project** or activity. syn: **funding agency**

spouse *n* - [ME, fr OF *espous* (masc) & *espouse* (fem), fr L *sponsus* betrothed man, groom & *sponsa* betrothed woman, bride, both fr *sponsus*, pp of *spondēre* to promise, betroth; akin to Gk *spendein* to make a libation, promise, *spondē* libation (pl, treaty)] One's partner in marriage; one's husband or wife.

spread, **spreading**, **spreads** *v* - [ME *spreden*, fr OE *spǣdan*; akin to OHG *spreiten* to spread, OE *-sprūtan* to sprout] To open or expand over a large area; to stretch out or extend; to distribute over an area.

spreadsheet *n* - [fr *spreadsheet* oversized page used by accountants] 1. A **two-way table**, typically in **landscape orientation**, used to display **data**. 2. A **computer program** used for entering, processing, and displaying spreadsheet data.

spurious *adj* - [LL & L; LL *spurius* false, fr L, of illegitimate birth, fr *spurius*, n bastard] Outwardly similar or corresponding to something without having genuine qualities; **false**; fictitious.

spurious correlation *n* - A **correlation** (**positive** or **negative**) that arises from or is the result of some artifact or irrelevant peculiarity in the **data**.

square *n* - [ME, fr MF *esquarre*, fr (assumed) VL *exquadra*, fr *exquadrare* to square, fr L *ex-* + *quadrare* to square] The product of a number multiplied by itself.

square root *n* - A factor of a number, that when squared, gives that number (eg, 3 is the square root of 9).

square root transformation *n* - A **variance** stabilizing **transformation** of the form

$$y = \sqrt{x} \qquad or \qquad \sqrt{x+1}$$

applied to **data** having or believed to have a **Poisson distribution**.[146] See **inverse sine transformation** for corresponding transformation for **proportions**.

stage *n* - [ME, fr MF *estage*, fr (assumed) VL *staticum*, fr L *stare* to stand] A period or step in a development, process, or procedure.

stage of trial *n* - A defined set of activities performed during a specified period in a **trial**; herein **initial design stage**, **protocol development stage**, **patient recruitment stage**, **treatment and followup stage**, **followup stage**, **patient close-out stage**, **termination stage**, and **post-trial followup stage**. *Usage note*: Not to be confused with **phase of trial**. The phase of a trial is determined by its purpose and order in the sequence of trials done in developing a treatment for use in human beings. Stage pertains to a class of activities within a trial as it proceeds from beginning to end.

standard *n* - [ME, fr OF *estandard* rallying point, standard, of Gmc origin; akin to OE *standan* to stand and to OE *ord* point] 1. Something established by authority, custom, **consent**, convention, or **calculation** that is used as a basis of **comparison** or judgment. 2. An acknowledged base for **comparison** or contrast. 3. **criterion** 4. An object that, under specified conditions, defines, represents, or records a **unit** of a **measure**.

standard care *n* - [**medicine**] **Care** that conforms to established norms or **standards**.

standard control *n* - **standard control treatment**

standard control treatment *n* - A form of **active control treatment** in which the **treatment** is designed and administered to correspond to the present-day norm or standard of care or treatment.

standard deviation (SD, sd) *n* - [**statistics**] a **measure of dispersion** of a **frequency distribution** that is the **square root** of the **arithmetic mean** of the squares of the **deviations** of the values represented in the distribution from the mean of the distribution; a similar quantity using n - 1 rather than n as a divisor; a measure of dispersion that is equal to the square root of the **variance**. syn: root-mean square deviation, **root-mean square error** rt: **variance**

standard distribution *n* - 1. A **distribution** used for **rate adjustment**. 2. A distribution assumed, imposed, or derived used as a **standard** for a **comparison** or **calculation**.

standard error (SE, se) *n* - [**statistics**] The **standard deviation** of the **sampling distribution** of a **statistic**; eg, the standard error of the **mean** for a **variable** is the **standard deviation** for that variable divided by the **square root** of the number of **observations** represented in the mean.

standard medical care *n* - **Medical care** conforming to or in accordance with accepted **norms** or **standards**.

standard medical treatment *n* - A **standard treatment** involving **medicines**, eg, as distinct from **surgical treatment**. rt: **standard surgical treatment**

standard normal distribution *n* - A **normal distribution** with **mean**, $\mu = 0$ and **variance**, $\sigma^2 = 1$.

standard operating procedure (SoP, SOP) *n* - 1. A **procedure** performed under specified conditions. 2. A procedure performed as specified in a **manual of operations**.

standard population *n* - A defined (actual or contrived) **population** used for **comparison**, **adjustment**, or **standardization** of results from one or more **study populations**; **reference population**. rt: **reference population, target population**

standard score *n* - A **score** derived from a **transformation** in which the transformed score corresponds to a **variable** having known distributional properties, eg, a **normalized score** or one resulting from a **T-** or **Z-transformation**. rt: **data transformation, normalized standard score, T-score, Z-score**

standard surgical treatment *n* - A **standard treatment** involving surgery. rt: **standard medical treatment**

standard treatment *n* - A **treatment** widely practiced and routinely applied for **treatment** of a specified **disease** or health condition; **standard care**. *Usage note*: Often used in a loose inferential sense with the inference being based on limited observations or suppositions regarding typical practice procedures. On occasions, the designation may be the result of a decree by some agency, body, or society. Do not use in settings where the normal practice is to not treat. Do not use in relation to **placebo treatments**. There are differences in connotation between not treating at all and administering a placebo treatment.

standard unit *n* - [**data transformation**] A type of **unit** resulting from a **transformation** in which **data** for a given **variable** are converted to a form having **mean** 0 (zero) and **variance** 1 (one); done by subtracting the observed mean for the variable from each value in the **dataset** and dividing the difference by the **standard deviation** for the variable. rt: **data transformation, normalized standard score, T-score, Z-score**

standardization *n* - [**epidemiology**] The process of bringing an observed set of results into conformity with another via a series of arithmetic or mathematical maneuvers for the purpose of **comparison**, as in **direct rate adjustment**. rt: **direct standardization, indirect standardization**

standardize, standardized, standardizing, standardizes *v* - To compare with or bring into conformity with a **standard**.

standardized morbidity ratio *n* - The **ratio** (usually multiplied by 100) of the number of **morbid events** due to some **disease** or condition observed in a specified **study group** or **population** to the number expected if that group or **population** had demographic characteristics corresponding to those of a specified **standard population**; a method of **adjustment**. rt: **standardization, standardized mortality ratio**

standardized mortality ratio (SMR) *n* - The **ratio** (usually multiplied by 100) of the number of deaths observed in a specified **study group** or **population** to the number expected if that group or population had demographic characteristics corresponding to those of a specified **standard population**; a method of **adjustment**. rt: **standardization, standardized morbidity ratio**

standardized normal deviate *n* - A **normal deviate** divided by its **standard deviation**.

standardized random variable *n* - A **random variable** transformed to have **mean** 0 and **variance** 1. rt: **data transformation, T-score, standard unit, Z-score**

standardized rate *n* - A **rate** derived by **direct** or **indirect standardization**. rt: **crude rate, observed rate**

standardized score *n* - A **score** indicating one's performance relative to a defined or hypothetical **standard population**; the score may correspond to a **percentile** (such as the percent of people scoring at or below one's score) or may measure the extent to which the score departs from the **mean** as measured by the number of **standard deviations** one's score departs from the **mean** of the standard population.

standardized test *n* - 1. A **test** (defn 1), such as one used for measuring intelligence, developed using a defined **standard population**. 2. A test that yields a **standardized score**.

start *n* - The beginning point as defined in relation to motion, an activity, or development, eg, **random start** in relation to a **randomization process**.

start-up *n* - The act or instance of setting in operation or motion.

start-up patient *n* - 1. The first patient **enrolled** into a **trial**. 2. The first patient enrolled at each **clinic** in a **multicenter trial** (defn 1 or 3). 3. **vanguard patient** 4. **test patient** *Usage note*: See **start-up patients**.

start-up patients *n* - The collective set of **patients** designated as constituting a start-up set for some purpose or function. rt: **test patients, vanguard patients** *Usage note*: Avoid, except when there is some operational meaning or importance given to the designation, as in relation to the way such patients are treated or handled relative to trial-proper patients. See also notes for **test patients** and **vanguard patients**.

statement *n* - The act or process of stating or presenting orally or on paper; something stated or reported.

statistic *n* - [back-formation fr *statistics*] 1. A quantity, such as a **mean** or **variance**, derived or computed from **observed data**. 2. A mathematical formula for computing such a statistic. 3. A **random variable** that takes on the possible values of a statistic. 4. A single number or **datum** in a collection of statistics.

statistical *adj* - Of, relating to, or using the principles of **statistics**.

statistical association *n* - 1. An **association** of two **variables** considered to be beyond the realm of **chance**. 2. An association not likely to be due to chance; especially one judged to be **statistically significant** using a **test of significance**. rt: **statistical correlation** *Usage note*: Sometimes used in contradistinction to **clinical significance**, especially when the association is of questionable or unknown biological or medical importance.

statistical center *n* - 1. A **center** in **multicenter** structures responsible for **analysis** and interpretation of **data** generated within the structure. 2. **data center** 3. **data coordinating center** 4. **coordinating center** syn: **biostatistical center**

statistical correlation *n* - 1. A **correlation** of two **variables** considered to be beyond the realm of **chance**. 2. A correlation not likely to be due to chance; especially one judged to be **statistically significant** using a **test of significance**. rt: **statistical association** *Usage note*: See **statistical association**.

statistical difference *n* - An **observed difference** with an appropriately small **p-value**, say, ≤ 0.05.

statistical inference *n* - **Inference** to a general **population** based on sample **data** or **estimates** from that **population**; broadly, any generalization, **prediction, estimate**, or decision based on a **sampling**.

statistical interaction *n* - An **interaction** that is considered to be **statistically significant**; may or may not be biologically or clinically meaningful. *Usage note*: See **statistical association**.

statistical power *n* - **power**

statistical significance *n* - 1. **p-value** 2. An observed **result** that yields an appropriately small **p-value**, say ≤0.05, when evaluated against the **null hypothesis** using a specified **test of significance**.

statistical test *n* - **test of significance**

statistics *n* - [pl but sing or pl in constr; G *statistik* study of political facts and figures, fr NL *statisticus* of politics, fr L *status* state] 1. A branch of mathematics concerned with variation in **data generation** and **data collection** processes, with the development of strategies for eliminating, reducing, or dealing with that variability, and with the **analysis** and interpretation of such data. 2. A collection of facts.

status *n* - The state, condition, or standing of a person or thing with regard to some measure or criterion, eg, the **vital status** of a person.

steer, steered, steering, steers *v* - [ME *steren*, fr OE *stīeran*; akin to OE *stēor*- steering oar; Gk *stauros* stake, cross, *stylos* pillar, Skt *sthavira*, *sthūra* stout, thick, L *stare* to stand] To direct the course of; guide.

steering committee (SC) *n* - A **committee** responsible for directing or guiding activities. In **multicenter trials**, the committee responsible for conduct of the **trial** and to which all other committees report, except, perhaps, the **treatment effects monitoring committee** and **advisory-review committee** or **advisory-review and treatment effects monitoring committee**. Usually headed by the **study chair** and consisting of the directors of some or all the functioning **centers** or consisting of a combination of designated and elected representatives of the entire **investigative group**. One of the **key committees** in **multicenter** structures. rt: **executive committee** *Usage note*: Sometimes used interchangeably with **executive committee**; not recommended (see **executive committee** for comment).

step *n* - [ME, fr OE *stæpe*; akin to OHG *stapfo* step, *stampfōn* to stamp] 1. One of a **series** of specified actions or procedures carried out in **order**. 2. One of a series of increments or

elevations. *Usage note*: Avoid as a characterization of acts or processes not preceded or followed by one or more steps.

stepped *adj* - Of, relating to, or being a **step**.

stepped treatment *n* - **Treatment** that proceeds in **steps** or increments according to some **protocol** or algorithm as dictated by the need or condition of the person being treated.

stepped treatment protocol *n* - A **treatment protocol** providing for **stepped treatment**. The stepping process may involve increments in the **dosage** of the same **drug** or use of additional drugs or more powerful drugs.

stepwise *adj* - Marked by or proceeding in **steps**.

stepwise adjustment *n* - **Adjustment** involving **stepwise regression**; in distinction to **simultaneous adjustment**.

stepwise regression *n* - **Multiple regression** involving a defined set of **regressors**, x_1, x_2, x_3, ..., x_r, performed in a **series** of **steps** each one of which consists of adding (**forward stepwise regression**) or deleting (**backward stepwise regression**) a **regressor** to or from the **model** based on measures of changes in **residual variation**, as indicated by **p-values** associated with the indicated regressors. Nonautomated procedures may involve reconsideration of regressors already accepted or rejected in previous steps. The process is aimed at finding a suitably small set of regressors while still being able to account for most of the variation explained by the r regressors. Traditionally, in **computer** automated procedures based on p-values, a regressor is added to the set (forward selection) if it has the smallest p-value (among regressors not already in the set) below a specified **cutpoint** (eg, p = 0,05); a regressor is deleted from the set (backward selection) if it has the largest p-value (among regressors in the set) above a specified cutpoint (eg, p = 0.05). As distinct from **simultaneous regression**.

stochastic *adj* - [Gk *stochastikos* skillful in aiming, fr *stochazesthai* to aim at, guess at, fr *stochos* target, aim, guess] **Random**; involving a **random variable**; involving **chance** or **probability**.

stochastic curtailment *n* - [trials] **Curtailment** based on the **likelihood** of obtaining a **result** different than the one observed if the trial were to continue to its appointed end (eg, the likelihood of an observed **positive result** being reduced to a **nil result** or the likelihood of a nil result being elevated to a positive result); typically based on calculations of **conditional power** or **conditional or type I error** assuming a specified **treatment effect** from the point of assessment to the appointed end of the trial. The decision may be to stop the trial if the assessment suggests that continuing is unlikely to produce a result different from the one observed.

stochastic process *n* - A process involving **chance** or probabilistic events or processes.

stochastic variable *n* - **random variable**

stop *n* - 1. The **cessation**, end, or finish of. 2. Something that impedes, obstructs, limits, or brings to a halt. 3. The act of **stopping**.

stop, stopped, stopping, stops *v* - [ME *stoppen*, fr OE -*stoppian*, fr (assumed) VL *stuppare* to stop with tow, fr L *stppa* tow, fr Gk *styppē*] 1. To cause to **cease**, halt, or discontinue. 2. To hinder or prevent the passage of. 3. To close or block up.

stop condition *n* - 1. A **condition** (defn 1 or 2) that signals the need to **stop** (defn 1), eg, the **cessation** of a **drug treatment** in the face of serious toxicity. 2. A condition signaling the absence of a need to continue, as in an ordered **screening process** once an exclusion condition is encountered. 3. A condition signaling the need to hold or halt an activity, eg, a hold in the evaluation of a person for **enrollment** into a **trial** because of illness). 4. A defined condition that, when encountered for a person **enrolled** in a **trial**, requires or permits **clinic** personnel to take some action related to that person, such as instituting a change in **treatment** or terminating **followup** of that person. rt: **stop item**

stop item *n* - An **item** (defn 1) or **response category** on a **data form** that, when checked or completed, indicates the presence of a **stop condition**. rt: **stop condition**

stop trial *n* - 1. The state of **stopping** a **trial**. 2. The state of stopping a trial before its scheduled or normal end, as in an **early** or **premature stop**. rt: **trial stop** *Usage note*: Jargon; not informative without accompanying detail indicating the reason for the **stop** and specifics of what, in fact, is being stopped. See **trial stop**.

stopped trial *n* - A **trial** that has been **stopped** before reaching its scheduled or normal end. syn: **early stop, premature stop** *Usage note*: See comments for **early stopping** and **trial stop**.

stopping boundary *n* - [**trials**] 1. The set of **boundary** values formed by a **line**, or pair of lines, as determined for **sequential designs**, which, if exceeded, cause investigators to **stop** the trial. 2. The set of **boundary** values formed by a line or pair of lines for a **fixed sample size design**, usually specified before or shortly after the start of **enrollment**, which, if exceeded, indicate the existence of a **treatment difference** that satisfies certain statistical properties (eg, has a **p-value** of less than a certain size), whether or not used as a strict **stopping rule**.

stopping rule *n* - [**trials**] A **rule**, based on some **test statistic** or other function, specified by the **design** in the case of **sequential trials** and that is established by **investigators** before or shortly after the start of **enrollment**, in trials having **fixed sample size designs**, that specifies a limit for the observed **treatment difference** for the **primary outcome measure**, which, if exceeded, automatically leads to **termination of trial** or one of the **study treatments**, depending on the nature and direction of the **observed treatment difference**. rt: **early stopping**

stopping the trial *n* - The act of stopping a **trial**; especially in relation to a **trial stop**. rt: **early stop, early stopping, premature stop** *Usage note*: Jargon; avoid without accompanying detail to indicate sense of use as discussed for **trial stop**.

storage *n* - 1. A place or space for storing, such as **memory** in a **computer** for storing **data**. 2. The act of storing. 3. The state of being stored, especially for safekeeping.

strata pl, **stratum** sing *n* - [NL, fr L spread, layer, bed, fr neut of *stratus*, pp of *sternere* to spread out] A series of distinct levels or layers. In **trials**, generally **subgroups** of persons formed by classification on some **variable** or set of variables, usually **baseline variables**. Not to be confused with **blocks** (defns 2 and 3).

stratification *n* - 1. Broadly, the act or process of **stratifying** (defn 2 or 3). 2. An active ongoing process of **stratifying**, as in the sense of defn 2, as in placing **patients** into **strata** as they arrive at a **clinic** as a prelude to **enrollment** and **randomization** to **treatment** in a **trial**. 3. The act or process of classifying **treatment units** or **observations** into strata after **enrollment** or collection for a **subgroup analysis; post-stratification**. rt: **classification** *Usage note*: Stratification is done as a means of **controlling** sources of **variation** related to or assumed to be related to the **outcome**. Stratification (defn 2) and **blocking** in the **treatment assignment** process serve different purposes. Blocking is imposed as a means of ensuring that the **assignment ratio** will be satisfied or nearly satisfied; stratification is done to ensure the comparability of the treatment groups with regard to the variable(s) used in stratification. There is confusion regarding the meaning and impact of stratification on the design and operation of a trial. Often the act of stratification is taken as evidence of the need to perform **treatment comparisons** within the various strata represented in the stratification. Although that may be desirable, such comparisons are not necessary. Valid comparisons of the **treatment groups** can be performed by pooling across strata. As a rule, the mix of persons enrolled into a trial is determined by the mix of persons seen and ultimately judged eligible for **enrollment**. Hence, the numbers to be represented in the various strata will be **variables** having values known only after completion of enrollment. The imposition of a **sample size requirement** for one or more of the strata (see **recruitment quota**), in addition to one for the trial, extends the time required for **recruitment** and should not be imposed unless there are valid scientific or practical reasons for doing so. Confusion also arises from use of the term **stratification** in two distinctly different contexts, as suggested in defn 2 and 3 above. Use **post-stratification** for uses in the sense of defn 3, especially when in settings, such as trials, where both forms of stratification are used.

stratification variable *n* - 1. A **variable** used to classify **treatment units** into **strata** in relation to **treatment assignment**. 2. A variable used to classify **observation units** into strata in relation to **data analysis**.

stratified assignment *n* - **stratified treatment assignment**

stratified random assignment *n* - **stratified random treatment assignment**

stratified random sample *n* - 1. A **random sample** that arises from a sampling scheme based on **strata**. 2. A method of sampling in which **sampling units** are identified within strata for a designated **variable** or variables (eg, age and sex) and sampled within those strata using selection **probabilities** specified to achieve a desired mix of sampling units. rt: **simple random sample**

stratified random sampling *v* - **Random sampling** within defined **strata**; done to ensure a specified mix of **units** in the sample; mix being determined by the sampling fractions used for the various strata. For example, if chosen to be proportionate to those of the **parent population**, the sample will have the same **expected** mix as in that population.

stratified random treatment assignment *n* - **Random treatment assignment** within defined **assignment strata**.

stratified randomization *n* - A **treatment assignment process** using **stratified random treatment assignment**.

stratified sampling *n* - **Sampling** taking place within defined **strata**; **stratified random sampling** when the sampling involves **randomization**.

stratified treatment assignment *n* - [**trials**] **Treatment assignment** performed within **strata** defined by one or more demographic characteristics (eg, sex and age) or **baseline variables** (eg, body weight and systolic blood pressure); the **assignment schedule** within a stratum is constructed to satisfy a specified **assignment ratio**. Done as a means of **controlling** for the variables used in the stratification. **Stratified random treatment assignment** if assignments are **randomized**.

stratify, stratified, stratifying, stratifies *v* - [NL *stratificare*, fr *stratum* + L *-ificare -ify*] 1. Broadly, to divide or arrange into **classes** or **groups**. 2. To so divide or arrange in an active, ongoing way as a prelude to some act or process, as in arranging **patients** into **strata** as they arrive at a **clinic** for **enrollment** and **randomization** to **treatment** in a **trial**. 3. To so divide or arrange an assembled group of **observation units** or **treatment units** and associated **data** as a prelude to a **subgroup analysis** or for some other purpose related to **data analysis**; **post-stratify**. *Usage note*: See **stratification**.

stratum, pl **strata** *n* - [NL, fr L, spread, bed, fr neut of *stratus*, pp of *sternere* to spread out] 1. A layer or level. 2. A particular **subgroup** defined by a **stratification variable** or variables.

structure *n* - [ME, fr L *structura*, fr *structus*, pp of *struere* to heap up, build] 1. Something made up of a number of parts put together in a particular way. 2. The particular way in which parts are put together to form a whole. 3. Something arranged in a particular way, eg, a **factorial structure**.

Student *n* - Pseudonym of **William S Gosset**.

Student's t *n* - **t test**

Student's t distribution *n* - **t distribution**

study *adj* - Of or relating to one or something being evaluated or studied. *Usage note*: Used primarily as a general descriptor, as in **study candidate**, when other more precise terms are not appropriate or have undesirable connotations (as in trial candidate). See usage note for **study** *n* for additional notes.

study *n* - [ME *studie*, fr OF *estudie*, fr L *studium*, akin to L *studēre* to study, *tundere* to beat] 1. An **experimental** or **nonexperimental investigation** or **analysis** of a question, process, or phenomenon. 2. Any one of a variety of activities involving the **collection**, **analysis**, or interpretation of **data**. 3. **Clinical trial**, especially in a setting where there is a desire or need to de-emphasize the experimental nature of the investigation. 4. An investigation involving both a trial and nonexperimental investigation (as in the Coronary Artery Surgery Study, comprised of a clinical trial and a **followup study**[21, 22]). *Usage note*: Widely and loosely used. Avoid in favor of more informative, less generic terms whenever possible (eg, use trial rather than study when appropriate). As a label, limit use to defined sets of activities involving **data collection** not ordinarily characterized with a more informative, design-specific term (such as trial or followup study), or where a general term is needed to characterize a collection of activities involving a number of different designs (eg, referring to a mix of trials and **observational studies**). Avoid as a synonym for a specified kind of investigation having a recognized term (as in referring to an investigation as a trial in the title or abstract of a paper and study in the body of the paper).

study, studied, studying, studies *v* - To investigate or evaluate through use of defined procedures, eg, outlined in a **study plan** or **study protocol**.

study candidate *n* - One who is being considered or evaluated for **enrollment** into a **study**.

study center *n* - [trials] 1. **data collection site**; **study clinic** 2. **Data collection** or **data genera-**

tion site. 3. The **center** (defn 3 or 4) from which activities are directed; **coordinating center**; **project office**. 4. An operational unit in the structure of a **study**, especially a **multicenter** structure, separate and distinct from other such units in the structure, responsible for performing specified functions in one or more stages of the study; eg, a **clinical center** or **resource center**. *Usage note*: Avoid usage in the sense of defn 1 in **multicenter trials** for reasons stated in the usage note for **center**. Restrict usage as a collective term to uses in the sense of defn 4; use an appropriately modified term when the reference is to a specific subset of centers. For example, use **study clinic** or simply **clinic** when referring to the subset of centers responsible for enrolling and treating **study patients**.

study center director *n* - 1. The scientific head of a **study center**. 2. The administrative and scientific head of such a center. 3. The administrative head of such a center.

study chair *n* - **Chair** of the **investigative group**; chair of the **steering committee** of an investigative group. rt: **study vice-chair**

study clinic *n* - A **clinic** responsible for the **recruitment**, **enrollment**, **followup**, or **treatment** of **patients** and related **examinations** and **data collection** procedures, as required in a specified **study**.

study clinic coordinator *n* - 1. An individual in a **study clinic** responsible for coordinating the **data collection** activities for that **clinic** and for expediting the flow of **data** and related **records** from the clinic to the **data center**, **data coordinating center**, or **coordinating center**. 2. An individual in the data center, data coordinating center, or coordinating center responsible for coordinating the receipt of data from study clinics and for communicating with clinics regarding data flow; **data coordinator**.

study clinic director *n* - The administrative or administrative and scientific head of a **study clinic**.

study clinic monitor *n* - 1. An individual, in the **treatment coordinating center**, **data center**, **data coordinating center**, **coordinating center**, or **sponsoring agency**, responsible for monitoring **data collection** and data flow procedures at associated **clinics**. 2. A person located within a clinic and responsible for monitoring data collection and data flow procedures for that clinic;

field monitor. rt: **circuit rider**, **study clinic coordinator**

study clinic personnel *n* - **Personnel** associated with a **study clinic** and responsible for performing the duties and activities involved in a **study**.

study clinic visit *n* - Any **visit** by a **patient** to a **study clinic** in relation to study activities or related care procedures. In **trials**, visits related to **enrollment**, **followup** or **treatment** and typically involving **examination** and **data collection**.

study committee *n* - 1. A **committee** with responsibility for the **design**, conduct, or **analysis** of a **study**. 2. Any one of the several committees in a **multicenter study**, especially **key committees**.

study coordinator *n* - 1. A person responsible for coordinating or directing activities related to a **study**. 2. **clinic coordinator** 3. **data coordinator**

study data *n* - 1. **Data** generated from a **study**. 2. Data being **studied**.

study database *n* - 1. The entire set of **data**, whether or not codified and keyed for electronic storage, collected on **observation units** in a study and contained on study **data forms**; exclusive of data contained on **medical records**, except when such records are a required part of **data collection** for a study. 2. **Study data** comprising the **electronic database** of a study.

study design *n* - The general **plan** by which a **study** was or is to be carried out, including details on the nature of the **study population** and **data collection** procedures and, when appropriate, other details, such as for **treatment** procedures, in the case of **trials**. rt: **experimental design**

study examination *n* - Any **examination** (defns 3 or 4) of a person performed in relation a **study protocol**; includes examinations performed for evaluation or assessment, administering **treatment** or care, **data collection**, and **followup**. rt: **study visit**

study form *n* - 1. Any of the various **forms** used for operation of a **study**. 2. Any of the various forms used for **data collection** in a study.

study group *n* - 1. Any defined group of **observation units** on whom specified **data** are collected. 2. The entire group of observation units included in a **study**. 3. **treatment group** 4. The group of investigators carrying out a study. 5. **investi-**

gative group *Usage note*: Subject to confusion. Note that defns 1, 2, and 3 refer to the focus of study, whereas defns 4 and 5 refer to those doing the study. Avoid confusion by reserving the term for uses in the sense of defns 1, 2, and 3; use some other term, such as **research group** or **investigative group** for uses in the sense of defns 4 and 5. Use **treatment group** rather than **study group** for uses in the sense of defn 3.

study handbook *n* - A **book** of tables, charts, figures, and pages containing details regarding design and operating features of a **study**, largely without use of written narrative. rt: **handbook**, **study manual** *Usage note*: See **study manual of operations**.

study home visit *n* - A **study visit** taking place in a person's home. syn: **home visit**, **patient home visit**

study identification number *n* - 1. A **number** used for **identification** of a **study**. 2. **patient identification number** rt: **identification number**

study investigator *n* - 1. A person having a key role in the **design**, conduct, or **analysis** of a **study**. 2. One involved in a **study** as an **investigator**; **clinical investigator**. 3. A member of the **investigative group**. rt: **co-investigator**, **co-principal investigator** *Usage note*: See **investigator**.

study manual *n* - 1. **study manual of operations** 2. **study handbook**

study manual of operations *n* - 1. A **document** or collection of documents, largely in narrative form, describing the procedures used in a **center** or set of centers in a **study** (eg, **study clinics**, **coordinating center**, or **reading center**) for performing defined functions. 2. **study handbook** *Usage note*: Manual and **handbook** are sometimes used interchangeably; however, there are differences between the two types of documents. Use **manual** to characterize a document organized much like a book with a series of chapters and written narrative. Use **handbook** for a collection of tables, lists, charts, etc, arranged in some organized manner, largely devoid of written narrative.

study, off *adj* - **off study**

study, on *adj* - **on study**

study participant *n* - 1. A person **enrolled** into a **study**; **study subject**; **research subject**. 2.

study investigator (not recommended) rt: **study candidate** *Usage note*: Used in place of **study patient** for studies involving well people to avoid the connotation of illness, as in a **primary prevention trial**.

study patient *n* - 1. One who has a specified health condition or **disease** and is **enrolled** into a **study**; **study subject**; **research subject**. 2. One enrolled into a study, even if not a **patient** in the true sense; **study subject**. 3. A **patient** being considered for **enrollment** into a study (not recommended; use **study candidate**). rt: **study participant** *Usage note*: Limit use to settings involving persons with an illness or disease; avoid in settings involving well people or when there is a need to avoid connotations of illness or of medical care by using a medically neutral term, such as **study participant**.

study physician *n* - A **physician** associated with a **study**, eg, one in a **study clinic** in a **clinical trial**, responsible for the **diagnosis**, **treatment**, or evaluation of **study candidates**, **study patients**, or **study participants** according to plans and procedures set forth in the **study protocol**, **study manual**, or **study handbook**.

study plan *n* - 1. **study design** 2. **study protocol**

study population *n* - 1. The set of persons or **observation units enrolled** or to be enrolled into a **study**. 2. The entire set of persons or observation units considered for **enrollment** into a study, regardless of whether or not enrolled. 3. **parent population**

study protocol *n* - 1. General rules and procedures for carrying out a **study**; usually written. 2. **treatment protocol** 3. **study plan** *Usage note*: Subject to varying usages ranging from loose to rigorous; when used loosely, usually refers to a general plan, not in writing. Usage in formal research settings, such as for **trials**, normally refers to a written plan that is part of a **funding application**, **study manual of operations**, or **study handbook**.

study re-entry *n* - 1. The **re-entry** of a **study patient** or **study participant** into a **study** in which they were previously **enrolled** but from which they were separated because of being ineligible or because the aspect of the study relating to them was completed or temporarily halted. 2. The reinstatement to active status of a person previously enrolled into a **study** but who **dropped out** or was unable to continue

participation because of extenuating circumstances (eg, because of a change of residence); especially, with resumption of required **treatment** and **data collection** procedures in relation to **trials**.

study review visit *n* - 1. A **visit** of a **review group** to a **study site**, to the **sponsoring agency**, or to a third site chosen for its convenience, for the purpose of **review** of a proposed or ongoing **study**. 2. **study site visit** (defn 2) syn: **site visit** *Usage note*: Typically referred to as **study site visit** when the location of the visit is at a study site and **reverse study site visit** when the location is elsewhere. However, the latter term is not recommended for reasons stated in a usage note for that term.

study section *n* - 1. Any one of several different **review groups** of the **National Institutes of Health**; chartered to carry out reviews of **research proposals** in a general area of **research** and meeting at regular intervals to perform those reviews. 2. A group of individuals, normally recruited by the **sponsoring agency**, charged with the review of a specific research proposal or set of research proposals for scientific merit. syn: **review group**

study site *n* - 1. The **site** at which a **study** is or is to be performed. 2. One of the sites of a **multicenter study**, eg, the site of a **clinic** or of a **resource center** in such a study; **study center**.

study site visit *n* - 1. **site visit** (defn 1) 2. A **visit** to an established functioning **study site**, by representatives of the **sponsoring agency** or by personnel from other functioning study sites, to evaluate **performance** and to help identify and address problems affecting performance. rt: **on-site audit**, **on-site record audit**

study subject *n* - 1. A person being or to be studied, especially in an **experimental** or other **investigational** setting. 2. An animal being studied in a laboratory or other experimental settings (not common usage). *Usage note*: See **subject** for usage note in the setting of **trials**.

study treatment *n* - 1. A **treatment** that is the focus of **study**, especially in an **experimental** setting; **test treatment**. 2. Any treatment, including a **control treatment**, applied in a **trial** as part of a **study protocol**; **treatment arm**. *Usage note*: Note that defn 2 includes **control treatment** (see usage note for that term), that **treatment** is used in the sense of defns 4 or 5, and that **treatment**, in this usage, may be devoid of medical connotations. See **treatment** and page xx for additional comments.

study validity *n* - 1. **internal study validity** 2. **external study validity** rt: **test validity**

study vice-chair *n* - A person elected or designated to perform the functions of a **vice-chair**, especially one who performs or is expected to perform the functions of the **chair** in the absence or incapacitation of that person. syn: vice study chair rt: **study chair**

study visit *n* - 1. Any **visit** by a **study candidate** or **study participant** to a **study site** for the purpose of assessment, **treatment**, care, or **data collection** in relation to a **study protocol**. 2. **study clinic visit** rt: **study examination**

sub- *prefix* - [ME, fr L under, below, secretly, from below, up, near, fr *sub* under, close to] 1. Under, beneath, or below. 2. Subordinate or secondary to; next lower or inferior to. 3. Less than complete; containing less than the complete or full amount or count.

subcontract *n* - 1. A **contract** with a prime **contractor**. 2. Such a contract consummated with a party not **funded** via a contract, eg, in the case of contracts with **clinics** in a **multicenter trial** initiated by and consummated with a **coordinating center**, funded via a **grant** (not recommended usage). *Usage note*: The term **subcontract** should be reserved for usages in the sense of defn 1 and should not be used in the sense of defn 2. The appropriate term for usages in the sense of defn 2 is **contract**, not subcontract, since the party initiating and consummating the contract is not itself funded via a contract. Nevertheless, **business offices** in academic institutions may refer to any contract initiated and consummated by them as a subcontract, regardless of whether their own funding from a **sponsor** is via a contract or grant. See **contract** and **grant** for additional comments.

subcontractor *n* - 1. One who agrees to provide specified goods or services to a **contractor** for specified payments or considerations. 2. A person or party subordinate to a party other than the primary payer, eg, a **clinic** in a **trial** funded via a **contract** with a **coordinating center** funded via a contract, **grant**, or **cooperative agreement** with the **sponsoring agency** (not recommended usage). rt: **contractor** *Usage note*: See **subcontract**, **contract**, and **grant**.

subgroup *n* - 1. [general] A subordinate **group** whose members share some differentiating or distinguishing trait or feature. 2. [research] A subpart or subset of a **study population** distinguished by a particular characteristic or set of characteristics (eg, males under age 45 at entry). rt: **cluster**

subgroup analysis *n* - 1. Any **data analysis** focused on a selected **subgroup** (defn 2). 2. Analysis aimed at characterizing **observed differences** among different subgroups, eg, **comparison** of **treatment differences** in a **trial** for different subgroups of **patients** defined by sex and age at entry. 3. A form of **exploratory data analysis** aimed at trying to identify a subgroup of persons that account for an observed difference, eg, such an analysis in a trial to determine whether or not an observed **treatment difference** can be accounted for by some **subgroup**. See also **data dredging**.

subgrouping *v* - 1. The process of separating **observation units** into **subgroups** on the basis of specified characteristics (eg, age and sex) or designated **cutpoints** for **variables** used for making the separations. 2. The process of identifying subgroups through **subgroup analyses**.

subgrouping cutpoint *n* - The value of a **subgrouping variable** used to separate **observation units** or **treatment units** into **subgroups**; eg, formation of subgroups of patients less than 35 years of age, 35 through 54 years of age, and 55 years of age or older requires use of cutpoints at 35 and 55 years of age.

subgrouping variable *n* - A **variable**, such as age, used to classify **observation units** or **treatment units** into **subgroups**; a **baseline characteristic** for most **subgroup analyses** in **trials**.

subject *n* - [ME, fr MF, fr L *subjectus* one under authority & *subjectum* subject of a proposition, fr masc & neut, respectively, of *subjectus*, pp of *subiere* to subject, lit to throw under, fr *sub-* + *jacere* to throw] [general] One under authority or control of some institution, such as the state, eg, a subject of the United Kingdom. [research] 1. A person under **study**, especially one **enrolled** in a **study**; **study subject**. 2. An animal under study in a laboratory or other experimental settings (not common usage). *Usage note*: The term is widely used in research involving human beings, especially in settings emphasizing the experimental nature of some **investigation**, procedure, or **treatment**. The primary difficulty with the term as a generic label for a person being studied in the setting of **trials** has to do with the implication that the person is being *used* as a research object. Further, the term carries the connotation of subjugation and, thus, is at odds with the voluntary nature of the participation and requirements of **consent**. In addition, it carries the connotation of use without **benefit**; a misleading connotation in many trials and, assuredly, in most **treatment trials**. Even if such a connotation is correct, the term suggests a passive relationship with study investigators when, in fact, the relationship is more likely to be akin to a partnership involving active cooperation. Avoid by using more humanistic terms, such as human being, person, patient, or participant. If used at all, limit to settings where participation is for the sole benefit of the investigation and does not carry **benefit** (other than remunerative) for the person being studied.

subprotocol *n* - A **study protocol** for a **substudy** or **ancillary study**.

subscript *n* - [L *subscriptus*, pp of *subscribere*] 1. A distinguishing symbol, such as a letter or number, positioned slightly below and immediately preceding or following the expression of interest, eg, the quantities *i, j*, and *125*, as in y_i, y_{ij}, $_{125}I$, and $_iy_j$; used to characterize or denote a specific value or feature of a quantity or entity. 2. Any symbol having the function of a subscript regardless of position, eg, the quantity *i* in a(*i*) as used in a **computer program**. ant: **superscript**

substance *n* - [ME, fr MF, fr L *substantia*, fr *substant-*, *substans*, prp of *substare* to stand under, fr *sub-* + *stare* to stand] A physical material from which something is made; matter of particular or definite chemical composition. rt: **active substance**, **biological tracer substance**, **inactive substance**, **tracer substance**

substudy *n* - A **study** subordinate to another; **ancillary study**.

subtract, subtracted, subtracting, subtracts *v* - [L *subtractus*, pp of *subtrahere* to draw from beneath, withdraw, fr *sub-* + *trahere* to draw] 1. To take away by deducting. 2. To perform **subtraction**. ant: **add**

subtraction *n* - [ME *subtraccion*, fr LL *subtraction-*, *subtractio*, fr L *subtractus*, pp] 1. The result of **subtracting**. 2. The operation of deducting one **number** from another. ant: **addition**

sufficient *adj* - [ME, fr L *sufficient-*, *sufficiens*, fr prp of *sufficere*] Enough to meet the needs of a situation or proposed end; adequate.

sufficient condition *n* - 1. A **condition** that is adequate for establishing the truth or falseness of something. 2. A condition from which a given statement logically follows. rt: **necessary condition**, **necessary and sufficient condition**

sum *n* - [ME *summe*, fr OF, fr L *summa*, fr fem of *summus* highest; akin to L *super* over] 1. The whole amount; aggregate; **total**. 2. The result of addition (defn 1).

sum of squares *n* - The **sum** of a set of squared **numbers**.

super- *prefix* - [L, over, above, in addition, fr *super* over, above, on top of] Over and above; higher in quality, quantity, or degree than.

supercomputer *n* - A **computer** with speed, **memory**, and **storage** capacities far in excess of that for an ordinary **mainframe** central facility and used for scientific purposes. rt: **computer**, **mainframe**

superminicomputer *n* - A **minicomputer** having markedly more speed, **memory**, and **storage** capacity than that of an ordinary minicomputer. rt: **minicomputer**

superscript *n* - [L *superscriptus*, pp of *superscribere*] A distinguishing symbol, such as a letter or **number**, written in a position superior to that immediately preceding or following, eg, y^x. ant: **subscript**

support center *n* - **resource center**

surgery *n* - [ME *surgerie*, fr MF *cirurgie*, *surgerie*, fr L *chirugia* fr Gk *cheirourgia*, fr *cheirourgos* surgeon, fr *cheirourgos* working with hands, fr *cheir* hand + *ergon* work] 1. A branch of **medicine** concerned with conditions and **diseases** amenable to **treatment** with operative procedures. 2. An operation performed by a surgeon.

surgical *adj* - Of or relating to surgeons or **surgery**; used in conjunction with surgery; following or resulting from surgery.

surgical treatment *n* - A **treatment** involving **surgery** or use of a surgical procedure. ant: **medical treatment**

surgical trial *n* - 1. A **trial** in which the **test treatment** is administered by surgeons. 2. A trial in which the test treatment is a form of **surgery**. ant: **medical trial**

surrogate *adj* - Of or relating to a **surrogate**.

surrogate *n* - One or something that substitutes for another or something else.

surrogate endpoint *n* - **surrogate outcome**

surrogate outcome *n* - 1. An **outcome** serving as a substitute for a higher order, more clinically relevant, outcome, eg, a laboratory result known or presumed to be **predictive** of **morbidity**. 2. An **observed outcome** for a **surrogate outcome measure**. rt: **intermediate outcome** *Usage note*: Subject to varying usage; often used to denote some outcome assumed to be predictive of the outcome of interest based on biological rationale. To be useful as a **design variable**, the outcome should be **predictive** of the outcome for which it substitutes. **Correlation** with the outcome of interest is a **necessary** but not **sufficient** condition. The correlation must be the result of the surrogate being in the causal chain leading to the **clinical event** or **disease**. The clinical relevance of change in a surrogate outcome measure, such as a laboratory test, is difficult to gauge, without the causality link. Designers of trials gravitate to surrogate outcomes because they allow them to develop trials with smaller sample sizes and shorter periods of followup than would be the case using clinical events as design variables. See papers by Boissel et al,[11] Prentice,[128] and Wittes and Lakatos.[166]

surrogate outcome measure *n* - 1. An **outcome measure** used as a substitute for some other **outcome**. In **trials**, usually one that is known to be or presumed to be predictive of a **clinical event** and that, when used as a basis for designing a trial, leads to an estimated **sample size** or duration of **followup** less than that required for detecting a **meaningful difference** using the clinical event as an outcome measure; eg, use of photographic evidence of retinitis as opposed to change in visual acuity. 2. **surrogate outcome** (defn 2)

surrogate outcome variable *n* - A **test, measurement, score**, or some other similar **variable** that is used in place of a **clinical event** (eg, use of blood pressure change in place of onset of clinical hypertension) in the design of a **trial**, or in summarizing results from it. Used because the variable is believed to be **predictive** of the clinical event of interest and because of its perceived utility in yielding detectable **treatment differences**.

surveillance *n* - [F, fr *survellier* to watch over, fr *sur-* + *veiller* to watch, fr L *vigilare*, fr *vigil* watchful] Close watch kept over something or someone.

survey *n* - 1. A **nonexperimental study** involving some form of **sampling** and systematic **data collection**; the latter typically done via **interview** (face-to-face or telephone), mailed questionnaire, or some other appropriate means. Distinguished from **census** by use of **sampling**. 2. The act or instance of **surveying**, or something surveyed. rt: **census**

survey, surveyed, surveying, surveys *v* - [ME *surveyen*, fr MF *surveeir* to look over, fr *sur-* + *veeir* to see] To systematically query to collect **data** for use in achieving some end or in addressing some question.

survey instrument *n* - **Questionnaire** used in a **census** or **survey**.

survival *n* - 1. The continuation of life or existence; living or continuing longer than another person or thing. 2. Continued existence or being in the absence of some defined state or **event**.

survival analysis *n* - 1. Any method of **data analysis** based on length of **survival** (defn 1 or 2) of the **observational units**. 2. **lifetable analysis**

survival curve *n* - 1. A **curve** plotted in **Cartesian coordinates** having an **x-axis** corresponding to time measured from some designated zero point (eg, the initiation of **treatment** in a **clinical trial**) and a **y-axis** corresponding to the number surviving (or to **survival rate**) that starts from a **number** on the y-axis corresponding to the total number in a designated **population** (actual number or a relative number, such as unity or a multiplier of unity) at time zero, and that decreases (as a smooth function or in a series of discrete steps) as deaths occur over time. The complement of a **mortality curve**. 2. Such a display for any discrete nonfatal event as implied for defn 2 of **survival**, such as onset of **disease** or occurrence of some health related event, such as a heart attack or stroke.

survival probability *n* - 1. The **probability** that a person entering a defined time **interval** survives

Survival curve

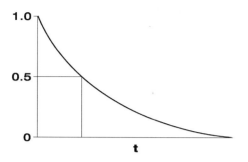

to the end of that time interval. 2. **conditional survival rate**

survival rate *n* - 1. The **product** of **survival probabilities** over a defined series of time **intervals**; **cumulative survival rate**. 2. One minus the **proportion** not **surviving** (defn 2). 3. The fraction of a group surviving. rt: **conditional survival rate** *Usage note*: Technically, not a **rate** because the unit of time is unspecified or mixed (ie, the composite of differing periods of **followup**). See also usage note for **rate**.

survive, survived, surviving, survives *v* - [ME *surviven*, fr MF *survivre* to outlive, fr L *supervivere* fr *super-* + *vivere* to live] 1. To remain alive or in existence; to live on; to remain alive after the death of another or others. 2. To remain free of some condition or **event**.

susceptible *adj* - [LL *susceptibilis*, fr L *susceptus*, pp of *suscipere* to take up, admit, fr *sub-* up + *capere* to take] Open, subject, or unresistant to some agent, stimulus, or influence, not **immune**, eg, being susceptible to an infectious agent.

suspend, suspended, suspending, suspends *v* - [ME *suspenden*, fr OF *suspendre* to hang up, interrupt, fr L *suspendere*, fr *sub-*, *sus-*, up + *pendere* to cause to hang] 1. To cause to stop temporarily. 2. interrupt 3. To hold in abeyance indefinitely.

suspension *n* - [LL *supension-*, *supensio*, fr L *suspensus*, pp of *supendere*] The act of **suspending**; the state or period of being suspended.

suspension of enrollment *n* - **enrollment suspension**

suspension of treatment *n* - **treatment suspension**

suspension of treatment protocol *n* - **treatment protocol suspension**

switch *n* - [perh, fr MD *swijch* twig] To shift from one to another; a shift or transfer; **change**.

switchback *n* - An arrangement involving a series of reversals in direction or **sequence** to achieve some end.

switchback crossover design *n* - A type of **crossover treatment design** in which the **treatment units** are exposed to the same **treatment** more than once; eg, the sequences ABA and BAB in a three-period crossover design; the sequences involve forms of **switchbacks** because they start and end with the same treatment.

symbol *n* - [fr L *symbolum* fr Gk token, sign, symbol, fr Gk *symbolon*, lit token of identity verified by comparing its other half, fr *symballein* to throw together, compare, fr *syn-* + *ballein* to throw] Something that stands for or suggests something else by reason, **relationship**, **association**, convention, or resemblance.

symmetrical *adj* - Having or involving **symmetry**.

symmetry *n* - [L *symmetria*, fr Gk, fr *symmetros* symmetrical, fr *syn-* + *metron* measure] Balanced proportions; the property of being **symmetrical**, especially as relating to size, shape, and relative position of parts on opposite sides of a dividing line, median plane, or about the center **axis**.

symptom *n* - [LL *symptomat-*, *symptoma*, fr Gk *symptōmat-*, *symptōma* happening, attribute, symptom, fr *sympiptein* to happen, fr *syn-* + *pipetin* to fall] 1. [general] Any circumstance or phenomenon regarded as indicating or that is characteristic of some condition or event. 2. [**medicine**] Subjective evidence of **disease** or bodily malfunction; phenomenon experienced and reported by a **patient** indicative of or consistent with some disease process or bodily malfunction. rt: **sign**

syndrome *n* - [NL, fr Gk *syndromē* combination, syndrome, fr *syn-* + *dramein* to run] A group of **signs** and **symptoms** that occur together and that characterize a particular abnormality or health condition, eg, acquired immune deficiency syndrome (AIDS).

synergist *n* - [**medicine**] A **substance**, such as a **drug**, that aids or enhances the action of another substance; an **adjuvant**. ant: **antagonist**

synergistic treatment effect *n* - An **effect** produced by use of two or more **agents** (eg, **drugs**) in combination that is greater than the **sum** of the effects for those agents acting alone.

synthetic *n* - Something resulting from synthesis rather than arising or occurring naturally; not real.

synthetic case-control study *n* - **case-cohort study**

synthetic retrospective study *n* - [term coined by Mantel[96]] **case-cohort study**

system *n* - [LL *systemat-*, *systema*, fr Gk *systēmat-*, *systēma*, fr *synistanai* to combine, fr *syn-* + *histanai* to cause to stand] 1. A regularly interacting or interdependent group of items forming a unified whole, such as a number system. 2. A group of body organs that together perform one or more vital functions. 3. A collection of interrelated devices or procedures for performing some function or process, such as **data collection** or **data processing**.

systematic *adj* - [LL *systematicus*, fr Gk *systēmatikos*, fr *systēmat-*, *systēma*] 1. Of or relating to a **system**. 2. Marked by regularity. 3. Marked by thoroughness of approach or execution.

systematic error *n* - **Error** due to some **systematic** process or **bias**; not to be confused with **random error**. rt: **random error**

systematic random sample *n* - A **systematic sample** as drawn using a **random** starting point.

systematic sample *n* - A **sample** selected by first ordering the objects, elements, or units in the **population** to be sampled and then selecting every **k**th object, element, or unit; **k** corresponds to the sampling fraction and the starting point in the sampling process is arbitrarily determined or chosen at **random**.

systematic treatment assignment *n* - **Nonrandom treatment assignment** in which **assignment** is based on some known or observable fact or phenomenon, as in **alternation treatment assignment**, eg, a scheme in which every other person arriving at a **clinic** is given the **test treatment**.

T

t *n* - [20th letter of the English alphabet] 1. Symbol denoting the numerical value of a **t test**. 2. A **variable** having a **t distribution**.

t distribution *n* - A **probability density function**, due to Gosset, of the form:

$$f(x) = \frac{\Gamma[1/2(n+1)]}{\sqrt{n\pi}\ \Gamma(n/2)}(1+x^2/n)^{-(n+1)/2}$$

where Γ is the **gamma function** and **n** corresponds to the number of **degrees of freedom**; the distribution has **mean** 0 for **n** > 1 and **variance** n/(n - 2) for **n** > 2. Used primarily for inferences concerning means of **normal distributions** whose variances are unknown. syn: **Student's-t distribution**

t distribution

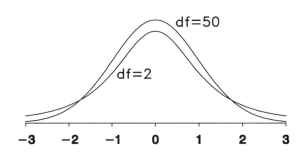

t test *n* - **Test of significance** based on the **t distribution**.

T-score *n* - A **score** based on a **T-transformation**.

T-transformation *n* - A type of **data transformation** in which the resulting **variable** is **normally distributed** (or approximately so) with **mean** 50 and **standard deviation** 10; used in construction of **standardized tests** in education and psychology. rt: **T-score**

table *n* - [often attrib; ME, fr OE *tabule* & OF *table*; both fr L *tabula* board, tablet, list] 1. A systematic arrangement of **data** usually into

rows and **columns** for display or ready use. 2. A condensed enumeration; **list**. rt: **contingency table, frequency table, spreadsheet, two-by-two table, two-way table**

table shell *n* - 1. A **table** intended for **data display**; usually complete with title and **row** and **column** labels and with cells containing symbolic or factitious data. 2. A data table with empty data cells. syn: **dummy table, mock table**

tabular *adj* - [L *tabularis* of boards, fr *tabula* board, tablet] 1. Of or relating to **data** arranged in a systematic fashion, such as in a **table**. 2. Of or relating to data that have been codified for the purpose of **analysis**. 3. Derived or computed using data from a table.

tabulate, tabulated, tabulating, tabulates *v* - [L *tabula* tablet] To put into **tabular** form; to count.

tabulation *n* - The act of **tabulating**.

tail *n* - [often attrib; ME, fr OE *tagel*; akin to OHG *zagal* tail, Olr *dūal* lock of hair] That portion of a **distribution** at the **left** or **right** extreme; **left tail, right tail**.

target *n* - [often attrib ME, fr MF *targette*, dim of *targe* light shield, of Gmc origin; akin to ON *targa* shield] 1. A goal to achieve. 2. A focus of some activity or **inference**. 3. Someone or something to be affected by an action or development.

target population *n* - The general **population** of interest; especially one that is the focus of an **inference** or generalization or the one that is of interest in planning for dissemination of information (eg, those with hypertension) or for administration of a **treatment** or **vaccine**. rt: **reference population**

tau *n* - [Gk, of Sem origin; akin to Heb *tāw* taw] The 19th letter of the **Greek alphabet**, uppercase T, lowercase τ.

team *n* - [ME *teme*, fr OE *tēam* offspring, lineage, group of draft animals; akin to OE *tēon* to draw, pull] Two or more persons working together in relation to a specified activity and interacting for the purpose of achieving some common end or goal. rt: **investigative team**

technical *adj* - [Gk *technikos* of art, skillful, fr *technē* art, craft, skill; akin to Gk *tektōn* builder, carpenter, L *texere* to weave, OHG *dahs* badger] Of or relating to **technique**; marked or characterized by specialization.

technical group *n* - **investigative group**

technique *n* - [F, fr *technique* technical, fr Gk *tecknikos*] A method of accomplishing a desired end.

telephone *n* - An instrument for transmitting sound signals from one location to another and for reproducing those sound signals on receipt at their destination, especially such an instrument connected to others by wires.

telephone randomization *n* - **Randomization** performed by **telephone**.

TEMC *n* - **treatment effects monitoring committee**

temporal *adj* - [ME, fr L *temporalis*, fr *tempor-*, *tempus* time; akin to Lith *tempti* to stretch, and prob to L *tendere* to stretch] Of or relating to time (as opposed to eternity); of or relating to time as opposed to space; of or relating to the sequence of time or to a particular time. rt: **secular**

temporal trend *n* - A **trend** that is time-related; **secular trend**.

temporal variation *n* - **Variation** in some biological process, **measurement**, **observation**, or **reading** that is time-related. rt: **circadian variation**, **seasonal variation**

tendency *n* - [ML *tendentia*, fr L *tendent-*, *tendens*, prp of *tendere*] Direction or approach toward a place, object, effect, or limit; inclination toward.

teratogen *n* - A **teratogenic** agent.

teratogenic *adj* - Causing **fetal** malformations.

teratogenic risk category rating of approved drugs - A use-in-pregnancy rating (introduced in 1979) applied by the **Food and Drug Administration** to **approved drugs** and included in **label inserts**; based on information regarding known risks of **teratogenicity**. The rating categories, as detailed by the Teratology Society Public Affairs Committee,[152] are as follows: Category A: *Controlled studies show no risk. Adequate, well-controlled studies in pregnant women have failed to demonstrate risk to the fetus.* Category B: *No evidence of risk in humans. Either animal findings show no risk, but human findings do not; or, if no adequate human studies have been done, animal findings are negative.* Category C: *Risk cannot be ruled out. Human studies are lacking, and animal studies are either positive for fetal risk or lacking as well. However, potential benefits may justify the potential risk.* Category D: *Positive evidence of risk. Investigational or post-marketing data show risk to the fetus. Nevertheless, potential benefits may outweigh the potential risk.* Category X: *Contraindicated in pregnancy. Studies in animals or humans, or investigational or post-marketing reports, have shown fetal risk which clearly outweighs any possible benefit to the patient.* Based on a review of drugs listed in the 1992 *Physicians' Desk Reference*,[95] about two-thirds of the 1,033 listed drugs were in category C; 19% were in category B, 0.7% were in category A, 7% were in category D, and 7% were in category X.

teratogenicity *n* - The state or quality of causing fetal malformations.

teratology *n* - The study of malformations, monstrosities, or serious deviations from the normal type in organisms.

tercile *n* - One of a contiguous set of **ranges** of values that accounts for one-third of the total **counts** represented in a **frequency distribution**. rt: **centile**, **decile**, **fractile**, **quintile**, **quartile**, **quantile**

term *n* - [ME *terme* boundary, end, fr OF, fr L *terminus* akin to Gk *termōn* boundary, end, Skt *tarati* he crosses over] 1. A limited or definite extent of time. 2. A word or expression that has a precise meaning in some uses or is particular to a science, art, profession, or subject.

terminal *n* - 1. A part that forms the end. 2. A device, such as a **CRT**, by which **data** enter or exit a communication **network**; **computer terminal**.

terminate, terminated, terminating, terminates *v* - To extend to a **limit** or **end**; to form an end; to come to an end in **time**.

termination *n* - 1. End in time or existence; conclusion; finish. 2. The act of **terminating**. 3. Limit in space or extent.

termination of trial *n* - **trial termination**

termination stage *n* - The sixth and usually last stage of a **clinical trial**; concerned primarily with **analysis** of **results** and paper writing. See **stage of trial** for list.

tertiary *n* - 1. Of or being third in **order**. 2. Of or being the third stage or step, as in **tertiary care**.

tertiary care *n* - [medicine] 1. **Care** of a **patient** at or by a **tertiary care center**. 2. **Referred care** as performed by a subspecialist at a **secondary** or tertiary care center. rt: **primary care, secondary care**

tertiary care center *n* - [medicine] A **center**, such as a **clinic** or hospital, that provides diagnostic services and care for persons referred from a **primary** or **secondary care center**. rt: **primary care center, secondary care center**

tertiary prevention *n* - 1. **Prevention** aimed at the sequela of a **disease** or adverse health condition (eg, treatment of diabetics to prevent the retinopathy typically seen in the later stages of the disease). 2. Efforts at the reduction of disabilities and impairments resulting from disease; broadly, from the perspective of **epidemiology**, as given by Last:[84] *Measures available to reduce or eliminate long-term impairments and disabilities, minimize suffering caused by existing departures from good health, and to promote the patient's adjustment to irremediable conditions.* rt: **primary prevention, secondary prevention**

test *n* - [ME, vessel in which metals were assayed, cupel, fr MF, fr L *testum* earthen vessel; akin to L *testa* earthen pot, shell, *texere* to weave] 1. A procedure performed on a person for **screening, diagnosis,** or evaluation. 2. An **analysis** of a biological specimen, such as blood, urine, or body tissue, obtained or collected from a person for the purpose of **diagnosis** or **treatment** of that person's disease or health condition. 3. **test of significance** 4. A **result** or value obtained or determined by testing. 5. A critical evaluation or **examination**. 6. The act or process of testing, as in a **trial** (defn 1) or **experiment**. 7. **test treatment** 8. A series of questions (written or oral) administered to determine a person's level of understanding of a defined area of study for the purpose of assigning a grade or determining whether the person should be passed. 9. Assessment of the proficiency of a person in performing some procedure or routine (eg, as determined from a driving test in relation to an application for a license to drive).

test, tested, testing, tests *v* - 1. To put to or undergo a **test**; to subject to **test**; to subject to critical **analysis; examine**. 2. To apply a test as a means of evaluation or **analysis**. 3. To **assay** or **measure**. 4. To determine the presence or properties of. 5. To administer a test to **diagnose**. 6. To achieve as a score or rating through testing.

test for randomness *n* - A **test of statistical significance** performed on **data** presumed to be or hypothesized to be the result of some **random process** to determine if the presumption or **hypothesis** is plausible. *Usage note*: Such tests in **trials** are often used in relation to **analysis** of the **distribution** of **baseline variables** among the different **treatment groups** represented in the trial in assessing the baseline comparability of the treatment groups. Often, in such settings, a **comparison** resulting in an arbitrarily small **p-value**, say ≤ 0.05, is taken as evidence of a breakdown in the way the **randomization** was done. However, such thinking overlooks the fact that the process of randomization, by its very nature, is designed to yield extreme results on occasions, in the same way that an infinite sequence of flips of an **unbiased** coin will, at times, yield long uninterrupted runs of heads or tails. Hence, tests of significance and p-values are useful in quantifying the degree of baseline comparability present in the treatment groups, but are not, per se, indicators of a randomization process gone bad or of breakdowns in the administration of the process. Breakdowns due to tampering or inadequate safeguards in the administration of the randomization process can be identified only by examination of the randomization process itself and by checking to see whether or not the schedule, as constructed, was followed.

test group *n* - [trials] 1. A group of **treatment units** assigned to receive a **test treatment** and contrasted with another test group or a **control group** to form a judgment or conclusion regarding the **treatment; test-assigned group**. 2. A group having received or receiving an assigned test treatment. rt: **comparison group, control group**

test of hypothesis *n* - A procedure involving a **test statistic** and rules for deciding whether to accept the **null** or **alternative hypothesis** using the value obtained from the test; also **hypothesis test**.

test of significance *n* - [**statistics**] 1. The evaluation of **observed data** by calculating a specified **test statistic** and then using the **result** to decide whether to accept the **null hypothesis** and reject the **alternative hypothesis** or to reject the null hypothesis and accept the alternative hypothesis, as determined by whether or not the observed result lies in the **acceptance** or **rejection region** for the test, as defined by **critical values** for the test. 2. The evaluation of observed data by calculating a specified test statistic and then deriving the associated **p-value** for the statistic under the **null hypothesis**.

test patient *n* - 1. Broadly, a **patient** on whom something is tried or tested to determine feasibility. 2. The exposure of a patient to some procedure or **treatment** to assess feasibility or acceptability of use in a proposed **research project**; **start-up patient**. 3. **study patient** 4. A patient assigned to a **test treatment** in a trial. rt: **vanguard patient** *Usage note*: See **test patients**.

test patients *n* - [**trials**] 1. The collective set of **patients** on whom something has been or is being tested. 2. **start-up patients**; **vanguard patients** *Usage note*: Avoid in the sense of defns 3 and 4 for **test patient**. In the setting of trials, use should be limited to instances in which there is a need to differentiate between **trial-proper patients** and test patients, eg, because results from test patients are not to be combined with results from trial-proper patients. See also usage notes for **start-up patients** and **vanguard patients**.

test result *n* - 1. The **result** (defn 6) of a **test** performed for **screening**, **diagnosis**, or evaluation. 2. The result of a **test of significance**.

test run *n* - A **test** to determine readiness for opening some facility or starting some activity; typically undertaken solely for testing purposes, not designed or intended to produce a usable product or deliverable service but performed under conditions intended to approximate those applying when the facility is opened or the activity is undertaken in earnest. syn: **dry run**, **pilot test**, **pretest** rt: **pilot study** *Usage note*: Generally, in the context of **trials**, used in relation to tests not intended to produce usable results, eg, a test run of a set of **data forms** on **test patients** to identify glitches in the forms or in a test run of an automated **randomization** process to detect problems in the process.

test statistic *n* - 1. The formula or computing algorithm used to carry out a **test of significance**. 2. The numerical value provided by the formula or computing algorithm for a specified **test of significance** using a defined **dataset**.

test treatment *n* - 1. Any of the **study treatments** in a **trial**, except those designated as **control treatments**. 2. The treatment or one of the treatments (except **control treatments**) being or to be evaluated in a trial. 3. **treatment variable** *Usage note*: Typically, in medical settings the term refers to a **drug**, **device**, or **procedure** administered or performed for its presumed therapeutic or diagnostic value. However, the term can also be used in broader settings as implied in usages corresponding to defns 2 and 5 for **treatment** (see usage note for **treatment**). Hence, it may refer to nontherapeutic schemes or regimens applied to well people in nonmedical settings, eg, in a **prevention trial** involving counseling schemes intended to produce lifestyle changes. rt: **control treatment, experimental treatment, study treatment, treatment arm, treatment variable**

test validity *n* - The extent to which a **test**, such as a psychological test, measures what it purports to measure. rt: **study validity**

test variable *n* - **treatment variable, experimental variable**

test-assigned *adj* - [**trials**] Of, relating to, or being **assigned** to a **test treatment**. rt: **control-assigned, test-treated** *Usage note*: Used to characterize the **assignment** of a **treatment unit** (usually a person) or group of such units to a test treatment, as in **test-assigned patient** or **test-assigned group**.

test-assigned group *n* - [**trials**] The **group** assigned to receive a **test treatment**. rt: **control-assigned group, test-treated group** *Usage note*: See note for **test-assigned**.

test-assigned patient *n* - [**trials**] A **patient** assigned to receive a **test treatment**. rt: **control-assigned patient, test-treated group** *Usage note*: See note for **test-assigned**.

test-control *adj* - Of, relating to, or concerned with a **comparison** of the **test** and **control groups**.

test-control difference *n* - **test-control treatment difference**

test-control treatment difference *n* - The postulated or **observed difference** between the **test** and **control treatment groups** with regard to a specified **outcome measure**.

test-treated *adj* - [**trials**] 1. Of, relating to, concerned with, or being treated with a **test treatment**. 2. Of, relating to, or being **assigned** to a test treatment. rt: **control-treated, test-assigned** *Usage note*: Sometimes used as a synonym for **test-assigned** (defn 2), but not recommended, except perhaps when there is a one-to-one correspondence between **assignment** and **treatment**; often not the case.

test-treated group *n* - [**trials**] 1. The **group** of persons or **treatment units** that have received a particular **test treatment**, whether or not originally assigned to that treatment. 2. The group of persons or treatment units assigned to a particular test treatment; **test-assigned group**. rt: **control-treated group** *Usage note*: Not recommended in the sense of defn 2; obscures the difference between an assigned and administered treatment. Use **test-assigned** instead of **test-treated** for uses in the sense of defn 2.

test-treated patient *n* - [**trials**] 1. A **patient** who has received a particular **test treatment**, whether or not originally assigned to that treatment. 2. A patient assigned to a particular test treatment; **test-assigned patient**. rt: **control-treated patient** *Usage note*: Not recommended in the sense of defn 2; obscures the difference between an assigned and administered treatment. Use **test-assigned** instead of **test-treated** for uses in the sense of defn 2.

theorem *n* - [LL *theorema*, fr Gk *theōrēma*, fr *theōrein* to look at, fr *theōros* spectator, fr *thea* act of seeing] A formula, proposition, or statement in mathematics or logic deduced from other formulas or propositions. rt: **law**

theory *n* - [LL *theoria*, fr Gk *theōria*, fr *theōrein*] 1. The general or abstract principles of a body of facts or of a science. 2. An ideal or hypothetical set of facts, principles, or circumstances. 3. A plausible or scientifically acceptable general principle or body of principles serving to or offered to explain a phenomenon. 4. A **hypothesis** assumed for the sake of argument or **investigation**. 5. An unproved assumption; conjecture.

therapeutic *adj* - [Gk *therapeutikos*, fr *therapeuein* to attend, treat, fr *theraps* attendant] Of, relating to, or concerned with the **treatment** of **disease** or disorder by remedial agents or methods.

therapeutic effect *n* - An **effect** produced in relation to the **treatment** of some **disease** or disorder that is palliative or curative, or otherwise beneficial. rt: **treatment effect**

therapeutic index *n* - Broadly, an **index** for a given **drug** that gives the relationship of unwanted to wanted therapeutic effects expressed as a **ratio** of a **toxic dose** over a therapeutically **effective dose**; in animal studies, often expressed as the ratio of the **median lethal dose** over the median effective dose; the larger the index the greater the margin of **safety** for the drug in question. rt: **therapeutic range**

therapeutic range *n* - The **range** of concentrations or **doses** of a **drug** having the highest **probability** of producing a beneficial **therapeutic effect** and over which the probability of serious adverse effects is acceptably low; especially that range over which said probabilities are relatively **uniform**. syn: therapeutic window rt: **therapeutic index**

therapeutic trial *n* - A **trial** designed to **test** the **safety** and **efficacy** of a particular **drug, device**, or procedure considered to have a **therapeutic effect**. syn: **treatment trial** ant: **prevention trial, prophylactic trial**

therapeutic window *n* - **therapeutic range**

therapy *n* - [NL *therapia*, fr Gk *therapeia*, fr *therapeuein*] Remedial **treatment** of a bodily, mental, or psychological disorder.

therapy withdrawal trial *n* - **treatment withdrawal trial**

theta *n* - [Gk *thēta*, of Sem origin; akin to Heb *tēth* teth] The 8th letter of the **Greek alphabet**, uppercase Θ, lowercase θ.

throwaway *adj* - Designed or intended to be thrown away; of or relating to something not valued.

throwaway medical journal *n* - A periodical catering to the professional interests of a specific segment of the medical community (eg, internists or those involved in treating a specific **disease**) and distributed free of charge to members of that community; especially one supported by revenues derived from advertising of products relevant to the presumed readership. Typically in tabloid form, distributed weekly, and containing relevant medical news, digests of information contained in indexed medical journals, and commentaries and reviews produced by contributors to or editors of the periodical. *Usage note*: Pejorative.

tier *n* - [MF *tire* rank, fr OF] A series of **rows, ranks**, or layers placed one above another; **class** or **category**.

time *n* - [ME, fr OE *tīma*, akin to ON *tīmi*, OE *tid*] 1. The measured or measurable **period** during which an action, process, or condition exists or continues. 2. The **point** or period when something occurs. rt: **time interval, time measure, time point, time period, time window** *Usage note*: See **time measure**.

time interval *n* - An **open** or **closed interval** of **time**, such as represented by a **time window**. rt: **time measure, time point, time period, time window** *Usage note*: See **time measure**.

time measure *n* - 1. Any of several **measures** of **time**, such as **hour, day, week, month**, or **year**. 2. **time interval; time period, time point** rt: **time window** *Usage note*: The progression of time and its measurement is the essence of **clinical trials** and **followup studies** in general. Most of what is done in those settings is according to specified time schedules. **Patients** in trials are seen on entry and at specified intervals thereafter. Their **treatment** is usually regimented by clocks and calendars. The **manuals of operations** and **handbooks** for trials will contain details regarding essential timing requirements for the various **data collection** and evaluation procedures to be performed over time. Often, those instructions, unless carefully crafted, are subject to varying interpretations and uses, especially instructions using everyday terms that are subject to varying definitions, as with **day, daily, week, weekly, month**, and **monthly**. Avoid vagueness by providing accompanying definitions or details as to meaning. See notes for **day, week**, and **month**.

time of enrollment *n* - [trials] The **time point** at which a person or **treatment unit** is regarded as having officially entered a **trial** and is regarded to be part of the **study population**. *Usage note*: Typically defined by some act; usually in **randomized trials**, the act of **treatment assignment**, as denoted by the point at which the assignment is revealed to clinic staff. In trials not involving treatment assignment, the time of enrollment may be defined by the point of

consent (as denoted by the act of the **enrollee** signing the consent) or by the point at which treatment is initiated.

time period *n* - A **period** (defn 1) marked by a defined **interval** of **time**; a **time interval** that is **closed**. rt: **time interval, time measure, time point, time window** *Usage note*: See **time measure**.

time point *n* - A designated **point** in **time** within some **interval** or **range**, such as the **midpoint** of a **time window**. rt: **time interval, time measure, time period, time window** *Usage note*: See **time measure**.

time series *n* - A collection of **data** for a designated **measure** or set of measures observed or recorded at designated **time points** or **intervals**.

time series analysis *n* - **Analysis** of **data** representing a **time series** and performed with the aim of identifying the **factors** or **components** influencing the series or of decomposing the series into its component parts.

time window *n* - The permissible **time interval** for performing a specified activity or procedure. In **trials** and other **followup studies**, usually the **window** for performing a specified **examination** or type of **data collection**, such as for **baseline** or **followup**. rt: **time interval, time measure, time point, time period** *Usage note*: See **time measure**.

time-dependent covariate *n* - 1. A **covariate** measured or observed at two or more **points** in **time**. 2. A covariate not **invariant** with regard to **time**; any covariate capable of assuming different values at different points in time. ant: **time-independent covariate**

time-independent covariate *n* - A **covariate invariant** with regard to **time**. ant: **time-dependent covariate**

time-invariant covariate *n* - A **covariate**, such as blood type or **sex** (defn 2) for a person, that is **invariant** over **time**. ant: **time-independent covariate**

tissue *n* - [ME *tissu*, a rich fabric, fr OF, fr pp of *tistre* to weave, fr L *texere*] An aggregate of cells, usually of a particular kind that, together with their intercellular substance, form one of the structural materials of a plant or an animal. rt: **fetal tissue**

titer *n* - [F *titre* title, proportion of gold or silver in a coin, fr OF *title* inscription, title] The strength of a solution or the concentration of a substance or entity (such as a specific type of antibody) in a solution, as determined by **titration**. Also titre.

titrate, titrated, titrating, titrates *v* - To subject to **titration**.

titration *n* - 1. A method or process of determining the strength of a solution or the concentration of some **agent** or entity in a solution in terms of the smallest amount of a reagent of known concentration required to bring about a given **effect**. The result is said to be the **titer** of the solution or of the agent. 2. The process of determining the desired or required amount or concentration of a substance or agent needed to produce a desired effect, eg, the amount of **drug** needed for a **patient** to lower blood glucose by a specified amount or to a specified level.

titration period *n* - [**medicine**] A **period** of **time** in the **treatment** of a person marked by changes in the **dosage** or concentration of that being administered or applied in order to arrive at a desired dosage or concentration. Most common at the start of treatment or at a change of treatment in relation to drugs given to achieve a desired end, such as in relation to hypoglycemic agents given to achieve a desired blood glucose level.

tolerable *adj* - Capable of being borne or endured.

tolerance *n* - 1. Permissible or acceptable **deviation** from some **standard**. 2. The ability to endure the **effects** of a **drug** or agent in relation to **treatment**.

tolerance limits *n* - The **limits** within which some **measure** or process is expected to or required to lie for the measure to be accepted or for the process to produce acceptable results.

total *n* - 1. The result of **addition**; **sum**. 2. An entire quantity or amount, a whole; **count**.

total cost *n* - [general] The entire **cost** of something after adding all costs. [**research**] 1. The **sum** of all **direct costs**. 2. The sum of direct and **indirect costs**. rt: **direct cost, indirect cost**

total research cost *n* - **Total cost** expected or incurred in relation to a **research project**. rt: **direct research cost, indirect research cost**

total sum of squares *n* - In **analysis of variance**, the **sum of squares** for all **observations** from the overall **mean**.

toxic *adj* - [LL *toxicus*, fr L *toxicum*, poison, fr Gk *toxikon*, arrow poison, fr neut of *toxikos*, of a bow, fr *toxon*, bow, arrow; prob akin to L *taxus*, yew] Of or relating to a poison or toxin.

toxic drug reaction *n* - An **adverse drug reaction** that results in **morbidity** or **mortality**. *Usage note*: See **drug reaction**.

toxic side effect *n* - An **adverse side effect** that results in or is likely to result in **morbidity** or **mortality**. *Usage note*: See notes for **drug reaction** and **side effect**.

trace *n* - [ME, fr MF, fr *tracier* to trace] A minute and often barely detectable amount or quantity.

trace, traced, tracing, traces *v* - To seek, find, or locate.

tracer *n* - Someone or something that **traces**. rt: **tracer substance**

tracer substance *n* - 1. A **substance**, such as a labeled element, used to **trace** the course of a chemical or biological process. 2. A substance which, when introduced into a biological organism, can be detected and used to draw **inferences** regarding some action or underlying process (eg, about the ingestion or metabolism of a **drug** by presence of the **tracer substance** in urine or blood, or about blood flow in angiography). rt: **biological marker, biological tracer substance**

track, tracked, tracking, tracks *v* - To search for until found; **trace**; to **follow**.

tradition *n* - [ME *tradicioun*, fr MF & L; MF *tradition*, fr L *tradition-, traditio*, action of handing over, tradition] 1. Established or customary pattern of thought, action, or practice. 2. Characteristic manner or style.

traditional *adj* - Of, pertaining to, or in accord with **tradition**.

traditional sequential dosage design *n* - A **sequential dosage design** used in **phase I/II trials** of chemoprophylactic agents in which **patients** are **enrolled** in groups of three using a **dosage** determined by the experience of the preceding group of patients in regard to presence or absence of unacceptable or intolerable **side effects**. If none of the three patients experience such effects, the next group of three patients is given a higher dose, according to a **modified Fibbonaci sequence dosage design**. If one or more of the three patients experience such an effect, the next three patients enrolled receive the same dosage as the preceding group. Dose escalation ceases if one or more of the three patients in that group experience an unacceptable or intolerable side effect. The aim is to find the **maximum tolerable dose**. rt: **dosage design, continual assessment dosage design, up-down sequential dosage design**

trail *n* - A chain of **events** or consequences. rt: **audit trail**

train, trained, training, trains *v* - [ME *trainen*, fr MF *trainer*, fr OF, fr (assumed) VL *traginare*; akin to L *trahere* to draw] 1. To form by instruction, discipline, or drill. 2. To teach so as to make fit, qualified, or proficient.

trait *n* - [MF, lit act of drawing, fr L *tractus*] A distinguishing quality or feature.

transcribe, transcribed, transcribing, transcribes *v* - [L *tanscibere*, fr *trans-* + *scribere*, to write] To write down or record.

transcription *n* - The process, act, or instance of transcribing, eg, writing down or recording using paper and pencil.

transform, transformed, transforming, transforms *v* - [ME *tansformen*, fr L *tansformare*, fr *trans-* + *formare*, to form, fr *forma*, form] To change in form, composition, or structure.

transformation *n* - An act, process, or instance of **transforming** or of being transformed. See **arcsine transformation, inverse sine transformation, log transformation, square root transformation, T-transformation,** and **Z-transformation** for types of numeric transformations.

treat, treated, treating, treats *v* - [ME *treten*, fr OF *traitier*, fr L *tractare*, to handle, deal with, fr *tractus*, pp of *trahere*, to draw] [general] To deal with or handle. [**medicine**] To care for, deal with, or handle medically or surgically.

treater *n* - One who **treats**.

treater mask *n* - [**trials**] 1. A condition or procedure imposed to keep persons involved in **treatment** from knowing the identity of the treatment being administered. 2. A condition or procedure imposed to keep persons involved in treatment from knowing the identity of the **treatment assignment**. rt: **data analyst mask, data collector mask, mask, reader mask**

treatment *n* - 1. The act of **treating**, as in caring for a **patient**. 2. The specific regimen(s), method(s), or procedure(s) being tested in a **trial**; **test treatment**. 3. An application of a prescribed

regimen to a person. 4. **prescribed treatment** 5. Any condition or **variable** that is purposely varied in an **experiment** to investigate its role in determining or influencing some **measurement** or **outcome**; may be a variable in a simulation process, level of a fertilizer in an agriculture experiment, type or combination of substances or factors (eg, by using different **drugs** or different levels of the same drug) in an experiment involving animals or human beings, etc. *Usage note*: The term, **treatment**, in references to **design**, such as in defn 5, refers to the handling, technique, or action customarily applied in a specified instance. It does not necessarily carry medical connotations, as implied by defn 1. Hence, **control treatment** in a trial may be devoid of "treatment" in the medical sense of usage. See page xx for additional comments.

treatment adherence *n* - The degree to which a person or the person's **treater** follows the **assigned treatment** regimen. syn: **treatment compliance**

treatment adherence level *n* - The degree of **adherence** achieved to the **assigned treatment** for a person or group of persons **enrolled** in a **trial**. syn: level of treatment adherence

treatment adjustment followup visit *n* - **treatment application and adjustment followup visit**

treatment adjustment visit *n* - **treatment application and adjustment followup visit**

treatment administered *n* - **administered treatment**

treatment administration *n* - The act of administering a **treatment**.

treatment allocation *n* - **treatment assignment**

treatment and followup stage *n* - The fifth stage of a **clinical trial**, concerned with **treatment administration** and **followup**. See **stage of trial** for list of stages.

treatment application and adjustment followup visit *n* - A **followup visit** made to enable study personnel to apply or adjust **treatment**, depending on the needs of the person being treated and the **study protocol**.

treatment application and adjustment visit *n* - **treatment application and adjustment followup visit**

treatment application followup visit *n* - **treatment application and adjustment followup visit** treatment application visit *n* - **treatment application and adjustment followup visit**

treatment arm *n* - 1. **study treatment** 2. **treatment group** *Usage note*: Not recommended, although often used in cancer trials. Avoid; use **study treatment** or **treatment group**. Use can lead to confusion in designs involving several **test treatments** or in designs involving a **comparison treatment** that is itself a treatment in the medical sense.

treatment assignment *n* - 1. The process of assigning **treatment units** (usually persons) to **treatment**, as in the construction of a **treatment assignment schedule** for a **trial**. 2. The treatment assigned to a particular person or treatment unit in a trial, eg, as revealed when opening the envelope containing the assignment. 3. The treatment to be administered to a **treatment unit** as indicated in the **treatment assignment schedule**.

treatment assignment bias *n* - 1. **Bias** that influences the way in which **treatment assignments** are made; **selection bias** related to treatment assignment. 2. Any departure from the **treatment assignment design** having the potential of biasing **treatment comparisons**.

treatment assignment block *n* - A **block** (defn 2) consisting of a specified sequence of treatments (as in a **crossover treatment design**) or number of **treatment assignments**, such that, when considered together, satisfy a specified design condition (eg, the **assignment ratio** in a **parallel treatment design**). rt: treatment assignment block size *Usage note*: See **block**.

treatment assignment block effect *n* - [trials] The amount of **variance** accounted for by **treatment assignment blocks** in an **experimental design**. syn: **block effect**

treatment assignment block size *n* - The number of **treatment assignments** required or issued for a specified **treatment assignment block** in a **parallel treatment design**, eg, 8, 12, or 16 in a **design** involving blocks of those sizes arranged in **random order** and where the **sequence** of assignments represented in a block is constrained so as to satisfy the **assignment ratio**.

treatment assignment blocking interval *n* - **treatment assignment block size**

treatment assignment clinic visit *n* - A **clinic visit** at which a **study candidate** is or is to be assigned to **treatment**. rt: **randomization examination, randomization visit, treatment assignment examination**

treatment assignment design *n* - The **plan** for assigning **treatment units** (usually persons) to **treatment**, as indicated by details concerning the way in which **treatment assignments** are generated and issued.

treatment assignment examination *n* - An **examination** that is done or is to be done as part of the **treatment assignment visit**; same as **randomization examination** in **trials** involving **randomization**.

treatment assignment probability *n* - The **probability** value associated with a specified **treatment assignment**. The value is fixed over the course of **enrollment** in **trials** with **fixed assignment designs** and allowed to change in trials having **adaptive assignment designs**.

treatment assignment process *n* - The process of assigning **treatment units** (usually persons) to **treatment** in a **trial**.

treatment assignment ratio *n* - 1. The **ratio** of the number of **treatment units** (usually persons) to be or actually in one **treatment group** relative to another, eg, a ratio of 1:2 for a particular **test-treated group** relative to the **control-treated group**. 2. The ratio of one group relative to all others, eg, a ratio of 1:1:1:1:1:2.5 for a trial with five **test treatments** and a **control-assigned group** that is or is to be 2.5 times larger than any of the **test-assigned groups**.

treatment assignment schedule *n* - The **schedule** used for issuing **treatment assignments**.

treatment assignment stratum *n* - A **stratum**, designated prior to the start of **enrollment** and defined by a geographic variable, such as **clinic** site, or by one or more **baseline characteristic**(s) of those to be enrolled (eg, age upon entry and gender), within which **treatment assignments** are in the same proportionate mix as in all other strata. Such variables are said to be **controlled** in the assignment process because their **distribution** is, within the limits of the **stratification**, the same for all **treatment groups** represented.

treatment assignment unit *n* - The **unit** to which **treatment assignments** relate; **treatment unit**; usually a person, but may be a part of a person (eg, eye) or multiple persons (eg, members of a household or a community). Equivalent to **randomization unit** in trials involving **random** assignment. rt: **group treatment assignment**, **unit treatment assignment**

treatment assignment visit *n* - A **visit** of a **patient** to a **study clinic** at which the **treatment assignment** is or is to be issued or announced.

treatment break *n* - [**trials**] An interruption of **protocol** designated **treatment** for reasons above and beyond the control of treatment personnel, eg, a temporary move of a **patient** from the **clinic** area, elective surgery, intercurrent illness, or troubling **side effects** presumably due to the **assigned treatment**. Generally the interruption is temporary. Use of the assigned treatment is resumed after the condition requiring the interruption resolves.

treatment cessation *n* - 1. **Cessation** of **treatment** of a **patient**, especially that due to lack of **benefit** or intolerable or undesirable **side effects** associated with treatment. 2. Cessation of a designated **treatment regimen** in a **trial**. 3. **treatment termination** (defn 2) rt: **protocol suspension, trial termination, treatment suspension, treatment termination**

treatment change *n* - [**trials**] 1. Any **change** in the **treatment** of a **treatment unit** mandated by or consistent with the **treatment protocol**. 2. Any such change, whether or not mandated by or consistent with the treatment protocol. rt: **treatment switch**

treatment comparison *n* - Any **comparison** involving two or more of the **study treatment groups** based on a designated **outcome** or **followup variable**. rt: **treatment group comparison**

treatment compliance *n* - The degree to which a person or the person's treater follows the **assigned treatment** regimen. syn: **treatment adherence**

treatment compliance variable *n* - A **variable** used for characterizing **treatment compliance**; a **followup variable** relating to treatment compliance.

treatment coordinating center *n* - 1. A **center** in a **clinical trial** responsible for coordinating the development and administration of the **treatment protocol**; usually present with some other **coordinating center**, such as a **data coordinating center**, having responsibilities for coordinating other aspects of the trial. Typically found only in **multicenter trials** and usually only in relation to complicated **treatment protocols**. 2. **clinical**

coordinating center See also **coordinating center**.

treatment cross-contamination *n* - [**trials**] The exposure of a **treatment unit** to a **treatment** other than the one indicated by the **treatment assignment**.

treatment crossover *n* - 1. A **change** in **treatment** that is part of the **study protocol**, as in a **crossover trial**. 2. The use of one of the other **study treatments** on a **treatment unit** in a trial having a **parallel treatment design**; also **treatment cross-contamination** and **treatment switch**. rt: **crossover treatment** *Usage note*: Distinguish usage in the sense of defn 1 from that of defn 2. The two usages carry different implications. In defn 1 the change is a part of the study protocol. It is not in defn 2.

treatment crossover design *n* - **crossover treatment design**

treatment crossover trial *n* - A **trial** having a **crossover treatment design**.

treatment dependent covariate *n* - 1. A **covariate** influenced by **treatment** or capable of being so influenced. 2. A covariate observed after initiation of treatment. 3. A covariate observed after **treatment assignment**. 4. Any measure of **treatment compliance**. ant: **treatment independent covariate**

treatment design *n* - [**trials**] The portion of the **study design** that specifies the **treatments** to be evaluated, the nature of the **treatment structure**, the **treatment assignment design**, and the way in which the treatments are to be administered. rt: **treatment protocol**

treatment difference *n* - 1. A **difference** observed between two or more **treatments** for some specified **outcome measure**, eg, a **test-control treatment difference** for mortality or morbidity. 2. Any specified or observed difference for a designated **outcome** or **followup variable** involving two or more **treatment groups** in a **trial**. rt: **effect size**

treatment dosage *n* - The **doses** of **treatment administered** or that are to be administered over a defined time period, measured by number of applications, volume, intensity, or the like.

treatment dose *n* - The **dose** of **treatment administered** or to be administered at one time.

treatment effect *n* - 1. A quantity representing the **change** in **response** produced by a **treatment**, as in models for **analysis of variance**. 2. An **effect** (**adverse** or **beneficial**) attributed to the **test treatment**; in **trials**, usually inferred or **estimated** from a **comparison** of the **test-** and **control-assigned groups**. 3. The effect (adverse or beneficial) produced or assumed to be produced by a treatment in a **treatment unit**, usually assessed by **measurements** made before and after administration of the treatment in that unit. rt: **adverse treatment effect, beneficial treatment effect, therapeutic effect**

treatment effects and performance monitoring committee *n* - A **committee** having responsibility for **treatment effects** and **performance monitoring**. See **performance monitoring committee** and **treatment effects monitoring committee**.

treatment effects monitoring *n* - 1. In **trials**, the act of or an instance of reviewing accumulated **outcome data** by **treatment group** to determine if the trial should continue unaltered. 2. The act or an instance of watching for **treatment effects** in an individual **patient**. syn (not recommended): **data monitoring, safety monitoring, data and safety monitoring** rt: **administrative review, efficacy monitoring, multiple looks, safety monitoring, treatment effects monitoring** *Usage note*: See note for **treatment effects monitoring** *v* and notes for **administrative review, efficacy monitoring**, and **safety monitoring**.

treatment effects monitoring *v* - **Monitoring** done to assess the **effects** of **treatments** used in a **trial** as measured by designated **treatment comparisons** and for the purpose of deciding whether the trial should continue unaltered. Typically, a process starting early in the course of the trial and continuing to its planned end or until a decision is made to stop it as a result of the monitoring. The monitoring may be done in **masked** or **unmasked** fashion and may be done by a single individual or a formally constituted **treatment effects monitoring committee**. In **multicenter trials**, usually performed by such a committee using **treatment effects monitoring reports** prepared by the **data center, data coordinating center**, or **coordinating center**. syn (not recommended): **data monitoring, safety monitoring, data and safety monitoring** *Usage note*: Harm, in the context of trials, can arise from use of a bad treatment or failure to use a good one. *Safety* in **safety monitoring** or **data**

and safety monitoring suggests that the monitoring is concerned primarily with preventing harm arising from use of a bad treatment. The terms are largely silent on the aspect of harm arising from failure to use a good treatment. **Treatment effects monitoring** provides a better description of the process involved by keying on the focus of the monitoring (**treatment effects**) and avoids the one-sided emphasis by neutrality. The term **data monitoring**, while also neutral, is not informative. Technically, any ongoing process involving periodic assessments of **data** of any kind constitutes a form of data monitoring.

treatment effects monitoring and analysis committee *n* - A **committee** having responsibility for **treatment effects monitoring** and **data analysis**. See **treatment effects monitoring committee** and **analysis committee**.

treatment effects monitoring committee (TEMC) *n* - [**trials**] A standing **committee** in the structure of **single** or **multicenter trials** responsible for the periodic review of accumulated **data** for evidence of **adverse** or **beneficial treatment effects** during the **trial** and for making recommendations for modification of a **study treatment**, including termination, when appropriate. One of the **key committees** in the organizational structure of a multicenter trial. Usually constituted such that voting privileges are restricted to members not directly involved in the execution of the trial and not associated with participating **centers** or **sponsors** of the trial. Others, such as **officers of the study** or other key **study investigators**, if included as members, serve without vote. Voting members are appointed by the **sponsor** (defn 2) or **research group**, often with the advice and consent of the other party. The committee reports to the appointing authority and usually to the other party via the appointing authority or directly. syn (not recommended): **data monitoring committee, data and safety monitoring committee**, ethical committee, **ethics committee, safety monitoring committee** rt: **advisory-review and treatment effects monitoring committee** *Usage note*: The committee may be variously named. One of the more common synonyms is **data monitoring committee**. Though acceptable, it is not recommended because of its nondescript nature and possible confusion with other types of monitoring. Also common is the name **safety monitoring commit-**

tee; not recommended because of the implied emphasis on **safety**. The committee may have a compound name when the treatment monitoring function is vested in a committee having other broad responsibilities, eg, **advisory-review and treatment effects monitoring committee** or **data and safety monitoring committee** (not recommended).

treatment effects monitoring report *n* - A **report**, prepared during the course of a **trial** that uses accumulated **data** and provides a **comparison** of the various **treatment groups** represented in the trial for the **outcomes** of interest. It is used by those reviewing it as a vehicle for deciding whether the trial should continue unaltered. Typically prepared by the **coordinating center**, **data coordinating center**, or **data center** and reviewed by the **treatment effects monitoring committee** in the case of **multicenter trials**.

treatment failure *n* - [**trials**] 1. The **failure** of a **treatment**, as administered to a person or **treatment unit** in a trial, to produce the desired **effect** or **result**. 2. Such a failure as observed, inferred, or declared by a **study physician** or other study personnel from measurements, evaluations, or **observations** on the person or treatment unit in question and accompanied by **cessation** of that treatment or a **treatment switch**. 3. A person or treatment unit **enrolled** in a **trial** no longer receiving the **assigned treatment**; especially when the cessation occurred because of concerns regarding the **safety** or **efficacy** of the treatment. *Usage note*: The term should be used with caution because of the implied conclusion regarding the treatment itself. Its use should be limited to settings where there is supporting evidence indicating a failure. It should not be used simply as a synonym for **treatment cessation** regardless of reason, eg, in relation to defn 3. See note for **value laden term** for additional comments.

treatment group *n* - 1. The group of persons or **treatment units assigned** to receive a specified **treatment** in a **trial**. 2. That group so **enrolled** or still to be enrolled. syn: **study group** (not recommended)

treatment group comparison *n* - Any **comparison** involving two or more of the **study treatment groups** based on a **baseline** or **followup variable**. rt: **treatment comparison**

treatment hypothesis *n* - 1. A **hypothesis** (defn 3) put forward as an explanation of how a **treatment** may exert its effect. 2. The size of the **treatment effect** postulated in the **alternative** to the **null treatment hypothesis**. rt: **research hypothesis**

treatment IND *n* - **treatment investigational new drug**

treatment independent covariate *n* - 1. A **covariate** not influenced by **treatment**; a covariate not capable of being influenced by treatment. 2. A covariate observed at or prior to initiation of **treatment**. 3. A covariate observed at or prior to **treatment assignment**. 4. Any **time invariant covariate**. ant: **treatment dependent covariate**

treatment initiation *n* - The start of **treatment**; in **trials** generally at the **treatment initiation visit**.

treatment initiation visit *n* - [**trials**] 1. The **clinic visit** at which **treatment** is **initiated**. 2. The visit at which **treatment** is **assigned**, even if not administered or started on the day of the visit.

treatment interaction *n* - [**trials**] Interaction (**qualitative** or **quantitative**) of **treatment** and some characteristic or **variable** (or combinations thereof) observed on the **treatment units** that is **independent** of **treatment assignment**. Broadly, a situation in which the effect exerted by a **treatment** is influenced by the level, or presence or absence, of some other **factor** or condition not related to treatment (eg, one would say there is a treatment by gender interaction if the **test-control treatment difference** in a trial indicates an effect for one gender group and none for the other gender group, is in one direction for one gender group and in the other direction for the other gender group, or is of a different order of magnitude for the two gender groups).

treatment interaction effect *n* - The observed **effect** associated with a **treatment interaction**.

treatment investigational new drug *n* - A mechanism, under the control of the **FDA**, used for allowing access to an unapproved **drug**; mechanism typically limited to drugs considered to offer significant promise in caring for or treating the desperately ill; holders of such INDs are allowed, within limits of the treatment IND, to dispense or to obtain the indicated drug for use in caring for or treating specified patients; use of the mechanism has been criticized by trialists because of its potential for slowing recruitment for **trials** needed for an **NDA** and by AIDS activists, in particular those associated with the AIDS Coalition to Unleash Power (ACTUP), because of vagueness in the FDA regulations for obtaining and administering such INDs and because of the time and effort involved in obtaining and maintaining them. Concerns of AIDS activists ultimately led to the creation of the so-called **parallel track** as an alternative vehicle for **expanded availability**. rt **compassionate use, expanded availability, parallel track, investigational new drug**

treatment lag *n* - The time required, or assumed to be required, for a **treatment** to exert its full effect.

treatment mask *n* - 1. A **mask** imposed in relation to **treatment**, in the form of a **single** or **double mask**. 2. A mask of **treatment assignment**.

treatment masking *n* - 1. A process in which **treatments** are administered in a **single-** or **double-masked** fashion. 2. Any process that is designed to withhold information on **treatment assignment** from some individual or group of individuals in a **trial**.

treatment monitoring *v* - **treatment effects monitoring**

treatment monitoring report *n* - **treatment effects monitoring report**

treatment period *n* - 1. The **period** of **time** over which **treatment** is to be administered to persons or **treatment units** in a **study**. 2. The period of time in a study in which treatment is actually administered to a person or treatment unit.

treatment plan *n* - [**trials**] A **plan** that specifies the **treatments** to be administered, conditions under which they are to be administered, schedule of treatment, and treatment **doses**. rt: **treatment protocol**

treatment preference design *n* - **preference treatment design**

treatment prescription *n* - 1. **Prescription** (defn 1) of **treatment**, as given by one authorized or licensed to write such orders, eg, a **physician**. 2. **prescribed treatment** 3. **treatment assignment** (not a recommended use)

treatment procedure *n* - The **procedure** for or method of applying a particular **treatment**, eg, as specified in the **treatment plan** or **treatment protocol**.

treatment protocol *n* - A description, usually written, of the **treatments** and **treatment procedures** used or to be used in a **trial**. rt: **data collection protocol, study protocol**

treatment protocol suspension *n* - **Suspension** of the **treatment protocol** or elements of it during the course of a **trial**; especially when based on **treatment effects monitoring** or recommendations of a **treatment effects monitoring committee** because of concerns regarding **safety** or **efficacy** or because of the presumed **benefits** or harm associated with one or more of the **study treatments**. rt: **enrollment suspension, trial termination, treatment cessation, treatment suspension, treatment termination** *Usage note*: Not to be confused with **trial termination, treatment cessation**, or **protocol suspension**. Usage generally implies that other elements of the **protocol** remain in force, eg, those having to do with **followup** and **data collection**. Hence, **patients** may continue to be seen according to the **data collection protocol** of the trial and be treated according to best medical judgment. See also usage notes for **enrollment suspension** and **protocol suspension**.

treatment protocol violation *n* - A departure from the **treatment protocol**.

treatment regimen *n* - 1. **treatment assignment** 2. **treatment schedule** 3. **treatment plan**

treatment related bias *n* - 1. **Bias** related to **treatment**. 2. Bias related to **treatment assignment**.

treatment related selection bias *n* - Broadly, **bias** related to **treatment assignment** introduced during the selection and **enrollment** of persons or **treatment units** into a **trial**. Often, **selection bias** due to knowing treatment assignments in advance of use and using that information in the selection process. The **risk** of the bias is greatest in **unmasked trials** involving **systematic** assignment schemes (eg, one in which assignments are based on order or day of arrival of **patients** at a **clinic**). It is **nil** in trials involving **simple (unrestricted) randomization** but can arise in relation to **blocked randomization** if the blocking scheme is known or deduced. For example, one would be able to correctly predict one-half of the assignments before use in an unmasked trial of two **study treatments** arranged in blocks of size two, if the blocking was known or deduced. The chance of the bias operating, even if the blocking scheme is simple, is minimal in **double-masked trials** (because correct guesses are not likely to translate into a treatment related selection bias when the treatments are masked).

treatment result mask *n* - A **mask** of **treatment group** when evaluating **results** of the trial, eg, in a **treatment effects monitoring report** with **treatment groups** identified by letter or number code, rather than by their true identity.

treatment schedule *n* - The **schedule** according to which **treatment** is administered or is to be administered in a **trial**.

treatment side effect *n* - An **effect** of treatment **secondary** to its intended or desired effect; expected or unexpected; desired or undesired. The effect may be minor and transient or major and sustained. It may be easily tolerated and devoid of known health **risks**, or may require **cessation** or modification of treatment. In extreme cases, it may require treatment and may result in identifiable morbidity or even death. rt: **adverse side effect, toxic side effect** *Usage note*: Use with caution for the same reasons as stated in the usage note for **treatment failure**. Use of the term as a label in **trials** should be limited to settings in which there is a clear difference in the frequency of specific side effects by **treatment group**.

treatment site *n* - 1. A **site** at which **treatments** are administered, such as a **clinic**. 2. The focus or target of treatment, eg, the site of irradiation for a tumor.

treatment structure *n* - The interrelation of **treatments** used in a **trial**, eg, as characterized by treatments arranged in a **factorial treatment structure**.

treatment suspension *n* - 1. The temporary **cessation** of **treatment** of a **patient** because of intercurrent illness or other conditions or events making treatment ill-advised or impossible. 2. **treatment protocol suspension** rt: **treatment cessation, treatment termination, trial termination**

treatment switch *n* - [trials] 1. A **change** of **treatment modality** or **regimen** during the course of **treatment**, especially such a change indicated by **protocol** or **best medical judgment**. 2. The **administration** of a treatment other than the one **assigned**, especially such an administration as a result of an **error** or mixup.

rt: **crossover treatment, treatment change**

treatment termination *n* - 1. The **termination** of **treatment** of a **patient** because of intercurrent illness or other conditions or events making treatment ill-advised or impossible. 2. The termination of a designated **treatment regimen** in a trial because of lack of **efficacy** or because of the possibility of harmful effects. rt: **protocol suspension, treatment cessation, treatment suspension, trial termination**

treatment trial *n* - 1. A **clinical trial** involving **treatment** (defn 1); generally in settings characterized by **enrollment** of **patients** having a **disease** or health condition requiring treatment or considered to be likely to benefit from treatment; usually involving **study treatments** already in general use (or likely to come into general use in the near future) and treatment procedures approximating (to the extent feasible given design constraints, such as **treatment masking**) those used in routine clinical practice, and in which all (or nearly all) scheduled **patient clinic visits** and related procedures are essential to good patient care. 2. A **trial** in which the **test treatments** consist of procedures used for **treatment** of a specific **disease** or health condition. syn: **therapeutic trial** rt: **pragmatic trial**

treatment unit *n* - [trials] The smallest **unit** to which **treatment** is assigned or administered; usually a person, but may be a subpart of a person in some **designs** or an aggregate of persons, such as members of a household, patients in a hospital ward, or members of a **community** or region, in other designs. rt: **design unit, group treatment assignment, observation unit, treatment assignment unit**

treatment variable *n* - 1. The **independent variable** in a designed **experiment**. 2. [trials] **treatment assignment** (defn 2) rt: **experimental variable**

treatment withdrawal *n* - The act or instance of **withdrawing** or stopping **treatment**, eg, in a **treatment withdrawal trial**.

treatment withdrawal trial *n* - A **trial** designed or performed to **measure** the **effects** of **treatment withdrawal**; often done by simply observing and measuring effects before, during, and after **cessation** of **treatment**. syn: therapy withdrawal trial

trend *n* - 1. A general direction or course of movement. 2. A prevailing tendency or inclination.　3. The general course of a detectable **change** over time.

trend, trended, trending, trends *v* - [ME *trenden* to turn, revolve, fr OE *trendan*; akin to MHG *trendel* disk, spinning top, OE *tetan* to tear] 1. To extend in a general direction; to follow a general course.　2. To show a tendency or inclination, eg, *the data are trending in a positive direction.*

triage *n* - [F, sorting, sifting, fr *trier* to sort, fr OF] 1. The sorting of victims of battlefield injuries or of some manmade or natural disaster and allocating **treatment** with the aim of maximizing survivors.　2. **Classification** on the basis of need for treatment in a medical setting.

trial *adj* - 1. Of, relating to, or used in a **trial**. 2. Made or done as a **test** or an **experiment**. 3. Used or tried out in a test or experiment.

trial *n* - [AF, fr *trier* to try] 1. An **experiment** designed and carried out to provide information on the merits of one **treatment** or procedure relative to another treatment or procedure; **controlled trial**. 2. Any tentative or experimental **procedure** or **treatment** carried out, performed, or administered to obtain **data** to arrive at some judgment or conclusion concerning the procedure or treatment. 3. One of a number of **replications** of an **experiment**, process, or procedure, eg, **Bernoulli trial**. 4. The action or process of putting something to a test or proof. 5. Something tried.　*Usage note*: The term is subject to varying uses with different meanings, eg, when used in the sense of defn 1 as compared to defn 4.　Other modifiers, such as **controlled** or **randomized** (when appropriate), help distinguish **experimental** processes, as in defns 1 or 2, from **observational** ones, as in defns 4 and 5.　See also usage note for **clinical trial**.

trial and error *n* - The process of solving a problem or of developing something by trying, one-by-one, a number of approaches, noting, with each one tried, **errors** or deficiencies made or observed and using that information for fashioning the next try. The process is continued until a satisfactory solution is reached or obtained.

trial close *n* - **close of trial**

trial phase *n* - **phase of trial**

trial proper *n* - That portion of a **trial** defined by **trial-proper patients**.

trial stage *n* - **stage of trial**

trial stop *n* - [**trials**, defn 1)] 1. **Cessation** of all activities in a trial, eg, after completion of the **termination stage** or as a result of termination of **funding**. 2. Cessation of **treatment**; cessation of treatment under the **treatment protocol**. 3. Cessation of **followup**. 4. Cessation of treatment but continuation of followup. 5. Cessation of **enrollment**.　rt: **stop trial**　*Usage note*: Not informative in the absence of detail indicating sense of use.

trial termination *n* - 1. The **cessation** of **enrollment**, **treatment**, and **data collection** in a **trial**. 2. The cessation of all activities related to a trial, including **data analysis**, eg, in relation to the cessation of **funding**.　syn: termination of trial　rt: **protocol suspension, termination stage, treatment cessation, treatment suspension, treatment termination**　*Usage note*: See **trial stop**.

trial-proper *adj* - Of, relating to, or concerned with that portion of the **trial** concerned with **trial-proper patients**; typically that set designated at the outset to comprise the **treatment groups** for use in assessing **treatment effects** in **primary data analyses**; may be exclusive of **start-up patients**.

trial-proper patient *n* - A **patient enrolled** into the **trial proper**.

trial-proper patients *n* - The collective set of **patients enrolled** into the **trial proper**.

trialist *n* - One who specializes in the **design** and conduct of **trials**; one who so specializes and who is concerned with procedural issues related to their design, conduct, or **analysis**.　rt: **methodologist**

trim *n* - Something that is **trimmed** or cut out or off.

trim, trimmed, trimming, trims *v* - [(assumed) ME *trimmen* to prepare, put in order, fr OE *trymian, trymman* to strengthen, arrange, fr *trum* strong, firm; akin to Skt *dāru* wood] 1. To make free of excess. 2. To eliminate something not wanted, needed, or desired.　rt: **censoring, Winsorization**

triple *adj* - [MF or L; MF, fr L *triplus*, fr tri- + -*plus* multiplied by] Being three in number or three times as great or as many; having three numbers or relationships; having a threefold relation or character.　rt: **double, single**

triple blind, triple blinded *n* - **triple mask, triple masked** *Usage note*: See **blind**. In **trials**, sometimes used in a jocular fashion to denote settings where neither the **patient**, **physician**, nor **statistician** knows what is happening.

triple mask, triple masked *n* - [**trials**] An arrangement involving a **double mask** plus masking for the individual (or group of individuals) responsible for **treatment effects monitoring**.

triple-blind *adj* - **triple-mask** *Usage note*: See **blind**.

triple-blinded clinical trial *n* - **triple-masked clinical trial**

triple-mask, triple-masked *adj* - [**experiments**] Of, relating to, or being a procedure in which neither the experimenters, the people being experimented upon, nor those responsible for **treatment effects monitoring** know the identity of the **treatments** being applied during the course of the experiment. syn: triple-blind (not recommended; see **mask, masked** *adj* for reasons) rt: **single-mask, double-mask, nonmask**

triple-masked trial *n* - A **double-masked trial** in which **data analyses** done for **treatment effects monitoring** are presented to the individual or group responsible for such **monitoring** in a way that conceals the identity of the **treatment groups**.

trohoc *adj* - [**Cohort** spelled backward; due to Feinstein [1973][44] and characterized by him as "the name for a group of people who are followed backward from 'effect' (or 'noneffect') toward cause".] **case-control** *Usage note*: Not recommended because of its esoteric and jocular connotations.

trohoc study *n* - **case-control study**

true *adj* - [ME *trewe*, fr OE *trēowe* faithful; akin to OHG *gitriuwi* faithful] 1. Honest, truthful, genuine. 2. Being in accordance with the actual state or condition. 3. Not intended to deceive or mislead 4. Not **false**; consistent with the facts. ant: **false**

true mean *n* - **population mean; expected mean**

truncate, truncated, truncating, truncates *v* - To shorten by or as if cutting off. rt: **censor**

truncated *adj* - Cut short; curtailed.

truncated data *n* - 1. **Continuous data** or **counts** exceeding or falling below a specified value that are recorded or treated as belonging to an **open class interval**, eg, recording body weights for persons weighing more than 250 lbs simply as >250 lbs. 2. Data not observed or recorded because of being so extreme so as to not be of interest.

truncated distribution *n* - 1. A **distribution** in which the lower or upper **interval** is **open**. 2. A distribution in which values exceeding a specified value or less than some value are excluded from the distribution.

truncation *n* - The act of **truncating** or instance of being truncated.

tube *n* - [F, fr L *tubus*; akin to L *tuba* trumpet] A hollow elongated cylinder or cylinder-like object; such an object filled with gases and used for operation of an electronic device; **cathode ray tube**

turnaround *n* - 1. An act or instance of turning about and facing or proceeding in the opposite direction. 2. The time spent in preparing or processing a document for return to its place of origin.

turnaround document *n* - A **document** intended for **turnaround**, eg, a written **edit query** originating at a **coordinating center** and directed to a **clinic** for redress and then to be returned to the coordinating center with a written reply intended to resolve the query or that leads to further query.

turnkey *adj* - Of or being ready for use.

turnkey system *n* - A **computer** system and related **software** package ready for immediate use on delivery or installation.

two *adj* - [ME *twa*, *two*, fr OE *twā* (fem & neut); akin to OE *twēgen* two (masc), *tū* (neut), OHG *zwēne*, L *duo*, Gk *dyo*] Being or comprised of two units, entities, or objects; being or relating to something that is second in **order** or place.

two-armed bandit *adj* - Of, relating to, or concerned with two **stochastic processes** occurring in sequence. rt: **bandit, one-armed bandit**

two-armed bandit outcome adaptive assignment *n* - A method of **outcome adaptive assignment** in which the **treatment assignment probability** for a particular **treatment** is a function of the observed **treatment difference** in **outcomes** of those already **enrolled** in the **trial**; motivation being to minimize the number assigned to the inferior treatment [Zelen, 1969;[171] Smith and Pyke, 1965;[144] Robbins, 1956;[130] 1952[131]].

two-by-two table *n* - [Also 2x2 table] A type of **contingency table** involving two **variables**, each having two **classes** or **categories** (eg, gender and age < 55 and ≥ 55 years). The cells in the body of the **table** represent **joint frequencies** for the different combinations of the two variables. Summing across cells for rows yields the **marginal frequency distribution** for the one variable and summing across columns yields the marginal frequency distribution for the other variable. So named because of the number of cells in the body of the table.

two-period crossover design *n* - A **crossover treatment design** that involves administration of two **treatments** to each person in a **crossover trial**, one after the other in some specified or **random order**; the second administration is typically preceded by a **washout period**.[78, 62] rt: **n-period crossover design**

two-sided alternative *n* - **two-tailed alternative hypothesis**

two-sided alternative hypothesis *n* - **two-tailed alternative hypothesis**

two-sided test *n* - [**statistics**] **two-tailed test**

two-stage design *n* - A **multi-stage design** having two **stages**.

two-tailed *adj* - [**statistics**] Having, or characterized by two **tails**, eg, a **two-tailed alternative hypothesis**; also **two-sided**. ant: **one-tailed**

two-tailed alternative hypothesis *n* - A **composite hypothesis** serving as an **alternative** to the **null hypothesis** that specifies a **range** of permissible values of a **parameter**, symmetrically arrayed about the **null** value (eg, $H_0:\mu_1 = \mu_2$ versus $H_A:\mu_1 \neq \mu_2$). rt: **one-tailed alternative hypothesis**

two-tailed test *n* - [**statistics**] A **test of significance** based on the **null hypothesis** versus a **two-tailed alternative hypothesis**. rt: **one-tailed test**

two-way *adj* - 1. Of, relating to, or having two directions of movement or allowing movement in two directions. 2. Of, relating to, or having two dimensions. 3. **Simultaneous classification** using two **characteristics** or **variables**.

two-way analysis of variance *n* - **Analysis of variance** involving a **model** having a single **continuous dependent outcome measure** and two **independent categorical variables**, eg, one for **treatment group** and the other for **block**

(defn 1); in **trials**, usually the **analysis** focuses on **treatment effect** (adjusted for blocks) and **block effect** (adjusted for treatment effect) or treatment by block **interaction effect**.

two-way classification *n* - A **classification** into **categories** defined by a combination of two **variables**, eg, a classification based on gender and age. rt: **one-way classification**, **two-way table**

two-way table *n* - A **table** having **rows** and **columns** defined by values of two (usually) **independent variables**, eg, one containing counts for the various gender and age intervals represented in a tabulation of the gender and age makeup of a **population**. rt: **two-by-two table**, **spreadsheet**

type I error *n* - [**statistics**] The **probability** of rejecting the **null hypothesis** when it is **true**, usually denoted by the Greek symbol α. rt: **significance level**

type II error *n* - [**statistics**] The **probability** of accepting the **null hypothesis** when it is **false**, usually denoted by the Greek symbol β. rt: **power**

U

u, **U** *n* - [21st letter of the English alphabet] Something shaped like the letter U.

u-shaped *adj* - Having the form or profile of the letter **u**; characterized by having zeniths at the two ends of a tracing and a single nadir somewhere in between.

u-shaped curve *n* - A **curve** having the shape of the letter **u**; a curve having modal values near its two extremes and its nadir near the **midpoint** of the extremes   rt: **j-shaped curve, s-shaped curve**

u-shaped distribution *n* - A **distribution** resembling the letter **u**; one having local **modes** at or near the terminuses of the distribution.   rt: **j-shaped distribution**

un- *prefix* - [ME, fr OE *un-*, *on-*, alter of *and-* against] 1. Do the opposite of; in reverse of a specified action. 2. Deprive of, remove from.

unadjusted *adj* - 1. Not modified or accommodated to a set of conditions or specifications. 2. Of or relating to an **estimate** that is **raw** or **crude**. ant: **adjusted**

unbalanced *adj* - Relating to or having the quality of being out of **balance**; not **balanced**; imbalanced. ant: **balanced** *Usage note*: In **trials**, often used in characterizations of the **baseline composition** of the **treatment groups**, eg, *the treatment groups are unbalanced*, or *patients in the test treated group were sicker on entry than those assigned to the control treatment*; when used as a claim or assertion, usually intended to suggest that the perceived lack of balance is evidence of a **breakdown** in the **assignment process** (see **randomization breakdown** for comment) or, if compatible with **chance variation**, that it is, nonetheless, large enough to explain a **treatment difference** or to cause one to moderate interpretation of a **crude (unadjusted)** treatment difference. Most such claims or assertions should be viewed with a healthy dose of skepticism, especially those made in the context of trials involving **bias free treatment assignment** schemes in the absence of evidence indicating breakdowns in the assignment processes. Most baseline differences are inconsequential in regard to impact on **observed treatment differences** for **outcomes** of interest. They are irrelevant if the baseline variables examined do not influence those outcomes. Even if they do influence outcomes, the effect in regard to the size of the observed treatment differences is usually small. Differences of import between **adjusted** and **unadjusted** treatment comparisons are rare. In other words, the conclusion reached regarding a treatment is usually the same, whether based on adjusted or unadjusted **treatment comparisons**. See **balanced** for additional comments.

unbalanced block *n* - A **block** that is not **balanced**. ant: **balanced block**

unbalanced block design *n* - A **block design** involving **blocks** not **balanced**. ant: **balanced block design**

unbalanced design *n* - 1. **unbalanced treatment design** 2. **unbalanced block design**

unbalanced treatment assignment block *n* - A **treatment assignment block** that is not or will not be **balanced**. syn: **unbalanced block** ant: **balanced block, balanced treatment assignment block**

unbalanced treatment assignment block design *n* - A **treatment design** involving **treatment assignment blocks** that are not **balanced**. syn: **unbalanced block design** ant: **balanced block design, balanced treatment assignment block design**

unbalanced treatment design *n* - A **treatment design** having or designed to have **imbalance** in the **treatments** assigned or administered, eg, as produced by designs involving **incomplete blocks**. ant: **balanced treatment design**

unbiased *n* - Free of **bias**; not **biased**. ant: **biased**

unbiased estimator *n* - An **estimator** having an **expected value** equalling the **parameter** or quantity it is intended to **estimate**. ant: **biased estimator**

unconditional *adj* - Not subject to or **dependent** upon. ant: **conditional** rt: **unrestricted**

unconditional distribution *n* - The **distribution** of a **variable**, not subject to **conditions** or constrained or conditioned by other **variables**. ant: **conditional distribution**

unconditional life expectancy *n* - **Life expectancy** not subject to conditioning assumptions; life expectancy as estimated at birth. rt: **life expectancy, conditional life expectancy, lifetable**

unconditional probability *n* - The **probability** of an **event** or **outcome**, not subject to conditioning assumptions or constraints. ant: **conditional probability**

uncontrolled *adj* - 1. Not **controlled**. 2. Lacking a basis for **comparison**. 3. Not **monitored**. ant: **controlled** *Usage note*: The term in relation to **trials** and **treatment assignments**, is generally used to indicate the lack of an appropriate **comparison** or **control group**. See **controlled** for additional notes.

uncontrolled clinical trial *n* - 1. A **clinical trial** (defn 4) involving a single **test treatment** and not having a **control** or **comparison treatment**. 2. A clinical trial not having a **concurrent control** or **comparison group**, eg, one using **historical controls**. 3. A clinical trial not having a **control treatment**. *Usage note*: See usage notes for **controlled, uncontrolled trial,** and **clinical trial**.

uncontrolled randomization *n* - Uncontrolled **treatment assignment** using **randomization**. ant: **controlled randomization**

uncontrolled treatment assignment *n* - 1. Any **treatment assignment scheme** in which **assignments** may be obtained by personnel responsible for **treatment** without any intervening checks or safeguards to reduce or preclude possibilities of generating or releasing assignments before the persons or **units** to be treated have been judged eligible for **enrollment** and ready for treatment (eg, a series of numbered envelopes that clinic personnel are free to draw as needed without intervening checks). ant: **controlled treatment assignment** 2. Treatment chosen by the person to be treated or that person's physician.

uncontrolled trial *n* - 1. A **trial** involving a single **test treatment** and no **control** or **comparison treatment**. 2. A trial not having a **concurrent control** or **comparison group**, eg, a trial based on **historical controls**. 3. A **trial** involving two or more **test treatments** but no **control treatment**. *Usage note*: Usage in the sense of

defn 3 should be avoided; such trials meet the general definition of controlled. See **controlled** for reason.

uncontrolled variable *n* - 1. A **baseline observation variable** not **controlled** in the **treatment assignment** process by **stratification** or in some other way; a variable baseline not used in **adjustment** of the observed **treatment effect** during **data analysis**. 2. A variable not **monitored** or watched during the **data collection** process. 3. An unobserved variable.

uncrossed *adj* - Of or relating to not being mixed or not being **crossed**. ant: **crossed**

uncrossed treatments *n* - 1. A **treatment structure** not involving a **crossover treatment design**; **parallel treatments**. 2. **nonfactorial treatment structure**

under *adj* - Lower than usual, proper, or desired in amount, quality, or degree.

undermatch, undermatched, undermatching, undermatches *v* - To **match** to a lesser degree or amount than desired or required. rt: **overmatch** *Usage note*: See overmatch *n* for note.

underrepresent, underrepresented, underrepresenting, underrepresents *v* - To **represent** in lower or lesser amount or degree than desired or required. ant: **overrepresent** rt: **understudy** *Usage note*: Use with caution; **value-laden** or **vacuous** when used as a claim or assertion in the absence of definition or supporting **data**, eg, *women have been underrepresented in heart trials*. (Underrepresented in what sense? Is it in terms of the proportionate mix of men and women studied compared to some desired mix as represented in a **population** at large, and if so, what is that population? Or is it in terms of the impact of heart disease on women relative to men, and if so then in what sense? Is it in relation to the number of deaths due to heart disease in women relative to men, in terms of years of life lost due to heart disease for women versus men, or is it in terms of some morbidity measure, such as the incidence of myocardial infarctions in women versus men?) The notion of representation has a host of possible meanings. Hence, it is incumbent on the user to define sense of use. See note for **understudy** for added comments. See also notes for **vacuous term** and for **value-laden term**.

understudy, understudied, understudying, understudies *v* - To **study** less than desired or required. ant: **overstudy** rt: **underrepresent** *Usage note*: Use with caution; **value-laden** or **vacuous** when used as a claim or assertion in the absence of definition or supporting **data**, eg, *women and their diseases have been understudied relative to those of men.* The notion of **understudying** is predicated on the supposition that there is a proper amount of studying and that something less than that amount represents **understudying** and that something more than that amount represents **overstudying**. However, in reality there is no way to define the proper amount of study. In the statement above, is the use in the sense of **representation** and if so then in what sense (see note for **underrepresent**)? Or is it in the sense of number of studies done? Or in the sense of dollars spent? And if so what is the measure being used to define the proper amount of studying? If used, accompany with supporting definition or data to indicate sense of usage. See note for **underrepresent** for added comments. See also notes for **vacuous term** and for **value-laden term**.

unexpected *adj* - Not foreseen; not expected.

unexpected adverse drug experience *n* - An **adverse drug experience** that is **unexpected**. In the parlance of the FDA: *Any adverse experience that is not identified in nature, severity, or frequency in the current investigator brochure; or, if an investigator brochure is not required, that is not identified in nature, severity, or frequency in the risk information described in the general investigational plan or elsewhere in the current application, as amended.*[48] rt: **serious adverse drug experience, safety report**

uni- *prefix* - [ME, fr MF, fr L, fr *unus*] One, single, alone.

uniform *adj* - [MF *uniforme*, fr L *uniformis*, fr *uni-* + *-formis* -form] 1. Having or designed to have the same number. 2. Having always the same form, manner, or degree; not varying or **variable**. ant: **nonuniform**

uniform assignment ratio *n* - **uniform treatment assignment ratio**

uniform distribution *n* - 1. A **distribution**, rectangular in form; (**discrete data**) one for which the **probability** of observing any one of a **range** of **discrete** values is the same; (**continuous data**) one that has a **constant density probability** over a defined **range**.

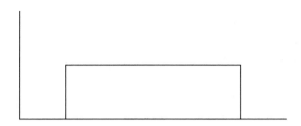

Uniform distribution

uniform treatment assignment *n* - **Treatment assignment** in which the **probability** of assignment to any given **treatment group** is the same as for all others. syn: **equal treatment assignment**

uniform treatment assignment ratio *n* - 1. A **treatment assignment ratio** intended to provide the same number of assignments to the various **treatment groups** represented; an **expected treatment assignment ratio** that is **uniform**. 2. An **observed treatment assignment ratio** that is **uniform** (defn 1), ie, one that produces the same number of **assignments** to each **treatment group**. ant: **nonuniform treatment assignment ratio**

uniformly most powerful test *n* - A **test of significance** for a given **hypothesis** that is as or more powerful than another over the range of **parameters** under consideration, eg, such a test for the null hypothesis $\theta = 0$ vs the **one-sided alternative** $\theta > 0$.

unimodal *adj* - Of, relating to, or having a single **mode**. rt: **mode, multimodal**

union *n* - [ME, fr MF, fr LL *union-*, *unio* oneness, union, fr L *unus* one] An act or instance of joining or fusing two or more things into one.

unique *adj* - [F, fr L *unicus*, fr *unus* one] 1. Being the only one, sole. 2. Being without a like or equal. 3. original; unusual rt: **original** *Usage note*: Use sparingly. Often that which is claimed to be unique (in the sense of original) is not. Self-laudatory when used in relations to one's own work. See also **original**.

unit *n* - [back-formation fr *unity*] A single thing, person, or group that is considered as a whole for some purpose.

unit randomization *n* - [**trials**] **Treatment assignment** via **randomization** in which the **randomization unit** is the **treatment unit**. rt: **unit treatment assignment, group randomization**

unit sequential *adj* - Of, relating to, or concerned with a **sequential** process in which the **unit** defining the **sequence** is a single **observation** or **treatment unit**. ant: **group sequential** (defn 1)

unit sequential design *n* - [**trials**] A **sequential design** (**open** or **closed**) that is **unit sequential**, ie, one in which **treatment comparisons** are made after **enrollment** and **observation** of each new unit. ant: **group sequential** *Usage note*: See **sequential design data analysis**.

unit treatment assignment *n* - [**trials**] **Treatment assignment** in which the **assignment unit** is also the **treatment unit**. rt: **group treatment assignment, unit randomization**

United States Public Health Service (USPHS) *n* - A part of the **Department of Health and Human Services** with the mission of protecting and advancing the health of peoples of the United States of America; consists of seven major agencies: Agency for Toxic Substances and Disease Registry; Alcohol, Drug Abuse, and Mental Health Administration; **Centers for Disease Control and Prevention**; **Food and Drug Administration**; Health Resources and Service Administration; Indian Health Service; and the **National Institutes of Health**. The Assistant Secretary for Health, with the assistance of the Surgeon General, heads the Service. syn: **Public Health Service**

univariate *adj* - Of, relating to, or being a single **variable**. ant: **multivariate** rt: **bivariate**

univariate distribution *n* - The **distribution** of a single **variable**, without regard to any other. rt: **bivariate distribution, multivariate distribution**

universe *n* - [L *universum*, fr neut of *universus* entire, whole, fr *uni-* + *versus* turned toward, fr pp of *vertere* to turn] A set that contains all elements relevant to a particular discussion or problem; **population**.

unmask, unmasked *adj* - 1. Of, related to, or concerned with not being **masked**. 2. Of, related to, or concerned with no longer being masked. 3. Of, related to, or concerned with removal of a mask. *Usage note*: Not to be confused with **nonmasked**.

unmask, unmasked, unmasking, unmasks *v* - 1. To reveal the **treatment assignment** of a person or group of persons to an individual or group of individuals associated with a **trial** (eg, **study physicians**) who have heretofore been **masked**. 2. To reveal the treatment assignment to a person **enrolled** in a trial heretofore masked. ant: **mask**

unmasked randomization *n* - Unmasked **treatment assignment** (defn 2) involving **randomization**. syn: open randomization ant: blind randomization, **masked randomization** rt: **partially masked randomization**

unmasked treatment *n* - **Treatment** that is not **masked**.

unmasked treatment assignment *n* - 1. A **treatment assignment** that reveals the identity of the **treatment** to be administered, as in the case of an **unmasked trial** (defn 1). 2. Any **treatment assignment scheme** in which assignments are known by personnel responsible for **treatment administration** or **data collection** in advance of need or use, eg, most systematic schemes based on the sequence in which persons arrive at the **clinic** or on the day of the **visit**. 3. Any treatment assignment scheme in which assignments are known by or made known to study personnel before a **treatment unit** has been judged eligible for **enrollment** and ready for **treatment**. 4. Any treatment assignment scheme in which assignments may be known in advance of the decision as to whether to enroll a person or treatment unit, regardless of whether they are known in fact, eg, one where a record of the assignment sequence is kept at the clinic and is available for anyone to see. syn: **open treatment assignment** (except for defn 1) ant: blind treatment assignment, closed treatment assignment, **masked treatment assignment** rt: **partially masked treatment assignment** *Usage note*: Note that defn 1 relates to treatment administration, whereas the others relate to the treatment assignment scheme. Note also that defn 4 is the strictest. Use with caution because of different meanings; provide sufficient supporting details to make sense of usage clear.

unmasked trial *n* - 1. A **trial** not involving **masked** administration of **treatment**; **nonmasked trial**. 2. A trial involving **open treatment assignment**.

unmasking bias *n* - 1. A preferential tendency or inclination to **unmask** persons **assigned** to one **treatment** at a higher **rate** than those assigned to another treatment. 2. A preferential tendency or inclination to unmask the treatment of some persons or **treatment units enrolled** into a **trial** versus others.

unnatural *adj* - Not being in accordance with nature or consistent with a normal course of events. ant: **natural** *Usage note*: See **natural**.

unrestricted *adj* - Not **restricted**; not constrained. ant: **restricted**

unrestricted random assignment *n* - Any **unrestricted** scheme for **treatment assignment** using **randomization**. ant: **restricted random assignment**

unrestricted randomization *n* - **complete randomization**

unrestricted treatment assignment *n* - 1. Any system of **treatment assignment** not involving the imposition of **restrictions** on the **assignment process**; **simple treatment assignment**. 2. Use of **assignment schedules** within **clinics** in a **multicenter trial**, or **strata** within a clinic, but not involving **blocking**. ant: **restricted treatment assignment**

unrestricted treatment assignment schedule *n* - An **assignment schedule** constructed using **unrestricted assignment**. ant: **restricted treatment assignment schedule**

unscheduled followup *n* - **Followup** that is not part of that **required**; not **scheduled followup**; **interim followup**. ant: **scheduled followup**

unscheduled followup visit *n* - interim followup visit, also **nonrequired followup visit** ant: **scheduled followup visit**

unscheduled interim followup visit *n* - **interim followup visit**

up *adj* - Directed or moving from a lower to a higher position. ant: **down**

up *adv* - [partly fr ME *up* upward, fr OE ūp; partly fr ME *uppe* on high, fr OE; both akin to OHG *ūf* up, L *sub* under, Gk *hypo* under, *hyper* over] In or into a higher position or level; to or at the top.

up-down sequential dosage design *n* - A type of **unit sequential dosage design** for testing at or near a particular **dosage**, eg, the **maximum tolerable dose** (MTD). In the context of **phase I/II trials** of chemoprophylactic agents, dosages to be tested are chosen to cover a specified **range** and are typically evenly spaced over that range. A person (or **treatment unit**) is given a particular **dosage** of the agent being tested and if the dosage produces an intolerable or undesired **side effect** or **reaction**, the dosage given to the next person (or treatment unit) is the adjoining lower dose. If the unit does not experience an intolerable or undesired side effect or reaction, the unit is retested at the adjoining higher dose, or the next unit receives the higher dose. The process continues until a specified number of units have been tested. Original work by Dixon and Mood (1948)[37] in relation to estimating the 50% response point for a **binary variable** (as applied to fuses for explosives); subsequently generalized by Wetherill[163] for use in estimating any response point. rt: **dosage design, continual assessment dosage design, traditional sequential dosage design**

update, updated, updating, updates *v* - To bring up to date.

upsilon *n* - [MGk *y psilon*, lit, simple *y*; fr the desire to distinguish it from *oi*, which was pronounced the same in later Greek] The 20th letter of the **Greek alphabet**, uppercase Υ, lowercase υ.

urn *n* - [ME *urne*, fr L *urna*] 1. An ornamental vessel, typically placed on a pedestal and used for various functional or ceremonial purposes. 2. Any vessel used for **sampling experiments** or for demonstrations or applications in that regard.

urn model *n* - A **model** involving the concept of an **urn** containing a specified number of **sampling units** (eg, balls of different colors); eg, a model used to illustrate the properties of some **random sampling** or **assignment scheme** [eg, as discussed by Friedman, 1949].[55]

urn model randomization *n* - **Randomization** based on an **urn model**, as proposed by Wei [1977][160] and Wei and Lachin [1988];[161] involves the concept of an urn model in which the **probability** of **assigning** a unit (eg, person) to a given **treatment** is made to diminish or increase depending on the direction of the **imbalance** observed in the **assignment ratio** for all previous **assignments**. A member of the family of **biased coin randomization** schemes.

urn model treatment assignment *n* - Treatment **assignment** based on **urn model randomization**.

use *n* - [ME *us*, fr OF, fr L *usus*, fr *usus*, pp of *uti* to use] The fact or state of being applied or employed; a method or manner of applying or employing.

use, **used**, **using**, **uses** *v* - To put into action or service; avail oneself of; employ or apply.

USPHS *n* - **United States Public Health Service**

utility *adj* - Of or relating to **use**.

utility *n* - [ME *utilite*, fr MF *utilité*, fr L *utilitat-*, *utilitas*, fr *utilis* useful, fr *uti* to use] Fitness for some purpose or worth to some end or **use**.

V

VA *n* - **Veterans Administration**

vaccine *n* - [L *vaccinus*, adj, of or from cows, fr *vacca* cow;. akin to Skt *vaśa* cow] A preparation of killed microorganisms, living attenuated organisms, or living, fully virulent organisms, administered to produce or artificially increase immunity to a particular **disease** or disease state. rt: **biologic**

vacuous *adj* - [L *vacuus*] Emptied of or lacking content.

vacuous term *n* - 1. A **term** lacking in content or meaning. 2. A term used to convey an implied meaning without definition or supporting **data**, eg, **understudied** in the claim that *women and their diseases have been understudied relative to those of men*. rt: **currency term, value-laden term, weasel term** *Usage note*: Terms used to connote departure, as with **over** in **overmatch** or **under understudy** or **underrepresent**, are **value-laden** or **vacuous** when used as claims or assertions in the absence of definition or supporting **data**. See also notes for **value-laden term** and for **overmatch, underrepresent**, and **understudy**.

valid *adj* - [MF or ML; MF *valide*, fr ML, *validus*, fr L strong, fr *valēre*] Sound, well-founded, justified.

valid analysis *n* - 1. An **analysis** having or presumed to have **validity**. 2. A **design** capable of yielding an analysis having validity. 3. An analysis having adequate **power** for detecting an indicated effect. 4. A design allowing one to perform an indicated analysis, eg, a design involving both males and females allowing one to estimate **treatment effects** for males and females. *Usage note*: Use with caution, especially as a label or requirement. Support with details indicating sense of use. Note that the requirement for use in the sense of defn 3 is far more stringent than for use in the sense of defn 4. The term arises in the **National Institutes of Health Revitalization Act of 1993** in relation to **trials** and the ability to detect gender and ethnic origin by **treatment interactions**. *In the case of any clinical trial in which women or members of minority groups will under subsection (a) be included as subjects, the Director of the NIH shall ensure that the trial is designed and carried out in a manner sufficient to provide for a valid analysis of whether the variables being studied in the trial affect women or members of minority groups, as the case may be, differently than other subjects in the trial.*[154] Its use in that setting, without definition, gives rise to various interpretations. The guideline issued by the NIH for implementation of the legislation[114] defines valid analysis to mean an unbiased design and assessment. According to the guideline, *such an assessment will, on average, yield the correct estimate of the difference in outcomes between two groups of subjects. Valid analysis can and should be conducted for both small and large studies. A valid analysis does not need to have a high statistical power for detecting a stated effect. The principal requirements for ensuring a valid analysis of the question of interest are: Allocation of study participants of both genders and from different racial/ethnic groups to the intervention and control groups by an unbiased process such as randomization; Unbiased evaluation of the outcome(s) of study participants; Use of unbiased statistical analyses and proper methods of inference to estimate and compare the intervention effects among the gender and racial/ethnic groups.*

validate, validated, validating, validates *v* - [ML *validatus*, pp of *validare*, to validate, fr *validus*] 1. To confirm the **validity** of. 2. To support or corroborate on some sound or authoritative basis. *Usage note*: A **currency word**. Use with caution and only with accompanying details as to procedures and methods employed to validate. Avoid as a vacuous claim or promise, eg, *we intend to validate the results*. Often used in connotations suggesting truth or **veracity** when, in fact, the only thing known is that two sources of information agree. The emphasis in usage should be on soundness or plausibility of information rather than on truth. See also **validation**.

validation *n* - 1. The act, process, or instance of **validating**. 2. A process involving attempts to

verify the accuracy of information (eg, medication use) obtained from one source (eg, **patient**) with that from another source (eg, **physician**). *Usage note*: Use with caution to avoid implying more than done or intended. Corroboration is different than validation. The fact that two pieces of information, collected from different sources, agree does not necessarily mean the information is valid in the sense of being sound or true. For example, a check of a patient's **medical record** to determine whether it contains information consistent with the **disease** or health condition the **patient** purports to have does not mean the person has that disease or health condition.

validity *n* - 1. The state or quality of being **valid**. 2. **test validity** 3. **study validity** *Usage note*: The validity of a **trial** (defn 1) is internal (see **internal study validity**). It derives from the **design** and the extent to which it, and associated procedures for execution of the trial, provide reliable bases for comparing treatments. Such **comparisons** are considered to be valid if the most likely explanation of the **observed differences** is the **experimental variable**, ie, **treatment**. Most of the design maneuvers, such as **randomization** and **masking**, and ongoing **quality assurance** procedures implemented and maintained over the course of a trial, are for the express purpose of establishing and maintaining the internal validity of the trial. The notions of validity and **generalizability** in the context of trials are different and should not be confused. Validity relates to comparisons within a trial. Generalizability relates to the extent to which the conclusions derived from a trial can be generalized beyond the setting of the trial and the particular people studied in the trial. See usage note for **generalizability**.

value *n* - [ME, fr MF, fr (assumed) VL *valuta*, fr fem of *valutus*, pp of L *valēre*, to be worth, be strong] 1. A numerical quantity that is assigned or derived by **calculation**, **measurement**, or **observation**. 2. Relative worth, utility, or importance.

value-laden term *n* - A **term** carrying an implied **value** or conveying an implied value judgment (in the sense of good or bad, desired or undesired); candidate terms include **treatment failure**, **underrepresent**, **understudy**, **overrepresent**, **overstudy**, and **overmatch**. rt: **currency term**, **vacuous term**, **weasel term**

Usage note: Good trialists take pains to avoid value-laden language in the discourse of their work. Success at avoidance requires constant vigilance over the course of a trial. The window of opportunity for avoidance is narrow, once a language convention is introduced into the lexicon of a trial. See also note for **vacuous term**.

vanguard *n* - [ME *vantgard*, fr MF *avant-garde*, fr OF, fr *avant-* fore- (fr *avant* before, fr L *abante*) + *garde* guard] 1. Those occupying a foremost position; those in the lead or out in front. 2. **vanguard patient**

vanguard patient *n* - [trials] A **patient** within the set of **vanguard patients**. rt: **start-up patient**, **test patient** *Usage note*: See **vanguard patients**.

vanguard patients *n* - [trials] The set of **patients** designated as **vanguard** and on whom the various procedures of the different **visits** called for in the **treatment** and **data collection schedule** of the trial are tested in advance of **trial-proper patients**. rt: **start-up patients**, **test patients** *Usage note*: Not synonymous with **start-up** or **test patients**, except when those terms are used in the sense above. Limit use to settings where specific patients are designated as being in a vanguard set (eg, the set represented by the first two patients **enrolled** at each **clinic** in a **multicenter trial**) and where information from that set is intended for use in modifying or adjusting methods or procedures. See also usage notes for **start-up patients** and **test patients**.

variability *n* - The state or condition of being **variable**.

variable *adj* - [ME, fr MF, fr L *variablilis*, fr *variare*, to vary] 1. Able or apt to **vary**; subject to **variation** or change; characterized by variation. 2. Having the characteristics of a **variable**.

variable *n* - 1. A quantity, **trait**, **characteristic**, or **measure** that may assume any one of a set of **values**. 2. **observed variable** 3. **random variable** 4. A symbol representing a variable. 5. Something that is variable. rt: **observation variable**, **random variable**, **stochastic variable**

variance *n* - [MF *variaunce*, fr MF, fr L *varianita*, fr *variant-*, *varians*, prp of *variare* to vary] 1. A **parameter** equal to the second **moment** of the underlying **variable** (or associated distribution function) about its **mean**. 2. The mean of the square differences about the mean of a **frequen-**

cy distribution; a similar quantity using **n** - 1 rather than **n** as a divisor. 3. The square of the **standard deviation**. rt: **standard deviation**

variance control *v* - Reducing or eliminating **variance** in some process or procedure; such reduction or elimination arising from **bias control**, **matching**, **stratification**, **monitoring**, or **adjustment**. rt: **bias control**

variance ratio *n* - The **ratio** of two **independent estimates** of a **population variance**.

variance-components model *n* - **random-effects model**

variance-covariance matrix *n* - A **matrix** giving the **variances** and **covariances** of **estimates** for the various **parameters** represented in a **model** having two or more parameters; the element represented in the ith **row** and jth **column** correspond to the **covariance** of the estimates for the ith and jth parameters when i ≠ j and to the **variance** of the estimate of the ith parameter when i = j. rt: **correlation matrix**

variance-ratio distribution *n* - **F distribution**

variant *adj* - 1. Being **variable**. 2. Manifesting or showing **variance** or **variation**. ant: **invariant**

variant *n* - One of two or more persons, places, or things showing differences.

variate *n* - 1. **variable** 2. **random variable**

variation *n* - [ME *varicioun*, fr MF or L; MF *variation*, fr L *variation-*, *variatio*, fr *variatus*, pp of *variare* to vary] 1. The act or process of **varying**; the state or fact of being varied; an instance of varying. 2. The extent to which a **variable** or set of **observations vary** or are spread. 3. A **measure** of change in a **function**, **variable**, or **data**. rt: **variance**

variation, coefficient of *n* - **coefficient of variation**

variation measure *n* - Any **measure** of spread or dispersion of **data**, such as **standard deviation**, **variance**, **range**, or **mean deviation**. syn: measure of variation

vary, varied, varying, varies *v* - [ME *varien*, fr MF or L; MF *varier*, fr L *variare*, fr *varius*, various] To make or cause **change** or **difference**; to undergo or show change or difference.

VDT *n* - **video display terminal**

Venn diagram *n* - A **diagram** in which geometrical forms are used to represent logical relationships among the **factors**, conditions, or sets

represented by the forms; after John Venn (1824 - 1923), English logician.

Venn diagram

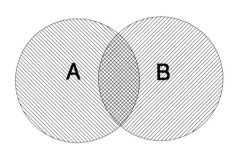

veracity *n* - [NL *veracitas*, fr L *verac-*, *verax*] 1. Devotion to the truth; truthfulness. 2. Power of conveying or perceiving the truth. 3. Conforming to truth or fact; **accuracy**. rt: **accuracy**

verbal *adj* - [MF, fr LL; MF, fr LL *verbalis*, fr L *verbum* word] 1. Of, relating to, or consisting of words written or spoken. 2. Spoken rather than written; **oral**. *Usage note*: Often used as a synonym for **oral** (defn 2 above), eg, *patients gave verbal consents*. Oral refers to spoken words; verbal refers to words, written or spoken. Use oral for uses in the sense of defn 2.

verbal assent *n* - 1. **oral assent** 2. **written assent** (defn 1) 3. **Assent** occurring without the documenting signature of the assenting party, ie, not a **signed assent**. *Usage note*: Avoid because of dual meaning; both oral and written assents are **verbal**. See **verbal**.

verbal consent *n* - 1. **oral consent** 2. **written consent** (defn 2) 3. **Consent** occurring without the documenting signature of the consenting party, ie, not a **signed consent**. *Usage note*: Avoid because of dual meaning; both oral and written consents are **verbal**. See **verbal**.

verification *n* - The act, process, or instance of **verifying**; the state of being verified.

verify, verified, verifying, verifies *v* - [ME *verifien*, fr MF *verifier*, fr ML *verificare*, fr L *verus* true] To confirm or substantiate; to establish the truth or accuracy of.

Veterans Administration (VA) *n* - An agency of the United States government having responsibility for administering benefits mandated by law for war veterans, their dependents, and beneficiaries, including medical and hospital care.

Veterans Administration Cooperative Studies Program (VACSP) *n* - A **research program** sponsored by the **Veterans Administration** concerned with the development and execution of **multicenter studies**.

vice study chair *n* - **study vice-chair**

vice-chair *n* - 1. One who is second in position to head an organization. 2. One who serves as presiding officer of a group or organization in the absence or incapacitation of the **chair**. rt: **chair** *Usage note*: See **chair**.

vice-chairperson *n* - **vice-chair**

vice-chairwoman *n* - **vice-chair**

video *adj* - [L *vidēre* to see + E *-o* (as in audio)] Being, relating to, or involving images on a **screen** such as on that of a television or **computer**.

video display *n* - A **display** as presented on a **screen**, such as on that of a television or **computer**.

video display terminal (VDT) *n* - A **device** having a **screen** for displaying **input** and **output** from a **computer**. rt: **cathode ray tube**

video screen *n* - A **screen** for displaying images created electronically, such as those seen on television or on a **video display terminal**.

violate, violated, violating, violates *v* - [ME *violaten*, fr L *violatus*, pp of *violare*; akin to L *violentus* violent, *vis* strength] 1. To break, intentionally or unintentionally; disregard; transgress. 2. To harm or desecrate.

violation *n* - [ME *violacioun*, fr L *violation-*, *violatio*, fr *violatus*, pp] The act or instance of **violating**; an infringement of **rules** or **procedures**, eg, **protocol violation**.

virus *n* - [L, slimy liquid, poison, stench, akin to OE *wāse* marsh, Gk *ios* poison, Skt *visa*] [**computer**] Broadly, something that poisons or corrupts after importation or invasion; more specifically a set of **program** instructions or commands introduced into an operating system or program that has the potential of causing the system or program to malfunction; typically imported via shared **software**. rt: **bug**

visit *n* - 1. A short stay. 2. **clinic visit**

visit, visited, visiting, visits *v* - [ME *visiten*, fr OF *visiter*, fr L *visitare*, freq of *visere* to go to see, fr *vidēre* to see] To come or go to.

vitae *n* - **curriculum vitae**

vital *adj* - [ME, fr MF fr L *vitalis* of life, fr *vita* life; akin to L *vivere* to live] 1. Characteristic of **life** or living beings. 2. Concerned with or necessary to the maintenance of life. 3. Of utmost importance; essential.

vital records *n* - **Records** and certificates related to major **life events**, such as births, deaths, marriages, divorces, and occurrences of certain diseases.

vital signs *n* - [**medicine**] Basic **signs** of life; in **medicine** specifically pulse, respiratory rate, body temperature, and blood pressure.

vital statistics *n* - **Statistics** relating to births, deaths, marriages, divorces, health, and **diseases** of a defined **population**.

vital status *n* - The state of being alive or dead.

volunteer *n* - [obs F *voluntaire* (now *volontaire*), fr *voluntaire*, *adj* voluntary, fr L *voluntarius*] One who enters into or offers oneself for service of one's own free will without coercion or force.

W

walk *n* - The path or course followed in traversing from one point to another; **random walk**.

washout *n* - To remove some extraneous or foreign substance from a biological system.

washout period *n* - 1. The **interval** of time considered necessary for a biological system to remove a foreign substance and to be free of its influence. 2. The period of time in a **crossover trial** between cessation of one **drug treatment** and the start of a new one considered adequate for **washout**.

weasel *n* - [ME *wesele*, fr OE *weosule*; akin to OHG *wisula* weasel, and prob to L *virus* slimy liquid, stench] 1. Any of various small slender active carnivorous mammals known for their stealth and that consume small animals such as mice, rats, and birds; usually reddish brown with white or yellow underparts; white in winter months in northern climates. 2. One who has the quality of stealth.

weasel, weaseled, weaseling, weasels *v* - 1. To avoid or evade by cunning or stealth; to escape from or evade an obligation or responsibility by cunning or stealth. 2. To avoid or evade making a definitive spoken or written statement by use of qualifiers or **weasel terms** for equivocation. *Usage note*: See note for **weasel term**.

weasel term *n* - [fr the weasel's reputed reputation of sucking the contents out of an egg while leaving its shell largely intact] A **term** (word or phrase) used to equivocate some statement or position in order to retreat from or avoid taking a direct position or making a forthright statement. rt: **currency term, vacuous term, value-laden term** *Usage note: One of our defects as a nation is a tendency to use what have been called weasel words. When a weasel sucks eggs the meat is sucked out of the eggs. If you use a weasel word after another there is nothing left of the other* (Theodore Roosevelt, St Louis, 31 May 1916). The language of the researcher is sprinkled with terms intended to qualify or equivocate. Terms such as *maybe, perhaps, possibly,* or *probably* are useful in conveying doubt or uncertainty and, to that extent, have legitimate

functions. However, they can also be used for equivocating. Avoid in tandem, eg, with *perhaps possibly* in *perhaps possibly the results are due to chance*. See also note for **vacuous term**.

week *n* - [ME *weke*, fr OE *wicu, wucu*; akin to OHG *wehha* week, L *vicis* change, alternation] 1. One of a series of seven-**day** periods used in various calendars. 2. A seven-day period beginning with a specified day of the week, eg, Sunday. 3. Seven consecutive days. 4. A series of regular working, business, or school days during a seven-day calendar period, generally five. 5. Monday through Friday. rt: **weekly, day, month, year** *Usage note*: Subject to varying usage; may refer to seven- or five-day period depending on usage. Be explicit if not clear from context. Do not use interchangeably with **month**, as in equating four weeks to a month. See usage notes for **month** and **day**. See also notes for **biweekly, semiweekly,** and **time measure**.

weekday *n* - 1. A **day** of the **week**, except Sunday. 2. A day of the week, except Saturday or Sunday. rt: **day, week, workweek** *Usage note*: See **week** and **time measure**.

weekly *adj* - Occurring, appearing, or done once a **week**. rt: **week, daily, monthly, yearly** *Usage note*: See **week** and **time measure**.

weight *n* - [ME *wight, weght*, fr OE *wiht*; akin to ON *voett* weight, OE *wegan* weigh] A multiplier of an **observed value** that indicates the importance or influence that value has in some **calculation** or **analysis**, as in deriving a **weighted mean**. rt: **weighted**

weighted *adj* - Having a **weight** attached. rt: **weight**

weighted mean *n* - A **mean** derived using **weighted** values, eg, the weighted mean age for a group having four persons aged 50 years and two persons aged 60 years is $[(4)50 + (2)60]/6 = 53.3$ years.

well *adj* - Being in satisfactory condition or circumstance; satisfactory.

well-controlled *adj* - **controlled**; especially in experimental settings employing **randomization** of **treatment** and **masking**. *Usage note*: Modifier, **well**, often unnecessary; adds little to the root term, **controlled**, except emphasis. See **controlled** for additional notes.

what you see is what you get (WYSIWYG) - [**computers**] Jargon used to indicate that the appearance of a document displayed on the **video screen** of a **computer** will be the same as the printed version of that document; generally considered to be a desirable quality of word processing packages.

WHO *n* - **World Health Organization**

Wilcoxon test *n* - A **nonparametric test** alternative to the **t test** for paired **observations**; based on **rank** values of the observed **absolute differences** of the paired observations.[165] See also **Mann-Whitney test**.

win, won, winning, wins *v* - [ME *winnen*, fr OE *winnan* to struggle; akin to OHG *winnan* to struggle, L *venus* love, charm] 1. To succeed in arriving at a place or state. 2. To obtain by effort or by good fortune. 3. To receive something as a result of having engaged in a game of **chance**. 4. To receive a return greater than that invested. ant: **lose** rt: **free** *Usage note*: Subject to misuse, especially in everyday usage. One may win in the sense of defns 2 or 3 but **lose** in the sense of defn 4. Use with caution and with sufficient detail as to the sense of usage. See also note for **free**.

window *n* - [often attrib ME *windowe*, fr ON *vindauga*, fr *vindr* wind (akin to OE *wind*) + *auga* eye; akin to OE *ēage* eye] [**data collection**] A **range** of **time** within which something is allowed or possible, as in **time window**.

winner *n* - One or something that **wins**; one who wins.

Winsorization *n* - A procedure for reducing the influence of extreme values of a **continuous variable** on distribution-dependent **statistics**, such as **means** and **variances**; performed by ordering the observed values and then establishing **limits** defining the **right** and **left tails** of the **distribution** (eg, limits defined by the upper value of the first **decile** and the lower value of the tenth decile of the distribution) below which values are considered extreme. All values to the left of the lower limit are assigned the value of the lower limit or the nearest **observed value** to

the right of the limit; all values to the right of the upper limit are assigned the value of the upper limit or the nearest observed value to the left of the limit. Named for Charles P Winsor (1895 - 1951). See Hoaglin et al [1983][67] or Huber [1981][68] for details.

Winsorize, winsorizing, Winsorized *v* - **Trimming** via use of a **Winsorization** procedure.

with *prep* - [ME, against, from, with, fr OE; akin to OE *wither* against, OHG *widar* against, back, Skt apart] 1. A function word used to indicate the presence of something or some condition; ant: **without**. 2. against

withdraw, withdrew, withdrawn, withdrawing, withdraws *v* - [ME *withdrawen*, fr *with* from + *drawen* to draw] 1. To take back or away; remove. 2. To cease or terminate. 3. To remove from consideration by setting aside.

withdrawal *n* - 1. The act of **withdrawing**. 2. The removal of a person or **observation unit** from a **lifetable analysis** for a designated **event** at the cessation of **followup** for that person or **observation unit** or at the occurrence of the **event** of interest; removal due to cessation of followup may occur as a consequence of when the person or unit was **enrolled** (eg, calculation of a three-year event **rate** of necessity is based on **data** provided by those who were enrolled at least three years prior to the date of the analysis) or because the person or unit dropped out. 3. **dropout** (not a recommended synonym) 4. [**trials**] One who has been removed from **treatment** (not recommended usage). *Usage note*: Usage should be limited to those implied in defns 1 and 2. The term should not be used as a synonym for **dropout** for reasons discussed in the usage note for that term. rt: **censor**

withdrawn *adj* - To be removed from.

within *prep* - 1. A function word used to indicate enclosure or containment. 2. Not beyond the quantity, degree, or limitation of.

within-group sum of squares *n* - **Error sum of squares** in a one-way **analysis of variance**.

within-patient *adj* - **within-person**

within-person *adj* - Being, consisting of, or relating to that done or **observed** on a person at the same time or at different points in time; of or relating to **designs** and **analyses** involving **comparisons** within persons. ant: **between-person**

within-person study *n* - A **study** in which the **comparisons** of interest are based on **data** derived from **within persons** (as in a **crossover trial** or **n of 1 trial**). ant: **between-person study**

within-person treatment comparison *n* - A **treatment comparison** that involves the same person, eg, a **crossover trial** or **n of 1 trial**.

within-person treatment design *n* - **crossover treatment design**

within-person trial *n* - 1. **crossover trial** 2. **n of 1 trial** 3. A **trial** involving **treatment groups** comprised of the same **persons**. ant: **between-person trial**

without *prep* - [ME *withoute*, fr OE *withūtan*, fr *with* + *ūtan* outside, fr *ūt* out] 1. A function word used to indicate the absence of or lack of something. ant: **with** 2. outside

witness *n* - [ME *witnesse*, fr OE *witnes* knowledge, testimony, witness, fr *wit* intelligence] 1. One asked to be present at a transaction so as to be able to testify to the transaction having taken place. 2. One who has personal knowledge of something. 3. Attestation of a fact or event; testimony.

witness, witnessed, witnessing, witnesses *v* - 1. To testify or attest to. 2. To have a personal or direct cognizance of; see for oneself. 3. To be present at so as to be able to attest to some fact or action.

witnessed assent *n* - 1. **Assent** given by a **study subject** in the presence of a 3rd party. 2. The act of obtaining a **signed assent** in the presence of a **witness**, especially one in which the witness affixes his or her signature to the **assent form** below the signature of the **study subject** to attest to the fact of assent. rt: **documented assent**

witnessed consent *n* - 1. **Consent** given by a **study subject** in the presence of a 3rd party. 2. The act of obtaining a **signed consent** in the presence of a **witness**, especially one in which the witness affixes his or her signature to the **consent form** below the signature of the **study subject** to attest to the fact of consent. rt: **documented consent**

word *n* - [ME, fr OE; akin to OHG *wort* word, L *verbum*, Gk *eirein* to say, speak] [**computer**] A fixed number of adjacent **bits** defined in the architecture of a **computer** and used in its operations, such as for addressing memory

locations and in performing arithmetic operations. rt: **word size**

word size *n* - [**computers**] The number of **bits** required to form a **word** in a computing system, typically some power of 2, eg, 4, 8, 16, or 32. rt: **word**

work, worked, working, works *v* - [ME *werken*, *worken*, fr OE *wyrcan*; akin to OE *weorc*] 1. To bring to pass. 2. To fashion or create a useful or desired product by purposeful effort.

worker *n* - One who **works**.

working *adj* - Assumed or adopted to permit an activity or exploration.

working hypothesis *n* - **research hypothesis**

workup *n* - 1. A detailed evaluation of a **patient** to establish a **diagnosis** as a prelude to **treatment**. 2. Any such detailed evaluation as a prelude to performing some **procedure** or **step**, such as **enrollment** into a **study** or the like.

workweek *n* - 1. The number of **hours** worked or required to be worked in a **week**. 2. Monday through Friday. 3. The days of a week for normal business activities. rt: **week, weekday, work** *Usage note*: See **week** and **time measure**.

World Health Organization (WHO) *n* - An agency of the United Nations, with headquarters in Geneva and devoted to the improvement of health through multinational **research** and training.

World Medical Association *n* - Federation of medical associations, formed in 1947. Dedicated to promoting better understanding and care of people worldwide. Responsible for the **Helsinki Declaration** and subsequent revisions of the Declaration. Offices located in Ferney-Voltaire, France.

World Medical Association Declaration of Helsinki *n* - A set of **guidelines** and standards for the ethical conduct of **research** on human beings, adopted at the 18th assembly of the **World Medical Association** in Helsinki, June 1964; modified periodically since then. The declaration, as modified by the 29th assembly of the World Medical Association in Tokyo in 1975, may be found in Levine [1986].[88] The original resolution and all subsequent modifications are referred to as the **Declaration of Helsinki**. rt: **Nuremberg Code**

worst *adj* - [ME *werste, worste*, fr OE *wierresta, wyrsta*, superl of the root of OE *wiersa* worse] 1.

Most unfavorable in relation to a stated **hypothesis** or position. 2. Most difficult. 3. Most unsuitable. 4. Most defective or faulty. ant: **best**

worst case *n* - The **case** (defn 1) that is **worst** in some sense or aspect. ant: **best case**

worst case analysis *n* - An **analysis** based on **worst case assumptions**, eg, an analysis of mortality from a **followup study** in which one **assumes** that all persons not known to be alive at the time of the analysis were in fact dead; an analysis of a **drug effect** in which one assumes that all observed or reported **events** are due to the drug. ant: **best case analysis** rt: **destructive data analysis**

worst case assumption *n* - **Assumption** of the **worst case** in regard to some event, condition, or **dataset** having varying interpretations or meanings, eg, assumption that **events** observed during the course of **treatment** with an **experimental drug** are due to the **drug**. ant: **best case assumption** rt: **worst case analysis**

write, wrote, written, writing, writes *v* - [ME *writen*, fr OE *writan* to scratch, draw, inscribe; akin to OHG *rizan* to tear, Gk *rhine* file, rasp] To draw or draft; to be an **author**.

writing committee *n* - 1. **publication committee** 2. **paper writing committee**; **writing team**

writing team *n* - A **team** of **investigators** from a **study** appointed or designated to **write** a study **manuscript** as agents or representatives of the **investigative group**. syn: **writing committee**

written assent *n* - 1. An **assent statement** that is written. 2. Such a statement presented to a person being asked to **assent**. 3. **signed assent**

written consent *n* - 1. A **consent statement** that is written. 2. Such a statement presented to a person being asked to **consent**. 3. **signed consent**

When you are up to your rear end in alligators, it's hard to remember you started out to drain the swamp

Sign over mechanic's bench

X, Y, and Z

x, X *n* - [24th letter of the English alphabet] Often the letter used, along with a unique identifying subscript, to designate an **independent variable** in a **regression model**.

x-axis *n* - 1. The horizontal **axis** in a plane **Cartesian coordinate** system. 2. The horizontal axis of a two-dimensional **graphic display** of **data**. rt: **y-axis**

x-coordinate *n* - The value on the **x-axis** intersected by a **line** drawn **parallel** to the **y-axis** from a designated point in a plane **Cartesian coordinate** system.

xi *n* - [Gk *xei*] The 14th letter of the **Greek alphabet**, uppercase Ξ, lowercase ξ.

xy-coordinate *n* - The x- and y-**coordinates** of a point in a plane **Cartesian coordinate** system.

y, Y *n* - [25th letter of the English alphabet] Often the letter used to designate the **dependent variable** in a **regression model**.

y-axis *n* - 1. The vertical **axis** in a plane **Cartesian coordinate** system. 2. The vertical axis of a two dimensional **graphic display** of **data**. rt: **x-axis**

y-coordinate *n* - The value on the **y-axis** intersected by a **line** drawn **parallel** to the **x-axis** from a designated point in a plane **Cartesian coordinate** system. rt: **x-coordinate**

Yates' continuity correction *n* - A **continuity correction** applied to the values represented in a **2x2 contingency table** when using the **chi-square distribution** for **analysis** of the **relationship** represented in the **table**. The correction reduces the **difference** between the **observed** and **expected frequencies** for each cell in the table by 0.5 [Yates, 1934].[167] Used when some cells would otherwise be zero.

year *n* - [ME *yere*, fr OE *gēar*; akin to OHG *jār* year, Gk *hōros* year, *hōra* season, hour, L *ire* to go] 1. A period of time approximately equal to 365.25 **days** and representing the **time** required for the earth to make one revolution of the sun. 2. A cycle in the Gregorian calendar of 365 or 366 days beginning with 1 January and ending with 31 December. 3. A **period** of time equal to a Gregorian year beginning on any given day and ending 365 or 366 days hence, eg, a **fiscal year** beginning on July 1 and ending on June 30. rt: **yearly**, **day**, **week**, **month** *Usage note*: See **time measure**.

yearly *adj* - 1. Occurring or appearing every year; occurring or appearing once a year. 2. Occurring once every other year. 3. Reckoned by the year. 4. Lasting a year. rt: **year**, **daily**, **weekly**, **monthly** *Usage note*: See **time measure**.

years of age *n* - 1. A person's **age** measured by the number of birthday anniversaries having passed since that person's **date of birth** to the present. 2. Age as measured from some event or date in the past. rt: **age**, **birthdate**, **date of birth**

yoke *n* - [ME *yok*, fr OE *geoc*; akin to OHG *joh* yoke, L *jugum*, Gk *zygon*, Skt *yuga*, L *jungere* to join] Something that connects or joins.

yoked *adj* - Being joined or being held or kept together by some constraint or condition.

yoked, yoking, yokes *v* - To become connected, joined, or bound together.

yoked control *n* - A person serving as a **control** by virtue of being **yoked** to another, eg, the twin sibling of a control receiving the same care and **treatment** as the control.

z, Z *n* - [26th and last letter of the English alphabet] **Z-score**

Z distribution *n* - The **distribution** of a logarithmic **transformation** of a **variance ratio**.

Z-score *n* - A **score** (value) resulting from a **Z-transformation**. rt: **standard score**, **T-score**

Z test *n* - 1. A **test of significance** based on the **normal distribution** with Z representing a **standardized normal deviate**. 2. A test based on the **Z distribution**.

Z-transformation *n* - A type of **data transformation** performed on observed values of a defined **dataset** in which the **mean** for that dataset is subtracted from the individual values of the dataset and the resulting differences divided by

the observed **standard deviation**. syn: **Z-score**
rt: **standard score**, **T-transformation**

Zelen consent *n* - **postassignment consent**

zeta *n* - [Gk *zēta*] The 6th letter of the **Greek alphabet**, uppercase Z, lowercase ζ.

References

1 Aickin M: A program for balancing the allocation of subjects to treatment in a clinical trial. <u>Computers</u> <u>and</u> <u>Biomedical</u> <u>Research</u> 15:519 - 524, **1982**. (Aickin, 1982)
. . . . **158**

2 *The American Heritage Dictionary, 2nd College Edition*. Houghton Mifflin Company, Boston, **1991**. (American Heritage, 1991)
. . . . **xxi, xliii, 13**

3 Anderson LK, Hendershot RA, Schoolmaker RC: Self-checking digit concepts. <u>J</u> <u>Systems</u> <u>Management</u> 25:36 - 42, **1974**. (Anderson et al, 1974)
. . . . **39**

4 Armitage P, Berry G: *Statistical Methods in Medical Research*. Blackwell Scientific Publications, London, **1994**. (Armitage and Berry, 1994)
. . . . **xxi**

5 Bartlett MS: The use of transformations. <u>Biometrics</u> 3:39 - 52, **1947**. (Bartlett, 1947)
. . . . **148**

6 Bayes T: *An essay towards solving a problem in the doctrine of chances.* (Reproduced in <u>Biometrika</u> 45:296 - 315**1958**.) <u>Philos</u> <u>Trans</u> <u>Roy</u> <u>Soc</u> <u>Lond</u> 53: - 370 - 418, **1763**. (Bayes, 1763)
. . . . **21**

7 Begg CB: Advances in statistical methodology for diagnostics medicine in the 1980's. <u>Statistics</u> <u>in</u> <u>Medicine</u> 10:1,887 - 1,895, **1991**. (Begg, 1991)
. . . . **224**

8 Berkson J: Limitations of the application of fourfold table analysis to hospital data. <u>Biometrics</u> <u>Bull</u> 2:47 - 53, **1946**. (Berkson, 1946)
. . . . **23**

9 Bernoulli J: *Ars Conjectandi*. (Reprinted in Latin by Culture et Civilisation, 1968) Belgium, **1713**. (Bernoulli, 1713)
. . . . **23**

10 *Black's Law Dictionary*. West Publishing Company, St Paul, Minnesota, **1990**. (Black's, 1990)
. . . . **xxi, 104**

11 Boissel J-P, Collet J-P, Moleur P, Haugh M: Surrogate endpoints: A basis for a rational approach. <u>Eur</u> <u>J</u> <u>Clin</u> <u>Pharmacol</u> 43:235 - 244, **1992**. (Boissel et al, 1992)
. . . . **265**

12 Bradley C: Designing medical and educational intervention studies: A review of some alternatives to conventional randomized controlled trials. <u>Diabetes</u> <u>Care</u> 16:509 - 518, **1993**. (Bradley, 1993)
. . . . **204**

13 Brain Resuscitation Clinical Trial II Study Group: A randomized clinical trial of calcium entry blocker administration to comatose survivors of cardiac arrest: Design, methods and patient characteristics. <u>Controlled</u> <u>Clin</u> <u>Trials</u> 12:525 - 545, **1991**. (Brain Study Group, 1991)
. . . . **69**

14 Breslow NE, Day NE: *Statistical Methods in Cancer Research, Vol 1*. International Agency for Research on Cancer, Lyon, **1980**. (Breslow and Day, 1980)
. . . . **xxi**

15 Brewin CR, Bradley C: Patient preferences and randomised clinical trials. <u>BMJ</u> 299:313 - 315, **1989**. (Brewin and Bradley, 1989)
. . . . **204**

16 Brittain E, Wittes J: The run-in period in clinical trials. <u>Controlled</u> <u>Clin</u> <u>Trials</u> 11:327 - 338, **1990**. (Brittain and Wittes, 1990)
. . . . **143, 196**

17 Buchwald H, Varco RL, Matts JP, Long JM, Fitch LL, Campbell GS, Pearce MB, Yellin AE, Edmiston WA, Smink Jr RD, Sawin HS, Campos CT, Hansen BJ, Tuna N, Karnegis JN, Sanmarco ME, Amplatz K, Castaneda-Zuniga WR, Hunter DW, Bissett JK, Weber FJ, Stevenson JW, Leon AS, Chalmers TC, and the POSCH Group: Effect of partial ileal

bypass surgery on mortality and morbidity from coronary heart disease in patients with hypercholesterolemia: Report of the Program on the Surgical Control of the Hyperlipidemias (POSCH). N Engl J Med 323:946 - 955, **1990**. (Buchwald et al, 1990)

. . . . **79**

18 Buyse ME, Staquet MJ, Sylvester RJ (eds): *Cancer Clinical Trials: Methods and Practice*. Oxford University Press, Oxford, **1984**. (Buyse et al, 1984)

. . . . **xxi**

19 Cardiac Arrhythmia Suppression Trial (CAST) Investigators: Preliminary report: Effect of encainide and flecainide on mortality in a randomized trial of arrhythmia suppression after myocardial infarction. N Engl J Med 321:406 - 412, **1989**. (CAST Investigators, 1989)

. . . . **143**

20 Carter SK: Clinical trials in cancer chemotherapy. Cancer 40:544 - 557, **1977**. (Carter, 1977)

. . . . **155**

21 CASS Principal Investigators and their Associates: Coronary Artery Surgery Study (CASS): A randomized trial of coronary artery bypass surgery: Comparability of entry characteristics and survival in randomized patients and nonrandomized patients meeting randomization criteria. J Am Coll Cariol 3:114 - 128, **1984**. (CASS PIs and Associates, 1984)

. . . . **260**

22 CASS Principal Investigators and their Associates: National Heart, Lung, and Blood Institute Coronary Artery Surgery Study (CASS): A multicenter comparison of the effects of randomized medical and surgical treatment of mildly symptomatic patients with coronary artery disease, and a registry of consecutive patients undergoing coronary angiography. Circulation 63 (monograph 79) (Part II):I-1 - I-81, **1981**. (CASS PIs and Associates, 1981)

. . . . **260**

23 Chalmers TC, Smith H Jr, Blackburn B, Silverman B, Schroeder B, Reitman D, Ambroz A: A method for assessing the quality of a randomized control trial. Controlled Clin Trials 2:31 - 49, **1981**. (Chalmers et al, 1981)

. . . . **221**

24 Chandor A: *The Facts on File Dictionary of Microcomputers*. Facts on File, Inc, New York, **1981**. (Chandor, 1981)

. . . . **xxi**

25 Cochran WG, Cox GM: *Experimental Designs (2nd ed)*. John Wiley and Sons, Inc, New York, **1957**. (Cochran and Cox, 1957)

. . . . **xxi**

26 Coordinating Center Models Project Research Group: *Coordinating Center Models Project: A Study of Coordinating Centers in Multicenter Clinical Trials: I. Design and Methods (in two parts)*. Division of Heart and Vascular Diseases, National Heart, Lung, and Blood Institute, Bethesda, MD, **1979a**. (CCMP Research Group, 1979a)

. . . . **x**

27 Coordinating Center Models Project Research Group: *Coordinating Center Models Project: A Study of Coordinating Centers in Multicenter Clinical Trials: IV. Terminology*. Division of Heart and Vascular Diseases, National Heart, Lung, and Blood Institute, Bethesda, MD, **1979b**. (CCMP Research Group, 1979b)

. . . . **x**

28 Cornfield J: The Bayesian outlook and its application (including discussion by S Geisser, HO Hartley, O Kempthrone, H Rubin). Biometrics 25:617 - 657, **1969**. (Cornfield, 1969)

. . . . **22**

29 Cornfield J: Sequential trials, sequential analysis and the likelihood principle. Am Statistician 20:18 - 23, **1966**. (Cornfield, 1966)

. . . . **22, 146, 229**

30 Coronary Drug Project Research Group: The Coronary Drug Project: Design, Methods, and Baseline Results. <u>Circulation</u> 47 (suppl 1):I-1 - I-50, **1973**. (CDP Research Group, 1973)

   . . . . **48, 143, 163, 185, 196, 244, 251, 254**

31 Cox DR: Regression models and life tables (including discussion). <u>JRSS</u> 34(series B):187 - 220, **1972**. (Cox, 1972)

   . . . . **62**

32 DeMets DL, Ware JH: Group sequential methods for clinical trials with a one-sided hypothesis. <u>Biometrika</u> 67:651 - 660, **1980**. (DeMets and Ware, 1980)

   . . . . **112**

33 Department of Health and Human Services: Expanded availability of investigational new drugs through a parallel track mechanism for people with AIDS and other HIV-related disease. <u>Federal</u> <u>Register</u> 57:13,250 - 13,259, **1992**. (DHHS, 1992)

   . . . . **186**

34 Department of Health and Human Services: *Public Health Service Grants Policy Statement*. Publ no (OASH) 82-50,000(rev), Washington, **1982**. (DHHS, 1982)

   . . . . **56, 109**

35 Department of Health, Education, and Welfare: *The Negotiated Contracting Process: A Guide for Project Officers*. Washington, Oct, **1977**. (DHEW, 1977)

   . . . . **56, 109**

36 Diaconis P, Efron B: Computer-intensive methods in statistics. <u>Scientific</u> <u>American</u> 248:116 - 130, **1983**. (Diaconis and Efron, 1983)

   . . . . **30, 137**

37 Dixon WJ, Mood AM: A method for obtaining and analyzing sensitivity data. <u>JASA</u> 43:109 - 126, **1948**. (Dixon and Mood, 1948)

   . . . . **291**

38 *Dorland's Illustrated Medical Dictionary (24th ed)*. WB Saunders Co, Philadelphia, **1965**. (Dorland, 1965)

   . . . . **xxi**

39 DuBois D, DuBois EF: A formula to estimate the approximate surface area if height and weight are known. <u>Arch</u> <u>Intern</u> <u>Med</u> 17:863 - 871, **1916**. (DuBois and DuBois, 1916)

   . . . . **170**

40 Dupont WD: Sequential stopping rules and sequentially adjusted p-values; Does one require the other?. <u>Controlled</u> <u>Clin</u> <u>Trials</u> 4:3 - 10, **1983**. (Dupont, 1983)

   . . . . **146**

41 Edwards AWF: *Likelihood: An account of the Statistical Likelihood Concept of Likelihood and its Application to Scientific Inference*. Cambridge University Press, Cambridge, **1972**. (Edwards, 1972)

   . . . . **146**

42 Efron B: Forcing a sequential experiment to be balanced. <u>Biometrics</u> 58:403 - 417, **1971**. (Efron, 1971)

   . . . . **3**

43 Federer WT: *Experimental Design, Theory and Application*. Oxford and India Book House, Calcutta, **1967**. (Federer, 1967)

   . . . . **xxi**

44 Feinstein AR: XX. The epidemiologic trohoc, the ablative risk ratio, and 'retrospective' research. <u>Clin</u> <u>Pharmarol</u> <u>Ther</u> 14:291 - 307, **1973**. (Feinstein, 1973)

   . . . . **34, 284**

45 Fellegi IP, Sunter A: A theory for record linkage. <u>JASA</u> 64:1,183 - 1,210, **1969**. (Fellegi and Sunter, 1969)

   . . . . **39**

46 Feller W: *An Introduction to Probability Theory and Its Applications (Vol 1, 3rd ed)*. John Wiley & Sons, New York, **1968**. (Feller, 1968)

   . . . . **xxi, 23, 29**

47 Fisher RA: *The Design of Experiments.* Oliver & Boyd, Edinburgh, **1935**. (Fisher, 1935)
. . . . **97, 100**

48 Food and Drug Administration: *Code of Federal Regulations; 21, parts 300 to 499, Revised as of April 1, 1992.* Office of the Federal Register, National Archives and Records Administration, Washington, **1992**. (FDA, 1992)
. . . . **7, 12, 134, 247, 289**

49 Food and Drug Administration: *FDA Regulatory Manual Series, Vol 1, James T O'Reilly.* McGraw-Hill, New York, **1984**. (FDA, 1984)
. . . . **107**

50 Food and Drug Administration: *National Center for Devices and Radiological Health: Regulatory Requirements for Medical Devices: A Workshop Manual, Publ no FDA 83-4,165.* Rockville, Md, **1983**. (FDA, 1983)
. . . . **133, 156, 203**

51 Food and Drug Administration: *General Considerations for the Clinical Evaluation of Drugs.* Publ no HEW (FDA) 77-3040, Rockville, Md, **1977**. (FDA, 1977)
. . . . **193, 194**

52 Food and Drug Administration: Applicability of Drug Efficacy Study Implementation notices and notices of opportunity for hearing to identical, related, and similar drug products. <u>Federal Register</u> 39:11,681 - 11,682, **29 March 1974**. (FDA, 1974)
. . . . **80, 107**

53 Fost N, Robertson JA: Deferring consent with incompetent patients in an intensive care unit. <u>IRB: A Review of Human Subject Research</u> 2(7):5 - 6, **1980**. (Fost and Robertson, 1980)
. . . . **69**

54 Freund FE, Williams FJ: *Dictionary/Outline of Basic Statistics.* McGraw-Hill Book Company, New York, **1966**. (Freund and Williams, 1966)
. . . . **xxi**

55 Friedman B: A simple urn model. <u>Communications on Pure and Applied Mathematics</u> 2:59 - 70, **1949**. (Friedman, 1949)
. . . . **291**

56 Friedman LM, Furberg CD, DeMets DL: *Fundamentals of Clinical Trials (2nd ed).* PSG Publishing Co, Inc, Boston, Massachusetts, **1985**. (Friedman et al, 1985)
. . . . **xxi**

57 Galton F: Regression towards mediocrity in hereditary stature. <u>Anthropological Institute</u> 15:246 - 263, **1886**. (Galton, 1886)
. . . . **228**

58 Gill JL: *Design and Analysis of Experiments in the Animal and Medical Sciences (vol 2).* Iowa State University Press, Ames, **1978**. (Gill, 1978)
. . . . **xxi**

59 Glass GV: Primary, secondary and meta-analysis of research. <u>Educational Researcher</u> 5:3 - 8, **1976**. (Glass, 1976)
. . . . **157**

60 Glaucoma Laser Trial Research Group: The Glaucoma Laser Trial (GLT): 3. Design and methods. <u>Controlled Clin Trials</u> 12:504 - 524, **1991**. (GLT Research Group, 1991)
. . . . **186**

61 Gompertz B: On the nature of the function expressive of the law of human mortality. <u>Phil Trans R Soc (A)</u> 115:513 - 583, **1825**. (Gompertz, 1825)
. . . . **109**

62 Grizzle JE: The two-period change-over design and its use in clinical trials. <u>Biometrics</u> 21:467 - 480, **1965**. (Grizzle, 1965)
. . . . **285**

63 Guyatt G, Sackett D, Taylor DW, Chong J, Roberts R, Pugsley S: Determining optimal therapy — Randomized trials in individual patients. <u>New Engl J Med</u> 314:889 - 892, **1986**. (Guyatt et al, 1986)
. . . . **165**

64 Hand DJ: Statistical expert systems: Design. The Statistician 33:351 - 369, **1984**. (Hand, 1984)
. . . . **93**

65 Hanley JA: Receiver operating characteristic (ROC) methodology: The state of the art. Critical Reviews in Diagnostic Imaging 29:307 - 335, **1989**. (Hanley, 1989)
. . . . **224**

66 Henneken CH, Eberlein K, for the Physicians' Health Study Research Group: A randomized trial of aspirin and β-carotene among US physicians. Prev Med 14:165 - 168, **1985**. (Henneken and Eberlein, 1985)
. . . . **25, 251**

67 Hoaglin DC, Mosteller F, Tukey JW: *Understanding Robust and Exploratory Data Analysis*. John Wiley & Sons, Inc, New York, **1983**. (Hoaglin et al, 1983)
. . . . **xxi, 298**

68 Huber PJ: *Robust statistics*. John Wiley & Sons, New York, **1981**. (Huber, 1981)
. . . . **298**

69 James G, James RC (eds): *Mathematics Dictionary (4th ed)*. Van Nostrand Reinhold Company, New York, **1976**. (James and James, 1976)
. . . . **xxi**

70 Jelliffe DB, Jelliffe EFP: Underappreciated pioneers. Am J Clin Nutr 32:2,519 - 2,521, **1979**. (Jelliffe and Jelliffe, 1979)
. . . . **217**

71 Johnson S: *A Dictionary of the English Language*. (in two vols). Printed by W Strahan, for J and P Knapton; T and T Longman; C Hitch and L Hawes; A Millar; and R and J Dodsley, **1755**. (Johnson, 1755)
. . . . **ix, 2**

72 Kahn HA, Sempos CT: *Statistical Methods in Epidemiology*. Oxford University Press, New York, **1989**. (Kahn and Sempos, 1989)
. . . . **74, 176**

73 Kaplan EL, Meier P: Nonparametric estimation from incomplete observations. JASA 53:457 - 481, **1958**. (Kaplan and Meier, 1958)
. . . . **138**

74 Kempthorne O: *The Design and Analysis of Experiments*. John Wiley & Sons, New York, **1952**. (Kempthorne, 1952)
. . . . **xxi**

75 Kendall MG: A new measure of rank correlation. Biometrika 30:81 - 93, **1938**. (Kendall, 1938)
. . . . **138**

76 Kendall MG, Buckland WR: *A Dictionary of Statistical Terms (2nd ed)*. Hafner Publishing Company, New York, **1960**. (Kendall and Buckland, 1960)
. . . . **xxi**

77 Kennedy D: A calm look at the "drug lag". JAMA 239:423 - 426, **1978**. (Kennedy, 1978)
. . . . **79**

78 Kenward MG, Jones B: The analysis of data from 2 x 2 cross-over trials with baseline measurements. Statistics in Medicine 6:911 - 926, **1987**. (Kenward and Jones, 1987)
. . . . **285**

79 Kirk RE: *Experimental Design: Procedures for Behavioral Sciences*. Brooks/Cole, Monterey, **1982**. (Kirk, 1982)
. . . . **xxi**

80 Klein E: *A Comprehensive Etymological Dictionary of the English Language*. Elsevier Scientific Publishing Co, Amsterdam, **1971**. (Klein, 1971)
. . . . **xxi**

81 Knuth DE: *Seminumerical Algorithms (vol 2; Art of Computer Programming)*. Addison-Wesley Publishing Co, Reading, Mass, **1969**. (Knuth, 1969)
. . . . **212**

82 Kotz S, Johnson NL, Read BC (eds): *Encyclopedia of Statistical Sciences.* Johns Wiley & Sons, New York, **1982**. (Kotz et al, 1982)
. . . . **xxi, 18**

83 Kruskal WH, Tanur JM (eds): *International Encyclopedia of Statistics (in 2 vols).* The Free Press, Macmillan Publishing Co, Inc, New York, **1978**. (Kruskal and Tanur, 1978)
. . . . **xxi**

84 Last JM (ed): *A Dictionary of Epidemiology (2nd ed).* Oxford University Press, New York, **1988**. (Last, 1988)
. . . . . **xxi, 35, 83, 116, 176, 206, 244, 271**

85 Last JM (ed): *A Dictionary of Epidemiology.* Oxford University Press, New York, **1983**. (Last, 1983)
. . . . **xxi, 53**

86 Lenter M, Bishop T: *Experimental Design and Analysis.* Valley, Blacksburg, Va, **1986**. (Lenter and Bishop, 1986)
. . . . **xxi**

87 Leventhal BG, Wittes RE: *Research Methods in Clinical Oncology.* Raven Press, New York, **1988**. (Leventhal and Wittes, 1988)
. . . . **xxi**

88 Levine RJ: *Ethics and Regulation of Clinical Research (2nd ed).* Yale University Press, New Haven, **1986**. (Levine, 1986)
. . . . . **xxi, 22, 47, 128, 138, 174, 233, 299**

89 Levine RJ: Deferred consent. Controlled Clin Trials 12:546 - 550, **1991**. (Levine, 1991)
. . . . **69**

90 Lilienfeld AM, Lilienfeld DE: *Foundations of Epidemiology (2nd ed).* Oxford University Press, New York, **1980**. (Lilienfeld & Lilienfeld, 1980)
. . . . **xxi**

91 Lind J: *A Treatise of the Scurvy.* (Reprinted in *Lind's Treatise on Scurvy.* Edited by CP Stewart, D Guthrie; Edinburgh University Press, Edinburgh, **1953**.) Sands, Murray, Cochran, Edinburgh, **1753**. (Lind, 1753)
. . . . **x, 146**

92 Macular Photocoagulation Study Group: Argon laser photocoagulation for ocular histoplasmosis: Results of a randomized clinical trial. Arch Ophthalmol 101:1,347 - 1,357, **1983**. (MPS Group, 1983)
. . . . **83, 162**

93 Macular Photocoagulation Study Group: Argon laser photocoagulation for senile macular degeneration: Results of a randomized clinical trial. Arch Ophthalmol 100:912 - 918, **1982**. (MPS Group, 1982)
. . . . **83, 162**

94 Mann HB, Whitney DR: On a test of whether one of two random variables is stochastically larger than the other. Ann Math Stat 18:50 - 60, **1947**. (Mann and Whitney, 1947)
. . . . **151**

95 Manson JM: *Testing of Pharmaceutical Agents for Reproductive Toxicity.* In *Developmental Toxicology* (2nd ed), CA Kimmel and J Buelke-Sam, eds, Raven Press, New York, **1994**. (Manson, 1994)
. . . . **270**

96 Mantel N: Synthetic retrospective studies and related topics. Biometrics 29:479 - 486, **1973**. (Mantel, 1973)
. . . . **34, 267**

97 Mantel N: Evaluation of survival data and two new rank order statistics arising in its consideration. Cancer Chemother Rep 50:163 - 170, **1966**. (Mantel, 1966)
. . . . **149**

98 Mantel N, Haenszel W: Statistical aspects of the analysis of data from retrospective studies of disease. J Natl Cancer Inst 22:719 - 748, **1959**. (Mantel and Haenszel, 1959)
. . . . **151**

99 Marriott FHC: *A Dictionary of Statistical Terms (5th ed).* Longham Scientific and

Technical, Essex, England, **1990**. (Marriott, 1990)
.... **xxi**

100 Meadows AJ: *Dictionary of New Information Technology*. Nichols Publishing Co, New York, **1982**. (Meadows, 1982)
.... **xxi**

101 Meinert CL: Terminology — A plea for standardization (editorial). Controlled Clin Trials 1:97 - 99, **1980**. (Meinert, 1980)
.... **x**

102 Meinert CL, Tonascia S: *Clinical Trials: Design, Conduct, and Analysis*. Oxford University Press, New York, **1986**. (Meinert and Tonascia, 1986)
.... **x, xxi, 11, 61**

103 Metz CE: Basic principles of ROC analysis. Seminars in Nuclear Medicine VIII:283 - 298, **1978**. (Metz, 1978)
.... **224**

104 Michael M, Boyce WT, Wilcox AJ: *Biomedical Bestiary: An Epidemiologic Guide to Flaws and Fallacies in the Medical Literature*. Little, Brown and Company, Boston, **1984**. (Michael et al, 1984)
.... **83**

105 Miller RG: The jackknife — A review. Biometrika 61:1 - 15, **1974**. (Miller, 1974)
.... **137**

106 Montgomery DC: *Design and Analysis of Experiments (2nd ed)*. John Wiley & Sons, New York, **1984**. (Montgomery, 1984)
.... **xxi**

107 Morganstern H, Bursic ES: A method for using epidemiologic data to estimate the potential impact of an intervention on the health status of a target population. J Community Health 7:292 - 309, **1982**. (Morganstern and Bursic, 1982)
.... **236**

108 Morris W (ed): *The American Heritage Dictionary of the English Language*. American Heritage Publishing Co, Inc and

Houghton Mifflin Co, New York, **1973**. (Morris, 1973)
.... **xxi**

109 Murray JAH, Bradley H, Craigie WA, Onion CT (eds): *The Oxford English Dictionary: A New English Dictionary on Historical Principles (in 13 vols)*. Clarendon Press, Oxford, **1970**. (Murray et al, 1970)
.... **x, xxi, 104**

110 Murray KME: *Caught in the Web of Words: James Murray and the Oxford English Dictionary*. Oxford University Press, Oxford, **1979**. (Murray, 1979)
.... **x**

111 National Center for Health Statistics: *National Death Index: User's Manual*. Publ no (PHS) 81-1148, Hyattsville, Md, **Sept, 1981**. (NCHS, 1981)
.... **165**

112 National Center for Health Statistics: *Vital Statistics of the United States, 1989; Vol II: Mortality, Part A*. US Government Printing Office (pub no (PHS) 93-1101), Washington, **1993a**. (NCHS, 1993a)
.... **145**

113 National Center for Health Statistics: *Health, United States, 1992*. DHHS pub no (PHS) 93-1232, Hyattsville, Md, **1993b**. (NCHS, 1993b)
.... **145**

114 National Institutes of Health: NIH Guidelines on the Inclusion of Women and Minorities as Subjects in Clinical Research. (Also in NIH Guide to Grants and Contracts 23: 2 - 10, 18 March 1994) Federal Register 59:14,508 - 14,513, **March 28, 1994**. (NIH, 1994)
.... **194, 293**

115 National Institutes of Health: Directory sources: The federal health tree. Jour NIH Research 6:67 - 69, **1994**. (NIH, 1994b)
.... **103, 166**

116 National Research Council, Division of Medical Sciences: *Drug Efficacy Study: Final Report to the Commissioner of Food and*

Drugs Food and Drug Administration. National Academy of Sciences, Washington, **1969**. (NRC, 1969)

.... **80, 107**

117 Office for Protection from Research Risks: *Code of Federal Regulations, Title 45: Public Welfare, Part 46: Protection of Human Subjects.* Department of Health and Human Services, National Institutes of Health, Bethesda, Md, **(revised) 18 June 1991**. (OPRR, 1991)

.... **91, 92, 135, 177, 232**

118 O'Quigley J, Pepe M, Fisher L: Continual reassessment method: A practical design for phase 1 clinical trials in cancer. Biometrics 46:33 - 48, **1990**. (O'Quigley et al, 1990)

.... **55**

119 Packard FR: *Life and Times of Ambroise Paré, 1510 - 1590.* Paul B Hoeber, New York, **1921**. (Packard, 1921)

.... **92**

120 Peto R, Peto J: Asymptotically efficient rank invariant test procedures (with discussion). J R Stat Soc A 135:185 - 206, **1972**. (Peto and Peto, 1972)

.... **149**

121 Peto R, Pike MC, Armitage P, Breslow NE, Cox DR, Howard SV, Mantel N, McPherson K, Peto J, Smith PG: Design and analysis of randomized clinical trials requiring prolonged observation of each patient: II. Analysis and examples. Br J Cancer 35:1 - 39, **1977**.

.... **183**

122 *Physicians' Desk Reference.* Medical Economics Data Production Co, Montvale, NJ, **1995**. (PDR, 1995)

.... **141**

123 Physicians' Health Study Research Group Steering Committee: Preliminary report: Findings from the aspirin component of the ongoing Physicians' Health Study. N Engl J Med 318:262 - 264, **1988**. (PHS, 1988)

.... **251**

124 Pines WL: *A Primer on New Drug Development.* Publ no 1980-311-254/83, Food and Drug Administration, Rockville, Md, **1980**. (Pines, 1980)

.... **193, 194**

125 Pocock SJ: Group sequential methods in the design and analysis of clinical trials. Biometrika 64:191 - 199, **1977**. (Pocock, 1977)

.... **112**

126 Pocock SJ: *Clinical Trials: A Practical Approach.* John Wiley and Sons, Chichester, **1983**. (Pocock, 1983)

.... **xxi, 158**

127 Prentice RL: A case-cohort design for epidemiologic cohort studies and disease prevention trials. Biometrika 73:1 - 11, **1986**. (Prentice, 1986)

.... **34**

128 Prentice RL: Surrogate endpoints in clinical trials: Definition and operational criteria. Statistics in Medicine 8:431 - 440, **1989**. (Prentice, 1989)

.... **265**

129 Quetelet A: *Sur l'Homme et el Dévloppement des Facultés.* Hauman, Brussels, **1836**. (Quetelet, 1836)

.... **217**

130 Robbins H: A sequential decision problem with finite memory. Proc Natl Acad Sci 42:920 - 923, **1956**. (Robbins, 1956)

.... **198, 284**

131 Robbins H: Some aspects of the sequential design of experiments. Bull Am Mathematics Soc 58:527 - 535, **1952**. (Robbins, 1952)

.... **198, 284**

132 Roethlisberger FJ, Dickson WJ: *Management and the Worker.* John Wiley & Sons, Inc, New York, **1964**. (Roethlisberger and Dickson, 1964)

.... **116**

133 Rothman KJ (ed): *Causal Inference*. Epidemiology Resources Inc, Chestnut Hill, Massachusetts, **1988**. (Rothman, 1988)
. . . . **35**

134 Rücker G: A two-stage trial design for testing treatment, self-selection and treatment preference effects. Statistics in Medicine 8:477 - 485, **1989**. (Rucker, 1989)
. . . . **204**

135 Sackett DL: The competing objectives of clinical trials. N Engl J Med 303:1,059 - 1,060, **1980**. (Sackett, 1980)
. . . . **93, 151, 202**

136 Sackett DL, Gent M: Controversy in counting and attributing events in clinical trials. N Engl J Med 301:1,410 - 1,412, **1979**. (Sackett and Gent, 1979)
. . . . **93, 151, 202**

137 Savage IR: Contributions to the theory of rank order statistics — The two sample case. Ann Math Stat 27:590 - 615, **1956**. (Savage IR, 1956)
. . . . **149**

138 Schlesselman JJ: *Case-Control Studies: Design, Conduct, and Analysis*. Oxford University Press, New York, **1982**. (Schlesselman, 1982)
. . . . **xxi**

139 Schwartz D, Lellouch J: Explanatory and pragmatic attitudes in therapeutic trials. J Chronic Dis 20:637 - 648, **1967**. (Schwartz and Lellouch, 1967)
. . . . **93, 151, 202, 204**

140 Selmer ES: Registration numbers in Norway: Some applied number theory and psychology. JRSS 130(series A):225 - 231, **1967**. (Selmer, 1967)
. . . . **39**

141 Senn S: n-of-1 trials. Controlled Clin Trials 14:1 - 5, **1993**. (Senn, 1993)
. . . . **165**

142 Simon R: Adaptive treatment assignment method and clinical trials. Biometrics 33:743 - 749, **1977**. (Simon, 1977)
. . . . **5**

143 Sippl CJ: *Computer Dictionary (4th ed)*. Howard W Sams & Co, Inc, Indianapolis, **1985**. (Sippl, 1985)
. . . . **xxi**

144 Smith CV, Pyke R: The Robbins-Isbell two-armed-bandit problem with finite memory. Ann Math Statistics 36:1,375 - 1,386, **1965**. (Smith and Pyke, 1965)
. . . . **284**

145 Smythe M: Record numbering(In *Record Linkage in Medicine*. HD Achison, editor) pages 179-187, The Williams and Wilkins Co, Baltimore, **1968**. (Smythe, 1968)
. . . . **39**

146 Snedecor GW, Cochran WG: *Statistical Methods (6th ed)*. The Iowa State University Press, , Ames, Iowa, **1967**. (Snedecor and Cochran, 1967)
. . . . **254**

147 Soukhanov AH (ed): *Webster's II New Riverside University Dictionary*. The Riverside Publishing Co, Houghton Mifflin Co, Boston, **1988**. (Soukhanov, 1988)
. . . . **xxi**

148 Stedman, TL: *Stedman's Medical Dictionary (25th ed)*. Williams & Wilkins, Baltimore, **1982**. (Stedman, 1982)
. . . . **xxi**

149 Stokes J, Noren J, Shindell S: Definition of terms and concepts applicable to clinical preventive medicine. J Community Health 8:33 - 41, **1982**. (Stokes et al, 1982)
. . . . **xxi**

150 Taves DR: Minimization: A new method of assigning patients to treatment and control groups. Clin Pharmacol Ther 15:443 - 453, **1974**. (Taves, 1974)
. . . . **158**

151 Taylor SH, Silke B, Ebbutt A, Sutton GC, Prout BJ, Burley DM: A long-term prevention study with oxprenolol in coronary heart disease. N Eng J Med 307:1,293 - 1,301, **1982**. (Taylor et al, 1982)
. . . . **244**

152 Teratology Society Public Affairs Committee: FDA classification of drugs for teratogenic risk. Teratology 49:446 - 447, **1994**. (Teratology Society, 1994)
. . . . **270**

153 Thomas CL (ed): *Taber's Cyclopedic Medical Dictionary (15th ed)*. FA Davis Co, Philadelphia, **1985**. (Thomas, 1985)
. . . . **xxi**

154 United States Congress: *NIH Revitalization Act of 1993, 42 USC § 131 (1993); Clinical Research Equity Regarding Women and Minorities; Part I: Women and Minorities as Subjects in Clinical Research.* **1993**. (United States Congress, 1993)
. . . . **xliv, 166, 177, 293**

155 University Group Diabetes Program Research Group: A Study of the effects of hypoglycemic agents on vascular complications in patients with adult-onset diabetes: V. Evaluation of Phenformin therapy. Diabetes 24 (suppl 1):65 - 184, **1975**. (UGDP Research Group, 1975)
. . . . **83**

156 University Group Diabetes Program Research Group: A Study of the effects of hypoglycemic agents on vascular complications in patients with adult-onset diabetes: I. Design, methods and baseline characteristics. Diabetes 19 (suppl 2):747 - 783, **1970a**. (UGDP Research Group, 1970a)
. . . . **iv, 139, 164, 195, 200, 209**

157 University Group Diabetes Program Research Group: A Study of the effects of hypoglycemic agents on vascular complications in patients with adult-onset diabetes: II. Mortality results. Diabetes 19 (suppl 2):785 - 830, **1970b**. (UGDP Research Group, 1970b)
. . . . **45, 77, 83**

158 Warner S: Randomized response: A survey technique for eliminating evasive answer bias. JASA 10:63 - 69, **1965**. (Warner, 1965)
. . . . **222**

159 *Webster's Ninth New Collegiate Dictionary.* Merriam-Webster Inc, Springfield, Mass, **1991**. (Webster's, 1991)
. . . . **xix, xx, xxi, xxxviii, 108**

160 Wei LJ: A class of designs for sequential clinical trials. JASA 72:382 - 386, **1977**. (Wei, 1977)
. . . . **291**

161 Wei LJ, Lachin JM: Properties of the urn randomization in clinical trials. Controlled Clin Trials 9:345 - 364, **1988**. (Wei and Lachin, 1988)
. . . . **291**

162 Weik MH: *Standard Dictionary of Computers and Information Processing.* Hayden Book Company, Inc, New York, **1970**. (Weik, 1970)
. . . . **xxi**

163 Wetherill GB: Sequential estimation of quantal response curves. J R Stat Soc 25 (series B):1 - 48, **1963**. (Wetherill, 1963)
. . . . **291**

164 Whitmore GA, Yalovsky M: A normalizing logarithmic transformation for inverse Gaussian random variables. Technometrics 20:207 - 208, **1978**. (Whitmore and Yalovsky, 1978)
. . . . **148**

165 Wilcoxon F: Individual comparisons by ranking methods. Biometrics Bulletin 1:80 - 83, **1945**. (Wilcoxon, 1945)
. . . . **151, 298**

166 Wittes J, Lakatos E: Surrogate endpoints in clinical trials: Cardiovascular diseases. Statistics in Medicine 8:415 - 425, **1989**. (Wittes and Lakatos, 1989)
. . . . **265**

167 Yates F: Contingency tables involving small number and the χ^2 test. J R Statist Soc 1(suppl):217 - 235, **1934**. (Yates, 1934)
. . . . **301**

168 Yusuf S, Simon R, Ellenberg S (eds): Proceedings of the workshop on methodologic issues in overviews of randomized clinical trials, May 1986. Stat Med 6:217 - 410, **1987**. (Yusuf et al, 1987)
. . . . **183**

169 Yusuf S, Peto R, Lewis J, Collins R, Sleight P: Beta blockade during and after myocardial infarction: An overview of the randomized trial. Prog Cariovasc Dis 27:335 - 371, **1985**. (Yusuf et al, 1985)
. . . . **183**

170 Zelen M: A new design for randomized clinical trials. N Engl J Med 300:1,242 - 1,245, **1979**. (Zelen, 1979)
. . . . **201**

171 Zelen M: Play the winner rule and the controlled clinical trial. JASA 64:131 - 146, **1969**. (Zelen, 1969)
. . . . **198, 284**

Index

F

FDA related terms

P

R

W

X, Y, and Z